Treatment Methods for Early and Advanced Prostate Cancer

Treatment Methods for Early and Advanced Prostate Cancer

Edited by

Roger S Kirby MD FRCS (Urol)
Professor, Directory
The Prostate Centre
Visiting Professor of Urology
St Georges Hospital
Healthcare Trust
Honorary Professor
Institute of Urology
University College London
London
UK

Alan W Partin MD
David Hall McConnell Professor and Director
The Brady Urological Institute
The Johns Hopkins Medical Institute
Baltimore, MD
USA

J Kellogg Parsons MD MHS
Assistant Professor of Surgery/Urology
Division of Urology
University of California
San Diego, CA
USA

Mark R Feneley MD (Cantab) FRCS (Urol) FRCS (Eng)
Senior Lecturer in Urological Oncological Surgery
Institute of Urology
University College London
Honorary Consultant Urologist
University College Hospital
London
UK

informa
healthcare

First published in the United Kingdom in 2008 by Informa Healthcare, Telephone House, 69-77 Paul Street, London EC2A 4LQ. Informa Healthcare is a trading division of Informa UK Ltd. Registered Office: 37/41 Mortimer Street, London W1T 3JH. Registered in England and Wales number 1072954.

Tel: +44 (0)20 7017 5000
Fax: +44 (0)20 7017 6699
Website: www.informahealthcare.com

A CIP record for this book is available from the British Library.
Library of Congress Cataloging-in-Publication Data

Data available on application

ISBN-10: 0 415 45893 5
ISBN-13: 978 0 415 45893 1

Distributed in North and South America by
Taylor & Francis
6000 Broken Sound Parkway, NW, (Suite 300)
Boca Raton, FL 33487, USA

Within Continental USA
Tel: 1 (800) 272 7737; Fax: 1 (800) 374 3401
Outside Continental USA
Tel: (561) 994 0555; Fax: (561) 361 6018
Email: orders@crcpress.com

Book orders in the rest of the world

Paul Abrahams
Tel: +44(0)20 7017 4036
Email: bookorders@informa.com

Composition by Exeter Premedia Services Pvt. Ltd., Chennai, India
Printed and bound in India by Replika Press Pvt. Ltd

Contents

Contributors

Michele Albert MD
Brigham and Women's Hospital and Dana Farber Cancer Institute
Department of Radiation Oncology
Boston, MA
USA

Peter C Albertsen MD MS
Professor of Surgery (Urology)
University of Connecticut Health Center
Farmington, CT
USA

Peter Amoroso
The Prostate Centre
London
UK

Chris Anderson
The Prostate Centre
London
UK

Andrew J Armstrong MD
Medical Oncology Fellow
Sidney Kimmel Comprehensive
Cancer Center at Johns Hopkins
Baltimore, MD
USA

Carlos Arroyo MD
Resident in Urology
Department of Urology
Institute Montsouris
University Rene Descartes
Paris
France

Vasily J Assikis MD
Assistant Professor of Oncology and Urology
Winship Cancer Institute
Emory University
Atlanta, GA
USA

Albaha Barqawi
Walter Reed Army Medical Center
Washington, DC
USA

Eric Barret MD
Senior Urologist
Department of Urology
Institute Montsouris
University Rene Descartes
Paris
France

Clair Beard MD
Assistant Professor in Radiation Oncology
Brigham and Women's Hospital and
Dana Farber Cancer Institute
Department of Radiation Oncology
Boston, MA
USA

Kathleen W Beekman MD
Lecturer
University of Michigan Comprehensive Cancer Center
Ann Arbor, MI
USA

Alberto Briganti MD
Resident in Training
Department of Urology
University Vita Salute San Raffaele
Milan
Italy

James A Brown MD FACS
Fellow
Vattikuti Urology Institute
Henry Ford Hospital
Detroit, MI
USA

Grant Buchanan PhD
Research Fellow
Dame Roma Mitchell Cancer Research Laboratories
University of Adelaide and Hanson Institute
Adelaide
Australia

Fiona C Burkhard MD
Staff member
Department of Urology
University Hospital of Bern
Bern
Switzerland

Michael A Carducci MD
Associate Professor of Oncology and Urology
Co-Leader, Prostate Cancer Program
Co-Director, Translational Drug Development
Kimmel Cancer Center
Johns Hopkins Baltimore
Baltimore, MD
USA

Xavier Cathelineau MD
Senior Urologist
Department of Urology
Institute Montsouris
Paris; University Rene Descartes
Paris
France

Jamie A Cesaretti MD MS
Assistant Professor
Mount Sinai School of Medicine
New York, NY
USA

Gerald W Chodak MD FACS
Midwest Urology Research Foundation
Chicago, IL
USA

Timothy S Collins MD
Medical Oncology Fellow
Duke University Medical Center
Durham, NC
USA

Robert A Cormack MD
Physicist
Brigham and Women's Hospital and
Dana Farber Cancer Institute
Department of Radiation Oncology
Boston, MA
USA

Jonathan P Coxon MD
Research Fellow
Department of Urology
St George's Hospital
London
UK

Anthony V D'Amico MD PhD
Professor and Chief of Genitourinary Radiation Oncology
Brigham and Women's Hospital
Dana Farber Cancer Institute
Harvard Medical School
Boston, MA
USA

Prokar Dasgupta
The Prostate Centre
London
UK

Jane Dawoodi RGN DN
Urology Specialist Nurse
London Clinic
London
UK

David P Dearnaley MA FRCP FRCR MD
Professor and Honorary Consultant in
Clinical Oncology
Head of Urology Unit
Royal Marsden Hospital
Sutton
UK

Serdar Deger MD
Department of Urology
Charite University Medicine
Berlin, Berlin
Germany

Jeffrey Demanes MD
Radiation Oncologist
California Endocurietherapy Center
Oakland, CA
USA

Theodore L DeWeese MD
Professor of Radiation Oncology
Urology and Oncology
Chair
Department of Radiation Oncology and
Molecular Radiation Sciences
Johns Hopkins University School of Medicine
Baltimore, MD
USA

Zach S Dovey MD
Resident Medical Officer
Department of Uro-oncology
Cromwell Hospital
London
UK

James A Eastham MD
Associate Professor
Memorial Sloan-Kettering Cancer Center
New York, NY
USA

Mario A Eisenberger MD
R Dale Hughes Professor of Oncology and Urology
Sidney Kimmel Comprehensive Cancer Center at
Johns Hopkins
Baltimore, MD
USA

Lars Ellison MD
Assistant Professor
Department of Urology
University of California
Davis, CA
USA

Steven J Feigenberg MD
Assistant Professor
Department of Radiation Oncology
Fox Chase Cancer Center
Philadelphia, PA
USA

Mark R Feneley MD (Cantab) FRCS (Urol) FRCS (Eng)
Senior Lecturer in Urological Oncological Surgery
Institute of Urology
University College London
Honorary Consultant Urologist
University College Hospital
London
UK

Marc Galiano MD
Department of Urology
Institute Montsouris
Paris; Universite Rene Descartes
Paris
France

Razvan Galalae MD
Radiation Oncologist
Kiel University
Kiel
Germany

Marc B Garnick MD
Chief Medical Officer
Praecis Pharmaceuticals Inc.
Clinical Professor of Medicine
Harvard Medical School
Beth Israel Deaconess Medical Center
Boston, MA
USA

Daniel J George MD
Associate Professor of Medicine and Surgery
Duke University Medical Center
Durham, NC
USA

Martin Gleave MD FRCSc
Director
Clinical Research
Prostate Center
Vancouver General Hospital
Vancouver
Canada

S Larry Goldenberg MD
Head of UBC Prostate Clinic
Vancouver General Hospital
Vancouver
Canada

Miles A Goldstraw
The Prostate Centre
London
UK

Jose Gonzalez MD
Urologist
William Beaumont Hospital
Department of Radiation Oncology
Royal Oak
Michigan, MI
USA

Gary Gustafson MD
William Beaumont Hospital
Department of Radiation Oncology
Royal Oak
Michigan, MI
USA

David M Hartke MD
Resident
Department of Urology
Case Western Reserve University School of Medicine
University Hospitals of Cleveland
Cleveland, OH
USA

Ashok K Hemal MD MCh FACS
Professor
Department of Urology
All India Institute of Medical Sciences
Ansari Nagar, New Delhi
India

Mitchell Hollander MD
Urologist, William Beaumont Hospital
Department of Radiation Oncology
Royal Oak
Michigan, MI
USA

Eric M Horwitz MD
Clinical Director and Associate Professor
Department of Radiation Oncology
Fox Chase Cancer Center
Philadelphia, PA
USA

Mark D Hurwitz MD
Assistant Professor in Radiation Oncology
Brigham and Women's Hospital and
Dana Farber Cancer Institute
Department of Radiation Oncology
Boston, MA
USA

Salma K Jabbour MD
Chief Resident
Department of Radiation Oncology and
Molecular Radiation Sciences
Johns Hopkins University School of Medicine
Baltimore, MD
USA

William Jonas MD
Fellow
Winship Cancer Institute
Emory University
Atlanta, GA
USA

Johnny Kao MD
Assistant Professor
Mount Sinai School of Medicine
New York, NY
USA

Vincent S Khoo MBBS FRACR FRCR MD
Consultant in Clinical Oncology
Royal Marsden Hospital
London
UK

Michael Kirby MBBS LRCP MRCS FRCP
Director
Hertfordshire Primary Care Research Network
Letchworth
UK

Roger S Kirby MD FRCS (Urol)
Professor, Directory
The Prostate Centre
Visiting Professor of Urology
St Georges Hospital
Healthcare Trust
Honorary Professor
Institute of Urology
University College London
London
UK

David Kirk DM FRCS
Consultant Urologist
Gartnavel General Hospital
Glasgow; Honorary Professor
University of Glasgow
Glasgow
UK

Laurence Klotz MD
Professor
Department of Surgery
University of Toronto
Chief
Division of Urology Sunnybrook and
Women's Health Sciences Center
Toronto, Ontario
Canada

Paul H Lange MD FACS
Professor and Chair
Department of Urology
University of Washington
Seattle, WA
USA

Dan Leibovici MD
Senior Urologist
Department of Urology
Assef-Harofeh Medical Center
Zerifin
Israel

Herbert Lepor MD
Professor and Martin Spatz Chairman
Department of Urology
New York University School of Medicine
New York, NY
USA

Murugesan Manoharan MD
Assistant Professor of Urology
University of Miami School of Medicine
Miami, FL
USA

Alvaro A Martinez MD FACR
William Beaumont Hospital
Department of Radiation Oncology
Royal Oak
Michigan, MI
USA

David G McLeod MD
Residency Program Director and Director
Urologic Oncology
Walter Reed Army Medical Center
Washington, DC
USA

Mani Menon MD FACS
Raj and Padma Vattikuti Distinguished Chair
Professor
Department of Urology
Case Western Reserve University School of Medicine
Cleveland, OH
Director
Vattikuti Urology Institute
Henry Ford Hospital
Detroit, MI
USA

David Miller MD
Health Services Research Fellow
Department of Urology
University of Michigan Urology Center
Ann Arbor, MI
USA

Leslie Moffat BSc MB MBA FRCS (Ed & Glas) FACS FRCP (Ed)
Senior Lecturer
University of Aberdeen
Department of Urology
Aberdeen Royal Infirmary
Aberdeen
UK

Francesco Montorsi MD
Associate Professor
Department of Urology
University Vita Salute San Raffaele
Milan
Italy

Camille Motta PhD
Professor
Department of Medical Information
Praecis Pharmaceuticals Inc.
Waltham, MA
USA

Mark A Moyad MD MPH
Phil F Jenkins Director of Complementary Medicine
Urologic Oncology
Clinical Cancer Researcher/Consultant
University of Michigan
Ann Arbor, MI
USA

Robert P Myers MD
Consultant
Department of Urology
Mayo Clinic
Rochester, MN
USA

Donald Newling
Medical Director (Urology)
AstraZeneca plc
Macclesfield
UK

Nils Nuernberg MD
Radiation Oncologist
Kiel University
Kiel
Germany

Jonathan R Osborn MB ChB MSc MRCS
Research Fellow
Midwest Urology Research Foundation
Chicago, IL
USA

Christopher Parker BA MRCP MD FRCP
Senior Lecturer and Honorary Consultant in
Clinical Oncology
Academic Urology Unit
Institute of Cancer Research and
Royal Marsden Hospital
Sutton
UK

J Kellogg Parsons MD MHS
Assistant Professor of Surgery/Urology
Division of Urology
University of California
San Diego, CA
USA

Alan W Partin MD
David Hall McConnell Professor and Director
The Brady Urological Institute
The Johns Hopkins Medical Institute
Baltimore, MD
USA

Krishna Patil
The Prostate Centre
London
UK

Jim Peabody
The Prostate Centre
London
UK

David F Penson MD MPH
Associate Professor of Urology and Preventive Medicine
Keck School of Medicine
University of Southern California
Los Angeles, CA
USA

Louis L Pisters MD
Associate Professor
The University of Texas MD Anderson Cancer Center
Houston, TX
USA

Alan Pollack MD
Chairman and Professor
The Gerald E Hanks Endowed Chair in
Radiation Oncology
Department of Radiation Oncology
Fox Chase Cancer Center
Philadelphia, PA
USA

Marcus L Quek MD
Urologic Oncology Fellow
Keck School of Medicine
University of Southern California
Los Angeles, CA
USA

Charlotte Rees BSc MEd PhD CPsychol
Senior Lecturer in Medical Education
Peninsula Medical School
Universities of Exeter and Plymouth
Devon
UK

Martin I Resnick MD
Lester Persky Professor and Chairman
Department of Urology
Case Western Reserve University School of Medicine
University Hospitals of Cleveland
Cleveland, OH
USA

Patrizio Rigatti MD
Professor and Chairman
Department of Urology
University Vita Salute San Raffaele
Milan
Italy

Rodney Rodriguez MD
Radiation Oncologist
California Endocurietherapy Center
Oakland, CA
USA

Francois Rozet MD
Senior Urologist
Department of Urology
Institute Montsouris
University Rene Descartes
Paris
France

Andrea Salonia MD
Fellow
Department of Urology
University Vita Salute San Raffaele
Milan
Italy

Paul P Schellhammer MD
Program Director, Virginia Prostate Center
Professor of Urology, Eastern Virginia Medical School
Norfolk, VA
USA

Howard I Scher MD
D Wayne Calloway Chair in Urologic Oncology
Attending Physician and Chief
Genitourinary Oncology Service
Department of Medicine
Sidney Kimmel Center for Prostate and
Urologic Cancers
Memorial Sloan-Kettering Cancer Center
New York, NY
USA

Martin Schumacher MD
Staff member
Department of Urology
University Hospital of Bern
Bern
Switzerland

William A See MD
Professor and Chairman
Department of Urology
Medical College of Wisconsin
Milwaukee, WI
USA

Jonathan W Simons MD
Director
Winship Cancer Institute
Emory University
Atlanta, GA
USA

Mark Soloway MD
Professor and Chairman
Department of Urology
University of Miami Miller School of Medicine
Miami, FL
USA

Danny Y Song MD
Assistant Professor of Radiation Oncology
Urology and Oncology
Department of Radiation Oncology and
Molecular Medicine
Johns Hopkins University School of Medicine
The Sidney Kimmel Comprehensive Cancer Center
Baltimore, MD
USA

Richard G Stock MD
Professor and Chairman of Radiation Oncology
Mount Sinai School of Medicine
New York, NY
USA

Nelson N Stone MD
Clinical Professor of Urology and Radiation Oncology
Mount Sinai School of Medicine
New York, NY
USA

Urs E Studer MD
Chairman and Professor
Department of Urology
University Hospital of Bern
Bern
Switzerland

Clare M Tempany MD
Professor of Radiology
Harvard Medical School
Director of Clinical MRI
Department of Radiology
Brigham and Women's Hospital and
Dana Farber Cancer Institute
Departments of Radiation Oncology and
Radiology
Boston, MA
USA

Wayne D Tilley PhD
Chair
Dame Roma Mitchell Chair in
Cancer Research Laboratories
University of Adelaide and Hanson Institute
Adelaide
Australia

Natalie Tschan
Department of Urology
University Hospital of Bern
Bern
Switzerland

Guy Vallancien MD
Professor
Department of Urology
Institute Montsouris
University Rene Descartes
Paris
France

Carlos Vargas MD
William Beaumont Hospital
Department of Radiation Oncology
Royal Oak
Michigan, MI
USA

Arnauld Villers MD PhD
Professor in Urology
Service d'Urologie
Hopital Huriez
Centre Hospitalier Regional University
Lille
France

Alessandro Volpe MD
Fellow Division of Urology
Department of Surgical Oncology
Sunnybrook and
Women's College Health Sciences Center
Toronto, Ontario
Canada

Patrick C Walsh
University Distinguished Service Professor of Urology
The James Buchanan Brady Urological Institute
Johns Hopkins Medical Institutions
Baltimore, MD
USA

John T Wei MD MS
Associate Professor
Director
Division of Clinical Research and Quality Assurance
University of Michigan Urology Center
Ann Arbor, MI
USA

Brian Wells MD FRCPsch
Consultant Psychiatrist
The Prostate Centre
London
UK

Ulrich K Fri Witzsch MD
Professor and Chair E Becht
Chief of Urology
Krankenhaus Nordwest Hospital for Urology and
Child Urology
Frankfurt
Germany

Preface

Prostate cancer is the most enigmatic of the common solid malignancies. Second only to lung cancer as a killer of men beyond middle age, it warrants more attention than it currently receives from governments, researchers and the general public worldwide. One major reason for this continuing neglect is the observation that the majority of men as they age harbour small foci of adenocarcinoma within their prostate that never become clinically significant. As a consequence, worries about over-diagnosis and over-treatment have surfaced and turned many doctors away from the task of identifying and treating earlier the more aggressive lesions that result in such significant morbidity and mortality. In fact, the time has come to abandon the prevalent attitude of nihilism about prostate cancer because, potentially, much suffering could be avoided and many lives saved.

Treatment for prostate cancer itself is evolving rapidly. For smaller 'low risk' tumors, active surveillance with selective delayed intervention is becoming increasingly popular; however, worries persist about the degree of accuracy with which we can detect local or distant progression. The Holy Grail for the management of localized prostate cancer is to eradicate the cancer effectively, while minimizing the collateral damage to adjacent structures such as the neurovascular bundles.

New technologies such as the da Vinci robot to facilitate laparoscopic radical prostatectomy and low dose brachytherapy both offer this prospect, and are rapidly becoming the dominant active treatment options in North America. By contrast, locally advanced prostate cancers are probably best managed by conformal external beam radiotherapy (EBRT) with pre- and sometimes posttreatment hormonal ablation, although high dose (HD) brachytherapy is looking very interesting.

Once prostate cancer has spread to either lymph nodes or bones, hormonal therapy is usually the first line of treatment and may be effective for many months or years. Eventually, however, hormone relapse develops and second line treatments need to be considered. Chemotherapy with taxotere has now been shown to improve survival and several newer therapies including endothelin A antagonists look promising in this context.

In this volume we have tried to cover all these rapidly evolving areas in a concise, informative and evidenced-based fashion. More and more patients and their families lives are touched by prostate cancer; we sincerely hope that this book will help those who care for them do their job with better, more readily accessible information.

Roger S Kirby

Section 1

General considerations affecting treatment options for patients with prostate cancer

1

Mortality trends in prostate cancer

Peter C Albertsen

With the exception of skin cancers, prostate cancer is the most commonly diagnosed cancer among men and the second leading cause of cancer death in many industrialized nations. In 2004, the American Cancer Society estimates that 29,900 American men will die from prostate cancer and 230,110 will be diagnosed with this disease.[1] Until the late 1980s the incidence and mortality of prostate cancer was rising in most western countries. During the past decade, death rates have declined in some parts of the world while rising in others (Table 1.1). Epidemiologists have closely followed these trends with great interest because they provide insight into the efficacy of screening for prostate cancer using prostate-specific antigen (PSA). Whether the decline in prostate cancer mortality can be attributed to early diagnosis and treatment is the subject of much controversy and debate. This chapter will examine recent trends in prostate cancer mortality and explore potential explanations for these changes.

Data collection, analysis, and presentation

Information regarding prostate cancer incidence and mortality often comes from different sources. Accurate incident rates require an organized tumor registry system in which all new diagnoses of cancers are recorded. In the US, information concerning newly diagnosed cancers is collected by the National Cancer Institute's Surveillance, Epidemiology, and End Results (SEER) program.[2] The SEER program was created following passage of the National Cancer Act in 1971 and is mandated to collect, analyze, and disseminate information that is useful in preventing, diagnosing, and treating cancer. The geographic area comprising the SEER program's database includes approximately 15% of the US population and consists of 11 population-based tumor registries located throughout the country. Similar tumor registries exist in other western countries. Some countries record 100% of cancer diagnoses, while others use an organized system to sample a representative portion of the population. A few tumor registries were organized before World War II; most have been organized more recently.

Information regarding prostate cancer deaths is obtained from death certificates. Several decades ago the World Health Organization (WHO) developed a standardized death certificate that is utilized by most industrialized countries (Figure 1.1). In the US, death certificates are collected and filed by state health departments and vital statistics offices. Each state subsequently forwards the information recorded on the certificate to the National Center for Health Statistics. The underlying cause of death is selected for tabulation

following procedures specified by the WHO in the relevant Manual of the International Classification of Diseases, Injuries, and Causes of Death.[3] Similar reporting mechanisms have been developed by most industrialized nations. The information compiled by each country is subsequently reported to the WHO for analysis.

Cancer incidence and mortality rates are often reported either as actual counts at a given point in time or are expressed as age-adjusted rates. Reporting the raw number of new cases annually provides some information concerning the magnitude of disease incidence and mortality within a country, but it does not take into account the demographic profile of the country. Since countries or regions within the US differ in the number of older men that reside within the geographic boundary of the tumor registry, absolute counts need to be divided by the number of men residing in a region who are at risk of developing prostate cancer. Western countries generally have a greater number of elderly men compared to most developing nations. As men live longer, their risk of developing prostate cancer increases. As a consequence, the absolute number of new cancer cases may increase, but the relative incidence or mortality rate may increase, decrease or remain the same.

To identify trends in cancer incidence and mortality, epidemiologists adjust rates by the age of the men at risk. This facilitates comparisons across differing geographic regions or time periods. In the US, the Bureau of Vital Statistics adjusts incidence and mortality rates to fit the US population age distribution present during a census year. Rates are usually reported as an age-adjusted rate per 100,000 men.

Although the systems for collecting and recording information vary throughout the world, the results can be viewed with a reasonable degree of confidence. In the US data collection takes approximately 3 to 4 years. The widely quoted projections reported annually by the American Cancer Society are derived from data available from the US Census Bureau and the cancer incidence rates collected by the SEER program. Estimates of new cancer cases are calculated using a three-step procedure. First, the annual age-specific cancer incidence rates for a 15-year period are multiplied by the age-appropriate US Census Bureau population projections for the same years to estimate the number of cancer cases diagnosed annually for a 15-year period. These annual cancer case estimates are then fitted to an autoregressive quadratic model. This method is used to predict the following year's rates, and the rates are subsequently extrapolated 3 to 4 years into the future.

Trends in prostate cancer mortality rates are frequently calculated using join-point regression techniques.[4,5] This is a form of regression analysis in which trend data can be described by a number of contiguous linear segments and "join points," a point at which trends change. Usually the statistics derived from these models are the annual percent change (APC) in rates associated with each line segment. Regression models are usually estimated using

Table 1.1 Contemporary trends in age-standardized prostate cancer mortality rates (age 50–79 years)

Increasing	Decreasing	Unchanged
Australia	Austria	Belgium
Bulgaria	Canada	Finland
Greece	France	Hungary
Ireland	Germany	Norway
Israel	Italy	
Japan	UK	
Netherlands	US	
New Zealand		
Poland		
Portugal		
Romania		
Spain		
Sweden		

weighted least squares. A full description of the use of join point regression in the analysis of trends in cancer rates, with special reference to prostate cancer, is given by Kim et al.[5]

International trends in prostate cancer mortality rates

Oliver et al have published age-standardized prostate cancer mortality rates for each of 24 countries (Figure 1.2).[6] The figures are derived from data compiled by the WHO between 1979 and 1997. There is a greater than five-fold difference between rates in Japan (15 prostate cancer deaths/100,000) and Sweden (82/100,000). The highest death rates are in Scandinavia and the lowest in Japan and southern Europe. There has been a constant increase in prostate cancer mortality during most of the period studied. Prostate cancer mortality rates have increased an average of 1% to 2% annually. Although, Japan has one of the lowest prostate cancer mortality rates, it has had one of the highest rates of increase. Downward trends in prostate cancer have been seen in Canada, the US, Austria, France, Germany, Italy, and the UK. Rates in Belgium and Hungary have remained static. Most of these downward trends became established around 1988 to 1991 and have generally decreased annually by 2.1% to 6.0%. Downward trends have been seen in all age groups in those countries experiencing a decrease in prostate cancer mortality with the exception of Germany and Austria, where decreases have been concentrated primarily in the age group 74 to 79 years (Figure 1.3).

Effect of PSA screening and resulting aggressive treatment

Researchers have advanced several theories to explain the observed changes in prostate cancer mortality during the past two decades. Proponents of PSA screening frequently cite the recent declines in prostate cancer mortality rates as proof that PSA testing and subsequent treatment is efficacious.[7-13] Unfortunately, some of the conclusions result from several biases and flawed analyses.[13] Others

hypothesize a cause-and-effect relationship that is too short considering the natural history of localized prostate cancer.[7] Even in the US it is difficult to attribute major population effects to treatment without making implausibly optimistic assumptions.[14]

The explanation that falling mortality rates are the result of PSA testing and aggressive treatment of localized disease does not account for the fact that prostate cancer mortality rates are falling both in regions where there is a high prevalence of screening and treatment and in regions were aggressive PSA testing is not practiced. The UK, for example, has recently witnessed declines in prostate cancer mortality during a period of time when there has been no widespread PSA testing.[15] We recently conducted a comparison of prostate cancer mortality rates in two SEER regions, Connecticut and Seattle.[16] We documented that the physicians in the greater Seattle/King County region were much more aggressive in adopting PSA testing in the late 1980s compared with their Connecticut colleagues. Despite much higher rates of screening, biopsy, and treatment with radical prostatectomy and radiation therapy in Seattle, no differences were noted in the prostate cancer mortality rates in the two regions during 10 years of follow-up. Interestingly, both regions showed similar declines in prostate cancer mortality beginning around 1991.

Effect of attribution bias

Feuer et al[17] explored the possibility that incorrect attribution of cause of death may have contributed to the recent trends in prostate cancer mortality. The large pool of undiagnosed prostate disease identified through autopsy studies makes the reported incidence of prostate cancer particularly susceptible to changes in the use of medical interventions such as PSA testing. The increased number of prostate cancer cases detected as a result of screening efforts drives up the observed pool of prevalent cases and yields a large population of men whose death may potentially be attributed to prostate cancer. Because prostate cancers are often slow growing and men with this disease commonly die of other causes, there is likely to be a certain number of men who die of causes other than prostate cancer but who mistakenly have had their underlying cause of death attributed to prostate cancer merely because they were labeled as having the disease as a result of screening.

To test this hypothesis Feuer et al[17] analyzed incidence-based mortality rates beginning before 1987, when PSA testing began in the US, and for several years afterwards. They noted that after 1987 incidence-based prostate cancer mortality rates rose above the baseline level, but returned to this level by 1994. They concluded that the rise and fall in prostate cancer mortality observed since the introduction of testing in the general population was consistent with the hypothesis that a fixed percent of the rising and falling pool of recently diagnosed patients who died of other causes were mislabeled as dying of prostate cancer.

In two separate studies, we explored the possibility of misattribution bias as a possible confounding effect when interpreting prostate cancer mortality rates. The first explored cause of death determination in Connecticut in two time periods, 1985 and 1995, dates that overlapped the introduction of PSA testing.[18] We found a high level of agreement concerning the underlying cause of death after a review of the information in hospital medical records and on death certificates for men who had previously been diagnosed with prostate cancer. The International Classification of Diseases-9 coding rules concerning cause of death attribution favored over- rather than under-reporting of prostate cancer deaths, but the effect was very

PART 1. DEATH WAS CAUSED BY (ENTER ONLY ONE CAUSE PER LINE FOR (a), (b) AND (c))		APPROXIMATE INTERVAL BETWEEN ONSET AND DEATH
30	IMMEDIATE CAUSE	
CONDITIONS, IF ANY WHICH GAVE RISE TO IMMEDIATE CAUSE (a) STATING THE UNDERLYING CAUSE LAST.	(a) _____ DUE TO, OR AS A CONSEQUENCE OF: (b) _____ DUE TO, OR AS A CONSEQUENCE OF: (c)	

PART II. OTHER SIGNIFICANT CONDITIONS: CONDITIONS CONTRIBUTING TO DEATH BUT NOT RELATED TO CAUSE	AUTOPSY ☐Y ☐N	IF YES, Were findings considered in determining cause of death
31	32	33

NURSE PRONOUNCEMENT TYPE OR PRINT NAME	DEGREE	SIGNATURE	DATE AND TIME PRONOUNCED				
			MONTH	DAY	YEAR	TIME	☐ A.M. ☐ P.M.

Figure 1.1
Death certificate.

modest. More importantly, the cause of death determination did not appear to have changed after the introduction of PSA testing.

A second study involving a review of clinical information and death certificates in King County, Washington confirmed these findings.[19] There was excellent agreement between the underlying cause of death from death certificates and medical records in prostate cancer patients. Prostate cancer patients with concurrent cardiovascular disease were less likely to be coded as having died of prostate cancer than if they had other co-morbidities. Patients with other cancers, such as colon or lung cancer, were also subject to misclassification, but there did not appear to be any systematic bias in either over- or under-diagnosing prostate cancer.

Effect of antiandrogen therapy

Another plausible explanation for the recent decline in prostate cancer mortality rates is the early use of antiandrogen therapy in the treatment of this disease. PSA has been used not only to screen for prostate cancer, but also to monitor disease recurrence following definitive surgery or radiation. Prior to the advent of PSA testing, urologists usually waited for symptomatic metastases before initiating antiandrogen therapy. Rising PSA values have alerted urologists to the presence of residual disease and have led many to initiate antiandrogen therapy before metastases can be identified. The report by Crawford et al in 1989[20] concerning the use of leuprolide and flutamide among men with very early metastatic disease, spurred an enormous increase in the use of antiandrogen therapy that has persisted throughout the past decade.[21]

The strongest evidence supporting the hypothesis that early antiandrogen therapy can increase survival, and thereby lower prostate cancer mortality rates, comes from the phase III EORTC

randomized trial comparing external radiation alone with external radiation combined with antiandrogen therapy in men with advanced localized disease. After a median follow-up of 66 months this trial has demonstrated a significant cancer-specific and all-cause survival advantage for men receiving 3 years of antiandrogen therapy.[22] Other evidence comes from the prospective trial conducted by the Eastern Cooperative Oncology Group that randomized 100 men with node-positive disease at the time of radical prostatectomy to receive either immediate or delayed antiandrogen therapy.[23] After a median follow-up of 7.1 years, men who received immediate antiandrogen therapy had a significant cause-specific and all-cause survival advantage.

The declines in prostate cancer mortality rates documented in several countries also support this hypothesis. Although screening for prostate cancer is not widely supported in the UK, the early use of antiandrogen therapy for men with evidence of systemic disease has paralleled practices in North America. Both geographic regions first witnessed a decline in prostate cancer mortality rates in 1991, shortly after the practice of maximum androgen blockade became widespread. The decline in prostate cancer mortality noted in Quebec is also difficult to ascribe to PSA screening when trends within birth cohorts are analyzed, but the results could be explained by the widespread early use of antiandrogen therapy.[24] Despite significantly different practice patterns in regard to PSA screening, we noted similar declines in prostate cancer mortality rates in Connecticut and Seattle, beginning in 1991.[16] Both regions adopted the practice of maximum androgen blockade around 1990. The evidence of declining prostate cancer mortality rates in Austria also support this hypothesis.[7] The time from the initiation of widespread PSA testing to the subsequent decline in prostate cancer mortality rates is too short to be explained by surgical intervention. The widespread use of early antiandrogen therapy, however, may have had an impact on mortality rates in a much shorter timeframe.

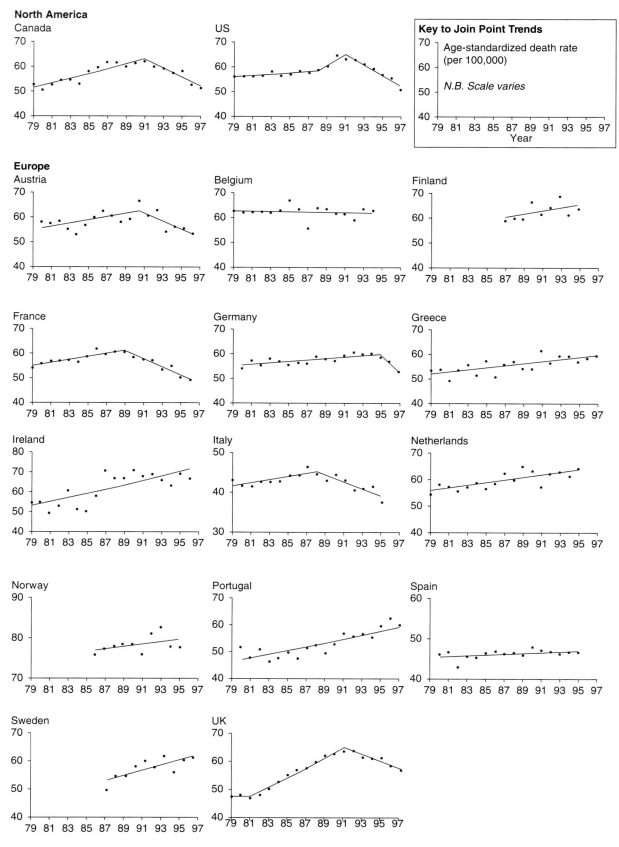

Figure 1.2
Age-standardized mortality rates (range 50–79) for prostate cancer in Europe and North America for the period 1979–1997, with line segments from join-point regression models.
From Oliver et al,[6] with permission.

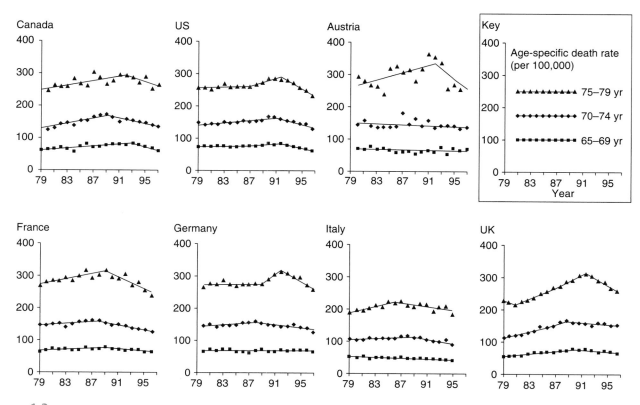

Figure 1.3
Age-specific mortality rates (range 50–79 years) for prostate cancer in countries with a downturn in mortality, with line segments from join-point regression models.
From Oliver et al,[6] with permission.

Summary

Before the 1980s prostate cancer mortality was increasing in most industrialized countries.[25] Between 1988 and 1991 rates began to turn downward in a number of different regions. Several hypotheses have been advanced to explain these findings.[26] Some believe that the downturn in prostate cancer mortality rates is a direct response to aggressive PSA screening and treatment with surgery or radiation. Arguing against this explanation is the observation that mortality rates have declined both in regions where screening is aggressively practiced, such as the US and Canada, *and* in regions were screening with PSA is not practiced, such as the UK. Furthermore, some regions with aggressive PSA screening programs, such as Australia, have not seen a subsequent decline in prostate cancer mortality rates. Even within the US, a region with very aggressive screening and treatment practices, Seattle, saw declines in prostate cancer mortality similar to a region, Connecticut, where PSA testing was not adopted as rapidly.

Another explanation for these findings is a possible systematic misattribution of prostate cancer to many men dying *with* this disease rather than *of* this disease. We have examined this problem and found that death certificates appear to be a reasonably accurate tool for identifying patients who die from prostate cancer. Problems arise in approximately 10% of cases and usually occur when men have other malignancies, such as lung or colon cancer, or suffer from significant co-morbidities, especially cardiac disease. Furthermore, we found no change in cause-of-death attribution when records from before and after the introduction of PSA testing were compared.

One potential explanation for the observed decline in prostate cancer mortality is the widespread use of early antiandrogen therapy. Two randomized trials have documented a survival benefit for those patients placed on antiandrogen therapy very early in the course of their disease. By prolonging life in an older male population many potential prostate cancer deaths may have been converted to deaths from other causes.

Unfortunately observational data are only capable of generating hypotheses. Linking declines in prostate cancer mortality with a specific cause requires a randomized trial. For this reason, clinical trials to determine whether PSA screening can reduce prostate cancer mortality continue in Europe and the US, and are expected to yield results by 2009. Should these trials prove negative, the efficacy of early antiandrogen therapy to lower prostate cancer mortality should be reinvestigated.

References

1. Jemal A, Tiwari RC, Murray T, et al. Cancer statistics, 2004. CA Cancer J Clin 2004;54:8–29.
2. Ries LAG, Kosary CL, Hankey BF, et al (eds). SEER Cancer Statistics Review, 1973–1995 (NIH Publication No. 98–2789). Bethesda, MD: National Cancer Institute, 1998.
3. World Health Organization. World Health Statistics Annual 1996. Geneva: World Health Organization, 1998.
4. Hinkley DV. Inference in two–phase regression. J Am Stat Assoc 1971;66:736–743.

5. Kim HJ, Fay MP, Feuer EJ, et al. Permutation tests for joinpoint regression with applications to cancer rates. Stat Med 2000;19:335–351.

6. Oliver SE, May MT, Gunnell D. International trends in prostate cancer mortality in the "PSA era". Int J Cancer 2001;92:893–898.

7. Bartsch G, Horninger W, Klocker H, et al. Prostate cancer mortality after introduction of prostate-specific antigen mass screening in the federal state of Tyrol, Austria. Urology 2001;58:417–424.

8. Hankey BF, Feuer EJ, Clegg LX, et al. Cancer surveillance series: Interpreting trends in prostate cancer – Part I: Evidence of the effects of screening in recent prostate cancer incidence, mortality and survival rates. J Natl Cancer Inst 1999;91:1017–1024.

9. Farkas A, Schneider D, Perrotti M, et al. National trends in the epidemiology of prostate cancer, to 1994: evidence for the effectiveness of PSA screening. Urology 1995;52:444–448.

10. Littrup PJ. Future benefits and cost-effectiveness of prostate carcinoma screening. Cancer 1997;80:1864–1870.

11. Hoeksema MJ, Law C. Cancer mortality rates fall: a turning point for the nation. J Natl Cancer Inst 1996;88:1706–1707.

12. Horninger W, Reissigl A, Rogatsch H, et al. Prostate cancer screening in the Tyrol, Austria: experience and results. Eur J Cancer 2000;36:1322–1335.

13. Labrie F, Candas B, Dupont A, et al. Screening decreases prostate cancer death. First analysis of the 1988 Quebec prospective randomized controlled trial. Prostate 1999;38:83–91.

14. Etzioni R, Legler JM, Feuer EJ, et al. Cancer surveillance series: Interpreting trends in prostate cancer – Part III: Quantifying the link between population prostate-specific antigen testing and recent declines in prostate cancer mortality. J Natl Cancer Inst 1999;91:1033–1039.

15. Oliver SE, Gunnell D, Donovan JL. Comparison of trends in prostate cancer mortality in England and Wales and the USA. Lancet 2000;355:1788–1789.

16. Lu-Yao G, Albertsen PC, Stanford JL, et al. Natural experiment examining the impact of aggressive screening and treatment on prostate cancer mortality in two fixed cohorts from Seattle area and Connecticut. BMJ 2002;325:740.

17. Feuer EJ, Merrill RM, Hankey BF. Cancer surveillance series: Interpreting trends in prostate cancer. Part II. Cause of death misclassification and the recent rise and fall in prostate cancer mortality. J Natl Cancer Inst 1999;91:1025–1032.

18. Albertsen PC, Walters S, Hanley JA. A comparison of cause of death determination in men previously diagnosed with prostate cancer who died in 1985 or 1995. J Urol 2000;163:519–523.

19. Penson DF, Albertsen PC, Nelson PS, et al. Determining cause of death in prostate cancer: are death certificates valid? J Natl Cancer Inst 2001;93:1822–1823.

20. Crawford ED, Eisenberger MA, McLeod DG, et al. A controlled trial of leuprolide with and without flutamide in prostatic cancer. N Engl J Med 1989;321:419–424.

21. Cooperberg MR, Grossfeld GD, Lubeck DP, et al. National practice patterns and time trends in androgen ablation for localized prostate cancer. J Natl Cancer Inst 2003;95:981–989.

22. Bolla M, Collette L, Blank L, et al. Long-term results with immediate androgen suppression and external radiation in patients with locally advanced prostate cancer (an EORTC study): a phase III randomized trial. Lancet 2002;360:103–108.

23. Messing EM, Manola J, Sarosdy M, et al. Immediate hormonal therapy compared with observation after radical prostatectomy and pelvic lymphadenectomy in men with node-positive prostate cancer. N Engl J Med 1999;341:1781–1788.

24. Perron L, Moore L, Bairati I, et al. PSA screening and prostate cancer mortality. Can Med Assoc J 2002;166:586–591.

25. Hsing A, Tsao L, Devesa SS. International trends and patterns of prostate cancer incidence and mortality. Int J Cancer 2000;85:60–67.

26. Frankel S, Smith GD, Donovan J, et al. Screening for prostate cancer. Lancet 2003;361:1122–1128.

2

Decision-making for men with prostate cancer

Mark R Feneley, Leslie Moffat, Charlotte Rees

Introduction

Decision-making is complex and involves processes comprising highly variable components; often these are unique to the individuals involved. It would be fair to say that the scientific analysis of decision-making by patients is in its infancy. Traditional expectations would pre-suppose that all patients receive the same factual information, that clinicians explaining treatment options would have only disinterested perceptions of best treatment, and that patients would have equivalent interests and expectations. Even in such rational and unbiased circumstances, decisions may be expected to differ. Outcomes, though notoriously variable for men with prostate cancer, are to some extent related to decisions and the factors that influence them. This chapter will consider factors that may influence decisions concerning prostate cancer management from medical, educational, and economic perspectives, as well as how "best" decisions may be facilitated.

Patient decision-making

Men with prostate cancer are faced with growing choices and increased involvement in decision-making for their disease management. There is a growing awareness that the "best choice" perceived by increasingly empowered patients may not necessarily be their physician's recommendation. Decisions regarding prostate cancer management should be reached by taking into consideration the best available evidence, but they are also influenced by other factors, such as the type of doctor–patient relationship, availability and use of information, individual circumstances, and personal values.

An expanding body of evidence, addressed in this chapter, indicates the importance of patient involvement in the medical decision-making process. Important (but often forgotten) issues that arise from facilitating such involvement relate to the ability of patients to make particular decisions, the extent of their willingness to engage in decisions, and the consequences arising when a patient's decisions differ from the recommendations of healthcare professionals. These considerations may influence substantially the presentation, content, and use of educational material required by patients.

Patient engagement in healthcare

For the patient with prostate cancer who is faced with therapeutic alternatives, involvement in decision-making is often not his first opportunity for choice in matters of prostate health, particularly when the disease was diagnosed through involvement in a healthcare program such as screening. Ethical consideration demands that prior to participation in a program of screening or early diagnosis, an individual should be reliably informed of the implications of test results.

Information and views acquired through the screening process may influence a patient's subsequent presentation to specialists after a diagnosis of prostate cancer. Hanna et al[1] observed that the specialty of the physician to whom patients were initially referred reflected subsequent treatment. Fowler et al[2] showed that individual oncologists and surgeons tend to favor the treatment they themselves deliver. These studies suggest potentially significant decisional bias. From the first healthcare contact, a patient's involvement in decision-making may be influenced significantly by the patient–doctor relationship.

Doctor–patient relationships

The importance of the doctor–patient relationship in decision-making is continually emphasized. Morgan[3] outlined four types of relationship—paternalism, mutuality, consumerism, and default—and describes them as follows. A *paternalistic* relationship involves high physician control over decision-making but low patient control. Here, the doctor acts as a trusted parent and makes decisions for the good of his/her patient. This relationship is vital in contexts such as emergency medicine where patients may be incapable of participating in decision-making processes. The *consumerist* relationship reverses this power association, and involves high patient control over decision-making but low physician control. This relationship is seen most keenly in settings such as private healthcare. A *mutual* relationship is characterized by a partnership between the patient and doctor, with the patient and doctor having active involvement in decisions. In this situation, the doctor and patient bring different expertise to the consultation. The patient comes as an expert on his experiences, beliefs, feelings, and expectations and the doctor brings his/her clinical experience to the consultation. The final type of doctor–patient relationship, *default*, occurs when doctors reduce their control within the consultation but patients continue to adopt a passive role in decision-making.

Shared decision-making

Shared decision-making is a widely used descriptive term, but the concept is often applied without precise definition. General definitions refer to increasing patient involvement in medical decisions,[4] and more specific definitions include the notion that professionals and patients contribute equally to decisions about treatment.[5] In shared decision-making, control is not vested entirely in the patient as in an informed choice model.[5]

Patients of course differ in their preferences for involvement in decision-making.[6] In a decision analysis study based in general practice, physical problems, older age, and lower social class were shown to be positively correlated with patients preferring a more directed approach over a shared approach.[7] However, other assumed factors, such as gender and perceived chronic health, were not found to predict preferences for a directed approach.[7] In addition, other studies emphasize a correlation between a preference for shared decision-making and a higher level of education. The value of the shared decision-making model and its various components requires further exploration and research, and the term should therefore be understood in the context of its given definition.

Information content

Patients' effective participation in decision-making requires that they are offered the most relevant information, and this is presented optimally for their understanding. Obligatory information must include the future impact of their disease, its likely response to treatment, and the potential side effects of treatment.[8] Details, however, may be perceived subjectively in relation to decision-making, and treatment outcomes cannot be predicted with absolute accuracy. There is large variation in the information required by individuals with early prostate cancer for decision-making, and this needs to be accommodated in the process of informing patients.[9]

The content utilized by individuals may vary according to the type of doctor–patient relationship, with more detailed information on treatments and impact on quality of life required in collaborative decision-making than if the patient takes an active or a passive role.[10] The conditions for balanced decisions will always be difficult to standardize. Also, the distinction between a patient's desire for information and his wish to assume responsibility for decision-making is important.[11] A patient's desire to participate actively in decision-making should therefore not be assumed on the basis of his need for information.

Information is frequently sought by patients following diagnosis and used in anticipation of specialist consultation. Davison et al[12] have shown that a computerized prostate cancer information program can provide men newly diagnosed with prostate cancer and their partners with individualized information that supports subsequent decision-making while also reducing psychological distress. This and other studies have shown that information provided at this early stage may empower the patient and facilitate his preferred more active or collaborative decision-making style within the consultation, as well as improving his subsequent recall of the consultation.[13–15]

The need for content and quality of standardized information resources to add benefit in terms of patient preferences and satisfaction has been pointed out by Rimer et al.[16] Importantly, but frequently assumed, the possible negative consequences of using standardized information should also be avoided.[16] As yet, the provision of information has not been linked to decisional regret following treatment, but this has not been evaluated sufficiently and further longitudinal study is required.[17,18] Appropriate tools for studying decisional regret need to be developed and validated,[19] particularly for long-term follow-up of prostate cancer decisions.

Patients now have access to vast amounts of information, selected and viewed from a wide variety of resources. The process tends to be nonsystematic and biased by individual interests. Content and quality may be inadequate, even in material prepared and provided by healthcare professionals.[20,21] Content generally considered imperative for men with prostate cancer includes prostate biology, anatomy, physiology, prostate specific antigen (PSA) testing, tumor biology, including grading and staging, description of standard management options, and outcomes. This medical information must be presented in a style appropriate to the patient in terms of educational level and literacy. Additional content helping the patient and his family to understand and live with the disease, cope with its potential impact on personal relationships, family, employment, and social life, as well as provide resources for support is essential, and must not be undervalued. The distinction between the need for information and the desire to participate in decision-making has been emphasized above,[11] and is important in the selection of content and its evaluation.

The particular sources and content of information that ultimately influence individual treatment decisions vary considerably. Healthcare professionals need to ensure that patients are appropriately informed of their choices and have a balanced understanding prior to decision-making. The patient's own views may nevertheless differ from a professional's assessment. This potential conflict emphasizes the need for a balance between a patient's quality of life, dignity, and autonomy on one side, and medical evidence and compassion on the other.

Educational material provided prior to consultation may be more effective when combined with additional individualized interventions. For instance, Davison and Degner[22] showed that an empowerment intervention supplementing the provision of brochures on prostate cancer resulted in patients taking a more active role during the consultation. This additional individualized and patient-orientated intervention included a review of a list of questions for discussion, an option to record on audiotape the subsequent consultation, and encouragement to bring significant others to accompany the patient.

Treatment decisions for men with prostate cancer

All patients do not perform equally in making choices, regardless of the value or a right or wrong attribute of an individual decision. Patients also vary in their desire to make choices and have different perceptions of what might constitute their best treatment choice. Patients differ in their self-interest and may be influenced by others, including the experiences of friends, relatives, significant others, and professionals.

Self-interested behavior has been described by Sen[23] to be characterised by three features:

- Self-centred welfare: a person's welfare depends only on his/her own consumption.
- Self-welfare goals: a person's goal is to maximize his/her own welfare and—given uncertainty—the probability-weighted expected value of that welfare.
- Self-goal choice: each act of choice of a person is guided immediately by the pursuit of his/her own goal.

Differences in self-interest may influence how individuals differently perceive risk versus benefit, and incorporate assessment of such trade-offs in deciding between available choices.

For men first diagnosed with early prostate cancer, immediate treatment choices include radical prostatectomy, various forms of radiation therapy, or active monitoring (with no immediate treatment). Alternatively, interventions employing developing technologies (i.e. those without long-term outcome data) may be considered. How the "best" medical decision is to be made will vary between patients. Its complexity is increased by the lack of any contemporary randomized trials demonstrating overall statistically significant survival differences between the three principal management choices (or the alternatives). Various trials of treatment are in progress, including the ProtecT (prostate testing for cancer and treatment) study in the UK, which importantly includes active monitoring in its randomization.[24]

Decisions may be strongly influenced, therefore, by the relative value placed on the impact of the disease versus the durability of treatment response, its side effects and impact on quality of life. Value assessments may reflect an individual's personality and experiences, and this may contribute to absolute differences in decision outcomes between patients and between patients and their healthcare advisors. For instance, the impact of incontinence may be over- or under-played by patient and doctor alike, depending on its impact, acceptability, and individual factors. Where none of the prospective options can be shown to be of comparative benefit by robust evidence, the predominating values of individuals and the nature of doctor–patient relationships will ultimately drive medical decisions.

An ethical view has arisen concerning the status of no immediate treatment (i.e. active monitoring) as an equivalent choice.[25–27] Views on equivalence may be influenced by information provided by healthcare professionals,[28] but there may be other considerations. Receiving no immediate treatment is not always considered objectively to be equivalent to effective treatment, either by the patient or by healthcare professionals. Furthermore, significant practical difficulties can face patients for whom watchful waiting may be a reasonable option.[29,30] The lack of perceived decisional equivalence may prevail in spite of the risk and implications of over-treatment (i.e. treatment of disease that would not impact the patient's future health). It seems likely that future studies will define increasing numbers of patients with early stage low-risk prostate cancer for whom active treatment may be appropriately deferred.

Wider ethical issues concern choices to which patients do not have equal opportunity, reflecting both individual entitlement and distribution of healthcare. Furthermore, given the finite budget of any healthcare system, there will be trade-offs between equity and efficiency endangering what could loosely be termed "fairness." Equity can be defined as equality of access for equal needs, whereas efficiency is the efficient allocation of resource where such resource is forced to be limited. The concept of efficiency is borrowed from the private sector.[31] If social and economic inequalities are to be arranged for an overall advantage to everyone, as suggested by the philosopher John Rawls, then ethical concerns will arise in healthcare.[32]

Decision tools

Decision tools may facilitate the complex process of decision-making. They must, however, be applied and integrated carefully within healthcare systems, and subjected to rigorous evaluation. Tools have been developed in a variety of settings for patients with prostate cancer, other malignancies, nonmalignant conditions, and prostate cancer screening.[33,34] Mostly, they have been evaluated for their

impact on decision-making itself, and few studies have examined their effect on subsequent outcomes.

The various components and processes in decision-making, and extrinsic factors that may influence decisions indirectly, give rise to a wide range in the utility of decision tools and other materials. Some tools are designed to facilitate the task of decision-making by reducing decisional conflict, mostly in an interactive setting.[35] These tools need to be distinguished from educational materials or programs that facilitate treatment decisions by other means. Any or all of these approaches need to be validated, and applied according to their specific design and purpose.

Educational material can be provided for patients with a variety of purposes, including as a decision-aid.[36] A wide range of information-containing media for use as decision aids has been described in relation to prostate cancer, but with limited evaluation of their utility. Indeed, much of the available patient educational material fails to address adequately components of decision-making other than disease, and therefore may perform poorly as decision aids.[20] Examples of the range of media include paper-based pamphlets, video tools,[13,37] CD-ROMs,[38] websites on the Internet,[39–41] and hypermedia programs.[42] Such products are widely distributed and supported by charities, government agencies, professional organizations, and other bodies.[43–45] Web-based programs can be accessed widely and updated appropriately. The information tends to be standardized rather than individualized.[12] Media that specifically allow patient interaction offer the means for individualized information requirements to be met, and they may be supported by print. Further research is required to assure the effectiveness and value of different approaches.

The facilitation of understanding via particular media varies between individuals, owing to differences in need, perception, and application (use) of the information offered. For example, patients differ significantly in their predisposition to monitoring (wanting voluminous information) or blunting (avoiding information) to facilitate coping processes.[46] Also, the degree of empowerment provided and its impact on the balance of the doctor–patient relationship may be highly variable.[47] The impact on decisions (and ultimately outcomes) of the availability of large volumes of information and various media is, however, poorly understood.[48]

Perceptions of prostate cancer diagnosis and involvement in treatment decisions may differ significantly between patients and their partners.[49] For example, Davison et al[50] found differences in the need for content-related information and preferences for decision-making, with patients preferring active roles and partners preferring collaborative roles. Appropriate information may also alter involvement of both patient and partner in decision-making.[12] These observations serve to illustrate the influence of relatives in decision-making and, therefore, their vital role.[51,52] This was exemplified in a Dutch study of shared decision-making in patients with prostate cancer.[53] Most patients (76%) were found to have had some influence in decision-making, and those who did not were more likely to be older and not to have a partner.[53]

Rees et al[44] examined the quality of 31 patient information leaflets widely available in the UK and which discuss treatment options. The leaflets were assessed for quality, readability, and suitability using the DISCERN instrument, Flesch formula, and Suitability Assessment of Materials (SAM) instrument. Despite scores on all measures varying between leaflets, it was possible to identity the best five leaflets across the conditions, including those produced for Cancer BACUP, the Prostate Cancer Charity, and the Covent Garden Cancer Research Trust. The study also examined their acceptability to patients, but not their effectiveness in aiding treatment decision-making.

Feldman-Stewart et al[54] reported on the use of a question-and-answer booklet aimed at addressing the distinct requirements of patients and their families wanting to understand early-stage prostate cancer. They showed that information is used differently by patients and family. Patients were more inclined to want help for decision-making and planning, while family tended to seek help for providing support. Due to the design of the study, however, it is impossible to say whether this booklet was effective in helping to make treatment decisions. Feldman-Stewart and Brundage[33] subsequently explored the challenges for designing and implementing decision aids with three illustrative examples. One of these was their decision aid to help patients with treatment decisions for early-stage prostate cancer. They observed that the design and implementation of such aids require critical assessment in definition of content, presentation of information, and application into decision-making, and may challenge preconceived assumptions.

Some educational programs aim to reduce anxiety associated with newly diagnosed cancer, particularly where ongoing distress may impair understanding and coping as well as decision-making itself.[55] Anxiety may also be influenced by personal relationships, educational background, and cultural differences.[56–59] Perceptions of "best" choice may also be significantly influenced by peer experience and opinion.[60] Conflict may also arise where decisions do not relate to the wider objectives of healthcare systems.

As mentioned above, important distinctions should be made between a patient's desire for information and his desire or ability to participate in decision-making. Understanding is essential for decision-making and this may be difficult to achieve when highly complex information is presented. Individual decision-making incorporates the utility of alternatives with characteristics of self-interested behavior. Patients' and doctors' judgements may also be biased, particularly by selective processing of information, and patients tend not to use available material either comprehensively or systematically.[61]

All these factors may have an unpredictable impact on patient-centered decision-making. For instance, in a study showing that paper-based decision aids increased men's knowledge of the advantages and disadvantages of screening, this benefit could not be related to men's decision to undergo screening.[34] This illustrates the importance of taking into consideration the many factors other than information that influence decision-making and outcomes, and the need to incorporate these in the critical evaluation of decision tools.

Evaluating an early prostate cancer treatment decision tool against disease-specific and quality-of-life outcomes is currently fraught with difficulties associated with lack of prospective data, changing clinical practice, and unavoidable bias in the observation of clinical outcomes. Decision tools to predict clinically useful endpoints have, however, been used for conditions other than prostate cancer. Dowding et al[62] reported on the development and preliminary evaluation of computerized decision aids for two nonmalignant conditions, including benign prostatic hyperplasia. This program is based on decision analysis using decision trees as a means to provide users with information about the probability of various outcomes and guidance on what might be the "best" option for the individual.[62]

Decision tools are likely to be developed and used by patients with prostate cancer at various stages of disease and may challenge medical recommendations and concepts in healthcare. Research and well-designed prospective longitudinal studies are required to exclude long-term negative impact from decisional regret, interpersonal conflict or discordance with professionals, as well as demonstrate reproducible advantages and benefits from the use of appropriately designed tools.

Conclusion

Educational material may be sought by patients, or provided by healthcare professionals, to give information necessary for patients to understand their condition and participate in medical decision-making. The balance between understanding and participation may vary considerably according to ability and desire, as well as personal values and relationships. Choices that face patients may not be equal, particularly in relation to inequalities in distribution and the therapeutic efficiency of alternative interventions, and thereby are subject to sociopolitical and ethical considerations.

Decision tools can facilitate specific aspects of medical decision-making and reduce anxiety or distress arising following diagnosis. The role and behavior of the patient and healthcare professional in specific decision-making may be altered with wider and longer-term potential benefits, such as concordance, and improved physical and psychological outcomes. Further research is needed to develop and validate programs to improve therapeutic decision-making and demonstrate advantage in long-term medical, physical, psychological, and social outcomes.

References

1. Hanna CL, Mason MD, Donovan JL, et al. Clinical oncologists favour radical radiotherapy for localized prostate cancer: a questionnaire survey. BJU Int 2002;90:558–560.
2. Fowler FJ Jr, McNaughton Collins M, et al. Comparison of recommendations by urologists and radiation oncologists for treatment of clinically localized prostate cancer. JAMA 2000;283:3217–3222.
3. Morgan M. The doctor–patient relationship. In Scambler G (ed): Sociology as Applied to Medicine, 4th ed. Edinburgh: WB Saunders, 1997, pp 47–62.
4. Malis R, Makoul G. Definitions of "shared decision making" evident in the medical literature. Paper presented at the International Conference on Communication in Healthcare, Sept 14–17, 2004, Bruges, Belgium.
5. Edwards A, Elwyn G. The potential benefits of decision aids in clinical medicine. JAMA 1999;282:779–780.
6. Degner LF, Kristjanson LJ, Bowman D, et al. Information needs and decisional preferences in women with breast cancer. JAMA 1997;277:1485–1492.
7. McKinstry B. Do patients wish to be involved in decision making in the consultation? A cross sectional survey with video vignettes. BMJ 2000;321:867–871.
8. Davison BJ, Keyes M, Elliott S, et al. Preferences for sexual information resources in patients treated for early-stage prostate cancer with either radical prostatectomy or brachytherapy. BJU Int 2004;93:965–969.
9. Feldman-Stewart D, Brundage MD, et al. The information required by patients with early-stage prostate cancer in choosing their treatment. BJU Int 2001;87:218–223.
10. Davison BJ, Parker PA, Goldenberg SL. Patients' preferences for communicating a prostate cancer diagnosis and participating in medical decision-making. BJU Int 2004;93:47–51.
11. Fallowfield L. Participation of patients in decisions about treatment for cancer. BMJ 2001;323:1144.
12. Davison BJ, Goldenberg SL, Gleave ME, et al. Provision of individualized information to men and their partners to facilitate treatment decision making in prostate cancer. Oncol Nurs Forum 2003;30:107–114.
13. McGregor S. Information on video format can help patients with localised prostate cancer to be partners in decision making. Patient Educ Couns 2003;49:279–283.
14. Schapira MM, Meade C, Nattinger AB. Enhanced decision-making: the use of a videotape decision-aid for patients with prostate cancer. Patient Educ Couns 1997;30:119–127.

15. Auvinen A, Hakama M, Ala-Opas M, et al. A randomized trial of choice of treatment in prostate cancer: the effect of intervention on the treatment chosen. BJU Int 2004;93:52–56.

16. Rimer BK, Briss PA, Zeller PK, et al. Informed decision making: what is its role in cancer screening? Cancer 2004;101(5 Suppl):1214–1228.

17. Davison BJ, Goldenberg SL. Decisional regret and quality of life after participating in medical decision-making for early-stage prostate cancer. BJU Int 2003;91:14–17.

18. Diefenbach MA, Dorsey J, Uzzo RG, et al. Decision-making strategies for patients with localized prostate cancer. Semin Urol Oncol 2002;20:55–62.

19. Brehaut JC, O'Connor AM, Wood TJ, et al. Validation of a decision regret scale. Med Decis Making 2003;23:281–292.

20. Fagerlin A, Rovner D, Stableford S, et al. Patient education materials about the treatment of early-stage prostate cancer: a critical review. Ann Intern Med 2004;140:721–728.

21. Walling AM, Maliski S, Bogorad A, et al. Assessment of content completeness and accuracy of prostate cancer patient education materials. Patient Educ Couns 2004;54:337–343.

22. Davison BJ, Degner LF. Empowerment of men newly diagnosed with prostate cancer. Cancer Nurs 1997;20:187–196.

23. Sen AK. On Ethics and Economics. Oxford: Blackwell, 1987.

24. Neal DE, Donovan JL. Prostate cancer: to screen or not to screen? Lancet Oncol 2000;1:17–24.

25. Lilford RJ. Ethics of clinical trials from a bayesian and decision analytic perspective: whose equipoise is it anyway? BMJ 2003;326:980–981.

26. Frankel S, Sterne J, Ebrahim S. Ethics of clinical trials from bayesian perspective: Medical decision making should use posteriors, not priors. BMJ 2003;326:1456.

27. Hamdy FC, Donovan JL, Lane JA, et al. Ethics of clinical trials from bayesian perspective: Randomisation to clinical trials may solve dilemma of treatment choice in prostate cancer. BMJ 2003;326:1456.

28. Donovan J, Mills N, Smith M, et al. Quality improvement report: Improving design and conduct of randomised trials by embedding them in qualitative research: ProtecT (prostate testing for cancer and treatment) study. Commentary: presenting unbiased information to patients can be difficult. BMJ 2002;325:766–770.

29. Chapple A, Ziebland S, Herxheimer A, et al. Is 'watchful waiting' a real choice for men with prostate cancer? A qualitative study. BJU Int 2002;90:257–264.

30. Holmboe ES, Concato J. Treatment decisions for localized prostate cancer: asking men what's important. J Gen Intern Med 2000;15:694–701.

31. Mooney G. Economics, Medicine and Health Care. London: Wheatsheaf, 1992.

32. Rawls J. A Theory of Justice. Oxford: Oxford University Press, 1999.

33. Feldman-Stewart D, Brundage MD. Challenges for designing and implementing decision aids. Patient Educ Couns 2004;54:265–273.

34. Sheridan SL, Felix K, Pignone MP, et al. Information needs of men regarding prostate cancer screening and the effect of a brief decision aid. Patient Educ Couns 2004;54:345–351.

35. Deyo RA. A key medical decision maker: the patient. BMJ 2001;323:466–467.

36. O'Connor AM, Stacey D, Entwistle V, et al. Decision aids for people facing health treatment or screening decisions. Cochrane Database Syst Rev 2003;(2):CD001431.

37. Gomella LG, Albertsen PC, Benson MC, et al. The use of video-based patient education for shared decision-making in the treatment of prostate cancer. Semin Urol Oncol 2000;18:182–187.

38. DePalma A. Prostate cancer shared decision: a CD-ROM educational and decision-assisting tool for men with prostate cancer. Semin Urol Oncol 2000;18:178–181.

39. Lipp ER. Web resources for patients with prostate cancer: a starting point. Semin Urol Oncol 2002;20:32-38.

40. Pautler SE, Tan JK, Dugas GR, et al. Use of the internet for self-education by patients with prostate cancer. Urology 2001;57:230–233.

41. Moul JW, Esther TA, Bauer JJ. Implementation of a web-based prostate cancer decision site. Semin Urol Oncol 2000;18:241–244.

42. Jenkinson J, Wilson-Pauwels L, Jewett MA, et al. Development of a hypermedia program designed to assist patients with localized prostate cancer in making treatment decisions. J Biocommun 1998;25:2–11.

43. Godolphin W, Towle A, McKendry R. Evaluation of the quality of patient information to support informed shared decision-making. Health Expect 2001;4:235–242.

44. Rees CE, Ford JE, Sheard CE. Patient information leaflets for prostate cancer: which leaflets should healthcare professionals recommend? Patient Educ Couns 2003;49:263–272.

45. Rees CE, Ford JE, Sheard CE. Evaluating the reliability of DISCERN: a tool for assessing the quality of written patient information on treatment choices. Patient Educ Couns 2002;47:273–275.

46. Miller SM. Monitoring versus blunting styles of coping with cancer influence the information patients want and need about their disease. Implications for cancer screening and management. Cancer 1995;76:167–177.

47. Wong F, Stewart DE, Dancey J, et al. Men with prostate cancer: influence of psychological factors on informational needs and decision making. J Psychosom Res 2000;49:13–19.

48. Patel HR, Mirsadraee S, Emberton M. The patient's dilemma: prostate cancer treatment choices. J Urol 2003;169:828–833.

49. Boehmer U, Clark JA. Married couples' perspectives on prostate cancer diagnosis and treatment decision-making. Psychooncology 2001;10:147–155.

50. Davison BJ, Gleave ME, Goldenberg SL, et al. Assessing information and decision preferences of men with prostate cancer and their partners. Cancer Nurs 2002;25:42–49.

51. Srirangam SJ, Pearson E, Grose C, et al. Partner's influence on patient preference for treatment in early prostate cancer. BJU Int 2003;92:365–369.

52. Carlson LE, Ottenbreit N, St Pierre M, et al. Partner understanding of the breast and prostate cancer experience. Cancer Nurs 2001;24:231–239.

53. Fischer MJ, Visser AP, Voerman B, et al. Who decides? Information and shared decision making in prostate cancer in the Netherlands. Paper presented at the International Conference on Communication in Healthcare, 14–17th Sept, 2004, Bruges, Belgium.

54. Feldman-Stewart D, Brundage MD, Van Manen L, et al. Evaluation of a question-and-answer booklet on early-stage prostate-cancer. Patient Educ Couns 2003;49:115–124.

55. Flynn D, Van Schaik P, Van Wersch A, et al. The utility of a multimedia education program for prostate cancer patients: a formative evaluation. Br J Cancer 2004;91:855–860.

56. Kim SP, Knight SJ, Tomori C, et al. Health literacy and shared decision making for prostate cancer patients with low socioeconomic status. Cancer Invest 2001;19:684–691.

57. Taylor KL, Turner RO, Davis JL, III, et al. Improving knowledge of the prostate cancer screening dilemma among African American men: an academic-community partnership in Washington, DC. Public Health Rep 2001;116:590–598.

58. Myers RE. African American men, prostate cancer early detection examination use, and informed decision-making. Semin Oncol 1999;26:375–381.

59. Guidry JJ, Aday LA, Zhang D, et al. Information sources and barriers to cancer treatment by racial/ethnic minority status of patients. J Cancer Educ 1998;13:43–48.

60. Berry DL, Ellis WJ, Woods NF, et al. Treatment decision-making by men with localized prostate cancer: the influence of personal factors. Urol Oncol 2003;21:93–100.

61. Steginga SK, Occhipinti S, Gardiner RA, et al. Making decisions about treatment for localized prostate cancer. BJU Int 2002;89:255–260.

62. Dowding D, Swanson V, Bland R, et al. The development and preliminary evaluation of a decision aid based on decision analysis for two treatment conditions: benign prostatic hyperplasia and hypertension. Patient Educ Couns 2004;52:209–215.

3

Practical and realistic lifestyle changes and supplements for the man concerned about prostate cancer: What do I tell my patients?

Mark A Moyad

Abstract

It is critical to remember that the primary cause of death in the United States and in most countries around the world is cardiovascular disease (CVD), and it is also the number 1 or 2 cause of death in prostate cancer prevention trials, and in untreated and treated prostate cancer patients. These findings serve to place the overall risk of death in men into its proper perspective, and it does not serve to belittle the seriousness of prostate cancer or another disease or condition. Generally speaking, what has been found to be heart healthy has been tantamount to prostate healthy, and there may even be a relationship between the two conditions. Therefore, clinicians need to provide a simplistic and realistic set of lifestyle changes to patients to not only attempt to reduce prostate cancer risk and mortality, but to attempt to impact all-cause mortality. A list of recommendations are provided in this chapter to assist the clinician and patient in their discussion of simple and practical changes that may not only be accomplished in a short period of time, but should provide at least some type of tangible overall benefit for the man concerned about prostate cancer.

Introduction

Some simplistic and practical observations need mentioning to place lifestyle recommendations in their proper perspective. Cardiovascular disease continues to be the number 1 cause of death in the United States and in other industrialized countries,[1] and it is now the primary cause of mortality worldwide. The World Health Organization (WHO) has documented that CVD is the number one cause of mortality in every region of the world with the exception of sub-Saharan Africa, and it is predicted that this disease will surpass the number 1 cause of death in that specific region, infectious disease, within the next decade.[2–5]

Recently the media was replete with reports indicating that cancer has now surpassed heart disease as the leading cause of death in Americans.[6] This was an interesting new finding, but it was not entirely correct. In 2002, the latest year for which mortality data are available, cancer was responsible for 478,082 deaths and heart disease was responsible for 446,727 deaths in individuals younger than the age of 85. Therefore, cancer was reported as the number 1 killer for Americans younger than 85 years of age. If this age consideration

was not categorized in this manner then heart disease is still the number 1 killer of Americans—in 2002, 696,947 individuals in the US died of heart disease versus 557,271 deaths from cancer. Heart disease is the primary cause or mortality in those aged 85 and older. In fact, in this older age group, heart disease was responsible for three times more deaths (>250,000) compared with cancer (~80,000 deaths) in 2002. Additionally, if one actually compares CVD (heart disease and diseases of the blood vessels, including strokes) with cancer, an entirely different picture of the situation is revealed. Cardiovascular disease is responsible for 38% of all deaths and is responsible for more deaths than the next five leading causes of death combined. Death rates from all cancers combined have been slowly declining over the past decade (1.5% per year since 1993 for men and 0.8% per year for women since 1992). However, the death rate from heart disease has been falling for a greater period of time, since the mid-1970s. Therefore, even in 1999, cancer deaths outnumbered heart disease deaths in individuals younger than 85 years. Even in individuals over the age of 85 years, heart disease deaths have declined compared with cancer. The notable improvements in mortality rates for both prominent diseases apparently were partially due to a decrease in smoking rates in the US. For example, in women, lung cancer deaths have stabilized after increasing for several decades, and death rates from breast and colorectal cancer have decreased. In men, the death rate has also continued to fall for the three most prevalent cancers (colorectal, lung, and prostate).

Some of the largest US cancer prevention trials and cancer screening studies demonstrate the impact of the observations presented above. The recent results of the Prostate Cancer Prevention Trial (PCPT) seem to have generated a lot of interest and controversy regarding the use of daily finasteride to reduce the risk of prostate cancer.[7–9] Finasteride was responsible for an approximate and significant 25% reduction in the number of prostate cancer cases during 7 years of study, but an apparent higher risk of aggressive prostate cancer was also found in the finasteride arm of the trial. Interestingly, as the debate over the advantages and disadvantages of finasteride continue, several important observations from this trial have not received much attention in the medical literature. Over 18,000 men were included in this randomized trial, and 5 men died from prostate cancer in the finasteride arm and 5 men died of prostate cancer in the placebo arm, but over 1100 men died in this study. Thus, prostate cancer was responsible for less than 1% of the deaths in this trial, while the majority of the deaths were apparently due to CVD. Thus, the results of the first large-scale prostate cancer prevention trial ever conducted in medicine demonstrated that CVD is indeed the primary cause of death in men, but again this finding has received little attention until now. Does this finding reduce the seriousness or impact of prostate cancer prevention utilizing a prostate-specific chemoprevention agent? Obviously not; but again it places the overall risk of mortality in it's proper perspective. Men inquiring about the benefits and detriments of finasteride for prostate cancer prevention should be told first that the number 1 risk to them, in general, is CVD, and then the potential prostate cancer risk-specific consultation should take place after the first point is discussed and emphasized.

Observations taken from the well-known selenium supplementation randomized trial that noted a significant reduction in the number of prostate cancer cases with the use of 200 µg/day selenium versus placebo seems to have generated much interest in utilizing selenium supplements to reduce the risk of prostate cancer. However, despite men in this trial having a higher mean risk of cancer, the number 1 cause of death in this randomized trial was still CVD.[10]

Additionally, the past and recent observation that the primary or secondary cause of death in patients with prostate cancer seems to be CVD[12] continues to emphasize the past non-emphasized discussion that clinicians and patients need to give more attention to the impact of CVD on overall mortality. Also, a study of the macrophage scavenging receptor gene 1 (MSR1) revealed that a mutation in this gene not only increases the risk of atherosclerosis, but it also appears to increase the risk of prostate cancer.[13] Some of the potential mechanisms involved in increasing a man's risk for heart disease may also increase his risk for prostate cancer,[14,15] and other chronic disease risk may also be increased with an abnormal cardiovascular risk[16,17] or lipid mutation, for example.[18] If the clinician were to highlight lifestyle changes that may impact one or ideally both conditions (CVD and cancer) favorably this would seem like the wisest and most practical and realistic clinical approach for the patient both before being diagnosed with prostate cancer and after being diagnosed or treated for this disease.[19]

These observations and general findings are not mentioned to belittle or reduce the seriousness of prostate cancer, but they place the average risk of death for a man in its proper perspective. Dietary or lifestyle changes to reduce the risk of CVD just make realistic and practical sense when examining the larger overall mortality picture. In other words a so-called "forest over the tree" approach seems most appropriate when discussing options with patients. Clinicians should not solely emphasize a prostate cancer-specific diet or prostate-specific lifestyle change only because this would ignore the previous important but seemingly unstressed findings from the past studies of prostate cancer. Heart healthy seems to be prostate healthy, and this should be constantly and consistently reiterated and emphasized to the man concerned about prostate cancer. The simplistic lifestyle recommendations proffered in this chapter serve not only to impact prostate cancer, but CVD as well. Therefore, patients may now be offered lifestyle changes that can potentially impact all-cause mortality rather than the more myopic focus or attention on disease-specific mortality.

Cardiovascular risks and assessment markers

Recommendation #1: Men should know their lipid profile, and other cardiovascular risks and assessment markers as well as they know their PSA values and the other results from their prostate exam.

In my experience, many patients seem to be well aware of their past prostate-specific antigen (PSA) values, but have either never had a cholesterol test, or are unaware of their latest values, or how to correctly construe these values. This observation seems initially frustrating, because again the number 1 or 2 cause of death in these patients is CVD.[1,7,10,11] This lack of comprehensive knowledge is not only prevalent in some prostate populations, but surveys of the general population indicate that a majority of individuals do not know their cholesterol values, or they have a lack of understanding of what they actually represent.[20] Clinicians need to emphasize the dual concern of CVD and cancer risk. In my experience, when this is emphasized, patients begin to become familiar with all of their clinical values or numbers. A simplistic clinical change and discussion or explanation seems to be very effective in these cases. Initially, it would seem appropriate to conduct a cholesterol/blood-pressure screening and prostate cancer screening on the same day at any institution. Second, patients should be educated regularly on the normal values of a cholesterol panel and blood pressure test, because these have recently been updated twice according to the expert panel from the National Cholesterol Education Program (NCEP).[21,22]

Ideally, for most men a total cholesterol (TC) level of less than 200 mg/dL and a low-density lipoprotein (LDL or "bad cholesterol") level of less than 100 mg/dL are optimal, but for some high-risk men (for example, those with documented CVD or a CVD past event), an LDL less than 70 mg/dL is optimal. A high-density lipoprotein (HDL or "good cholesterol") of 40 mg/dL or higher is good but 60 mg/dL or higher is optimal, and a triglyceride level of less than 150 mg/dL is optimal. It should also be kept in mind that a fasting (9–12 hours) cholesterol level is best, but in the case of prostate cancer screenings this is difficult, so a non-fasting test can be drawn and if certain levels of TC, HDL, or LDL are not ideal than a follow-up fasting test should be suggested.

Clinicians should also discuss other potential risks for CVD, which is also affected by lifestyle risk factors such as overweight and obesity, physical inactivity, and an atherogenic diet. Other emerging risk factors or risk markers should ideally be discussed because despite the cholesterol test being a good test for predicting future cardiovascular problems, it is not a perfect test. This should be similar to the clinician's approach to a PSA test—it is a good test for potential risk or recurrence following definitive therapy, but it is not a perfect test. Other newer cardiovascular markers, such as C-reactive protein (CRP),[21,23–26] homocysteine,[21,27] lipoprotein (a) or Lp(a),[21,28,29] impaired fasting glucose, or hemoglobin A1c,[21] and evidence of subclinical atherosclerotic disease[21] should also be discussed with the patient. A referral to a cardiologist may be appropriate in other cases because some of these markers may also be related to overall mortality as well as CVD risk. Several other advantages may occur for the patient and clinician that continue to follow these overall cardiovascular markers. For example, cholesterol levels are an excellent indicator of how well a patient may be adopting lifestyle changes following a PSA test or after definitive therapy. If these numbers improve, it may be more likely that the patient is adhering to a prostate-healthy lifestyle program. The HDL level may be a good indicator of the overall amount of exercise a patient is getting following a PSA test. The HDL tends to rise, and at times substantially, with a greater amount of physical activity,[30] and a higher HDL may be correlated with a lower risk of abnormal prostate conditions.[31]

On the other hand, in a minority of patients that follow a healthy lifestyle, a less than optimal change in cholesterol may occur, but these patients can then be referred to a specialist for potential drug and more aggressive lifestyle therapy. Blood pressure values should also be emphasized as much as the cholesterol and PSA values. Recently, the Joint National Committee on Prevention, Detection, Evaluation, and Treatment of High Blood Pressure also altered the criteria for what constitutes a healthy blood pressure.[32] Men should be informed that normal blood pressure is less than 120/80 mmHg and individuals with a systolic blood pressure of 120 to 139 mmHg or diastolic blood pressure of 80 to 89 mmHg are actually considered to be "prehypertensive," and lifestyle changes should be advocated in these individuals. Blood pressure tends to decrease with a healthier lifestyle[33] and again is a good indicator of lifestyle compliance; and a healthy blood pressure may also lower the risk of abnormal prostate conditions.[31] A minority of patients may not reduce their blood pressure with lifestyle changes, but these men can be referred to a specialist. Men that adopt lifestyle changes that do not result in a PSA change should still be given encouragement to continue these changes because of the other potential profound impacts these behaviors may have on overall health. For example, my experience has demonstrated that a man who does not reduce his PSA after lifestyle change still seems very much encouraged to continue these behaviors after he is told, for example, that his blood pressure has been reduced along with cholesterol values. In other words, the glass is very much half-full for patients who adopt healthy lifestyle changes and follow cardiovascular risk markers in addition to the PSA test.

There is one other recent pertinent example that highlights the problem with isolated PSA screenings without offering comprehensive screening and education. We conducted two large PSA screenings of African-American men in 2004 in two large metropolitan areas.[34] In the past, these screenings only offered PSA testing. However, we also offered cholesterol and other types of screenings in these settings and we were surprised to find that although PSA abnormalities were observed in less than 10% of these men, the rate of dyslipidemia was over 50% at both sites! Again, this drives home the point that more comprehensive screening and education seems to be the best potential approach for men concerned about prostate disease.

Body-fat indicators

Recommendation #2: The clinician needs to measure the patient's body mass index (BMI), and/or waist-to-hip ratio (WHR), or waist circumference (WC), and it should become a regular part of the clinical record.

The negative impact of being overweight or obese on overall health and mortality is well known. Less known is the impact of weight on prostate cancer risk, but it seems that its impact may be just as detrimental.[35] Body mass index is a fairly reliable and fast method to determine who may be overweight or obese.[36] It is defined as the weight in kilograms divided by the square of the height in meters (kg/m^2). Another method to calculate the BMI is to take weight in pounds and divide it by the height in inches squared and to multiply this number by 704 ($pounds/inches^2 \times 704$). A BMI of less than 25 is considered normal by the World Health Organization (WHO), whereas 25 to 29 is overweight, 30 or more than is defined as obese, and 35 or more is considered morbidly obese. Several recent large randomized trials have demonstrated that most individuals in these studies are overweight,[37] and this includes dietary trials to prevent prostate cancer or reduce PSA.[38]

Waist-to-hip ratio may be another simple measurement to determine obesity.[36] Individuals must stand during the entire measurement of WHR. This more precisely measures abdominal adipose circumference or tissue and fat distribution. The waist is defined as the abdominal circumference midway between the costal margin and the iliac crest. The hip is defined as the largest circumference just below the iliac crest. For men, a WHR of more than 0.90 is a fairly accurate indicator of an increased risk for obesity-related conditions, independent of BMI.

Waist circumference is perhaps the simplest and fastest method to currently access obesity. WC is rapidly gaining acceptance as one of the best predictors of a future cardiovascular event, regardless of the ethnic group studied.[39] Recent evidence also suggests that it may be a better predictor of early mortality from prostate cancer than other methods of weight measurement.[40] Regardless, WC has been one of the criteria to access metabolic syndrome. A WC of 35 inches or greater has been suggested as "overweight" and 40 or more is considered obese. Interestingly, a WC of 40 or more is also one of the five specific criteria of metabolic syndrome.

Also noteworthy is that dual energy X-ray absorptiometry (DEXA) has become the gold standard of measuring bone mineral density and determining the future risk of fracture in women and men.[41] However, in 2005 to 2006, it may be one of the most accurate predictors of body fat. Clinicians should advise patients who will be receiving a DEXA scan in the future for osteoporosis risk to also inquire about an overall body fat measurement. Utilizing the proper software, the DEXA scan allows an accurate determination of overall fat-free mass, but the ability to specifically quantify belly fat is more controversial.

Investigations of weight and prostate cancer are preliminary and not conclusive,[42] but some of the largest studies to date suggest a potential serious negative impact, especially post-diagnosis and treatment. For example, a large cohort study by Andersson et al followed 135,000 Swedish construction workers.[43] It included one of the largest numbers of prostate cancer cases (2368), prostate cancer deaths (708), and one of the longest follow-up periods to date (18 years). All of the anthropometric measurements were correlated with the risk of prostate cancer, but there was a stronger relation to mortality than to incidence. The risk of mortality from prostate cancer demonstrated statistical significance in all of the BMI subsets above the reference. This investigation represented a young cohort, because more than 50% of these men were under 40 years of age at entry into this investigation.

The Netherlands Cohort Study was one of the largest prospective studies to evaluate diet and lifestyle and the risk of prostate cancer.[44] This study found no associations between larger intakes of overall dietary fat and prostate cancer incidence; however, these same researchers also recorded BMIs, and it seems that this part of the study did not receive as much publicity.[45] A total of 58,279 men aged 55 to 69 years were followed. A total of 681 cases new cases of prostate cancer were diagnosed during 6.3 years of follow-up. There was a moderate association observed for BMI and prostate cancer (relative risk [RR] = 1.33) if a man was obese at a younger age, which was stronger for localized cancers than for advanced cancer.

One of the few large-scale randomized trials to report on obesity and prostate cancer risk was from a study whose primary endpoint was lung cancer incidence after taking vitamin E, β-carotene, both, or neither.[46,47] Prostate cancer incidence and mortality was a secondary endpoint of the trial. This study was known as the "Alpha-Tocopherol Beta-Carotene" (ATBC) Trial, and it documented 579 cases of prostate cancer with an 11-year follow-up. No relation between prostate cancer risk and BMI was noted in the moderate-to-overweight BMI ranges.[46] Researchers discovered later that men in the highest weight and BMI category had a 40% increased risk of developing prostate cancer compared with men with a normal BMI.[47] This was an interesting later discovery of the trial, because it was this same study that found that men consuming 50 mg/day vitamin E as a supplement had a 32% reduction in prostate cancer risk.[46] The results with the vitamin E supplement seemed to garner the most publicity in most major media outlets. Yet, another way of perceiving the results of this study was that the potential negative impact of being obese was greater than the positive impact of taking a vitamin E supplement, though few if any media sources have publicized this finding from the trial. Men were not only obese but smoked a mean of 20 cigarettes per day over several decades. This negative synergism of being obese and having a chronic heavy smoking history, or having other significant unhealthy habits, may lead to a greater risk and progression of prostate cancer. It seems critical for the clinician to explain to the patient that two of the largest dietary and supplement studies to analyze the risk of prostate cancer essentially both arrived at the same conclusion—that obesity can negatively impact prostate cancer risk or progression. This seems to provide a convincing argument that men need to maintain a healthy weight before or after a prostate cancer diagnosis.

One of the largest prospective epidemiologic investigations to evaluate the impact of obesity on cancer mortality was also published.[48] More than 900,000 US adults (404,576 men) who did not have cancer at baseline in 1982 were included in this 16-year follow-up study. Higher cancer mortality was associated with increasing BMIs and this included prostate cancer mortality. A significant (p < 0.001) increased risk of prostate cancer mortality was associated with increasing BMI from 25 to 29.9 (RR = 1.08), 30 to 34.9 (RR = 1.20), and 35 to 39.9 (RR = 1.34) for the 4004 deaths from prostate carcinoma that were documented.

Post-diagnosis studies are also providing some concerns for the man being treated for prostate cancer. Two large retrospective pooled multi-institutional analyses arrived at somewhat similar conclusions after evaluating patients following radical prostatectomy.[49,50] The first study included 3162 patients and found that a higher BMI was a significant independent predictor of a higher Gleason score, and a higher BMI was significantly associated with a higher risk of biochemical recurrence.[49] African-American men had significantly higher BMIs than white men, and also had significantly higher prostate cancer recurrence rates, which could provide a partial explanation of racial differences sometimes observed with this disease. The second study compared 1106 men treated with radical prostatectomy from 1998 to 2002. A BMI of over 35 was associated with a significant risk of biochemical recurrence after treatment even when controlling for surgical margin status.[50] Interestingly, the percentage of obese men undergoing surgery in this data set doubled in the last decade, and obesity was associated with higher-grade prostate cancers, a trend toward an increased risk of positive surgical margins, and higher biochemical failure rates.

Another recent epidemiologic study (Health Professionals Follow-Up Study) that published incidence but not mortality data from prostate cancer found a significantly lower risk of prostate cancer in men with higher BMIs if they were younger (<60 years) or had a family history of prostate cancer.[51] However, men with more sporadic cancers seemed to have a higher risk of prostate cancer with an increasing BMI. This observation led researchers of this study to hypothesize that, since obesity is associated with lower testosterone levels or partial androgen suppression, this could have resulted in a lower risk of prostate cancer in the early-onset or hereditary prostate cancers in these men compared with the more sporadic cancers. Obese men could theoretically also harbor prostate tumors, but have lower PSA levels, which could lead to the clinician falsely considering these men to be cancer free, and this may explain why some have been identified to have more advanced disease at the time of diagnosis and treatment.[49,50]

The proper perspective to the patient should be constantly emphasized, even if these recent alternative findings are accurate. Prostate cancer recurrence and mortality, and especially early mortality in general have been highly correlated with an increasing BMI. Whether or not obesity impacts just the incidence of prostate cancer should not be the primary focus for any man, because this observation simply fails to see the forest over the single tree when discussing the overall effect of obesity on general health.[35] For example, two of the largest prospective epidemiologic studies examining the issue of BMI and overall mortality had similar findings.[52,53] Both studies utilized data from the American Cancer Society. The first investigation was the American Cancer Society's Cancer Prevention Study I.[52] Over 62,000 men were included, and these men had no smoking history, no history of heart disease, stroke, or cancer (other than skin carcinoma), and no history of recent involuntary weight loss at baseline. Overall mortality was measured over 12 years. The second study was the Cancer Prevention Study II.[53] This was a study of 457,000 men observed for 14 years. Both studies documented that men with a BMI of approximately 25 to 30 had an increased mortality of 10% to 25%.[52,53] Individuals with a BMI of 30 or more had a 50% to 100% increased mortality compared with those with a BMI less than 25. The second study not only included more men but also looked at general cancer mortality.[53] The men within the highest BMI category (>35) had a 40% to 80% increased risk of mortality from cancer, and no evidence of any increased risk was found among the leanest individuals (BMI <20). Past studies completed in the US indicate that only a minority of adults (less than 8%) have a BMI of less than 20, and more than 50% of men in the US have a BMI over 25.[54]

Numerous cancers seem to be at least somewhat associated with a higher BMI, but renal cell carcinoma has demonstrated perhaps the strongest correlation with BMI compared with all the cancers studied to date.[55] Also, recent research suggesting increased risks of erectile dysfunction[56,57] and kidney stones[58] with obesity should be discussed with patients. Healthcare professionals working in the field of urology should constantly emphasize the negative overall impact of obesity. Clinicians need to let their patients know that maintaining a healthy weight should be one of the primary goals. For example, placing a BMI chart in the clinic office and always making BMI or WHR or WC a part of the individual clinical record should be a goal for every patient, regardless of his or her concern of a specific disease risk, because early mortality from all-causes is associated with increasing BMI. Clinicians should also refer patients on a regular basis to nutritionists, therapists, and to a variety of professional weight-loss programs. Clinicians should be able to provide the name and number of these individuals and organizations to the patient at the time of the urologic appointment in order to improve compliance, convey enthusiasm, and the immediacy or importance of this lifestyle change.

Fitness first

Recommendation #3: Always encourage fitness and overall health first in patients by telling them to get approximately 30 minutes of physical activity a day or more depending on individual need, and to lift weights or perform resistance exercises several times/week. Aerobic and resistance exercise should be emphasized equally; one is not more vital than the other. Weight loss should not be the initial goal.

The impact of exercise or regular physical activity on prostate cancer is controversial, but, like most lifestyle changes, it will always be deemed so due to the lack of long-term randomized trials, which will probably not be performed any time soon. A large review of the epidemiologic evidence pointed toward a "probable" reduction in risk with regular physical activity,[59] but keep in mind that prostate cancer mortality and obesity are related. Recently, higher levels of physical activity were associated with a lower risk of being diagnosed with a more aggressive prostate cancer, and a potential for improved survival in the Health Professionals Follow-up Study.[60]

Physical activity reduces CVD and mortality, and the data is profound, and weight lifting also seems to provide benefits. Additional data from the Health Professionals' Follow-up Study prospectively followed over 44,000 men for 12 years.[61] Men who ran for 1 hour or more per week had a 42% reduction (RR = 0.58; p < 0.001 for trend) in the risk of coronary heart disease (CHD), and those who just walked for 30 minutes or more per day or who were involved in other physical activities also had a risk reduction in CHD versus those who did not engage in these activities. Surprisingly, men who trained with weights for just 30 minutes or more per week experienced a 23% risk reduction (RR = 0.77; p = 0.03 for trend) in CHD. This was a unique observation because previous prospective studies have not addressed this issue. Weight training can increase fat-free mass, lean body weight, and resting metabolic rate, and potentially reduce the risk of abdominal fat deposition.[62] Weight training or resistance training also seems to improve glucose control or increase insulin sensitivity,[63] improve lipid levels,[64] and reduce hypertension.[65]

The first randomized study of resistance exercise for men receiving androgen deprivation therapy or luteinizing hormone-releasing hormone (LHRH) therapy for prostate cancer was completed several years ago.[66] The trial was only 12 weeks in duration (n = 155) and men either lifted weights 3 times per week, or were assigned to a non-lifting group. Body composition did not change during this short study, but the significant reduction in fatigue and improved quality of life with weight training should probably make this a standard lifestyle change for men receiving this type of treatment in the future, especially for those without bone metastasis. Men with bone metastasis should be told to check with several physicians in order to receive the approval of a resistance program due to the theoretical possibility of an increased risk for fracture with osteoblastic bone lesions.

Physical activity may reduce the risk of other urologic conditions, such as benign prostatic hyperplasia (BPH)[67] and erectile dysfunction (ED).[68] This unique and recent 2-year randomized trial of vigorous exercise to improve ED needs to garner more attention.[69] Approximately one third of the men reporting ED regained normal erectile function in this trial, but the majority of men experienced at least some tangible improvement in function and in reducing the risk of common CVD markers.[68] Also, the potential to impact the risk of several major cancers, such as colorectal carcinoma, should make exercise itself a lifelong priority for most men.[70]

Mental health benefits of physical activity seem to be just as acute preliminarily as the physical health benefits. A 6-month follow-up study of 156 adult volunteers with major depressive disorder (MDD) who were randomly assigned to a 4-month course of aerobic exercise (30 minutes 3 times/week), sertraline therapy, or a combination of exercise and sertraline was completed.[71,72] After 4 months, patients in all three groups demonstrated significant mental improvement. However, after 10 months, individuals in the exercise group had significantly lower recurrence rates than individuals in the medication arm of the study. Exercising during the follow-up period was associated with a 51% reduction in the risk of a diagnosis of depression at the end of the investigation. Men need to be instructed that regular physical activity and resistance training

have such profound physical and mental health benefits that not performing these activities certainly limits the potential for improved overall health. I often tell patients that if the overall results from physical activity studies were viewed similar to a pharmacologic intervention then it would have already garnered a Nobel prize in medicine.

Again, the initial goal for men should be to achieve fitness or wellness before assessing success in terms of weight loss. In other words, many men considered overweight or obese may reduce the risk of overall early mortality by just performing regular physical activity and not losing any weight. Men who exercise should be told that weight loss is not initially needed in order to obtain clinically relevant benefits. These findings have already been well documented in large prospective studies of women who have not lost weight, but who exercise on a regular basis.[73]

Lifestyle changes tailored to each person

Recommendation #4: Emphasize to patients that there is no single ideal weight loss diet or intervention. Help patients choose a diet or lifestyle change and interventions that are tailored to their own personality. Remember, the end result may actually justify the means, and most diets and interventions consist of several consistent and overall related healthy messages.

Low-fat diets, low-carbohydrate diets, drug therapy, surgery—the list of potential methods to reduce weight continues to abound, confuse, and at times frustrate many men.[36] The potential to lose sight of one of the primary goals is always a risk when dealing with a patient attempting to lose weight. A similar analogy exists for smoking cessation, whereby numerous potential credible interventions are now available rather than a single intervention.[74] Some dietary interventions involving men with prostate cancer, such as reducing overall dietary fat have been beneficial in terms of a PSA response,[75] while other longer randomized trials have not demonstrated such a benefit for men without prostate cancer.[38] Low-carbohydrate diets have provided some sustained weight loss in recent randomized trials, and it is a novel dietary method, but compliance rates in just 1 year approach 50% and PSA and prostate cancer risk data are needed.[76,77] Higher insulin or glucose levels from a variety of etiologies, such as diet and obesity, have been preliminarily associated with a higher prostate cancer risk, cancer-specific mortality, and overall mortality.[78–81]

A truly unique recently randomized published study comparing the effects of a variety of fad diets on weight loss and cardiovascular risk should provide the impetus for any clinician dealing with any patient attempting to lose weight with a more practical perspective on weight loss itself. A total of 160 overweight or obese men and women (mean BMI = 35) were randomized to one of the following diets for 1-year: low carbohydrate (Atkins®), low fat (Ornish®), low glycemic load (Zone®), or a calorie-restricted (Weight Watchers®) dietary program.[82] All of the diets were associated with weight loss and a reduced risk of coronary heart disease from Framingham risk scores in participants that were able to adhere to their respective allocated diets. However, drop-out rates within just 1 year of this study were notable. The drop out rates were 48% with the Atkins diet, 50% with the Ornish diet, 35% for the Zone diet, and 35% for Weight Watchers. Compliance is difficult, but for those who can adhere to these diets, the benefits may outweigh the negatives when considering the impact of obesity on all-cause mortality. All of these so-called "fad" diets carry consistent themes, such as reducing overall caloric intake and increasing physical activity levels. Most fad diets consist of a delicate balancing act between caloric control and additional exercise. The consistent simple mantra of caloric restriction should be emphasized. Food and beverage sizes have increased in recent years with obesity rates, and greater portion sizes and access to fast foods appear to at least encourage greater caloric intake.[83,84] Some studies have found an increased risk of prostate cancer in men with higher caloric intakes over time; regardless of whether these calories were mostly derived from fat, protein, or carbohydrate.[85] Simple caloric control may be one method of effective weight loss and disease prevention, and the research derived from the centenarians and schoolchildren on the island of Okinawa (Japan) have been a model for the benefits of caloric restriction and its potential impact on all-cause mortality.[86] Simply reducing total fat intake cannot be the only viable, realistic, or even practical solution, and the effectiveness over just caloric restriction has been questioned recently in meta-analysis,[87] especially since greater caloric concentrations can now be found in a variety of carbohydrate sources, for example.[88] Diet should indeed fit personality.

The most extensive animal studies to date examining the correlation between prostate cancer and fat and energy intakes may have revealed the most insight on energy restriction and cancer progression.[89] Researchers utilized androgen-sensitive prostate tumors from donor rats, transplanted them to other rats, and fed them either fat-restricted or carbohydrate-restricted diets. Severe combined immunodeficient mice (SCID) mice were injected with LNCaP human prostate cancer cells to generate tumors, and then ingested similar diets. Researchers restricted energy intake by reducing energy from fat or carbohydrate, or simply reducing total energy from all sources, while at all times keeping other nutrients constant. Cancer proliferation was observed to be independent of the percentage of fat in the diet, as long as the total energy was restricted. The reduction in cancer growth was even identical in all types of energy-restricted laboratory animals. The findings of this experiment suggest that a reduction in overall energy intake, and not just fat, reduced the risk or progression of prostate cancer.[89,90]

Again, another perspective on weight loss that can be proffered to patients is highlighted by the results of a unique recent prospective cohort. A total of 6391 overweight and obese individuals who were at least 35 years of age were followed for 9 years.[91] Compared with individuals not trying to lose weight and reporting no weight change, those individuals reporting intentional weight loss had a 24% reduced mortality rate. Mortality rates were reduced in individuals who reported attempting to lose weight compared with those not attempting to lose weight, independent of the actual weight change. Compared with individuals not attempting to lose weight and reporting no weight change, individuals attempting to lose weight had the following hazard rate ratios (HRR): no weight change (HRR = 0.80), lost weight (HRR = 0.76), and gained weight (HRR = 0.94). Attempted weight loss was associated with lower all-cause mortality; independent or regardless of the actual weight change. This study stresses an important overall issue; again weight loss is not necessarily the ultimate goal but at least attempting weight loss through whatever method seems to impact health. The current concern over which diet or exercise program has the most data, or which dietary method is best may not be the most effective realistic and practical approach. Men should be allowed to choose a fairly safe method of weight loss because the end may justify the means. A patient willing to simply attempt a weight loss program should provide encouragement to the clinician. In my practice, if a man is motivated to try a low-carbohydrate diet, low-fat, or another type of diet, drug therapy or even surgery; a proper review of the

data is provided but ultimately whatever method the patient ultimately chooses, we will work with them to achieve the first goal of becoming more healthy or fit, and hopefully the second goal of losing weight. If the second goal is not immediately, or ever, achieved then we do not believe that this is tantamount to a lack of success, because other cardiovascular markers have demonstrated that the first of the two goals is by far the most important. Effort counts, and the result may not ideally match the effort, but generally, in some capacity, the results are affected at least minimally by the effort. The concept of being overweight or obese and simultaneously healthy is plausible. Other individuals make no attempt or a feeble attempt to reduce weight regardless of their current status. It seems appropriate to encourage and applaud the consistent weight loss effort, and clinicians may play a primary role in monitoring and motivating patients, but only if regular contact between the patient and practitioner over a long duration is possible.[92] The clinician's role is to provide the range of possible of interventions, from least to most invasive, and the risks and benefits of each intervention. Ultimately the patient makes the choice and we monitor these patients and always encourage regular physical activity with the intervention to achieve the best potential result. I recommend certain dietary or lifestyle interventions more than others for most patients seeking advice, and they provide a foundation that other interventions can build upon and utilize to some degree. Some of these basic lifestyle interventions are listed in the rest of the following chapter.

Saturated, trans-fatty acids and cholesterol

Recommendation #5: Replace saturated, trans-fatty acids, and even cholesterol with more healthy types of monounsaturated or polyunsaturated fat. Total fat intake should not be the initial concern, but the specific types of dietary fat consumed. In addition, the utilization of commercial plant sterol/stanol products may also be heart and prostate healthy.

Saturated fat (SF) is also simply known as "hydrogenated fat," and it reduces LDL receptor expression and increases LDL serum levels[21]—LDL increases by 2% for every 1% increase in total calories from SF. The NCEP (Adult Treatment Panel III or ATP III) recommends that SF be reduced to less than 7% of total calories to reduce the risk of CVD. The average US adult intake of SF is 11% of total calories. Some non-lean meats, high-fat dairy products (whole milk, butter, cheese, ice cream, and cream), tropical oils (palm oil, coconut oil, and palm kernel oil), baked products, and mixed dishes with dairy fats and shortenings are some of the primary sources of SF. Many foods that contain high levels of SF also contain high levels of trans-fat ("partially hydrogenated fat").

Epidemiologic studies have found that the consumption of a high concentration of SF and cholesterol may significantly increase the risk for CHD.[93] A meta-analysis that included 6356 person-years of follow-up has documented that reducing serum cholesterol by reducing SF intake reduces the risk of CHD by 24%.[94,95] A 21% reduction in coronary mortality and a 6% reduction in total mortality were also observed. No increase in non-CVD mortality was observed.

Past lifestyle changes and prostate cancer risk studies revolve around primary prevention, but there have been several studies of men post-treatment, and these should also be discussed.[96] A Canadian prospective study of men with prostate cancer observed a total of 384 men for a median of 5.2 years.[97] Compared with the men consuming the lowest levels of SF, those consuming the highest amount had a significant increase in risk of mortality from prostate cancer (RR = 3.1). Total fat and other subtypes of fat (except saturated) did not show any correlation between prostate cancer and mortality. A collaborative analysis of five prospective studies compared death rates from diseases of vegetarians versus non-vegetarians with similar lifestyles.[98] Data on more than 76,000 men and women documented 8330 deaths with a mean of 10.6 years of follow-up. There were no significant differences in death between vegetarians and non-vegetarians from prostate cancer, breast cancer, colorectal cancer, lung cancer, stomach cancer, or all other causes combined. However, mortality from ischemic heart disease was significantly lowered by 24% in vegetarians. This lower mortality from ischemic heart disease was greater at younger ages and was limited to those who had followed this diet for a longer period of time (>5 years). Further subset analyses of vegetarian versus non-vegetarian diets found that ischemic heart disease was 20% lower in occasional meat eaters, 34% lower in those that ate fish but not meat, 34% lower in lactoovovegetarians, and 26% lower in vegans when compared with regular meat eaters. Reducing all saturated fat in an individual's diet is not necessarily a practical and healthy dietary lifestyle change. The current cardiovascular goal of obtaining less than 7% of calories from saturated fat seems almost ideal from past studies, because getting zero calories from saturated fat not only seems too excessive, but can actually decrease levels of HDL.[99] Therefore, the old adage "everything in moderation" applies to this lifestyle recommendation.

All three primary classes of fatty acids: saturated, monounsaturated, and polyunsaturated can increase HDL when they substitute for carbohydrates in the diet and this effect is slightly greater for saturated fat, and monounsaturated fat is slightly greater than polyunsaturated fat (saturated>monounsaturated>polyunsaturated).[100] Saturated fats increase LDL and monounsaturated and polyunsaturated fat slightly decrease LDL. Dietary fatty acids replaced by carbohydrates cause an increase in triglyceride levels. Replacing saturated fat with carbohydrates proportionally reduces both HDL and LDL, and has minimal impact on the LDL/HDL ratio and increases triglycerides. Thus, this type of dietary change would be expected to have a minimal impact on the risk of CHD. When mono- or polyunsaturated fats are utilized or replace saturated fat, LDL is reduced and HDL changes minimally. Additionally, utilizing polyunsaturated instead of saturated fat could have numerous health benefits, for example, increasing insulin sensitivity and decreasing the risk of type II diabetes.[101,102]

Trans-fatty acids are also known as "partially hydrogenated" fatty acids.[103,104] They are found in higher concentrations in a variety of foods such as doughnuts, cake mixes, fast foods, potato chips, and many other products. Many of these compounds were placed in the food supply over a decade ago to increase the shelf-life of numerous popular food items. Some trans-fats are also found naturally in other foods. However, recent cardiovascular investigations have demonstrated a general health concern with these types of fatty acids.[105–108] These compounds seem to demonstrate a unique and dual negative effect because not only do they raise levels of LDL, but they can also reduce levels of HDL. In fact, the increase in the ratio of total/HDL cholesterol for these fats are approximately double that found for saturated fat.[109] Some specific unhealthy changes associated with greater intakes of trans-fat are increases in lipoprotein a,[110,111] increases in triglycerides,[107] impaired vasodilation,[112] increases in sudden cardiac death,[105] increased insulin resistance[113] and type II diabetes,[112] and adverse effects on the metabolism of healthy polyunsaturated fats through the inhibition of delta-6 desaturase.[114,115]

The association of trans-fat with cancer is unknown because some past and recent epidemiologic studies have not found an association,[44,116] but interestingly some other recent studies have suggested that these fatty acids may encourage cancer growth[117–119] and increase the risk of prostate cancer, and so the simple rule of what is heart healthy/unhealthy is also prostate healthy/unhealthy may also be applicable to these specific types of fatty acids. The observation that trans-fat is heart unhealthy makes the recommendation to reduce the intake of these fatty acids a priority.

Some food manufacturers tend to include large concentrations of these trans-fats in their products and others tend to include small concentrations or none at all. Men should be generally encouraged to consume items low in trans- or saturated fat. The Danish government decided that oils and fat with more than 2% industrially produced trans-fatty acids would no longer be sold in Denmark after January 1, 2004,[120] and the United States Food and Drug Administration (FDA) will require that the actual amount of trans-fat be reported on all food labels by January 1, 2006.[121] The FDA predicts that by 3 years after that date, the labeling of trans-fat will have prevented from 600 to 1200 additional cases of CHD and approximately 250 to 500 deaths per year. When this occurs, patients should simply compare several similar food items and choose the one lower in trans-fat. Consumer and economic pressure should lead to a general reduction or elimination of these fatty acids in the diet.

It is a fairly simple method to just rapidly and simply compare food labels and choose a similar dietary item that has a reduced quantity of saturated fat. Patients should be instructed to compare several milks, meats, potato chips, and any other items and choose the one that is lower in saturated fat. For example, when comparing whole milk to 2% fat, 1% fat, and skim milk one will quickly learn that all of these milk types compared with skim milk contain many more grams of saturated fat, and a higher amount of overall calories.

Again, the simple past suggestion of just reducing overall dietary fat intake, instead of sub-types of fat has not been supported recently in the prostate cancer or CVD literature,[38,122,123] especially in regards to mortality data.[123] Clinicians need to emphasize that the types of fat ingested seem to influence disease risk overall more than just dietary fat intake. In the worst case scenario, this tends to decrease cholesterol and reduce the risk of CVD, which is why this recommendation makes the most practical sense to any man concerned about prostate cancer.

Dietary cholesterol increases serum cholesterol, but not as significantly as saturated fat. A total of 100 mg of dietary cholesterol increases serum cholesterol approximately 10 mg/dL per 1000 kcal.[21] Daily mean cholesterol intake is greater for men in the US (331 mg) than women (213 mg). Foods high in cholesterol include eggs, animal and dairy products, poultry, and shellfish. Sterols or the marine equivalent of cholesterol in shellfish and shrimp do not greatly impact human serum cholesterol unless cooked in butter, fried, or consumed in high quantities.[124,125] Dietary cholesterol ingestion should be encouraged to be less than 200 mg/day to impact or lower LDL cholesterol.[21] The impact of dietary cholesterol on prostate cancer is unknown, but it is known that prostate cancer cells tend to utilize large amounts of cholesterol in their cellular membranes,[126] and this is especially notable with a greater extent or progression (metastases) of the disease itself.[127] Reducing dietary cholesterol just makes practical sense from a cardiovascular risk standpoint.

Plant sterols/stanols or the plant equivalent of cholesterol is found in higher concentrations in vegetarian diets.[128,129] These compounds inhibit the intestinal absorption of dietary and biliary cholesterol and are most effective in individuals with high cholesterol absorption and low cholesterol synthesis. Patients with apolipoprotein (apo) E4 experience greater cholesterol absorption and may respond more favorably to these compounds.[130] A total of 2 to 3 g/day of plant-derived sterols/stanols decreases LDL cholesterol in most individuals by 6% to 15% without changing HDL or triglyceride levels.[21,131–137] These products are now available in grocery stores as regular and low-fat margarines (Benecol®, Take Charge®) and may soon be widely available in other products such as orange juice, yogurt, and some dietary supplements.[128,129] Clinicians can encourage patients with higher cholesterol levels to consume 2 to 3 g/day of these compounds, but the current high price of these products is an issue,[21] and their impact on prostate cancer is not known. Interestingly, one of the main sources of these compounds is actually soybean oil, so the utilization of this oil in cooking is theoretically another option.

Fruit and vegetables

Recommendation #6: Encourage the regular consumption of a diversity of fruits and vegetables for CVD risk reduction, and not just tomato products and lycopene. Lycopene dietary supplements should not be recommended at this time for most patients.

Few topics in prostate cancer prevention have garnered as much attention as lycopene, tomato products, and their potential benefits. Numerous studies support the intake of tomatoes and tomato products, but numerous other investigations have not found a relationship. For example, a well-referenced analysis of over 80 epidemiologic studies was completed on tomatoes and cancer risk several years ago.[138] Half of the studies analyzed support the consumption of tomato products at least once a day to reduce the risk of a variety of cancers including prostate cancer, but a large number of studies in this same analysis failed to detect a correlation. Another important finding was that no investigations to date have indicated that a greater consumption of tomato products significantly increases the risk of cancer, but the overall recommendation of the author was to increase the consumption of fruits and vegetables and not just tomato products! The ongoing research of tomatoes and lycopene continues to moderately support the potential for these products to impact prostate cancer risk or progression.[139–141]

One of the largest animal studies utilized lycopene or tomato powder or a calorie-restricted diet and found some interesting results.[142] The consumption of tomato powder but not lycopene inhibited prostate carcinogenesis, which suggests that tomato products contain compounds in addition to lycopene that can potentially inhibit the growth of prostate tumors. Reducing overall caloric intake also reduced the risk of prostate cancer and increased survival in these male rats.

Tomatoes are not the only source of lycopene. A variety of other healthy foods contain this compound, including apricots, guava, pink grapefruit, and watermelon.[96] Indeed, a recent dietary case-control study from China that observed one of the largest reductions in prostate cancer risk in the literature (odds ratio = 0.18) found watermelon consumption may have been partially responsible, but the impact of pumpkin, spinach, tomatoes, and citrus intake was also notable even after adjusting for a variety of confounders such as fat and total caloric intake.[143]

The initial focus and ongoing interest in lycopene and its sources may actually stem from a potential reduced risk of CVD with a greater intake of this compound from dietary sources.[144–147] Again, heart health seems to potentially promote prostate health.

However, a variety of fruits and especially vegetables have been associated with a reduced risk of prostate cancer.[148] For example, members of the Brassica vegetable group such as: broccoli, Brussels sprouts, cabbage, cauliflower, kale, watercress, and many others may reduce the risk of prostate cancer.[149] The Allium vegetables have also been associated with a reduced risk of prostate cancer, and this group includes chives, garlic, leeks, onions, and scallions.[150] The interpretation of the sum of the data thus far is lucid—it advocates the increased consumption of fruits and vegetables to potentially impact prostate cancer, but the data currently supports the reduction in CVD risk and mortality. If a patient desires to focus only on the consumption of tomato products, it represents a myopic and not necessarily plausible choice in many cases because compliance can become a major issue after a period of time, and this behavior is not consistent with the overall research that supports that many fruits and vegetables have combined unique and shared anticancer and anti-heart disease compounds that contribute to improved overall health.[148]

It is disappointing and surprising to many currently that the largest prospective epidemiologic studies recently have not found a correlation for the increased consumption of fruits and vegetables and a reduced risk of most cancers or mortality from cancer,[151–155] and this includes prostate cancer. Clinicians need to be candid with patients and explain that, currently at least, a CVD risk reduction may occur, but the data is not as profound in cancer or survival from cancer.

Lycopene dietary supplements always seem to draw attention, but long-term data with these pills are lacking. In addition, a recent 1-year pilot trial of small to large intakes (15–120 mg/day) of lycopene pills for rising PSA following failed local therapy in 36 men also failed to demonstrate any initial PSA or clinical benefits.[156] Therefore, intake from dietary sources at this time continues to remain the wisest and cheapest choice.

Dietary fiber

Recommendation #7: Encourage the consumption of more total dietary fiber (25–30 g/day) from food and even supplements, especially viscous ("soluble") fiber, but insoluble fiber is also beneficial.

The diverse health benefits derived from consuming dietary fiber have been well referenced in the medical literature and include a decrease in CHD risk.[157–161] Most recent pooled analysis of past cohort studies of dietary fiber for the reduction of CHD included data from 10 studies from the US and Europe.[162] Over a period of 6 to 10 years of follow-up, a total of 5249 total coronary cases and 2011 coronary deaths were observed among over 91,000 men and 245,000 women. After researchers adjusted for demographics, BMI, and behavioral changes, each 10 g/day increase of calorie-adjusted total dietary fiber was correlated with a 14% reduction in the risk of total coronary events (RR = 0.86) and a 27% reduction in risk of coronary death (RR = 0.73). Cereal, fruit, and vegetable fiber consumption demonstrated a relative risk reduction of 0.90, 0.84, and 1.00 for total coronary events, and 0.75, 0.70, and 1.00 for coronary deaths with each 10 g/day increase of calorie-adjusted total dietary fiber from these sources. The findings were similar for both sexes. There was obviously minimal support for an inverse relationship between vegetable fiber consumption and risk of CHD, which was potentially explained by these researchers by the potential of some vegetables to lack many nutrients and/or that have the ability to dramatically increase glucose levels (potatoes), especially with the common starchy and highly processed vegetables (corn, peas, etc). Researchers from the pooled analysis also attempted to determine whether the decrease in risk of CHD was from soluble (viscous) and/or insoluble fiber. Past studies have not found a consistent benefit with one class of fiber over the other.[163–166] However, in this recent pooled analysis,[162] inverse associations occurred for both soluble and insoluble fiber, but the reductions in risk were greater for soluble fiber (RR = 0.46) and coronary death for each 10-g increment in intake. Soluble fiber has the ability to increase the concentration of intraluminal viscosity of the small intestine, and this can reduce nutrient absorption and encourage binding to bile acids.[167] This impact may reduce insulin production and improve glucose control,[168] reduce serum cholesterol,[169] and may even reduce blood pressure.[170] Viscous or "soluble" fiber from oats, barley, guar, pectin, beans, and psyllium (Metamucil®, etc) for example, has consistently demonstrated the ability to reduce LDL cholesterol levels compared with insoluble fiber.[21]

The addition of only 15 g of psyllium (soluble fiber) daily with a 10 mg statin (simvastatin) was demonstrated to be as effective as 20 mg of statin alone in lowering cholesterol in a recent small pilot placebo study of 68 patients over 12 weeks.[171]

Another recent meta-analysis of 24 randomized placebo-controlled trials of fiber supplementation found a consistent impact on blood pressure.[172] Supplementation with just small amounts of fiber (mean dose, 11.5 g/day) reduced systolic blood pressure by 1.13 mmHg and diastolic pressure by 1.26 mmHg. These reductions were greater in individuals over the age of 40 years and in hypertensive individuals compared with younger and normotensive subjects. It is of interest that the daily intake of fiber in the US and many other Western countries is only around 15 g/day, which is approximately only 50% of the amount consistently recommended by the American Heart Association (25 to 30 g/day).[173]

The data on fiber intake and cancer prevention are not consistent or without controversy, especially in the area of polyp formation and colorectal cancer risk.[161,174,175] In addition, the impact of dietary fiber on PSA levels has not been thoroughly evaluated. A recent randomized trial of a combination of a low-fat and high fiber diet over a 4-year period failed to find a reduction in PSA and prostate cancer risk in white and African-American men.[38,176] However, one of the largest case-control studies was published from Italy and found a moderate reduced risk of prostate cancer with increased consumption of dietary fiber, especially soluble fiber, cellulose, and vegetable fiber.[177] One of the only clinical studies of soluble versus insoluble fiber only for PSA reduction was published several years ago.[178] This small study (n = 14) of short duration (4 months) included men with hyperlipidemia and without cancer. Researchers found a small but statistically lower PSA in men consuming soluble fiber compared with insoluble fiber (25–30 g per 1000 kcal). Similar minimal clinical benefits in another short clinical controlled study of men with prostate cancer was noteworthy when utilizing only foods with higher fiber intakes such as rye-bran bread,[179] but whether the soluble fiber in these foods or the synergistic interaction of other nutrients with and without fiber were the reason for the benefit is not known. Again, soluble fiber can reduce cholesterol levels (LDL) compared with insoluble fiber. Thus, the increase of fiber and especially viscous fiber to 25 to 30 g/day makes sense in terms of potentially lowering LDL and the risk of CHD,[21] and this can be achieved with the combination of foods and supplements, or with food by itself.

In my experience, costly commercial products that contain modified citrus pectin (MCP) are popular with some patients with prostate cancer because some laboratory studies,[180,181] and one small (n = 13) clinical study of limited duration has suggested that this compound may inhibit the growth of a variety of cancers and may increase PSA doubling time after recurrent prostate cancer.[182] It is notable that the vast majority of the MCP is composed of soluble fiber. Recommending MCP or in my opinion just increasing amounts of soluble fiber from food or cheaper supplements, for example psyllium, seems to make more sense.

"Plant estrogen" products

Recommendation #8: Encourage the use of moderate amounts of traditional cheap dietary soy and other so-called "plant estrogen" products, such as flaxseed, because they also contain much more than just "plant estrogens."

Ischemic heart disease reductions have been correlated with a higher consumption of traditional soy products. International comparison studies have observed a reduced rate of this disease in Asian countries along with a higher consumption of soy products versus Western countries.[183] Although this correlation is most likely confounded by other dietary and lifestyle factors, such as a lower overall intake of saturated fat; laboratory and clinical studies have been fairly consistent in supporting the cardiovascular benefits of soy.[184–189] Soy protein may increase LDL uptake and removal, and increase the activity of hydroxymethylglutaryl-coenzyme A reductase and cholesterol 7α-hydroxylase, which further eliminates cholesterol in bile acids. Soy may contain additional benefits beyond its protein and phytoestrogen content, such as an adequate concentration of omega fatty acids, fiber, and vitamin E.[190] A past and more recent meta-analysis of clinical studies suggests that 2 to 3 servings per day of soy protein (approximately 25 g) or greater may be sufficient to significantly decrease cholesterol levels in men and women.[191,192] Although, the FDA has supported this finding, it is important to understand that this benefit is enhanced when soy protein consumption is increased and saturated fat consumption is decreased because otherwise the beneficial effects may not be as tangible. The FDA did not provide support for the plant estrogen content of soy and cardiovascular protection because the majority of the evidence demonstrated that the soy protein content has been more closely related to cholesterol reduction.

Biochanin A, a genistein precursor (from soy), and genistein itself have demonstrated the ability to inhibit the proliferation of both hormone-sensitive and hormone-insensitive cancer cell lines,[193,194] and both compounds have decreased PSA levels of LNCaP cells in vitro.[195] Genistein may inhibit the growth of prostate cancer through a variety of mechanisms, such as interfering with tyrosine kinase growth factor and other similar growth factors and receptors,[196–199] affecting topoisomerase II,[200] inhibiting angiogenesis,[201] and promoting apoptosis.[202] However, significant reductions in testosterone have not been observed in Japanese men consuming these products.[203] Perhaps partial suppression of a variety of hormones over several months, years or even decades may be sufficient to delay the onset of clinically significant prostate cancer or a recurrence.[204] Other potential benefits of genistein and other soy compounds may occur because of their estrogenic activity, the ability to inhibit 5α-reductase and/or the aromatase enzyme, and overall antioxidant free radical scavenger properties.[205] Clinical trials utilizing soy and its various isolated compounds, such as genistein, at a variety of dosages are required to determine if the in-vitro and epidemiologic data correlate to an actual clinical response. Clinical trials utilizing soy or soy products are currently being conducted at numerous institutions.[206,207] Early results from some small pilot trials have observed some benefits for genistein supplementation in men with prostate cancer undergoing watchful waiting, but not as an adjunct to or after conventional treatment.[208] Another smaller randomized trial did not find a significant impact with soy isoflavones on PSA, but increasing dosages of soy protein were not studied.[209]

Soy was a part of a randomized trial of men undergoing a combination lifestyle and supplement regimen after being diagnosed with prostate cancer, and after 1 year of study the results have been encouraging in men with lower Gleason scores (less than 7) or well-differentiated tumors.[75] Men without prostate cancer or those with minimal and less aggressive disease may potentially have the most to gain from including soy in their diet. Regardless, the cardiovascular benefits of soy seem adequate to recommend these products to most men. For example, the cholesterol lowering benefits of incorporating soy products in the diet seem reason enough to encourage their consumption.[210] Clinicians should recommend products that are high in soy protein or that have retained the characteristics of the traditional soy products such as soybeans, tofu, tempeh, soy protein powder, soy oil, soy nuts that are low in saturated fats, and in some cases, soy milk.[96,211] Soy protein bars are popular but, in our opinion, most contain too many calories; therefore, most of these products should be avoided. Soy pills are also a concern since they have not demonstrated a consistent ability to reduce hot flashes,[212] which may be an indicator of poor potency, and they do not contain the numerous other compounds available in the traditional dietary sources of soy.[96]

Clinical research and recommendations should not be limited to soy, because of the potential benefit of numerous other phytoestrogens in nature.

Flaxseed, also known as "linseed" has demonstrated a fairly consistent ability to lower cholesterol in normolipidemic and hyperlipidemic individuals.[213–217] Flaxseed contains an unusually high content of plant estrogen called "lignans," an omega-3 fatty acid (α-linolenic acid [ALA]), and soluble fiber; and it is low in cost.[96] Interestingly, crushed or grounded flaxseed has also demonstrated an ability to reduce menopausal symptoms as well as moderate doses of estrogen and progesterone in a cross-over 4-month total study trial of hypercholesterolemic menopausal women.[218] This same study demonstrated a minimal impact on cholesterol, but an ability to reduce glucose and insulin levels.

Again, ALA is an omega-3 fatty acid found in high concentrations in flaxseed and flaxseed oil, canola oil, and soybean oils, and this compound can be partially converted to eicosapentaenoic acid (EPA) and docosahexaenoic acid (DHA) in humans; interestingly, EPA and DHA are the primary omega-3 oils found in fish, which have demonstrated past significant cardiovascular benefits.[219] Randomized trials utilizing foods high in ALA have consistently reduced the risk of CHD and have favorably impacted all-cause mortality despite no significant changes in serum cholesterol.[220–222]

Lignans, another type of phytoestrogen found in high concentrations in flaxseed, and other components in flaxseed (ALA) have demonstrated potent anticancer properties in laboratory studies utilizing breast and prostate cancer cell lines.[223,224] The largest cohort study examining the correlation between fat intake and prostate cancer risk was the Netherlands Cohort Study.[225] Approximately 58,000 men were followed for more than 6 years, and 642 cases of prostate cancer were documented. An extensive 150-item food frequency questionnaire was utilized. No correlations were found between total fat and other subtypes of fat and prostate cancer risk. There was an association between a reduced risk of prostate cancer and an increased intake of ALA. This was a notable observation because several past prospective investigations observed the opposite trend with this fatty acid.[226,227] The first trial of flaxseed in men with prostate cancer was published several years ago. This pilot study of men consuming flaxseed and a low-fat diet 4 weeks before

radical prostatectomy demonstrated that flaxseed (about 3 round tablespoons/day of ground seed) may have provided a clinical benefit via hormone suppression and via other mechanisms, such as reducing the proliferation index of cancer cells in the prostate and encouraging apoptosis, especially for men with lower Gleason scores (6 or less), before and after this conventional treatment versus historic controls.[228] Also, the mean reduction in total cholesterol over the 4-week study was an impressive 27 points. A similar and almost identical recent study was performed by some of the same researchers. Men at higher-risk for prostate cancer (negative biopsy patients) also observed an apparent risk reduction and decreased cholesterol with just a 6-month course of daily flaxseed powder and a low-fat diet.[229]

Clinicians need to remind patients that cheap ground flaxseed itself has received the most research, while straight flaxseed oil and pills have received little research in humans.[96] In addition, flaxseed should be ingested 2 to 3 hours before or after taking a prescription drug(s) or dietary supplement(s) because the high concentration of fiber could theoretically reduce the absorption of these agents, as is the potential case with any product or supplement high in fiber. Moderate intakes are also important (1–3 tablespoons/day) along with water consumption with flaxseed because of the potential for impaction and/or laxative effects. Again, the potential for CVD risk reduction should be emphasized because the prostate benefits are preliminary.

Fish

Recommendation #9: Encourage the consumption of moderate weekly intakes of canned, broiled, baked, and raw fish (not fried), and other healthy sources of omega-3 fatty acids (for example, fish oil supplements, nuts, and cooking oils), dietary selenium, vitamin D, and vitamin E.

Soy and especially flaxseed are good sources of omega-3 fatty acids, but fish also contain high concentrations of omega-3 fatty acids (EPA and DHA) and in addition, vitamin D.[96] These compounds have demonstrated numerous benefits in terms of reducing the risk of a variety of prevalent chronic diseases,[230] especially CVD.[231,232] Some of the observed mechanisms of action for fish and fish oil include a reduction in triglycerides,[233] blood pressure,[234] platelet aggregation,[235] and arrhythmias.[236] However, the primary focus of their benefit has been their potential ability to reduce the risk of sudden cardiac death.[237–239]

Fish oils have also been shown to inhibit the growth of prostate tumors in the laboratory.[240] Several epidemiologic and pilot studies also support the consumption of fish or fish oils to reduce the incidence and progression of prostate cancer,[241,242] and the ability to reduce cyclooxygenase II (COX2) in patients may be one of the many apparent benefits.[242] Although an epidemiologic review of fish and marine fatty acids concluded that no consistent reduction in prostate cancer risk has been observed in past studies,[243] the results of a large recent prospective study published after this analysis may tip the balance in favor of prevention. The Health Professionals Follow-up Study included over 47,000 men with 12-years of follow-up.[244] During this study, a total of 2482 cases of prostate cancer were diagnosed, and 617 of these cases were diagnosed as advanced prostate cancer, including 278 metastatic prostate cancers. Researchers found that consuming fish more than 3 times per week compared with less than twice per month was associated with a reduced risk of prostate cancer, and the strongest relationship was for metastatic disease (44% reduction). Fish consumption in this study consisted of canned tuna, dark meat fish (mackerel, salmon, sardines, bluefish, and swordfish), and other unspecified fish dishes. The consumption of seafood such as shrimp, lobster, and scallops were not associated with prostate cancer risk.

Clinicians need to tell their patients that many fish contain high levels of omega-3 fatty acids and vitamin D—salmon, tuna, sardines, and a variety of other baked, broiled, raw, but not fried fish are potentially beneficial.[96] Variety should be encouraged to increase compliance. Overall, the beneficial effects of fish consumption on prostate cancer risk remain to be proven, but its role in reducing cardiovascular risk or all-cause mortality is extremely strong as mentioned before and as observed from clinical trials encouraging fish[245] or fish oil consumption[246,247] in patients with a history of CHD. A recent concern over mercury levels of fish has been expressed by the FDA and in the overall medical literature, but the preliminary data is controversial, and it is not known at this time what kind of clinical impact these mercury levels may have on the individual.[248,249] Four types of large predatory fish (king mackerel, shark, swordfish, and tilefish) have caused most concern because these fish retain greater concentrations of methyl-mercury. Regardless, moderate consumption (2–3 times/week) of most fish should have little impact on overall human mercury serum levels, but more ongoing research in this area should soon provide better clarity of the clinical impact of this concern. Interestingly, a recent large investigation of moderate mercury serum levels in older individuals found little to no negative long-term impacts on neurobehavioral parameters.[250] In any event, the positive impact of consuming fish seems to outweigh the negative impact in the majority of individuals with the exception of women considering pregnancy or who are pregnant.

A variety of nuts share some similar clinical positive impacts to omega-3 oils found in fish. For example, a consistent reduction in the risk of CHD and/or sudden cardiac death has been associated with an increased consumption of nuts in prospective studies.[251–256] Nuts contain a variety of potential beneficial compounds, such as ALA, other polyunsaturated fats, mono-unsaturated fats, vitamin E, magnesium, potassium, flavonoids,[251] and potentially selenium, for example, from Brazil nuts.[96] Some of these and other compounds from a variety of foods, but not necessarily dietary supplement sources, have been associated with a lower risk of prostate cancer, for example, vitamin E,[257] ALA,[225] and selenium.[96] However, more research is needed in this area.

A variety of cooking oils such as soybean, canola, and olive oil also contain a high concentration of omega-3 fatty acids, monounsaturated fat, and numerous other vitamins and minerals including vitamin E.[96,219,258] Consumption of a variety of these nuts and oils could also be encouraged to the patient concerned about prostate cancer, but again most of the evidence surrounding their use is for cardiovascular protection. Patients need to keep in mind that most cooking oils contain 120 calories per tablespoon; therefore, moderation is again the foundation of good health.

Recent reviews of healthy omega-3 fatty acids can be found in the literature.[259,260] Reviews such as this one continue to emphasize the general health benefits of certain diets and supplements without just a focus on prostate cancer itself. These publications continue to suggest that heart healthy products have some of the best potential to produce a prostate healthy situation.

Common sense changes

Recommendation #10: Always emphasize the obvious changes such as smoking cessation, moderate alcohol consumption, daily multivitamin, reduced supplement intake, especially vitamin E, and appropriate heart healthy drug intervention when needed because of the potential impacts on prostate and general health.

Numerous other lifestyle modifications and supplements should be discussed by clinicians such as smoking cessation to reduce all-cause mortality including cancer,[261,262] and potentially to reduce the risk of prostate cancer,[263] or the risk of advanced or aggressive prostate cancer.[264,265] Alcohol consumption in moderation seems to reduce cardiovascular events,[266] and its impact at this level of consumption has not been positive or negative in regards to prostate cancer risk.[96]

Most men may derive a benefit from taking a cheap low-dose multivitamin daily to eliminate basic nutritional deficiencies and improve overall health, and a recent 7.5 year randomized trial confirmed the potential benefits of this simplistic recommendation.[267] In addition, patients that qualify for a low-dose aspirin,[268] statin,[269] or other heart protective medications for CVD reduction[270] may be surprised to learn that even these products have been associated with prostate health.[267–270] Along the same line of thinking, patients should currently stay away from individual vitamin E supplements (apart from the low-dose-50 IU or less in a multivitamin) due to recent concerning data observed in randomized cardiovascular,[271,272] and cancer trials.[273]

Conclusions

This chapter may provide a strong foundation for men with a desire to incorporate lifestyle changes to not only reduce the risk of prostate cancer, but, more importantly, to impact all-cause mortality. Minimal time is needed to suggest these changes in an office encounter. These recommendations may seem simplistic; nevertheless, past studies have clearly demonstrated that very few men (less than 5%) report adherence to numerous healthy behaviors at one time.[274] It seems to be more common in the past to follow one healthy change in excess, rather than multiple changes in moderation. This may be the result of past studies focusing on one lifestyle change to produce an overall impact on disease risk, poor compliance, lack of attention, time, or understanding, or a lack of motivation. Regardless of the multiple potential reasons for minimal adherence, investigations of combined moderate lifestyle changes continue to demonstrate that it is more the sum of what you do, rather than one or two specific behavioral changes, that can impact cardiovascular markers, cancer, and all-cause mortality.[275]

Recommending a pill is the simple answer, but few supplements for prostate cancer prevention or total mortality reduction can be recommended at this time.[96,276–278] Moreover, compliance is also an issue over a long period of time with any agent. Additionally, potential supplements that may increase the risk of prostate cancer or interfere with conventional treatment continues to be a concern,[273,279,280] and no dietary supplement has ever come close to matching the reduction in all-cause mortality observed in clinical trials of lifestyle changes.[96] The time seems more than ripe to redirect our attention toward lifestyle changes with regard to prostate cancer. Indeed, what is turning out to be heart healthy seems tantamount to prostate healthy, and this is the best potential practical and realistic recommendation that has worked in my consulting practice for over 10 years. It also seems that larger health organizations are beginning to apply this same concept,[281] and this is truly exciting, because "the forest has to take precedence over the tree" when it comes to this important subject.

References

1. Bonow RO, Smaha LA, Smith SC, et al. The international burden of cardiovascular disease: responding to the emerging epidemic. Circulation 2002;106:1602–1605.
2. World Heart Federation web site. Available at: http://www.world-heart.org/introduction/call_to_action.html. Accessed August 20, 2002.
3. World Health Report. Mental Health: New Understanding, New Hope. Geneva, Switzerland: World Health Organization, 2001, pp 144–149.
4. Michaud CM, Murray CJL, Bloom BR. Burden of disease: implications for future research. JAMA 2001;285:535–539.
5. Murray CJL, Lopez AD. Mortality by cause for eight regions of the world: Global Burden of Disease Study. Lancet 1997;349:1269–1276.
6. Twombly, R. Cancer surpasses heart disease as leading cause of death for all but the very elderly. J Natl Cancer Inst 2005;97:330–331.
7. Thompson IM, Goodman PJ, Tangen CM, et al. The influence of finasteride on the development of prostate cancer. N Engl J Med 2003;349:215–224.
8. Scardino PT. The prevention of prostate cancer-The dilemma continues. N Engl J Med 2003;349:297–299.
9. Reynolds T. Prostate cancer prevention trial yields positive results, but with a few cautions. J Natl Cancer Inst 2003;95:1030–1031.
10. Clark LC, Combs GF Jr, Turnbull BW, et al. Effects of selenium supplementation for cancer prevention in patients with carcinoma of the skin. A randomized controlled trial. Nutritional Prevention of Cancer Study Group. JAMA 1996; 276:1957–1963.
11. Newschaffer CJ, Otani K, McDonald MK, et al. Causes of death in elderly prostate cancer patients and in a comparison nonprostate cancer cohort. J Natl Cancer Inst 2000;92:613–621.
12. Groome PA, Rohland SL, Brundage MD, et al. The relative risk of early death from comorbid illnesses among prostate cancer patients receiving curative treatment. J Urol 2005;173 (Suppl.):53 [abstract 193].
13. Senior K. Atherosclerosis gene increases susceptibility to prostate cancer. Lancet 2002;360:928.
14. Neugut AI, Rosenberg DJ, Ahsan H, et al. Association between coronary heart disease and cancers of the breast, prostate, and colon. Cancer Epidemiol Biomarkers Prev 1998;7:869–873.
15. Peterson HI. Tumor angiogenesis inhibition by prostaglandin synthetase inhibitors. Anticancer Res 1986;6:251.
16. Sandfeldt L, Hahn RG. Cardiovascular risk factors correlate with prostate size in men with bladder outlet obstruction. BJU Intl 2003;92:64–68.
17. Solomon H, Man JW, Wierzbicki AS, et al. Relation of erectile dysfunction to angiographic coronary artery disease. Am J Cardiol 2003;91:230–231.
18. Clark CM, Karlawish JHT. Alzheimer disease: Current concepts and emerging diagnostic and therapeutic strategies. Ann Intern Med 2003;138:400–410.
19. Moyad MA. Emphasizing and promoting overall health and nontraditional treatments after a prostate cancer diagnosis. Semin Urol Oncol 1999;17:119–124.
20. Nash IS, Mosca L, Blumenthal RS, et al. Contemporary awareness and understanding of cholesterol as a risk factor: Results of an American Heart Association National Survey. Arch Intern Med 2003;163:1597–1600.
21. The Expert Panel. Executive summary of the Third Report of the National Cholesterol Education Program (NCEP). Expert Panel on Detection, Evaluation, and Treatment of High Blood Cholesterol in Adults (Adult Treatment Panel III). JAMA 2001;285:2486–2498.
22. Grundy SM, Cleeman JI, Marz NB, et al. Implications of recent clinical trials for the National Cholesterol Education Program Adult Treatment Panel III Guidelines. Circulation 2004;110:227–239.
23. Mosca L. C-reactive protein-to screen or not screen? N Engl J Med 2002;347:1615–1616.
24. Ridker PM. Clinical application of C-reactive protein for cardiovascular disease detection and prevention. Circulation 2003;107:363–369.
25. Nissen SE, Tuzcu EM, Schoenhagen P, et al. for the Reversal of Atherosclerosis with Aggressive Lipid Lowering (REVERSAL) Investigators. Statin therapy, LDL cholesterol, C-reactive protein, and coronary heart disease. N Engl J Med 2005;352:29–38.
26. Ridker PM, Cannon CP, Morrow D, et al. C-reactive protein levels and outcomes after statin therapy. N Engl J Med 2005;352:20–28.
27. The Homocysteine Studies Collaboration. Homocysteine and risk of ischemic heart disease and stroke. A meta-analysis. JAMA 2002; 288:2015–2022.
28. Kostner KM, Kostner GM. Lipoprotein(a): still an enigma? Curr Opin Lipidol 2002;13:391–396.
29. Ariyo AA, Thach C, Tracy R, for the Cardiovascular Health Study Investigators. Lp(a) lipoprotein, vascular disease, and mortality in the elderly. N Engl J Med 2003;349:2108–2115.
30. Kraus WE, Houmard JA, Duscha BD, et al. Effects of the amount and intensity of exercise on plasma lipoproteins. N Engl J Med 2002;347:1483–1492.
31. Hammarsten J, Hogstedt B. Hyperinsulinaemia as a risk factor for developing benign prostatic hyperplasia. Eur Urol 2001;39:151–158.
32. Chobanian AV, Bakris GL, Black HR, et al. for the Joint National Committee on Prevention, Detection, Evaluation, and Treatment of High Blood Pressure. National Heart, Lung, and Blood Institute; National High Blood Pressure Education Program Coordinating Committee. Hypertension 2003;42:1206–1252.
33. Whelton SP, Chin A, Xin X, et al. Effect of aerobic exercise on blood pressure: a meta-analysis of randomized, controlled trials. Ann Intern Med 2002; 136:493–503.
34. Moyad MA, Giacherio D, National Prostate Cancer Coalition (NPCC), Montie J. African-American men, high cholesterol & hs-CRP & alternative medicine use documented at a prostate cancer screening: A unique opportunity for a complete men's health intervention. Proceedings of the American Society of Clinical Oncology (ASCO) 2005;23(16S, part I of II):408s [abstract 4623].
35. Moyad MA. Is obesity a risk factor for prostate cancer, and does it even matter? A hypothesis and different perspective. Urology 2002; 59 (Suppl 4A):41–50.
36. Moyad MA. Current methods used for defining, measuring, and treating obesity. Semin Urol Oncol 2001;19:247–256.
37. Writing Group for the Women's Health Initiative Investigators. Risks and benefits of estrogen plus progestin in healthy postmenopausal women: principal results from the Women's Health Initiative randomized controlled trial. JAMA 2002;288:321–333.
38. Shike M, Latkany L, Riedel E, et al. Lack of effect of a low-fat, high-fruit, -vegetable, and -fiber diet on serum prostate-specific antigen of men without prostate cancer: results from a randomized trial. J Clin Oncol 2002;20:3592–3598.
39. Zhu S, Heymsfield SB, Toyoshima H, et al. Race-ethnicity-specific waist circumference cutoffs for identifying cardiovascular disease risk factors. Am J Clin Nutr 2005;81:409–415.
40. Marcella S, Rhoads GG. Waist size and mortality from prostate cancer. Proceedings of the American Society of Clinical Oncology (ASCO) 2005;23:409 [abstract 4626].
41. Moyad MA. Osteoporosis: a rapid review of risk factors and screening methods. Urol Oncol: Seminars and Original Investigations 2003;21:375–379.
42. Freedland SJ, Aronson WJ. Obesity and prostate cancer. Urology 2005;65:433–439.
43. Andersson SO, Wolk A, Bergstrom R, et al. Body size and prostate cancer: a 20-year follow-up study among 135,006 Swedish construction workers. J Natl Cancer Inst 1997;89:385–389.
44. Schuurman AG, van den Brandt PA, Dorant E, et al. Association of energy and fat intake with prostate carcinoma risk: results from the Netherlands Cohort Study. Cancer 1999;86:1019–1027.
45. Schuurman AG, Goldbohm RA, Dorant E, et al. Anthropometry in relation to prostate cancer risk in the Netherlands Cohort Study. Am J Epidemiol 2000;151:541–549.
46. Heinonen OP, Albanes D, Virtamo J, et al. Prostate cancer and supplementation with alpha-tocopherol and beta-carotene: incidence and mortality in a controlled trial. J Natl Cancer Inst 1998;90:440–446.

47. Aziz NM, Hartman T, Barrett M, et al. Weight and prostate cancer in the Alpha-Tocopherol Beta-Carotene Cancer Prevention (ATBC) Trial. ASCO 2000;19:647a.
48. Calle EE, Rodriguez C, Walker-Thurmond K, et al. Overweight, obesity, and mortality from cancer in a prospectively studied cohort of U.S. adults. N Engl J Med 2003;348:1625–1638.
49. Amling CL, Riffenburgh RH, Sun L, et al. Pathologic variables and recurrence rates as related to obesity and race in men with prostate cancer undergoing radical prostatectomy. J Clin Oncol 2004;22:439–445.
50. Freedland SJ, Aronson WJ, Kane CJ, et al. Impact of obesity on biochemical control after radical prostatectomy for clinically localized prostate cancer: A report by the Shared Equal Access Regional Cancer Hospital Database Study Group. J Clin Oncol 2004;22:446–453.
51. Giovannucci E, Rimm EB, Liu Y, et al. Body mass index and risk of prostate cancer in U.S. health professionals. J Natl Cancer Inst 2003;95:1240–1244.
52. Stevens J, Cai J, Pamuk ER, et al. The effect of age on the association between body-mass index and mortality. N Engl J Med 1998;338:1–7.
53. Calle EE, Thun MJ, Petrelli JM, et al. Body-mass index and mortality in a prospective cohort of US adults. N Engl J Med 1997;341:1097–1105.
54. Kuczmarski RJ, Carroll MD, Flegal KM, et al. Varying body mass index cutoff points to describe overweight prevalence among US adults: NHANES III (1988 to 1994). Obes Res 1997;5:542–548.
55. Moyad MA. Obesity, interrelated mechanisms, and exposures and kidney cancer. Semin Urol Oncol 2001;19:270–279.
56. Bacon CG, Mittleman MA, Kawachi I, et al. Sexual function in men older than 50 years of age: results from the Health Professionals Follow-up Study. Ann Intern Med 2003;139:161–168.
57. Walczak MK, Lokhandwala N, Hodge MB, et al. Prevalence of cardiovascular risk factors in erectile dysfunction. J Gend Specif Med 2002;5:19–24.
58. Taylor EN, Stampfer MJ, Curhan GC. Obesity, weight gain, and the risk of kidney stones. JAMA 2005;293:455–462.
59. Friedenreich CM. Physical activity and cancer prevention: from observational to intervention research. Cancer Epidemiol Biomark Prev 2001;10:287–301.
60. Giovannucci EL, Liu Y, Leitzmann MF, et al. A prospective study of physical activity and incident and fatal prostate cancer. Arch Intern Med 2005;165:1005–1010.
61. Tanasescu M, Leitzmann MF, Rimm EB, et al. Exercise type and intensity in relation to coronary heart disease in men. JAMA 2002; 288:1994–2000.
62. Poehlman ET, Melby C. Resistance training and energy balance. Int J Sport Nutr 1998;8:143–159.
63. Poehlman ET, Dvorak RV, DeNino WF, et al. Effects of resistance training and endurance training on insulin sensitivity in nonobese, young women. J Clin Endocrinol Metab 2000;85:2463–2468.
64. Prabhakaran B, Dowling EA, Branch JD, et al. Effect of 14 weeks of resistance training on lipid profile and body fat percentage in premenopausal women. Br J Sports Med 1999;33:190–195.
65. Hurley BF, Roth SM. Strength training in the elderly. Sports Med 2000;30:249-268.
66. Segal RJ, Reid RD, Courneya KS, et al. Resistance training in men receiving androgen deprivation therapy for prostate cancer. J Clin Oncol 2003;21:1653–1659.
67. Platz EA, Kawachi I, Rimm EB, et al. Physical activity and benign prostatic hyperplasia. Arch Intern Med 1998;158:2349–2356.
68. Esposito K, Giugliano F, Di Palo C, et al. Effect of lifestyle changes on erectile dysfunction in obese men: a randomized controlled trial. JAMA 2004;291:2978–2984.
69. Saigal CS. Obesity and erectile dysfunction: common problems, common solution? JAMA 2004;291:3011–3012.
70. Slattery ML, Edwards S, Curtin K, et al. Physical activity and colorectal cancer. Am J Epidemiol 2003;158:214–224.
71. Blumenthal JA, Babyak MA, Moore KA, et al. Effects of exercise training on older patients with major depression. Arch Intern Med 1999;159:2349–2356.
72. Babyak M, Blumenthal JA, Herman S, et al. Exercise treatment for major depression: maintenance of therapeutic benefit at 10 months. Psychosom Med 2000;62:633–638.
73. Hu FB, Willett WC, Li T, et al. Adiposity as compared with physical activity in predicting mortality among women. N Engl J Med 2004;351:2694–2703.
74. Grable JC, Ternullo S. Smoking cessation from office to bedside. An evidence-based, practical approach. Postgrad Med 2003;114:45–48,51–54.
75. Ornish D, Fair W, Pettengill E, et al. Can lifestyle changes reverse prostate cancer? J Urol 2003;169:74 [abstract 286].
76. Samaha FF, Iqbal N, Seshadri P, et al. A low-carbohydrate as compared with a low-fat diet in severe obesity. N Engl J Med 2003;348:2074–2081.
77. Foster GD, Wyatt HR, Hill JO, et al. A randomized trial of a low-carbohydrate diet for obesity. N Engl J Med 2003;348:2082–2090.
78. Hsing AW, Chua S Jr, Gao YT, et al. Prostate cancer risk and serum levels of insulin and leptin: a population-based study. J Natl Cancer Inst 2001;93:783–789.
79. Augustin LS, Franceschi S, Jenkins DJA, et al. Glycemic index in chronic disease: a review. Eur J Clin Nutr 2002;56:1049–1071.
80. Hsing AW, Gao Y-T, Chua S Jr, et al. Insulin resistance and prostate cancer risk. J Natl Cancer Inst 2003;95:67–71.
81. Jee SH, Ohrr H, Sull JW, et al. Fasting serum glucose level and cancer risk in Korean men and women. JAMA 2005;293:194–202.
82. Dansinger ML, Gleason JA, Griffith JL, et al. Comparison of the Atkins, Ornish, Weight Watchers, and Zone Diets for weight loss and heart disease risk reduction: a randomized trial. JAMA 2005;293:43–53.
83. Rolls BJ, Morris EL, Roe LS. Portion size of food affects energy intake in normal-weight and overweight men and women. Am J Clin Nutr 2002;76:1207–1213.
84. Pereira MA, Kartashov AI, Ebbeling CB, et al. Fast-food habits, weight gain, and insulin resistance (the CARDIA study): 15-year prospective analysis. Lancet 2005;365:36–42.
85. Hsieh LJ, Carter B, Landis PK, et al. Association of energy intake with prostate cancer in a long-term aging study: Baltimore Longitudinal Study of Aging (United States). Urology 2003;61:297–301.
86. Heilbronn LK, Ravussin E. Calorie restriction and aging: review of the literature and implications for studies in humans. Am J Clin Nutr 2003;78:361–369.
87. Pirozzo S, Summerbell C, Cameron C, et al. Advice on low-fat diets for obesity. Cochrane Database Syst Rev 2002;2:CD003640.
88. Hill JO, Peters JC. Environmental contributions to the obesity epidemic. Science 1998;280:1371–1374.
89. Mukherjee P, Sotnikov AV, Mangian HJ, et al. Energy intake and prostate tumor growth, angiogenesis, and vascular endothelial growth factor expression. J Natl Cancer Inst 1999;91:512–523.
90. Bosland MC, Oakley-Girvan I, Whittemore AS. Dietary fat, calories, and prostate cancer risk. J Natl Cancer Inst 1999;91:489–491.
91. Gregg EW, Gerzoff RB, Thompson TJ, et al. Intentional weight loss and death in overweight and obese U.S. adults 35 years of age and older. Ann Intern Med 2003;138:383–389.
92. Clinical guidelines on the identification, evaluation, and treatment of overweight and obesity in adults. www.nhlbi.nih.gov/guidelines/obesity/ob_home.htm. Accessed September 2002.
93. Keys A, Menotti A, Karvonen MJ, et al. The diet and 15-year death rate in the Seven Countries Study. Am J Epidemiol 1986;124:903–915.
94. Gordon DJ. Cholesterol and mortality: what can meta-analysis tell us? In: Gallo LL (ed.): Cardiovascular disease 2: cellular and molecular mechanisms, prevention, and treatment. New York: Plenum Press, 1995, pp 333–340.
95. Gordon DJ. Cholesterol lowering and total mortality. In: Rifkind BM (ed.): Lowering cholesterol in high-risk individuals and populations. New York: Marcel Dekker, 1995, pp 333–348.
96. Moyad MA. The ABCs of nutrition and supplements for prostate cancer. Ann Arbor, MI: JW Edwards Publishing, 2000.
97. Meyer F, Bairati I, Shadmani R, et al. Dietary fat and prostate cancer survival. Cancer Causes Control 1999;10:245–251.

98. Key TJ, Fraser GE, Thorogood M, et al. Mortality in vegetarians and non-vegetarians: detailed findings from a collaborative analysis of 5 prospective studies. Am J Clin Nutr 1999;70 (suppl):516S-524S.

99. Yu JN, Cunningham JA, Rosenberg Thouin S, et al. Hyperlipidemia. Primary Care 2000;27:541–587.

100. Mensink RP, Katan MB. Effect of dietary fatty acids on serum lipids and lipoproteins: a meta-analysis of 27 trials. Arterioscler Thromb 1992;12:911–919.

101. Hu FB, van Dam RM, Liu S. Diet and risk of type II diabetes: the role of types of fat and carbohydrate. Diabetologia 2001;44:805–817.

102. Salmeron J, Hu FB, Manson JE, et al. Dietary fat intake and risk of type 2 diabetes in women. Am J Clin Nutr 2001;73:1019–1026.

103. Innis SM, Green TJ, Halsey TK. Variability in the trans fatty acid content of foods within a food category: implications for estimation of dietary trans fatty acid intakes. J Am Coll Nutr 1999;18:255–260.

104. Clandinin MT, Wilke MS. Do trans fatty acids increase the incidence of type 2 diabetes? Am J Clin Nutr 2001;73:1001–1002.

105. Lemaitre RN, King IB, Raghunathan TE, et al. Cell membrane trans-fatty acids and the risk of primary cardiac arrest. Circulation 2002;105:697–701.

106. Nelson GJ. Dietary fat, trans fatty acids, and risk of coronary heart disease. Nutr Rev 1998;56:250–252.

107. Katan MB. Trans fatty acids and plasma lipoproteins. Nutr Rev 2000;58:188–191.

108. Mensink RP, Katan MB. Effect of dietary trans fatty acids on high-density and low-density lipoprotein cholesterol levels in healthy subjects. N Engl J Med 1990;323:439–445.

109. Ascherio A, Katan MB, Zock PL, et al. Trans fatty acids and coronary heart disease. N Engl J Med 1999;340:1994–1998.

110. Nestel P, Noakes M, Belling BE. Plasma lipoprotein and Lp(a) changes with substitution of elaidic acid for oleic acid in the diet. J Lipid Res 1992;33:1029–1036.

111. Sundram K, Ismail A, Hays KC, et al. Trans (elaidic) fatty acids adversely affect the lipoprotein profile relative to specific saturated fatty acids in humans. J Nutr 1997;127:514S–520S.

112. de Roos NM, Bots ML, Siebelink E, Schouten E, Katan MB. Flow-mediated vasodilation is not impaired when HDL-cholesterol is lowered by substituting carbohydrates for monounsaturated fat. Br J Nutr 2001;86:181–188.

113. Lovejoy JC. Dietary fatty acids and insulin resistance. Curr Atheroscler Rep 1999;1:215–220.

114. Kinsella JE, Bruckner G, Mai J, et al. Metabolism of trans fatty acids with emphasis on the effects of trans, trans-octadecadienoate on lipid composition, essential fatty acid, and prostaglandins: an overview. Am J Clin Nutr 1981;34:2307–2318.

115. Hill EG, Johnson SB, Lawson LD, et al. Perturbation of the metabolism of essential fatty acids by dietary hydrogenated vegetable oil. Proc Natl Acad Sci USA 1982;79:953–957.

116. Byrne C, Rockett H, Holmes MD. Dietary fat, fat subtypes, and breast cancer risk: lack of an association among postmenopausal women with no history of benign breast disease. Cancer Epidemiol Biomarkers Prev 2002;11:261–265.

117. Slattery ML, Benson J, Ma KN, et al. Trans-fatty acids and colon cancer. Nutr Cancer 2001; 39:170–175.

118. Voorrips LE, Brants HA, Kardinaal AF, et al. Intake of conjugated linoleic acid, fat, and other fatty acids in relation to postmenopausal breast cancer: the Netherlands Cohort Study on Diet and Cancer. Am J Clin Nutr 2002; 76:873–882.

119. King IB, Kristal AR, Schaffer S, et al. Serum trans-fatty acids are associated with risk of prostate cancer in beta-carotene and retinol efficacy trial. Cancer Epidemiol Biomarkers Prev 2005;14:988–992.

120. Stender S, Dyerberg J. Influence of trans fatty acids on health. Ann Nutr Metab 2004;48:61–66.

121. United States Food and Drug Administration web site. Available at: http://www.fda.gov/oc/initiatives/transfat. Accessed February 15, 2004.

122. Moyad MA. Dietary fat reduction to reduce prostate cancer risk: controlled enthusiasm, learning a lesson from breast or other cancers, and the big picture. Urology 2002;59 (Suppl 4A):51–62.

123. Laaksonen DE, Nyyssonen K, Niskanen L, et al. Prediction of cardio-vascular mortality in middle-aged men by dietary and serum linoleic and polyunsaturated fatty acids. Arch Intern Med 2005;165:193–199.

124. Connor WE, Lin DS. The effect of shellfish in the diet upon the plasma lipid levels in humans. Metabolism 1982;31:1046–1051.

125. Childs MT, Dorsett CS, Failor A, et al. Effect of shellfish consumption on cholesterol absorption in normolipidemic men. Metabolism 1987;36:31–35.

126. Zhuang L, Kim J, Adam RM, et al. Cholesterol targeting alters lipid raft composition and cell survival in prostate cancer cells and xenografts. J Clin Invest 2005;115:959–968.

127. Henriksson P, Eriksson M, Ericsson S, et al. Hypocholesterolaemia and increased elimination of low-density lipoproteins in metastatic cancer of the prostate. Lancet 1989;2:1178–1180.

128. Wong NCW. The beneficial effects of plant sterols on serum cholesterol. Can J Cardiol 2001;17:715–721.

129. Katan MB, Grundy SM, Jones P, et al. For the Stresa Workshop Participants. Efficacy and safety of plant stanols and sterols in the management of blood cholesterol levels. Mayo Clin Proc 2003;78:965–978.

130. Schaefer EJ. Lipoproteins, nutrition, and heart disease. Am J Clin Nutr 2002;75:191–212.

131. Vuorio AF, Gylling H, Turtola H, et al. Stanol ester margarine alone and with simvastatin lowers serum cholesterol in families with familial hypercholesterolemia caused by the FH-North Karelia mutation. Arterio Thromb Vasc Biol 2000;20:500–506.

132. Gylling H, Miettinen TA. Cholesterol reduction by different plant stanol mixtures and with variable fat intake. Metabolism 1999;48:575–580.

133. Hallikainen MA, Uusitupa MI. Effects of 2 low-fat stanol ester-containing margarines on serum cholesterol concentrations as part of a low-fat diet in hypercholesterolemic subjects. Am J Clin Nutr 1999;69:403–410.

134. Hendriks HFJ, Weststrate JA, van Vliet T, et al. Spreads enriched with three different levels of vegetable oil sterols and the degree of cholesterol lowering in normocholesterolaemic and mildly hypercholesterolaemic subjects. Eur J Clin Nutr 1999;53:319–327.

135. Gylling H, Radhakrishnan R, Miettinen TA. Reduction of serum cholesterol in postmenopausal women with previous myocardial infarction and cholesterol malabsorption induced by dietary sitostanol ester margarine: women and dietary sitostanol. Circulation 1997;96:4226–4231.

136. Miettinen TA, Puska P, Gylling H, et al. Reduction of serum cholesterol with sitostanol-ester margarine in a mildly hypercholesterolemic population. N Engl J Med 1995;333:1308–1312.

137. Vanhanen HT, Blomqvist S, Ehnholm C, et al. Serum cholesterol, cholesterol precursors, and plant sterols in hypercholesterolemic subjects with different apoE phenotypes during dietary sitostanol ester treatment. J Lipid Res 1993;34:1535–1544.

138. Giovannucci E. Tomatoes, tomato-based products, lycopene, and cancer: review of the epidemiologic literature. J Natl Cancer Inst 1999;91:317–331.

139. Mucci LA, Tamimi R, Lagiou P, et al. Are dietary influences on the risk of prostate cancer mediated through the insulin-like growth factor system? Brit J Urol Intl 2001;87:814–820.

140. Chen L, Stacewicz-Sapuntzakis M, Duncan C, et al. Oxidative DNA damage in prostate cancer patients consuming tomato sauce-based entrees as a whole-food intervention. J Natl Cancer Inst 2001;93:1872–1879.

141. Etminan M, Takkouche B, Caamano-Isorna F. The role of tomato products and lycopene in the prevention of prostate cancer: a meta-analysis of observational studies. Cancer Epidemiol Biomarkers Prev 2004;13:340–345.

142. Boileau TWM, Liao Z, Kim S, et al. Prostate carcinogenesis in N-methyl-N-nitrosurea (NMU)-testosterone-treated rats fed tomato powder, lycopene, or energy-restricted diets. J Natl Cancer Inst 2003;95:1578–1586.

143. Jian L, Du CJ, Lee AH, et al. Do dietary lycopene and other carotenoids protect against prostate cancer? Int J Cancer 2005;113:1010–1014.

144. Street DA, Comstock GW, Salkeld RM, et al. Serum antioxidants and myocardial infarction. Are low levels of carotenoids and alpha-tocopherol risk factors for myocardial infarction? Circulation 1994;90:1154–1161.

145. Arab L, Steck S. Lycopene and cardiovascular disease. Am J Clin Nutr 2000;71(suppl):1691S–1695S.

146. Rissanen TH, Voutilainen S, Nyyssonen K, et al. Serum lycopene concentrations and carotid atherosclerosis: the Kuopio Ischaemic Heart Disease Risk Factor Study. Am J Clin Nutr 2003;77:133–138.

147. Sesso HD, Buring JE, Norkus EP, et al. Plasma lycopene, other carotenoids, and retinol and the risk of cardiovascular disease in women. Am J Clin Nutr 2004;79:47–53.

148. Cohen JH, Kristal AR, Stanford JL. Fruit and vegetable intakes and prostate cancer risk. J Natl Cancer Inst 2000;92:61–68.

149. Kristal AR, Lampe JW. Brassica vegetables and prostate cancer risk: a review of the epidemiological evidence. Nutr Cancer 2002;42:1–9.

150. Hsing AW, Chokkalingam AP, Gao Y-T, et al. Allium vegetables and risk of prostate cancer: a population-based study. J Natl Cancer Inst 2002;94:1648–1651.

151. van Gils CH, Peeters PHM, Bueno-de-Mesquita HB, et al. Consumption of vegetables and fruits and risk of breast cancer. JAMA 2005;293:183–193.

152. Hung H-C, Joshipura KJ, Jiang R, et al. Fruit and vegetable intake and risk of major chronic disease. J Natl Cancer Inst 2004;96:1577–1584.

153. Sesso HD, Buring JE, Zhang SM, et al. Dietary and plasma lycopene and the risk of breast cancer. Cancer Epidemiol Biomarkers Prev 2005;14:1074–1081.

154. Vastag B. Recent studies show limited association of fruit and vegetable consumption and cancer risk. J Natl Cancer Inst 2005;97:474–475.

155. Michaud DS, Skinner HG, Wu K, et al. Dietary patterns and pancreatic cancer risk in men and women. J Natl Cancer Inst 2005;97:518–524.

156. Borden LS Jr., Clark PE, Miller A, et al. Prospective dose-escalation trial of lycopene in men with recurrent prostate cancer following definitive local therapy. Proceedings of the American Urologic Association Annual Meeting 2005;173:275 [abstract 1014].

157. Van Horn L. Fiber, lipids, and coronary heart disease. Nutrition Committee Advisory. Circulation 1997;95:2701–2704.

158. U.S. Department of Health and Human Services. Food and Drug Administration. Food labeling: health claims; soluble fiber from certain foods and coronary heart disease: final rule. Federal Register 1998;63:8103–8121.

159. U.S. Department of Health and Human Services. Food and Drug Administration. Food labeling: health claims; soluble fiber from certain foods and coronary heart disease: proposed rule. Federal Register 1997;62:28234–28245.

160. Brown L, Rosner B, Willett WW, et al. Cholesterol-lowering effects of dietary fiber: a meta-analysis. Am J Clin Nutr 1999;69:30–42.

161. Lieberman DA, Prindiville S, Weiss DG, et al. Risk factors for advanced colonic neoplasia and hyperplastic polyps in asymptomatic individuals. JAMA 2003;290:2959–2967.

162. Pereira MA, O'Reilly E, Augustsson K, et al. Dietary fiber and risk of coronary heart disease: a pooled analysis of cohort studies. Arch Intern Med 2004;164:370–376.

163. Liu S, Buring J, Sesso H, et al. A prospective study of dietary fiber intake and risk of cardiovascular disease among women. J Am Coll Cardiol 2002;39:49–56.

164. Wolk A, Manson ME, Stampfer MJ, et al. Long-term intake of dietary fiber and decreased risk of coronary heart disease among women. JAMA 1999;281:1998–2002.

165. Pietinen P, Rimm EB, Korhonen P, et al. Intake of dietary fiber and risk of coronary heart disease in a cohort of Finnish men: the Alpha-Tocopherol, Beta-Carotene Cancer Prevention Study. Circulation 1996;94:2720–2727.

166. Rimm EB, Ascherio A, Giovannucci E, et al. Vegetable, fruit, and cereal fiber intake and risk of coronary heart disease among men. JAMA 1996;275:447–451.

167. Marlett JA, Hosig KB, Vollendorf NW, et al. Mechanism of serum cholesterol reduction by oat bran. Hepatology 1994;20:1450–1457.

168. Chandalia M, Garg A, Lutjohann D, et al. Beneficial effects of high dietary fiber intake in patients with type 2 diabetes mellitus. N Engl J Med 2000;342:1392–1398.

169. Leinonen KS, Poutanen KS, Mykkanen HM. Rye bread decreases serum total and LDL cholesterol in men with moderately elevated serum cholesterol. J Nutr 2000;130:164–170

170. Keenan JM, Pins JJ, Frazel C, et al. Oat ingestion reduces systolic and diastolic blood pressure among moderate hypertensives: a pilot trial. J Fam Pract 2002;51:369.

171. Moreyra AE, Wilson AC, Koraym A. Effect of combining psyllium fiber with simvastatin in lowering cholesterol. Arch Intern Med 2005;165:1161–1166.

172. Streppel MT, Arends LR, van't Veer P, Grobbee DE, Geleijnse JM. Dietary fiber and blood pressure: a meta-analysis of randomized placebo-controlled trials. Arch Intern Med 2005;165:150–156.

173. Marlett JA, McBurney MI, Slavin JL, for the American Dietetic Association. Position of the American Dietetic Association: health implications of dietary fiber. J Am Diet Assoc 2002;102:993–1000.

174. Schatzkin A, Lanza E, Corle D, et al, and the Polyp Prevention Trial Study Group. Lack of effect of a low-fat, high-fiber diet on the recurrence of colorectal adenomas. N Engl J Med 2000;342:1149–1155.

175. Alberts DS, Martinez ME, Roe DJ, et al. Lack of effect of high-fiber cereal supplement on the recurrence of colorectal adenomas. N Engl J Med 2000;342:1156–1162.

176. Eastham JA, Riedel E, Latkany L, et al. for the Polyp Prevention Trial Study Group. Dietary manipulation, ethnicity, and serum PSA levels. Urology 2003;62:677–682.

177. Pelucchi C, Talamini R, Galeone C, et al. Fibre intake and prostate cancer risk. Int J Cancer 2004;109:278–280.

178. Tariq N, Jenkins DJ, Vidgen E, et al. Effect of soluble and insoluble fiber diets on serum prostate specific antigen in men. J Urol 2000;163:114–118.

179. Bylund A, Lundin E, Zhang JX, et al. Randomised controlled short-term intervention pilot study on rye bran bread in prostate cancer. Eur J Cancer Prev 2003;12:407–415.

180. Pienta KJ, Naik H, Akhtar A, et al. Inhibition of spontaneous metastasis in a rat prostate cancer model by oral administration of modified citrus pectin. J Natl Cancer Inst 1995;87:348–353.

181. Hayashi A, Gillen AC, Lott JR. Effects of daily oral administration of quercetin chalcone and modified citrus pectin on implanted colon-25 tumor growth in Balb-c mice. Altern Med Rev 2000;5:546–552.

182. Guess BW, Scholz MC, Strum SB, et al. Modified citrus pectin (MCP) increases the prostate-specific antigen doubling time in men with prostate cancer: a phase II pilot study. Prostate Cancer Prostatic Dis 2003;6:301–304.

183. Moyad MA, Sakr WA, Hirano D, et al. Complementary medicine for prostate cancer: effects of soy and fat consumption. Reviews in Urology 2001;3 (Suppl 2):S20–S30.

184. Sirtori CR, Galli G, Lovati MR, et al. Effects of dietary proteins on the regulation of liver lipoprotein receptors in rats. J Nutr 1984;114:1493–1500.

185. Khosla P, Sammam S, Carrol KK. Decreased receptor-mediated LDL catabolism in casein-fed rabbits precedes the increase in plasma cholesterol levels. J Nutr Biochem 1991;2:203–209.

186. Potter SM. Soy protein and serum lipids. Curr Opin Lipidol 1996;7:260–264.

187. Potter SM. Overview of possible mechanisms for the hypocholesterolemic effect of soy protein. J Nutr 1995;125:606S–611S.

188. U.S. Department of Health and Human Services. Food and Drug Administration. Food labeling: health claims; soy protein and coronary heart disease: proposed rule. Federal Register 1998;63:62977–63015.

189. U.S Department of Health and Human Services. Food and Drug Administration. Food labeling: health claims; soy protein and coronary heart disease: final rule. Federal Register 1999;64:57699–57733.

190. Potter SM. Soy protein and cardiovascular disease: the impact of bioactive components in soy. Nutr Rev 1998;56:231–235.

191. Anderson JW, Johnstone BM, Cook-Newell ME. Meta-analysis of the effects of soy protein intake on serum lipids. N Engl J Med 1995;333:276–282.

192. Zhan S, Ho SC. Meta-analysis of the effects of soy protein containing isoflavones on the lipid profile. Am J Clin Nutr 2005;81:397–408.

193. Peterson G, Barnes S. Genistein and biochanin-A inhibit the growth of human prostate cancer cells but not epidermal growth factor receptor tyrosine autophosphorylation. Prostate 1993; 22:335–345.

194. Rokhlin OW, Cohen MB. Differential sensitivity of human prostatic cancer cell lines to the effects of protein kinase and phosphatase inhibitors. Cancer Lett 1995;98:103–110.

195. Adlercreutz H, Makela S, Pylkkanen L, et al. Dietary phytoestrogens and prostate cancer. Proc Am Assoc Cancer Res 1995;36:687 [abstract 41].

196. Akiyama T, Ishida J, Nakagawa S, et al. Genistein, a specific inhibitor of tyrosine-specific protein kinases. J Biol Chem 1987;262:5592–5595.

197. Linnassier C, Pierre M, Le Pecq JB, et al. Mechanisms of action in NIH-3T3 cells of genistein, an inhibitor of EGF receptor kinase activity. Biochem Pharmacol 1990;39:187–193.

198. Nishimura J, Huang JS, Deuel TF. Platelet-derived growth factor stimulates tyrosine-specific protein kinase activity in Swiss mouse 3T3 cell membranes. Proc Natl Acad Sci USA 1982;79:4303–4307.

199. Rubin JB, Shia MA, Pilch PF. Stimulation of tyrosine-specific phosphorylation in vitro by insulin-like growth factor I. Nature 1983;305:438–440.

200. Okura A, Arakawa H, Oka H, et al. Effect of genistein on topoisomerase activity and on the growth of (VAL 12)Ha-ras-transformed NIH 3T3 cells. Biochem Biophys Res Commun 1988;157:183–189.

201. Fotsis T, Pepper M, Adlercreutz H, et al. Genistein, a dietary ingested isoflavonoid, inhibits cell proliferation and in vitro angiogenesis. J Nutr 1995;125:S790–S797.

202. Kyle E, Neckers L, Takimoto C, et al. Genistein-induced apoptosis of prostate cancer cells is preceded by a specific decrease in focal adhesion kinase activity. Mol Pharmacol 1997;51:193–200.

203. Nagata C, Inaba S, Kawakami N, et al. Inverse association of soy product intake with serum androgen and estrogen concentrations in Japanese men. Nutr Cancer 2000;36:14–18.

204. Moyad MA. Lifestyle/dietary supplement partial androgen suppression and/or estrogen manipulation: A novel PSA reducer and preventive/treatment option for prostate cancer? Urol Clin N Amer 2002;29:115–124.

205. Morton MS, Turkes A, Denis L, et al. Can dietary factors influence prostatic disease? BJU International 1999;84:549–554.

206. Ornish DM, Lee KL, Fair WR, et al. Dietary trial in prostate cancer: early experience and implications for clinical trial design. Urology 2001;57 (Suppl 4A):200–201.

207. Bosland MC, Kato I, Melamed J, et al. Chemoprevention trials in men with prostate-specific antigen failure or at high risk for recurrence after radical prostatectomy: application to efficacy assessment of soy protein. Urology 2001;57 (Suppl 4A):202–204.

208. DeVere White RW, Hackman RM, Soares SE, et al. Effects of a genistein-rich extract on PSA levels in men with a history of prostate cancer. Urology 2004;63:259–263.

209. Adams KF, Chen Chu, Newton KM, et al. Soy isoflavones do not modulate prostate-specific antigen concentrations in older men in a randomized controlled trial. Cancer Epidemiol Biomarkers Prev 2004;13:644–648.

210. Lichtenstein AH, Ausman LM, Jalbert SM, et al. Effects of different forms of dietary hydrogenated fats on serum lipoprotein cholesterol levels. N Engl J Med 1999;340:1933–1940.

211. Tham DM, Gardner CD, Haskell WL. Potential health benefits of dietary phytoestrogens: a review of the clinical, epidemiological, and mechanistic evidence. J Clin Endocrinol Metab 1998;83:2223–2235.

212. Kronenberg F, Fugh-Berman A. Complementary and alternative medicine for menopausal symptoms: a review of randomized, controlled trials. Ann Intern Med 2002;137:805–813.

213. Cunnane SC, Ganguli S, Menard C, et al. High alpha-linolenic acid flaxseed (Linum usitatissimum): Some nutritional properties in humans. Br J Nutr 1993;69:443–453.

214. Bierenbaum ML, Reichstein R, Watkins TR. Reducing atherogenic risk in hyperlipemic humans with flax seed supplementation: A preliminary report. J Am Coll Nutr 1993;12:501–504.

215. Arjmandi BH, Khan DA, Juma S, et al. Whole flaxseed consumption lowers serum LDL-cholesterol and lipoprotein(a) concentrations in postmenopausal women. Nutr Res 1998;18:1203–1214.

216. Jenkins DJ, Kendall CW, Vidgen E, et al. Health aspects of partially defatted flaxseed, including effects on serum lipids, oxidative measures, and ex vivo androgen and progestin activity: A controlled crossover trial. Am J Clin Nutr 1999;69:395–402.

217. Bloedon LT, Szapary PO. Flaxseed and cardiovascular risk. Nut Rev 2004;62:18–27.

218. Lemay A, Dodin S, Kadri N, et al. Flaxseed dietary supplement versus hormone replacement therapy in hypercholesterolemic menopausal women. Obstet Gynecol 2002;100:495–504.

219. Hu FB, Willett WC. Optimal diets for prevention of coronary heart disease. JAMA 2002;288:2569–2578.

220. Singh RB, Niaz MA, Sharma JP, et al. Randomized, double-blind, placebo-controlled trial of fish oil and mustard oil in patients with suspected acute myocardial infarction: the Indian Experiment of Infarct Survival 4. Cardiovasc Drugs Ther 1997;11:485–491.

221. de Lorgeril M, Renaud S, Mamelle N, et al. Mediterranean alpha-linolenic acid-rich diet in secondary prevention of coronary heart disease. Lancet 1994;343:1454–1459.

222. de Lorgeril M, Salen P, Martin JL, et al. Mediterrranean diet, traditional risk factors, and the rate of cardiovascular complications after myocardial infarction: final report of the Lyon Diet Heart Study. Circulation 1999;99:779–785.

223. Dabrosin C, Chen J, Wang L, et al. Flaxseed inhibits metastasis and decreases extracellular vascular endothelial growth factor in human breast cancer xenografts. Cancer Lett 2002;185:31–37.

224. Lin X, Gingrich JR, Bao W, et al. Effect of flaxseed supplementation on prostatic carcinoma in transgenic mice. Urology 2002;60:919–924.

225. Schuurman AG, van den Brandt PA, Dorant E, et al. Association of energy and fat intake with prostate carcinoma risk: results from the Netherlands Cohort Study. Cancer 1999;86:1019–1027.

226. Giovannucci E, Rimm EB, Colditz GA, et al. A prospective study of dietary fat and risk of prostate cancer. J Natl Cancer Inst 1993;85:1571–1579.

227. Gann PH, Hennekens CH, Sacks FM, et al. Prospective study of plasma fatty acids and risk of prostate cancer. J Natl Cancer Inst 1994;86:281–286.

228. Demark-Wahnefried W, Price DT, Polascik TJ, et al. Pilot study of dietary fat restriction and flaxseed supplementation in men with prostate cancer before surgery: exploring the effects on hormonal levels, prostate-specific antigen, and histopathologic features. Urology 2001;58:47–52.

229. Demark-Wahnefried W, Robertson CN, Walther PJ, et al. Pilot study to explore effects of low-fat, flaxseed-supplemented diet on proliferation of benign prostatic epithelium and prostate-specific antigen. Urology 2004;63:900–904.

230. Morris MC, Evans DA, Bienias JL, et al. Consumption of fish and n-3 fatty acids and risk of incident Alzheimer disease. Arch Neurol 2003;940–946.

231. Bucher HC, Hengstler P, Schindler C, et al. N-3 polyunsaturated fatty acids in coronary heart disease: a meta-analysis of randomized controlled trials. Am J Med 2002;112:298–304.

232. Kris-Etherton PM, Harris WS, Appel LJ, for the Nutrition Committee. Fish consumption, fish oil, omega-3 fatty acids, and cardiovascular disease. Circulation 2002;106:2747–2757.

233. Harris WS. N-3 fatty acids and serum lipoproteins: human studies. Am J Clin Nutr 1997;65(5 Suppl):1645S–1654S.

234. Morris MC, Sacks F, Rosner B. Does fish oil lower blood pressure? A meta-analysis of controlled trials. Circulation 1993;88:523–533.

235. Mori TA, Beilin LJ, Burke V, et al. Interactions between dietary fat, fish, and fish oils and their effects on platelet function in men at risk of cardiovascular disease. Arterioscler Thromb Vasc Biol 1997;17:279–286.

236. Christensen JH, Korup E, Aaroe J, et al. Fish consumption, n-3 fatty acids in cell membranes, and heart rate variability in survivors of myocardial infarction with left ventricular dysfunction. Am J Cardiol 1997;79:1670–1673.

237. Leaf A, Kang JX, Xiao Y-F, et al. Clinical prevention of sudden cardiac death by n-3 polyunsaturated fatty acids and mechanism of prevention of arrhythmias by n-3 fish oils. Circulation 2003;107:2646–2652.

238. Albert CM, Campos H, Stampfer MJ, et al. Blood levels of long-chain n-3 fatty acids and the risk of sudden death. N Engl J Med 2002;346:1113–1118.
239. Kromhout D. Fish consumption and sudden cardiac death. JAMA 1998;279:65–66.
240. Chung BH, Mitchell SH, Zhang SS, et al. Effects of docosahexaenoic acid and eicosapentaenoic acid on androgen-mediated cell growth and gene expression in LNCaP prostate cancer cells. Carcinogenesis 2001;22:1201–1206.
241. Terry P, Lichtenstein P, Feychting M, et al. Fatty fish consumption and risk of prostate cancer. Lancet 2001;357:1764–1766.
242. Aronson WJ, Glapsy JA, Reddy ST, et al. Modulation of omega-3/omega-6 polyunsaturated ratios with dietary fish oils in men with prostate cancer. Urology 2001;58:283–288.
243. Terry PD, Rohan TE, Wolk A. Intakes of fish and marine fatty acids and the risks of cancers of the breast and prostate and of other hormone-related cancers: a review of the epidemiologic evidence. Am J Clin Nutr 2003;77:532–543.
244. Augustsson K, Michaud DS, Rimm EB, et al. A prospective study of intake of fish and marine fatty acids and prostate cancer. Cancer Epidemiol Biomark Prev 2003;12:64–67.
245. Burr ML, Fehily AM, Gilbert JF, et al. Effects of changes in fat, fish, and fibre intakes on death and myocardial reinfarction: Diet and Reinfarction Trial (DART). Lancet 1989;2:757–761.
246. GISSI-Prevenzione Investigators. Dietary supplementation with n-3 polyunsaturated fatty acids and vitamin E after myocardial infarction: results from the GISSI-Prevenzione trial. Lancet 1999;354:447–455.
247. Marchioli R, Barzi F, Bomba E, et al. Early protection against sudden cardiac death by n-3 polyunsaturated fatty acids after myocardial infarction: time-course analysis of the results of the Gruppo Italiano per lo Studio della Sopravvivenza nell'Infarto Miocardico (GISSI)-Prevenzione. Circulation 2002;105:1897–1903.
248. Guallar E, Sanz-Gallardo MI, van't Veer P, et al. Mercury, fish oils, and the risk of myocardial infarction. N Engl J Med 2002;347:1747–1754.
249. Yoshizawa K, Rimm EB, Morris JJ, et al. Mercury and the risk of coronary heart disease in men. N Engl J Med 2002;347:1755–1760.
250. Weil M, Bressler J, Parsons P, et al. Blood mercury levels and neurobehavioral function. JAMA 2005;293:1875–1882.
251. Albert CM, Gaziano JM, Willett WC, et al. Nut consumption and decreased risk of sudden cardiac death in the physicians' health study. Arch Intern Med 2002;162:1382–1387.
252. Ellsworth JL, Kushi LH, Folsom AR. Frequent nut intake and risk of death from coronary heart disease and all causes in postmenopausal women: the Iowa Women's Health Study. Nutr Metab Cardiovasc Dis 2001;11:372–377.
253. Brown L, Sacks F, Rosner B, et al. Nut consumption and risk of coronary heart disease in patients with myocardial infarction. FASEB J 1999;13:A4332 [abstract].
254. Hu FB, Stampfer MJ, Manson JE, et al. Frequent nut consumption and risk of coronary heart disease: prospective cohort study. BMJ 1998;317:1341–1345.
255. Fraser GE, Shavlik DJ. Risk factors for all-cause and coronary heart disease mortality in the oldest-old: the Adventist Health Study. Arch Intern Med 1997;157:2249–2258.
256. Fraser GE, Sabate J, Beeson WL, et al. A possible protective effect of nut consumption on risk of coronary heart disease: the Adventist Health Study. Arch Intern Med 1992;152:1416–1424.
257. Helzlsouer KJ, Huang H-Y, Alberg AJ, et al. Association between alpha-tocopherol, gamma-tocopherol, selenium, and subsequent prostate cancer. J Natl Cancer Inst 2000;92:2018–2023.
258. Hu FB, Manson JE, Willett WC. Types of dietary fat and risk of coronary heart disease: A critical review. J Am Coll Nutr 2001;20:5–19.
259. Moyad MA. An introduction to dietary/supplemental omega-3 fatty acids for general health and prevention: Part I. Urol Oncol 2005;23:28–35.
260. Moyad MA. An introduction to dietary/supplemental omega-3 fatty acids for general health and prevention: Part II. Urol Oncol 2005;23:36–48.
261. Critchley JA, Capewell S. Mortality risk reduction associated with smoking cessation in patients with coronary heart disease: a systematic review. JAMA 2003;290:86–97.
262. Yu GP, Ostroff JS, Zhang ZF, et al. Smoking history and cancer patient survival: a hospital cancer registry study. Cancer Detect Prev 1997;21:497–509.
263. Plaskon LA, Penson DF, Vaughan TL, et al. Cigarette smoking and risk of prostate cancer in middle-aged men. Cancer Epidemiol Biomarkers Prev 2003;12:604–609.
264. Roberts WW, Platz EA, Walsh PC. Association of cigarette smoking with extraprostatic prostate cancer in young men. J Urol 2003;169:512–516.
265. Rodriguez C, Tatham LM, Thun MJ, et al. Smoking and fatal prostate cancer in a large cohort of adult men. Am J Epidemiol 1997;145:466–475.
266. Mukamal KJ, Conigrave KM, Mittleman MA, et al. Roles of drinking pattern and type of alcohol consumed in coronary heart disease in men. N Engl J Med 2003;348:109–118.
267. Hercberg S, Galan P, Preziosi P, et al. The SU.VI.MAX Study: a randomized, placebo-controlled trial of the health effects of antioxidant vitamins and minerals. Arch Intern Med 2004;164:2335–2342.
268. Basler JW, Piazza GA. Nonsteroidal anti-inflammatory drugs and cyclooxygenase-2 selective inhibitors for prostate cancer chemoprevention. J Urol 2004;171:S59–S63.
269. Moyad MA, Merrick GS. Statins and cholesterol lowering after a cancer diagnosis: Why not? Urol Oncol 2005;23:49–55.
270. Debes JD, Roberts RO, Jacobson DJ, et al. Inverse association between prostate cancer and the use of calcium channel blockers. Cancer Epidemiol Biomarkers Prev 2004;13:255–259.
271. The Hope and Hope-Too Trial Investigators. Effects of long-term vitamin E supplementation on cardiovascular events and cancer. JAMA 2005;293:1338–1347.
272. Miller ER III, Pastor-Barriuso R, Dalal D, et al. Meta-analysis: High-dosage vitamin E supplementation may increase all-cause mortality. Ann Intern Med 2005;142:37–46.
273. Bairati I, Meyer F, Gelinas M, et al. A randomized trial of antioxidant vitamins to prevent second primary cancers in head and neck cancer patients. J Natl Cancer Inst 2005;97:481–488.
274. Platz EA, Willet WC, Colditz GA, et al. Proportion of colon cancer risk that might be preventable in a cohort of middle-aged US men. Cancer Causes Control 2000;11:579–588.
275. Trichopoulou A, Costacou T, Bamia C, et al. Adherence to a Mediterranean diet and survival in a Greek population. N Engl J Med 2003;348:2599–2608.
276. Morris CD, Carson S. Routine vitamin supplementation to prevent cardiovascular disease: a summary of the evidence for the U.S. Preventive Services Task Force. Ann Intern Med 2003;139:56–70.
277. U.S. Preventive Services Task Force. Routine vitamin supplementation to prevent cancer and cardiovascular disease: Recommendations and rationale. Ann Intern Med 2003;139:51–55.
278. Leitzmann MF, Stampfer MJ, Wu K, et al. Zinc supplement use and risk of prostate cancer. J Natl Cancer Inst 2003;95:1004–1007.
279. Markowitz JS, Donovan JL, DeVane CL, et al. Effect of St John's wort on drug metabolism by induction of cytochrome P450 3A4 enzyme. JAMA 2003;290:1500–1504.
280. Ang-Lee MK, Moss J, Yuan C-S. Herbal medicines and perioperative care. JAMA 2001;286:208–216.
281. Eyre H, Kahn R, Robertson RM, et al. for the ACS/ADA/AHA Collaborative Writing Committee Members. Preventing cancer, cardiovascular disease, and diabetes: A common agenda for the American Cancer Society, the American Diabetes Association, and the American Heart Association. Circulation 2004;109:3244–3255.

4

Preservation of sexual function after treatment for prostate cancer

James A Eastham

Introduction

Patients diagnosed with a clinically localized prostate cancer face a daunting variety of management choices, including deferred treatment with observation, brachytherapy and/or external beam irradiation therapy with or without neoadjuvant hormonal therapy, cryotherapy, and radical prostatectomy. Physicians have long sought to guide patients through these choices based on their best judgment about the threat posed by the cancer, the effectiveness of treatment, the life-expectancy of the patient, as well as the potential for complications. Because screening programs have resulted in the identification of cancers much earlier in their natural history, the expection is that an individual patient will have a prolonged life-expectancy. In weighing treatment options, the patient and physician must consider the ability of the treatment to provide a durable cure while minimizing any negative impact on quality of life.

The most favorable outcome that can be achieved after local therapy for prostate cancer is complete eradication of the cancer with full recovery of urinary, bowel, and sexual function. These goals are inextricably linked and at times may appear to conflict with one another in that achieving one goal may occur at the expense of the others. The technical challenge of local treatment for prostate cancer is to treat sufficient periprostatic tissue to achieve cure, while at the same time preserving the cavernosal nerves required for erectile function, and the neuromusculature required for normal urinary and bowel function. This chapter will review the preservation of sexual function following local treatment for prostate cancer.

Radical prostatectomy

Potency is defined as the ability to obtain an erection that is sufficient for vaginal penetration and sexual intercourse. Before the 1980s, most patients permanently lost erectile function after radical prostatectomy. Then, Walsh et al[1,2] developed a technique for radical retropubic prostatectomy based on identification of the anatomic structures surrounding the prostate, including the autonomic nerves that control blood flow to the penis. Current surgical techniques are based on a more precise understanding of the autonomic innervation of the corpora cavernosa, allowing preservation of sexual function in the majority of men undergoing radical prostatectomy. Quinlan et al[3] demonstrated that recovery of potency is quantitatively related to the preservation of nerves. They identified three factors associated with recovery of potency after radical

prostatectomy: age, clinical and pathologic stage, and preservation of the neurovascular bundles. In their series, approximately 90% of men younger than 50 were potent if either one or both neurovascular bundles were preserved. For men older than 50, return of potency was more likely if both neurovascular bundles were preserved rather than only one. Catalona et al[4] reported potency in 68% of patients when both nerves were preserved and 47% when just one nerve was spared. They also demonstrated a strong correlation between preservation of potency and age.

Rabbani et al[5] have developed a nomogram to predict the return of potency based on a series of 314 previously potent patients treated since 1993 with radical prostatectomy for T1C to T3A prostate cancer (Table 4.1). Factors significantly associated with recovery of spontaneous erections satisfactory for intercourse included age of the patient, quality of erections before the operation, and degree of preservation of the neurovascular bundles. Time after surgery is also an important factor in the recovery of potency. The median time to recovery of an international index of erectile function (IIEF) score greater than or equal to 17 was 24 months, while 42 months was required to reach an IIEF of greater than or equal to 26 (Figure 4.1).

In addition to preservation of the autonomic innervation to the corpora cavernosa (i.e. the neurovascular bundles), preservation of the vascular branches to the corpora cavernosa has been reported to affect the recovery of erectile function after radical prostatectomy.[6-8] Accessory arterial branches that supply the corpora have been described.[7,8] When these branches are preserved, a normal arterial inflow to the penis will be maintained after surgery. Adequate arterial inflow may enable a patient to remain potent or, for a patient who is impotent, it will ensure an adequate response to medical treatment.

Preservation of the neurovascular bundles

Radical prostatectomy is among the most complex operations performed by urologists, and challenges surgeons because outcomes are highly sensitive to fine details in surgical technique. Modern outcomes research has repeatedly documented that the results and complications of this operation vary markedly, not only with surgeons' experience, but even more so among experienced surgeons. The elusive goals of modern radical prostatectomy are to remove the cancer completely with negative surgical margins, minimal

Table 4.1 Probability of recovery of potency by 24 and 36 months based on a combination of pre- and post-operative parameters.[5]

Preoperative potency	Probability (%) of recovery of potency by 24 months (36 months)		
	Age ≤60	Age 60.1–65	Age >65
Bilateral nerve sparing			
Full erection	70 (76)	49 (55)	43 (49)
Full erection, recently diminished	53 (59)	34 (39)	30 (35)
Partial erection	43 (49)	27 (31)	23 (27)
Unilateral or bilateral neurovascular bundle damage			
Full erection	60 (67)	40 (46)	35 (41)
Full erection, recently diminished	44 (50)	28 (32)	24 (28)
Partial erection	35 (40)	21 (25)	18 (21)
Unilateral neurovascular bundle resection			
Full erection	26 (30)	15 (18)	13 (15)
Full erection, recently diminished	17 (20)	10 (12)	8.5 (10)
Partial erection	13 (15)	7.5 (8.8)	6.3 (7.5)

used to gently sweep the nerves laterally away from the prostate. Denonvilliers' fascia must be deliberately incised, releasing the neurovascular bundle laterally and allowing a deep plane of dissection along the fat of the anterior rectal wall (see Figure 4.2C–E). The risk of a positive surgical margin will be greatly reduced if this layer of fascia is included in the excised specimen. This apical dissection is performed without a catheter in the prostate to give the prostate more mobility. Small clips placed parallel to the neurovascular bundle are used to control the small vascular bands that are usually present, particularly near the apex of the prostate. Once the neurovascular bundles have been mobilized off the prostate at the apex and mid gland, the urethra can be safely divided and the anastomotic sutures placed. The initial incisions in Denonvilliers' fascia are connected across the midline beneath the apex of the prostate.

Once the apex is completely mobilized, a catheter is placed through the urethra to facilitate dissection. Traction on this catheter allows the remaining neurovascular bundles to be dissected away bluntly as the prostate is dissected off the rectum, beneath Denonvilliers' fascia.

The nerves lie close to the prostate near the base. Dissection too close to the prostate will result in a positive margin in this area, shown to be associated with an increased risk of recurrence. We have been successful in preserving most or all of both neurovascular bundles in the majority of patients using this lateral approach, while still allowing a wider dissection around the apex of the prostate, especially posteriorly.

When resection of one or both neurovascular bundles is necessary, we use a technique for placing interposition grafts from the sural or genitofemoral nerve to one or both neurovascular bundles (Figure 4.3).[9,10] Surgeons have performed nerve grafts successfully for decades to replace damaged or transected peripheral sensorimotor nerves. The basis for nerve regeneration, and consequently for nerve grafting, is the ability of axons to produce axon sprouts. After nerve transection, axon sprouts will invariably grow, forming a neuroma if they do not come into contact with an environment that channels their growth. The cut end of a nerve sprouts minifascicles that contain axon sprouts, fibroblasts, Schwann cells, and capillaries. The minifascicles grow haphazardly for a limited distance and then form a neuroma. However, if the axons encounter an empty nerve sheath, growth becomes organized and directed, resulting in a new nerve. A nerve graft functions to

blood loss, no serious perioperative complications, and complete recovery of continence and potency. No surgeon achieves such results uniformly. This section provides surgeons with details about one approach to this operation, which has been modified frequently in a continual effort to improve results. The technique described here is not the only successful approach; various other techniques work as well. The hope is that the reader will discern the important anatomic and surgical principles that will allow him/her to improve his/her own technique and patient outcomes.

A lateral approach to the neurovascular bundles (Figure. 4.2) allows wide exposure of the apex so that the apical tissue can be completely resected. The lateral pelvic fascia over the neurovascular bundle can be incised more medially or laterally to the nerve, depending on the extent or location of the tumor and whether the nerves are to be preserved (see Figure 4.2A, B). A "peanut," or Kitner, dissector is

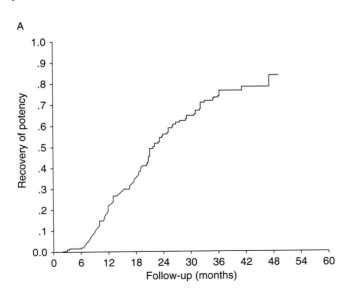

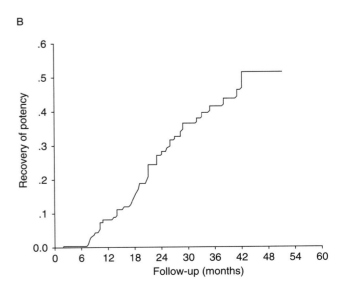

Figure 4.1
Probability of recovery of potency over time after bilateral nerve-sparing radical prostatectomy. *A*, International index of erectile function (IIEF) ≥17, and *B*, IIEF ≥26.

provide a conduit through which regenerating nerve fibers are directed to meet with the distal end of the transected nerve. These concepts support the hypothesis that cavernous nerve grafts may restore penile autonomic innervation and the ability to achieve spontaneous erections after deliberate neurovascular bundle resection during radical prostatectomy. With bilateral nerve grafts, one-third of patients with

bilateral nerve resection have had spontaneous, medically unassisted erections sufficient for sexual intercourse. The greatest return of function is observed 14 to 18 months after surgery. In our experience, nerve grafts provide one solution to a common surgical dilemma: in a patient with a large, high grade cancer located adjacent to the posterolateral capsule, should the surgeon dissect close to the prostate to

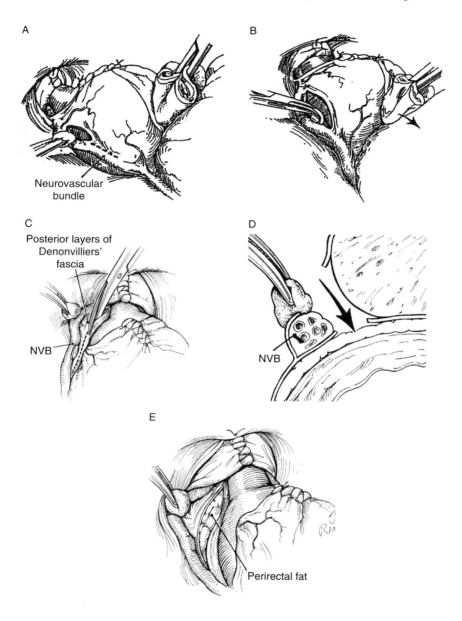

Figure 4.2

Preservation of left neurovascular bundle (NVB). After the dorsal vein complex has been divided and hemostasis attained, the prostate is rotated to the right with a sponge stick and any remaining levator ani muscle fibers are bluntly dessected away. The surgeon can examine the course of the neurovascular bundle in relation to the prostate and any palpable tumor. Frequently, a shallow groove defines the superior margin of dissection for the preservation of the NVB. A plane of division of the lateral prostatic fascia is then chosen to assure a negative surgical margin while at the same time preserving as much of the NVB as possible. Once the plane of dissection has been selected, the lateral prostatic fascia is sharply incised in the groove between the prostate and the neurovascular bundle. The neurovascular bundle is most easily dissected away from the apical third of the prostate (A, B). The small branches of the vascular pedicle to the apex are clipped and divided. Care must be taken to avoid electrocautery near this neural tissue. The NVB is then gently dissected and displaced laterally working from the spex toward the base. This should be done with either a Kitner (peanut) dissector and/or a right-angled clamp. Finger dissection should be avoided on the NVB. Denonvilliers' fascia is then incised in the angle between the NVB and urethra at the apex of the prostate, releasing the NVB from the prostate and urethra (C–E). The apperance of perirectal fat will assure the surgeon that the layer has been incised completely. The plane of dissection is then developed either sharply and/or bluntly. Special attention is paid to continuing the dissection of the NVB for a distance of almost 1 cm from the prostatourethreal junction so that the nerves will not be tethered when the urethral anastomotic sutures are tied.

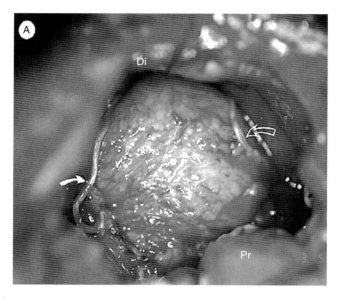

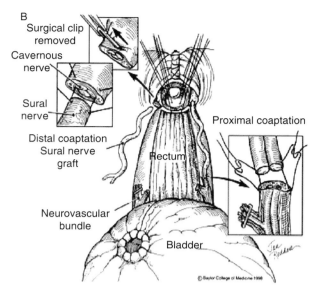

Figure 4.3
Sural nerve graft interposed between severed ends of each cavernosal nerve.

preserve the nerve or dissect close to the nerve, risking recovery of potency? Over the past 3 years, we have performed nerve grafts in about 15% of all previously untreated patients. The risks were very low: there was only one graft-related complication (cellulitis), and the overall operative time, blood loss, and hospital stays were identical in grafted and nongrafted patients. Final proof of the efficacy of nerve grafts must await completion of a prospective randomized trial comparing nerve grafts to no grafts after unilateral neurovascular bundle resection. Until then, surgeons must use sound judgment and informed consent to decide, along with their patients, whether a nerve graft is indicated when a neurovascular bundle is damaged or resected during radical prostatectomy.

Strategies to improve sexual function after radical prostatectomy

Early use of intracavernosal agents

Montorsi et al[11] prospectively assessed the effect of postoperative intracavernous injections of alprostadil on the recovery of spontaneous erectile function after nerve-sparing radical prostatectomy. Thirty preoperatively potent patients underwent bilateral nerve-sparing radical prostatectomy and were subsequently randomized to alprostadil injections three times per week for 12 weeks or observation without any treatment. Eight of 15 (53%) patients receiving alprostadil injections compared to 3 of 15 (20%) untreated men reported recovery of spontaneous erections at 6 months sufficient for satisfactory sexual intercourse. The investigators hypothesized that alprostadil injections improve cavernosal oxygenation, thereby limiting hypoxia-induced tissue damage.

Early use of phosphodiesterase-5 inhibitors

Levine et al[12] examined 54 men with normal preoperative erectile function who underwent bilateral nerve-sparing radical prostatectomy.

Patients were randomized to either sildenafil citrate (50 mg, n = 17; 100 mg, n = 18) or placebo (n = 19) 4 weeks post surgery and entered a 36-week, double-blind treatment period with nightly drug administration. Assessment 48 weeks after surgery demonstrated that 10 of 35 (29%) men given sildenafil citrate but only 5% of the control group had spontaneous erectile function as determined by nocturnal penile tumescence and rigidity testing. The investigators concluded that early postoperative treatment with a phosphodiesterase-5 inhibitor improves long-term recovery of erectile function and supports the concept of early rehabilitation of erectile function.

Perioperative immunophilin ligand therapy

Immunophilin ligands have shown neuroprotective activity in several animal models of nerve injury, including damage to sciatic, facial, and optic nerves assayed by nerve regeneration and/or functional recovery.[13,14] Histopathologically, axonal cross-sectional areas in animals with crushed nerves were significantly greater in those treated with immunophilin ligands compared to placebo. In addition, animals receiving placebo after nerve-crush injury had a greater than 90% decrease in myelination levels, while treated animals regained 30% to 40% of their original myelination levels.

Recently, the immunophilin ligand FK506 and its nonimmunosuppressive derivative GPI1046 have been investigated in a model of cavernous nerve injury.[15] In treated animals, the recovery of erections was significantly greater than in animals receiving placebo. Immunohistochemical studies demonstrated that the immunophilin ligand-treated animals had preserved cavernosal tissue histology. The authors suggested that the neurotrophic effects of these agents may decrease the extent of cavernosal nerve degeneration and improve the recovery of erectile function after radical prostatectomy. These agents are being evaluated in clinical trials to determine their potential role as neuroprotective agents following radical prostatectomy.

Cryosurgery

Technologic advances in cryosurgery as primary treatment for localized prostate cancer, including transrectal ultrasound guidance, urethral warmers, and argon-based cryomachines, have substantially reduced morbidity and improved quality-of-life outcomes after this procedure. Several years ago, erectile dysfunction was a universally expected outcome after cryosurgery, but current technology and treatment delivery permit a minority of men to regain potency after treatment. Ellis[16] reported results from his series of 75 patients with newly diagnosed, clinically localized prostate cancer treated between 2000 and 2001 by a double freeze–thaw cycle. Of the 34 patients who were potent preoperatively, 6 (18%) regained potency after surgery. Robinson et al[17] reported 3-year quality-of-life outcomes using patient-reported questionnaires after cryosurgery. At 36 months, 5 of 38 (13%) preoperatively potent patients had recovered erectile function. Bahn et al[18] reported their 7-year efficacy and safety results with targeted cryotherapy in 590 consecutive patients with newly diagnosed prostate cancer. Of the 373 men who were potent before the procedure, 95% were impotent after surgery. The average recovery time was 16.4 months. Clearly, the majority of men treated with cryosurgery will be impotent after the procedure, and potent men with clinically localized prostate cancer considering this option must be appropriately counseled.

Radiation therapy

The mechanism of erectile dysfunction after radiation therapy is not well defined. Radiation damage to the nerve bundles and vascular structures has been proposed as the cause.[19] However, the ability to decrease dose to these structures is limited by the proximity of the neurovascular bundles to the peripheral zone of the prostate, an area where cancer commonly is located and which thus requires the full prescription dose. In addition, total radiation dose, the use of concurrent/adjuvant hormonal therapy, and time since treatment may influence post-radiation potency. To date, there has been little study of neuroprotective agents or the early use of either intracavernosal injection therapy or phosphodiesterase type-5 inhibitors during and after radiation therapy, but these may improve outcomes in the future.

Prostate brachytherapy

Prostate brachytherapy is an increasingly common treatment for early-stage prostate cancer; its biochemical outcomes for low-risk patients are similar to those of external beam radiation therapy and radical prostatectomy at 5 and 10 years after treatment. As seen in radical prostatectomy, there is emerging evidence that erectile dysfunction induced by prostate brachytherapy is technique related and may be minimized by careful attention to source placement. Merrick and Butler[19] recently reviewed published reports to identify factors associated with post-brachytherapy erectile dysfunction. They found no data that either the radiation dose to the neurovascular bundle or choice of isotope was associated with brachytherapy-induced erectile dysfunction, while conflicting data have been reported regarding radiation dose to the prostate and the use of supplemental external beam radiation therapy. They concluded that the available data support the proximal penis as an important site-specific structure, and that refinements in implant technique will result in lower doses to this area with potential improvement in potency preservation.

In an attempt to improve preimplantation planning, Wright et al[20] examined factors associated with brachytherapy-induced erectile dysfunction. They concluded that increasing the dose to the penile bulb may increase the risk of erectile dysfunction, but

increasing the dose to the neurovascular bundle did not appear to. Similarly, Merrick et al[21] studied 46 potent men with clinically localized prostate cancer, 23 of whom developed post-brachytherapy erectile dysfunction. The mean volume of the penile bulb was greater in the potent men than in the impotent patients. Impotent men had received approximately twice the radiation dose of the potent men in each area of the bulb that was examined. While the penile bulb is not believed to play a role in the development of an erection,[22] it is easily recognized on prostate imaging and may serve as a surrogate for another structure involved in erectile function.

Reported rates of potency following prostate brachytherapy are summarized in Table 4.2.[23–25] Stock et al[23] treated 313 potent men with prostate brachytherapy alone between 1990 and 1998. The actuarial preservation of potency was 79% and 59% at 3 and 6 years, respectively. In this series, potency was assessed by physician interview and excluded the use of oral medications. Merrick et al[24] examined outcomes for 209 potent men following prostate brachytherapy. At 6-year follow-up, 39% maintained potency; including men using sildenafil citrate, this increased to 54%. Factors associated with postimplant erectile dysfunction were preimplant potency score, use of supplemental external beam radiation therapy, and diabetes. Potters et al[25] evaluated 482 men treated with prostate brachytherapy, including combination treatment with external beam radiation therapy and/or neoadjuvant hormonal therapy. Potency was preserved in 311 of the 482 patients, with a 5-year actuarial potency rate of 52.7%. The potency rate was better for those receiving monotherapy (76%) than those receiving combination therapy (see Table 4.2). Of 84 patients treated with sildenafil citrate, 52 had a successful result (62%), although the response to sildenafil citrate was significantly better in those patients not treated with neoadjuvant hormonal therapy. Taken together, these studies suggest that potency can be preserved in the majority of patients treated with prostate brachytherapy. Most patients with erectile dysfunction respond to oral medications such as sildenafil citrate. Potency outcomes appear to be worse when brachytherapy is combined with external beam radiation therapy and/or hormonal therapy. Lastly, time appears to be a critical factor as well, with potency rates decreasing over time.

External beam radiation therapy

As with prostate brachytherapy, both experimental and clinical evidence suggest that the radiation dose to the bulb of the penis is

Table 4.2 Potency rates following radiation therapy

Series	Type of radiation	Time after treatment	Potency (%)
Stock et al[23]	PPB	36 months	79
Stock et al[23]	PPB	72 months	59
Merrick et al[24]	PPB	6 year actuarial	54
Potters et al[25]	PPB	5 year actuarial	76
Potters et al[25]	PPB + EBT	5 year actuarial	56
Potters et al[25]	PPB + NAAD	5 year actuarial	52
Potters et al[25]	PPB + EBT + NAAD	5 year actuarial	29
Wilder et al[29]	EBT	3 year actuarial	63
Mantz et al[30]	EBT	5 year actuarial	53
Chen et al[31]	EBT	12 months	58

EBT, external beam radiation; NAAD, neoadjuvant androgen deprivation; PPB, permanent prostate brachytherapy.

critical to the maintenance of potency after external beam radiation therapy.[26–28] This again suggests that the technique used to deliver treatment, be it radical prostatectomy, prostate brachytherapy or external beam radiation therapy, significantly impacts recovery of erectile function after treatment. Careful pretreatment planning and treatment delivery will improve outcomes following any treatment for clinically localized prostate cancer.

Potency after external beam radiation therapy is shown in Table 4.2.[29–31] Wilder et al[29] reported potency preservation after three-dimensional conformal radiation therapy in 35 potent men with prostate cancer. Total dose to the prostate ranged from 66 to 79.2 Gy. Kaplan-Meier estimates of the potency preservation rates at 1, 2, and 3 years after treatment were 100%, 83%, and 63%, respectively. Mantz et al[30] performed a retrospective review of 287 men with clinically localized prostate cancer treated with conformal techniques to 62 to 73.8 Gy.[30] Actuarial potency rates at 40 and 60 months were 59% and 53%, respectively. Factors identified as significant predictors of erectile dysfunction after external beam radiation therapy included pretreatment potency status, diabetes, coronary artery disease, and antiandrogen usage. To further examine the potential effects of concomitant hormonal therapy and external beam radiation therapy, Chen et al[31] evaluated sexual function using self-administered patient questionnaires in 144 men (55 of whom also received hormonal therapy) before and after three-dimensional conformal radiation therapy for clinically localized prostate cancer. Before radiation therapy, 87 (60%) of the patients were potent compared to 47% at 12 months after treatment. Of 60 men who were completely potent before treatment and were followed for at least 1 year, 58% retained their baseline function. Patients who had radiation alone were more likely to be potent at 1 year than those receiving radiation and hormonal therapy (56% vs 31%, respectively).

Several studies have demonstrated that many men with erectile dysfunction after radiation therapy (brachytherapy or external beam) will respond to sildenafil citrate.[32–34] Incrocci et al[34] performed a randomized, double-blind, placebo-controlled cross-over study to determine the efficacy of sildenafil citrate in treating erectile dysfunction in men treated with three-dimensional conformal radiation therapy. The study included 60 patients who had completed radiation therapy at least 6 months earlier. They received 2 weeks' treatment with 50 mg of sildenafil citrate or placebo; at week 2 the dose was increased to 100 mg if there was an unsatisfactory response. At week 6, patients crossed over to the alternative treatment. Data were collected using the IIEF questionnaire. Successful intercourse was reported in 55% of patients after sildenafil citrate versus 18% after placebo. Most patients (90%) required an increase in the dose of sildenafil citrate to 100 mg. Whether or not earlier use of sildenafil citrate would improve these outcomes is unknown.

Conclusion

A better understanding of periprostatic anatomy and the factors associated with the development of post-treatment erectile dysfunction should result in a continued improvement in functional outcomes after radical prostatectomy, cryotherapy, prostate brachytherapy, and external beam radiation therapy for clinically localized prostate cancer. Each of these treatment options appears to be sensitive to the fine details of delivery of the therapy. While the technical aspects of neurovascular bundle preservation and the role of the surgeon in preserving potency at the time of radical prostatectomy have received considerable attention, outcomes after radiation

therapy also appear to be sensitive to how treatment is delivered. In particular, the dose of radiation delivered to the bulb of the penis appears to be intimately associated with the preservation of erectile function after both prostate brachytherapy and external beam radiation therapy. While the role of neoadjuvant and/or adjuvant phosphodiesterase-5 inhibitors or immunophilin ligands in preserving potency certainly needs further study, careful attention to the fine details of delivery of any of the treatment options should improve outcomes in the short term.

References

1. Walsh PC. Anatomic radical prostatectomy: evolution of the surgical technique. J Urol 1998;160:2418–2424.
2. Walsh PC, Donker PJ. Impotence following radical prostatectomy: insight into etiology and prevention. J Urol 1982;128:492–497.
3. Quinlan DM, Epstein JI, Carter BS, et al. Sexual function following radical prostatectomy: influence of preservation of neurovascular bundles. J Urol 1991;145:998–1003.
4. Catalona WJ, Carvalhal GF, Mager DE, et al. Potency, continence and complication rates in 1,870 consecutive radical retropubic prostatectomies. J Urol 1999;162:433–438.
5. Rabbani F, Stapleton AM, Kattan MW, et al. Factors predicting recovery of erections after radical prostatectomy. J Urol 2000;164:1929–1934.
6. Rogers CG, Trock BP, Walsh PC. Preservation of accessory pudendal arteries during radical retropubic prostatectomy: surgical technique and results. Urology 2004;64:148–151.
7. Bahnson RR, Catalona WJ. Papaverine testing of impotent patients following nerve sparing radical prostatectomy. J Urol 1988;139:773–774.
8. Breza J, Aboseif SR, Orvis BR, et al, Detailed anatomy of penile neurovascular structures: surgical significance. J Urol 1989;141:437–443.
9. Kim ED, Scardino PT, Hampel O, et al. Interposition of sural nerve restores function of cavernous nerves resected during radical prostatectomy. J Urol 1999;161:188–192.
10. Kim ED, Nath R, Slawin KM, et al. Bilateral nerve grafting during radical retropubic prostatectomy: extended follow-up. Urology 2001;8:983–987.
11. Montorsi F, Guazzoni G, Strambi LF, et al. Recovery of spontaneous erectile function after nerve-sparing radical retropubic prostatectomy with and without early intracavernous injections of alprostadil: results of a prospective, randomized trial. J Urol 1997;158:1408–1410.
12. Levine LA, McCullough AR, Padma-Nathan H. Longitudinal randomized placebo-controlled study of the return of nocturnal erections after nerve-sparing radical prostatectomy in men treated with nightly sildenafil citrate. J Urol 2004;171:231–232 (abstract).
13. Gold BG, Katoh K, Storm-Dickerson T. The immunosuppressant FK506 increases the rate of axonal regeneration in rat sciatic nerve. J Neurosci 1995;15:7509–7516.
14. Freeman EE, Grosskreutz CL. The effects of FK506 on retinal ganglion cells after optic nerve crush. Invest Ophthalmol Vis Sci 2000; 41:1111–1115.
15. Burnett AL, Becker RE. Immunophilin ligands promote penile neurogenesis and erection recovery after cavernous nerve injury. J Urol 2004;171:495–500.
16. Ellis DS. Cryosurgery as primary treatment for localized prostate cancer: a community hospital experience. Urology 2002;60:34–39.
17. Robinson JW, Donnelly BJ, Saliken JC, et al. Quality of life and sexuality of men with prostate cancer 3 years after cryosurgery. Urology 2002;60(2 Suppl 1):12–18.
18. Bahn DK, Lee F, Badalament R, et al. Targeted cryoablation of the prostate: 7-year outcomes in the primary treatment of prostate cancer. Urology 2002;60(2 Suppl 1):3–11.
19. Merrick GS, Butler WM. The dosimetry of brachytherapy-induced erectile dysfunction. Med Dosim 2003;28:271–274.
20. Wright JL, Newhouse JH, Laguna JL, et al. Localization of neurovascular bundles on pelvic CT and evaluation of radiation dose to structures

putatively involved in erectile dysfunction after prostate brachytherapy. Int J Radiat Oncol Biol Phys 2004;59:426–435.

21. Merrick GS, Butler WM, Wallner KE, et al. The importance of radiation doses to the penile bulb vs. crura in the development of post-brachytherapy erectile dysfunction. Int J Radiat Oncol Biol Phys 2002;54:1055–1062.

22. Mulhall JP, Yanover PM, Correlation of radiation dose and impotence risk after three-dimensional conformal radiotherapy for prostate cancer. Urology 2001;58:828.

23. Stock RG, Kao J, Stone NN. Penile erectile function after permanent radioactive seed implantation for treatment of prostate cancer. J Urol 2001;165:436–439.

24. Merrick GS, Butler WM, Galbreath RW, et al. Erectile function after permanent prostate brachytherapy. Int J Radiat Oncol Biol Phys 2002;52:893–902.

25. Potters L, Torre T, Fearn PA, et al. Potency after permanent prostate brachytherapy for localized prostate cancer. Int J Radiat Oncol Biol Phys 2001;50:1235–1242.

26. Carrier S, Hricak H, Lee SS, et al. Radiation-induced decrease in nitric oxide synthase-containing nerves in the rat penis. Radiology 1995;195:95–99.

27. Fisch BM, Pickett B, Weinberg V, et al. Dose of radiation received by the bulb of the penis correlates with risk of impotence after three-dimensional conformal radiotherapy for prostate cancer. Urology 2001;57:955–999.

28. Merrick GS, Wallner K, Butler WM, et al. A comparison of radiation dose to the bulb of the penis in men with and without prostate brachytherapy-induced erectile dysfunction. Int J Radiat Oncol Biol Phys 2001;50:597–604.

29. Wilder RB, Chou RH, Ryu JK, et al. Potency preservation after three-dimensional conformal radiotherapy for prostate cancer: preliminary results. Am J Clin Oncol 2000;23:330–333.

30. Mantz CA, Nautiyal J, Awan A, et al. Potency preservation following conformal radiotherapy for localized prostate cancer: impact of neoadjuvant androgen blockade, treatment technique, and patient-related factors. Cancer J Sci Am 1999;5:230–236.

31. Chen CT, Valicenti RK, Lu J, et al. Does hormonal therapy influence sexual function in men receiving 3D conformal radiation therapy for prostate cancer? Int J Radiat Oncol Biol Phys 2001; 50:591–595.

32. Zelefsky MJ, McKee AB, Lee H, et al. Efficacy of oral sildenafil in patients with erectile dysfunction after radiotherapy for carcinoma of the prostate. Urology 1999;53:775–778.

33. Weber DC, Bieri S, Kurtz JM, et al. Prospective pilot study of sildenafil for treatment of postradiotherapy erectile dysfunction in patients with prostate cancer. J Clin Oncol 1999;17:3444–3449.

34. Incrocci L, Koper PC, Hop WC, et al. Sildenafil citrate (Viagra) and erectile dysfunction following external beam radiotherapy for prostate cancer: a randomized, double-blind, placebo-controlled, cross-over study. Int J Radiat Oncol Biol Phys 2001;51:1190–1195.

5

Quality-of-life instruments for prostate cancer

Marcus L Quek, David F Penson

Introduction

Quality of life has become an increasingly important concern in clinical decision-making for patients with prostate cancer. With the advent of screening programs utilizing serum prostate-specific antigen (PSA) testing, prostate cancer appears to be diagnosed at an earlier stage than in the pre-PSA era. Whether early treatment has translated into improved survival rates or has increased the burden of treatment of clinically-insignificant cancers is debatable. What is certain, however, is that due to this stage migration, more patients are treated for prostate cancer and are thus living longer with their disease.[1]

Whereas traditional outcome measures of overall and recurrence-free survival rates have been used to directly compare various therapeutic modalities, focus on "non-traditional" quality-of-life outcomes may further allow patients to make truly informed decisions regarding their treatment. This is especially true for localized prostate cancer in which none of the standard therapies—radical prostatectomy, radiotherapy—has been shown to date to have a clear survival difference in observational studies,[2] and in which novel therapeutic modalities continue to emerge touting less impact on a patients' quality of life. In fact, the American Urological Association's practice guidelines committee has stressed the importance of measuring quality of life as an outcome in the management of this condition.[3]

For many patients, quality of life is the primary outcome of interest when selecting among the available options. Helgason et al asked 299 prostate cancer patients if they would undergo a treatment that could possibly lengthen life expectancy at the expense of complete loss of sexual function. Forty-seven percent were either unwilling to accept treatment regardless of the survival benefit or would only accept the treatment if it provided a greater than 10 year improvement in life expectancy over no treatment.[4] Obviously quality of life is an important factor that clinicians must recognize when discussing therapeutic options with their patients. In advanced disease, where hormone ablation remains the mainstay of therapy, quality of life issues are particularly salient, since hormone therapy does not offer cure and may significantly impact daily functioning and sense of well-being.

Health-related quality of life (HRQOL) is a novel variable from the field of public health research that encompasses a wide range of human experience, including necessities of daily living, intrapersonal and interpersonal responses to illness, and activities associated with professional fulfillment and personal happiness. Perhaps more importantly, HRQOL involves the patient's own perceptions of personal health, the ability to function in life, and the overall sense of satisfaction with life's experiences.[5] The degree of bother or distress associated with the functional limitations or symptoms resulting either from the disease itself or its treatment are also important

considerations in this concept of quality of life. Health-related quality of life is a patient-centered outcome that should not be estimated from a physician's report. The impact of quality of life on therapeutic decision-making is now considered so important that some suggest that clinical cancer trial design should routinely include an assessment of HRQOL as a measure of outcome.[6]

The goal of this chapter is to review the basic tenets of HRQOL assessment and introduce several established instruments currently in practice.

Measuring health-related quality of life in men with prostate cancer

Utilizing principles of psychometric test theory, standardized questionnaires (also known as "instruments" or "tools") are administered directly to patients (or a neutral third party interviewer) in order to objectively quantify HRQOL. These instruments typically contain questions, or items, that are organized into scales. Each scale measures a different aspect, or domain of HRQOL, which may be generic or disease-specific. Generic HRQOL domains address general aspects relevant to all persons regardless of their disease, and typically include overall sense of well-being and self-perceptions, and functionality in physical, emotional, and social arenas. Disease-specific HRQOL domains focus on the symptoms and/or concerns directly relevant to a particular condition or its treatment, such as anxiety about cancer recurrence, hot flashes, bladder irritability, bowel dysfunction, sexual dysfunction, and urinary incontinence.

Both generic and disease-specific domains need to be addressed in order to obtain the most complete "portrait" of the patient's experience. A recent study of men treated for early-stage prostate cancer noted that those who demonstrated dysfunction in the disease-specific domains also experienced small but significant changes in the generic domains, when compared with patients with no or minimal disease-specific dysfunction.[7] Hence, it is necessary to employ a multidimensional approach when assessing quality-of-life outcomes following prostate cancer treatment.

As HRQOL is a patient-centered outcome, it is critical that this outcome be measured directly from the patient, using either a self-administered survey or a third-party objective interviewer, as opposed to an invested healthcare provider. Many clinicians mistakenly underestimate the degree of symptoms and their impairment on HRQOL, introducing significant measurement error. In a large study of 2252 men, patients' self-assessment of HRQOL was compared with urologists' views, which significantly differed in all disease-specific domains, including urinary, sexual and bowel function, fatigue, and bone pain.[8] Other studies[9,10] have shown similar differences in assessment of HRQOL between patients and clinicians.

All HRQOL instruments must undergo arduous pilot testing and statistical analyses to ensure the psychometric properties of validity and reliability.[11] Reliability refers to the scale's reproducibility. In other words, what proportion of a patient's test score is true and what proportion is due to individual variation. There are different forms of reliability, which are routinely assessed during instrument development. Test-retest reliability is a measure of response stability over time. It is assessed by administering scales to patients at two separate time points, typically 1 month apart. The correlation coefficients between the two scores reflect the stability of responses. Internal consistency reliability is a measure of the similarity of an individual's responses across several items, indicating the homogeneity of a scale.[11]

Validity refers to how well the scale or instrument measures the attribute it is intended to measure. Validity provides evidence to support drawing inferences about HRQOL from the scale scores. Like reliability, there are different forms of validity, which are assessed during instrument development. Content validity involves a non-quantitative assessment of the scope and completeness of a proposed scale. Criterion validity is a more quantitative approach to assessing the performance of scales and instruments. It requires the correlation of scales scores with other measurable health outcomes (predictive validity) and with results from other established tests (concurrent validity). For example, the predictive validity of a new HRQOL scale for urinary incontinence might be correlated with the number of pads used per day. Alternatively, the concurrent validity of a new erectile dysfunction instrument might be correlated with an existing validated instrument, such as the International Index of Erectile Function.[12] Generally accepted standards dictate that validity statistics should exceed 0.70. Construct validity is a measure of how meaningful the scale or survey instrument is when in practical use. Often, it is not calculated as a quantifiable statistic. Rather, it is frequently seen as a gestalt of how well a survey instrument performs in a multitude of settings and populations over a number of years.

Given the fact the instrument development is quite an onerous task and that there are an increasing number of studies on HRQOL in urologic cancers, it is always preferable to use existing validated instruments that are established in the literature when assessing HRQOL in prostate cancer. In doing so, one can compare HRQOL from the current study cohort to prior reports and draw more meaningful conclusions that may ultimately assist patients when choosing therapy for this disease.

Health-related quality-of-life instruments in prostate cancer

Several HRQOL instruments have been developed for patients with prostate cancer (Table 5.1), including the University of California Los Angeles Prostate Cancer Index (UCLA PCI), the Expanded Prostate Cancer Index Composite (EPIC), the European Organization for Research and Treatment of Cancer Core Quality of Life Questionnaire (EORTC QLQ-C30) with its 25-item prostate cancer specific module (QLQ-PR25), the Functional Assessment of Cancer Therapy-Prostate Instrument (FACT-P), and the Prostate Cancer

Specific Quality of Life Instrument (PROSQOLI). All of these validated instruments provide an objective assessment of both generic and disease-specific domains. While this is not a complete list of the available validated HRQOL instruments for prostate cancer, it represents the most commonly used instruments and provides the reader with a reasonable overview of the available tools.

UCLA prostate cancer index

The UCLA PCI was the first validated instrument designed specifically to measure HRQOL in patients with localized prostate cancer.[13,14] General HRQOL domains are addressed in the first 36 questions, which are taken from the Medical Outcomes Study Short Form (SF-36), considered by many to be the "gold standard" questionnaire for general HRQOL.[15] The following 20 questions address six prostate-specific domains—urinary function and bother, sexual function and bother, and bowel function and bother. It has been applied to men with localized and metastatic disease and has been validated in other languages.[16] As the level of dysfunction does not necessarily correlate with the degree of bother experienced by the patient, the UCLA PCI attempts to distinguish between these two aspects of disease-specific quality of life.

Expanded prostate cancer index composite

Wei et al modified the UCLA-PCI to create the EPIC instrument which includes 12 generic HRQOL items as well as items that address the impact of hormone therapy and irritative voiding symptoms.[17] Whereas the UCLA-PCI urinary domain focuses primarily on incontinence, the EPIC also captures irritative voiding complaints, thereby expanding EPIC's utility in evaluating the impact of interstitial brachytherapy and external bean radiotherapy. Questions related to hot flashes and fatigue, commonly associated with hormone ablative therapy, are also included in the EPIC.

EORTC core quality of life questionnaire

The QLQ-C30 is a 30-item quality-of-life survey developed to assess domains significant to cancer patients, regardless of the site of the malignancy.[18] It incorporates five general function scales (physical, role, emotional, cognitive, and social), a global health scale, three symptom scales (fatigue, nausea/vomiting, and pain), and six items dealing with dyspnea, insomnia, appetite loss, constipation, diarrhea, and financial difficulties associated with the disease. In response to the lack of prostate-specific domains, the EORTC QLQ-PR25, an additional 25-item prostate cancer module was developed to include scales for bowel, urinary, and sexual symptoms.[19] The validity and reliability of this instrument has been tested in men with both localized and metastatic prostate cancer.[20–22] Although the EORTC QLQ-C30 and QLQ-PR25 do not distinguish between function and bother as in the UCLA PCI and the EPIC, the QLQ-C30 may be a better measure of HRQOL in patients with advanced disease given its unique symptom scales.

Table 5.1 Comparison of commonly utilized instruments to assess health-related quality of life in patients with prostate cancer

Instrument	Reference	Number of items	Mode of administration	Time recall	Est. completion time	Score report	Score direction	Bother assessed	Target population
UCLA-PCI (+ SF-36)	Litwin et al[12]	20 (+ 36)	Self	Past 4 wks	15–20 min	Individual domains	Higher = Better	Yes	Localized
EORTC QLQ-PR25 (+ EORTC QLQ-C30)	Borghede et al[19]	25 (+ 30)	Self	Past 1 wk	Not reported	Global summary	Lower = Better	No	Localized; metastatic
FACT-P (+ FACT-G)	Esper et al[23]	12 (+ 34)	Self	Past 1 wk	8–10 min	Global summary	Higher = Better	No	Metastatic
EPIC	Wei et al[16]	50	Self	Past 1 wk	15 min	Individual domains	Higher = Better	Yes	Localized; metastatic
PROSQOLI	Stockler et al[25]	10	Self	Past 24 hrs	Not reported	Global summary	Higher = Better	No	Hormone refractory

Functional assessment of cancer therapy–prostate

The generic portion of this instrument (FACT-G) contains 28 items covering four domains—physical, social/family, emotional, and functional well-being.[23] Like the EORTC QLQ-C30, the FACT-G also was developed to specifically assess HRQOL in cancer patients. The accompanying prostate-specific module (FACT-P) consists of a 12-item scale pertaining to appetite, weight loss, urinary difficulties, and erectile dysfunction.[24,25] A single summary score is generated, which unlike the UCLA PCI or EPIC does not capture symptom bother nor individual scores for specific areas, such as the urinary or sexual domain.

Prostate cancer specific quality-of-life instrument

This instrument utilizes linear analog self-assessment scales to measure pain, fatigue, appetite, constipation, physical activity, mood, family/marital relationships, urinary difficulty, and overall well-being. Designed specifically for use with advanced hormone-refractory prostate cancer, the PROSQOLI is relatively easy to administer and may be most suitable if the focus is on simple physical symptoms and function, rather than more complex psychosocial issues.[26]

Conclusion

Several validated and reliable disease-specific HRQOL instruments are now available for use in patients with all stages of prostate cancer. These instruments provide a means to quantify the effects of prostate cancer and its treatment on physical, emotional, and social functioning. As all current and emerging therapies have an effect on patients' quality of life, it is important that clinicians and researchers alike use these tools to assess outcomes in their patient with prostate cancer. By using these instruments and being aware of the literature on HRQOL outcomes in prostate cancer, clinicians will be better equipped to counsel their patients to make more informed treatment decisions.

References

1. Stephenson RF. Population-based prostate cancer trends in the PSA era: data from the SEER program. Monographs in Urology, vol. 91. 1998, pp 1.
2. Klein EA. Radiation therapy versus radical prostatectomy in the PSA era: a urologist's view. Semin Radiat Oncol 1998;8:87.
3. Schellhammer P, Cockett A, Boccon-Gibod L, et al. Assessment of endpoints for clinical trials for localized prostate cancer. Urology 1997;49(4A Suppl):27.
4. Helgason AR, Adolfsson J, Dickman P, et al. Waning sexual function—the most important disease-specific distress for patients with prostate cancer. Br J Cancer 1996;73:1417.
5. Patrick DL, Erickson P. Assessing health-related quality of life for clinical decision-making. In: Quality of Life Assessment: Key Issues in the 1990's. Walker SR, RM Rosser (eds): Boston: Kluwer Academic Publishers, 1993, pp 11.
6. Altwein J, Ekman P, Barry M, et al. How is quality of life in prostate cancer patients influenced by modern treatment? The Wallenberg Symposium. Urology 1997;49(4A Suppl):66.
7. Clark JA, Rieker P, Propert KJ, et al. Changes in quality of life following treatment for early prostate cancer. Urology 1999;53:161.
8. Litwin MS, Lubeck DP, Henning JM, et al. Differences in urologist and patient assessments of health related quality of life in men with prostate cancer: results from the Capsure database. J Urol 1998;159:1988.
9. Bennett CL, Chapman G, Elstein AS, et al. A comparison of perspectives on prostate cancer: analysis of utility assessments of patients and physicians. Eur Urol 1997;32 (Suppl 3):86.
10. Crawford ED, Bennett CL, Stone NN, et al. Comparison of perspectives on prostate cancer analyses of survey data. Urology 1997;50:366.
11. Tulsky DS. An introduction to test theory. Oncology 1990;4:43.
12. Rosen RC, Riley A, Wagner G, et al. The International Index of Erectile Function(IIEF): A Multidimensional Scale for Assessment of Erectile Dysfunction. Urology 1997;49:822.
13. Litwin MS, Hays RD, Fink A, et al. The UCLA Prostate Cancer Index: development, reliability, and validity of a health-related quality of life measure. Med Care 1998;36:1002.
14. Litwin MS, Hays RD, Fink A, et al. Quality-of-life outcomes in men treated for localized prostate cancer. JAMA 1995;273:129.
15. Ware JE. SF-36 Health Survey: Manual and Interpretation Guide, 2nd ed. Boston: The Health Institute, 1977.
16. Krongrad A, Perczek RE, Burke MA, et al. Reliability of Spanish translations of select urological quality of life instruments. J Urol 158: 493, 1997.
17. Wei JT, Dunn RL, Litwin MS, et al. Development and validation of the expanded prostate cancer index composite (EPIC) for comprehensive assessment of health-related quality of life in men with prostate cancer. Urology 2000;56:899.

18. Aaronson NK, Ahmedzai S, Bergman B, et al. The European Organization for Research and Treatment of Cancer QLQ-C30: a quality of life instrument for use in international clinical trials in oncology. J Natl Cancer Inst 1993;85:365.

19. Aaronson NK, van Andel G. EORTC Protocol 15011-30011: an international field study of the reliability and validity of the EORTC QLQ-C30 version 3 and a disease-specific questionnaire module (QLQ-PR25) for assessing the quality of life of patients with prostate cancer. Brussels: EORTC Data Center, 2001.

20. Borghede G, Sullivan M. Measurement of quality of life in localized prostatic cancer patients treated with radiotherapy. Development of a prostate cancer-specific module supplementing the EORTC QLQ-C30. Qual Life Res 1996;5:212.

21. Borghede G, Karlsson J, Sullivan M. Quality of life in patients with prostatic cancer: results from a Swedish population study. J Urol 1997;158:1477.

22. Albertsen PC, Aaronson NK, Muller MJ, et al. Health-related quality of life among patients with metastatic prostate cancer. Urology 1997;49:207.

23. Cella DF, Tulsky DS, Gray G, et al. The Functional Assessment of Cancer Therapy scale: development and validation of the general measure. J Clin Oncol 1993;11:570.

24. Esper P, Mo F, Chodak G, et al. Measuring quality of life in men with prostate cancer using the functional assessment of cancer therapy-prostate instrument. Urology 1997;50:920.

25. Esper P, Hampton JN, Smith DC, et al. Quality-of-life evaluation in patients receiving treatment for advanced prostate cancer. Oncol Nurs Forum 1999;26:107.

26. Stockler MR, Osoba D, Goodwin P, et al. Responsiveness to change in health-related quality of life in a randomized clinical trial: a comparison of the Prostate Cancer Specific Quality of Life Instrument (PROSQOLI) with analogous scales from the EORTC QLQ-C30 and a trial specific module. European Organization for Research and Treatment of Cancer. J Clin Epidemiol 1998;51:137.

Section 2

Treatment options for localized prostate cancer

6

Comparison of treatment modalities for localized prostate cancer using quality-of-life measures

David Miller, John T Wei

The physician's primary responsibility in caring for a patient with prostate cancer is to address the patient's concerns regarding treatment and prognosis. Currently, the most common therapeutic options for localized prostate cancer are radical prostatectomy, external radiation, and interstitial brachytherapy. Each of these interventions has undergone significant refinement in the past 10 years and can independently achieve higher than 95% cancer-specific survival at 5 years following primary treatment.[1–6] Therefore, the vast majority of patients with prostate cancer can anticipate post-therapy survival that is measured in years or even decades and, in many cases, prostate cancer can reasonably be characterized as a "chronic" disease of aging.[7] As with most chronic diseases, health-related quality of life (HRQOL) is often a primary concern for the patient and, as a result, there is now an increased emphasis on the importance of HRQOL outcomes after prostate cancer therapy. Indeed, the use of HRQOL endpoints is now commonplace in prostate cancer trials and research, and clinicians often identify HRQOL outcomes as a means for distinguishing between treatment options that are generally equivalent with regard to cancer control.[8–13] To date, studies of prostate cancer HRQOL have focused on two distinct, but complementary, priorities: 1) developing and utilizing validated instruments to more precisely and reliably characterize the prevalence and severity of adverse urinary, sexual, and bowel HRQOL effects after prostate cancer treatment; and 2) establishing patient-, rather than physician-, report data as the standard methodology for characterizing the HRQOL effects of prostate cancer and its treatment.[10,14–16]

Available instruments for measuring HRQOL among prostate cancer survivors, as well as their relative merits and pitfalls, are described in Chapter 69. The aim of this chapter is to review several "state of the art" concepts underlying the assessment of HRQOL and to summarize the contemporary literature that examines and compares patient-report HRQOL changes and outcomes following contemporary therapies for localized prostate cancer (e.g. radical prostatectomy, external beam radiation therapy, and brachytherapy), with emphasis on knowledge gained from studies that employ one or more validated HRQOL instruments.

functional effects and impairment that an illness or its therapies have on a patient as perceived by that patient. This definition is particularly appropriate given that it is usually the therapies for prostate cancer that negatively impact patient quality of life, rather than the manifestations of the disease. Increasingly, HRQOL endpoints are being included in clinical trials and studies. In many cases, funding agencies for large prostate cancer clinical research efforts require assessment of HRQOL, and a growing number of measures have been developed and validated to meet these demands.[18–24] Research over the past decade has laid the foundation for HRQOL assessments in prostate cancer, and the HRQOL literature on prostate cancer has grown exponentially. Consequently, clinicians and scientists alike must become familiar with this discipline.

The common goal of HRQOL assessment is to measure changes or differences in physical, functional, psychological, and social health. A frequent application of HRQOL assessments is the evaluation of new programs or interventions.[25] While the measurement of HRQOL is relevant to most clinical research, findings should be considered in the context of a broader research paradigm that includes clinical outcomes, such as biologic and physiologic measures.[26] As described by Wilson and Cleary,[26] health assessments should be considered on a continuum of biologic and physiologic factors that arise from the diagnosis and treatment of prostate cancer. Specifically, symptoms resulting from prostate cancer, or associated treatment, may affect physiologic functions (e.g. urinary or sexual function) that then lead to impairment of normal activities. In turn, these individual and collective processes will impact a patient's overall HRQOL. Hence, simultaneous assessment of symptoms, functions, and impairment will enhance the validity of HRQOL evaluations. Furthermore, various personal, motivational, and psychosocial factors may affect elements of this continuum. For example, post-prostatectomy urinary incontinence is quite distressing to most men; however, the use of adaptive behaviors such as a small continence pad may decrease the level of impairment associated with this symptom. As the goal of healthcare in general is to improve patient outcomes, the design of clinical research studies should attempt to identify the causal links within this continuum. As such, reliable assessments of HRQOL are necessary to complement traditional clinical endpoints, such as cancer control and survival.

Health-related quality of life

The utilization of rigorous HRQOL methods to evaluate prostate cancer outcomes is a relatively recent development.[12,15,17,18] The term "quality of life" in the urologic literature has been used as a "catch phrase" to include studies of urinary symptoms and health function; however, more appropriately, HRQOL should represent the

HRQOL and prostate cancer

Measurement and interpretation of HRQOL among men with prostate cancer is complex and should not be undertaken lightly.

One factor that must be considered when interpreting HRQOL outcomes among prostate cancer survivors is the timing of the assessment along the prostate cancer treatment continuum. Whereas prostate cancer typically has a slowly progressive natural history, most therapies will acutely alter HRQOL and health status. As a result, some effects are short-lived,[27] while others persist even among long-term survivors. In a longitudinal cohort study, Litwin et al[28] evaluated the rate of HRQOL recovery in men following RP. Using the University of California, Los Angeles prostate cancer index (UCLA PCI), they found that bowel function was the first symptom to return to baseline level (mean, 4.8 months); sexual function was the last (mean, 11.3 months); and urinary function was intermediate (mean, 7.7 months). Therefore, survey time point(s) should be based on the specific question being asked (e.g. early vs long-term recovery of function after RP).[29] As a corollary, the investigator should statistically adjust for the duration of follow-up after therapy if data are collected over a range of follow-up time points, to account for potential confounding effects.

Socioeconomic factors (e.g. patient age, race, education, income, insurance status, and marital status) must also be assessed concomitant with HRQOL. In addition to disease factors, various indicators of socioeconomic status have been found to be associated with HRQOL outcomes. Lubeck et al[30] have examined the question of racial disparity in prostate cancer HRQOL using the Cancer of the Prostate Strategic Urologic Research Endeavor (CaPSURE) dataset. They observed that black men generally had lower pretreatment HRQOL scores as measured by the SF-36 instrument and the UCLA PCI. Moreover, post-treatment recovery in a number of health domains was prolonged for black patients compared to white patients. Other social factors, including lower income and health insurance status, have also been associated with less favorable post-treatment HRQOL.[31] Eton et al[32] also explored the role of psychosocial factors on HRQOL among men who have recently completed therapy for prostate cancer. They observed that a higher level of spousal support was associated with better urinary and mental functioning in patients. In the same study, researchers evaluated demographic factors and found that African American men were more likely to report poorer urinary and sexual function following therapy, even after adjustment for age. In general, nonuniform distributions of these socioeconomic factors are likely to have an important impact on HRQOL, and adjustment for these potentially confounding factors must be undertaken in the analysis and interpretation of all HRQOL findings.

Finally, assessment of HRQOL among men with prostate cancer should be based on validated measures of generic HRQOL, cancer-specific aspects of quality of life, and prostate-specific quality of life.[33] The most common approach taken by researchers is to administer validated survey instruments (questionnaires or tools) that contain items (individual questions) that have been formulated to capture one or more of these aspects of a patient's quality of life (see Chapter 69). Whenever possible, HRQOL instruments should have demonstrable validity and reliability to ensure meaningful interpretation of the findings.[34] In survey work, *reliability* is an estimate of the consistency in the measurements. In other words, reliability is a measure of the likelihood an instrument will yield the same result on repeated trials without any significant changes in the clinical condition. *Validity* is the concept that an instrument will measure the attributes that it was designed to measure. The validity of a measure is more difficult to assess than reliability, particularly in the absence of an external criterion or "gold standard." There are several forms of validity (face validity, content validity, convergent validity, criterion validity, concurrent validity, and construct validity) and reliability (test–retest reliability, internal consistency, interobserver reliability, and intraobserver reliability). In the ideal sense, all survey instruments will have demonstrated all aspects of validity and reliability; however, this is seldom accomplished without years of instrument application and continued research. Practically speaking, a "valid" instrument is one that has demonstrated robust properties in several forms of validity and reliability, but not necessarily all.[34] Those reading the literature must be cognizant of the many HRQOL studies that are based on homegrown questionnaires that lack reliability and validity.[35] The practice of applying a subset of items from a previously validated instrument is fundamentally flawed, as the validity of the instrument will be necessarily reduced and the individual items may not perform reliably when taken out of context. Currently, all properly designed clinical protocols should strive to utilize only validated instruments and it is the results of such studies that will be emphasized in this chapter.

HRQOL in localized prostate cancer

Impact of radical prostatectomy

Data from the National Cancer Institute's Surveillance, Epidemiology and End Results (SEER) database, as well as from the American College of Surgeons National Cancer Database, consistently report surgery as the most commonly employed therapy for localized prostate cancer.[36–38] The composite results of existing studies have consistently shown that declines in both urinary incontinence and sexual HRQOL are common in the first 2 years after radical prostatectomy.[8,9,12,39] In contrast, radical prostatectomy has limited, if any, impact on urinary irritative and bowel HRQOL.[8,9]

In a cross-sectional study from our institution, the Expanded Prostate Cancer Index Composite (EPIC) instrument was employed to examine postsurgical HRQOL among 672 men treated with radical prostatectomy; outcomes for surgical patients were compared with concurrent HRQOL among an age-matched control group.[9] Based on the SF-36 instrument, general HRQOL scores did not differ between surgical patients and controls; however, EPIC urinary incontinence and sexual domain summary scores were significantly lower (poorer health state) for the radical prostatectomy group.[9]

In a longitudinal study of radical prostatectomy outcomes that employed the UCLA PCI, Litwin et al[28] prospectively observed that recovery of baseline urinary function occurred in only 56% of patients at 12 months postoperatively, with little additional recovery beyond 18 months. Sexual function had returned to baseline in only one-third of patients by 12 months post-radical prostatectomy; however, ongoing improvements in sexual HRQOL were noted beyond 24 months of follow-up as well.

In a population-based sample from the Prostate Cancer Outcomes Study (PCOS), Stanford et al[39] noted frequent leakage or no urinary control in 8.4% of men treated surgically; moreover, more than 20% of patients reported wearing one or more pads per day even up to 24 months after surgery. In this sample, post-radical prostatectomy sexual dysfunction was even more prevalent with nearly 60% of patients reporting the absence of erections adequate for intercourse at 24 months postoperatively. Based on the PCOS instrument, mean urinary incontinence and sexual function summary scores were significantly lower at 24 months post-radical prostatectomy compared with baseline levels of function.

More recently, Hu et al[40] prospectively studied 372 men from the CaPSURE database and reported that, 1 year after radical prostatectomy, only 63% and 20% of patients had returned to base-line continence and potency, respectively, based on the UCLA PCI urinary and sexual function domain summary scores. During this same interval, more than 80% of patients had returned to baseline physical and mental health. Notably, younger patient age was the most robust predictor of return to baseline urinary and sexual function.

Finally, in a recent randomized, controlled trial from Sweden, self-reported symptoms were compared among men treated with radical prostatectomy versus those managed expectantly.[41] The investigators demonstrated a significantly higher prevalence of distressful erectile dysfunction and urinary leakage among surgical patients versus those assigned to watchful waiting. However, measures of general HRQOL, including physical and psychological well-being and subjective quality of life were similar between the two groups.

Taken together, these data support the assertion that adverse sexual and urinary HRQOL outcomes are frequently observed following radical prostatectomy for localized prostate cancer.

In this context, nerve-sparing surgery has become a common practice among urologists in the hope of improving functional outcomes after prostatectomy (see Chapter 68).[42] This approach has been shown to decrease the time to recovery for both erectile function and urinary continence after RP.[39,42–44] Indeed, in the population-based PCOS sample, Stanford et al[39] reported that potency preservation was significantly more common among men receiving a bilateral nerve-sparing procedure versus a non-nerve sparing approach. The purported benefits of nerve-sparing techniques are further supported by a prospective observational study that examined the impact of nerve sparing on sexual function.[45] In this study, potency was defined as erection sufficient for intercourse, and a significant benefit was noted for the bilateral nerve-sparing technique (21% vs 0%). An effect of unilateral nerve sparing was not found at 12 months following surgery; however, the study was severely underpowered with an evaluable cohort size of only 49 subjects. In cases where nerve sparing cannot be performed for fear of compromising cancer control, sural nerve grafting has the theoretical ability to permit regeneration of the peripheral nerves necessary for erectile function.[46–48] In a study of 28 men who had undergone bilateral neurovascular bundle resection, 26% of patients had spontaneous return of erections sufficient for sexual intercourse at nearly 2 years of follow-up. Another 26% reported partial erections using a visual analog scale. Although this technique may have promise, further investigation using validated HRQOL instruments will be necessary before its widespread application.[46–48]

Recently, laparoscopic and robotic surgical techniques have emerged, with the purported potential for improving postoperative functional outcomes.[49–54] To date, implementation and utilization of these techniques has been driven by a combination of patient demand and individual surgeon interest. Notably, there remains a paucity of validated HRQOL data that demonstrate superior outcomes compared with conventional open radical prostatectomy. A preliminary study reported spontaneous erections in 45% of men who had preoperative erections, but a validated instrument was not used in this study.[55] Another group of investigators examined urinary continence at 1, 3, 6, and 12 months following laparoscopic prostatectomy.[56] As expected, urinary control improved over the course of the first year and daytime control, defined as needing no pads and reporting no leakage at all, was observed in 56.8% of patients at 12 months follow-up. These data suggest that recovery of urinary and sexual function is feasible with contemporary laparoscopic approaches; however, comparative HRQOL studies between laparoscopic and standard open radical prostatectomy techniques using validated instruments will be necessary to justify the increased expense that accompanies the use of this new technology. By and large, these data are immature and further experience with longer follow-up will be necessary for both sural nerve grafting and laparoscopic techniques in order to adequately determine the marginal benefit of these techniques over standard nerve-sparing techniques.

Impact of external beam radiation therapy

External beam radiation therapy (EBRT) is the second most commonly employed modality for the treatment of localized prostate cancer. Over the years, treatment techniques for EBRT have continued to evolve towards higher therapeutic doses, while minimizing concurrent toxicity to adjacent normal tissues.[57,58] A randomized trial comparing conformal to conventional EBRT demonstrated a lower incidence of proctitis and rectal bleeding in the conformal group at 2 years of follow-up.[59] Persistence of bladder and bowel symptoms was also evident with longer follow-up in one cross-sectional study of conformal EBRT.[60] Additional radiation to the entire pelvis was also found to decrease HRQOL in this study. Moreover, the manifestation of toxicities for EBRT patients may occur in a delayed fashion, and use of neoadjuvant and adjuvant androgen deprivation therapies are common.[61] Hence, there is a need to be mindful of the treatment technique and duration of follow-up in HRQOL studies of patients undergoing EBRT.

In a randomized trial of 108 men with localized-stage prostate cancer, EBRT was found to have significantly poorer outcomes for generic HRQOL (social functioning and limitations in daily activities) compared to expectant management as measured by the QLQ-C30 and QUFW94 instruments.[62,63] The median dose received in this study was only 64.8 Gy, and subjects received either conventional or conformal techniques. With a median follow-up of more than 30 months, urinary incontinence, hematuria, stool frequency, stool soilage, and other bowel symptoms were also found to be significantly higher in men receiving EBRT compared to expectant management. More immediate effects of EBRT on urinary, sexual, and bowel function, and cancer-specific HRQOL have been well documented.[63–66] Caffo et al[67] described the primary side effects of radiation therapy to be urinary and sexual impairment. More globally, physical and psychological functions were found to remain relatively high.

In a comprehensive evaluation based on the PCOS sample and HRQOL instrument, Hamilton et al[66] reported significant declines in disease-specific domains among 497 men with clinically localized disease treated with external beam radiation monotherapy. At 24 months of follow-up, 7.4% of men reported having frequent bowel movements on a daily basis, 14% reported pain on at least some days, and 8.9% described bowel function as being a moderate to severe problem. Urinary function was affected to a much lesser degree with severe urinary incontinence being an uncommon occurrence. Significant declines in sexual function are an additional important concern following EBRT, as the neurovascular bundles are immediately adjacent to the posterolateral limits of the prostate gland. To completely treat the peripheral zone where the prostate cancer is likely to be, EBRT must, by definition, also include the neurovascular bundles in the radiated field. The potential for collateral injury to the neurovascular bundle(s) is supported by HRQOL findings of decreased frequency of sexual activity, decreased penile rigidity, and decreased ability to maintain an erection following EBRT.[66] Moreover, 40% of men complained of a moderate to severe problem with sexual function at 24 months compared to 26% at baseline. An age effect of EBRT on post-treatment sexual HRQOL was also observed, with older men reporting significantly worse function in multiple sexual health domains. This finding may have particular clinical relevance, as the average age of men undergoing EBRT tends to be significantly older than for other active therapies. Overall, significant advances in EBRT techniques have improved HRQOL outcomes. Nonetheless, significant effects on disease-specific HRQOL remain apparent after EBRT.

Impact of brachytherapy

Brachytherapy, which is often presented as a less invasive alternative to radical prostatectomy and EBRT, is now recognized as a standard treatment option for men with low-risk prostate cancer.[68,69] Recently, HRQOL studies following contemporary brachytherapy techniques have identified urinary, bowel, and sexual HRQOL concerns among men treated with interstitial seed implantation.[9,70–73] With regard to post-brachytherapy urinary HRQOL, it is now increasingly recognized that urinary irritative and/or obstructive symptoms (e.g. pain/burning on urination, urinary frequency, hematuria, incomplete bladder emptying) are an important HRQOL concern following interstitial brachytherapy.[8,9,74,75] In general, this constellation of lower urinary tract symptoms, as measured by the American Urological Association symptom index (AUASI) or international prostate symptom score (IPSS), is most pronounced in the early postimplant period and tends to improve toward baseline with longer follow-up. Indeed, several prospective studies, using the AUASI/IPSS, have suggested that most brachytherapy patients experience new-onset or progressive urinary irritative and/or obstructive symptomatology, but that improvement in this domain may be anticipated within 1–2 years from the time of implantation.[75–77] Moreover, recent data from our institution suggest that significant and bothersome declines in urinary irritative/obstructive HRQOL (as measured by the EPIC instrument) may be primarily limited to the first 2 years after brachytherapy. With time, these post-brachytherapy urinary irritative and obstructive concerns diminish and, in fact, may continue to improve for up to 8 years following treatment.[9,78]

In addition to irritative/obstructive concerns, brachytherapy may also adversely affect urinary incontinence HRQOL. In a cross-sectional study with long-term (median, 5.2 years) follow-up, Talcott et al[70] observed that 40% of brachytherapy patients reported some degree of urinary leakage when queried regarding their urinary control during the prior week. However, this study has been criticized for its liberal definition of incontinence and, in contrast, Merrick et al[72] reported no differences in long-term (median follow-up, 64 months) urinary control, based on EPIC urinary incontinence domain summary scores, when brachytherapy survivors were compared with a group of newly diagnosed (but untreated) patients with prostate cancer. Ultimately, reconciliation of these disparate outcomes will require multi-institutional, prospective studies of post-brachytherapy urinary HRQOL that not only measure baseline urinary control, but also consider the potential impact of various technical factors, including treatment planning and urethral dosimetry.[72]

Deterioration in sexual and bowel HRQOL has also been reported following interstitial brachytherapy for adenocarcinoma of the prostate. Using an adaptation of a validated patient-report survey instrument, Talcott et al[70] observed that 73% of long-term brachytherapy survivors reported erections that were not firm enough for penetration without manual assistance. In a more recent study that utilized questions from the validated international index

of erectile function (IIEF), Merrick et al[79] noted that only 40% of patients treated with brachytherapy monotherapy reported satisfactory erectile function (IIEF score 11) at more than 5 years from the time of therapy. Similar findings have been noted at our institution, where men treated with brachytherapy (median follow-up, 5.4 years) reported significantly lower EPIC sexual domain summary scores compared with a sample of age-matched, prostate cancer-free controls.[78] Several studies have now demonstrated that bowel dysfunction, including diarrhea, painful bowel movements, and rectal bleeding, may also manifest as an important short-term HRQOL concern following seed implantation.[8,9] In general, however, post-brachytherapy rectal morbidity subsides with time and the long-term effects on bowel HRQOL may be less pronounced.[71]

An important caveat to the interpretation of studies evaluating post-brachytherapy HRQOL is the clinical reality that many patients classified as receiving brachytherapy may have actually been treated with a combination of brachytherapy and EBRT. This practice pattern is particularly common for patients considered "high risk" based on various pretreatment parameters, including clinical stage, prostate-specific antigen level, and biopsy Gleason sum. Among patients receiving such combination therapy, the administration of an EBRT "boost" may result in adverse HRQOL outcomes that cannot be uniquely attributed to seed implantation. Indeed, several investigators have identified supplemental EBRT as an important determinant of unfavorable HRQOL outcomes following brachytherapy.[70,71,80] In their cross-sectional study of long-term BT survivors, Talcott et al[70] observed that bowel dysfunction was both more prevalent and more severe among men treated with combination therapy (brachytherapy plus EBRT). Using the validated rectal function assessment score, Merrick et al[71] also noted an inverse association between post-brachytherapy rectal HRQOL and the use of supplemental EBRT. The use of supplemental EBRT has also been associated with increased urinary morbidity and sexual dysfunction following brachytherapy.[80] As a result, it is important to keep in mind that the validity and precision of post-brachytherapy HRQOL assessments will depend on the application of one or more methodologic techniques that adjust for the effect of concurrent EBRT.

Comparisons of treatment-specific HRQOLs

As mentioned above, patients with localized prostate cancer are faced with several treatment options and frequently ask their physician to discuss the side effect profiles of radical prostatectomy, EBRT, and brachytherapy. A number of recent studies have compared HRQOL outcomes following contemporary therapy for localized prostate cancer and may serve as a useful guide for addressing such concerns (Table 6.1). It is worth noting that, in many of these observational studies, men who receive EBRT are older and have less favorable cancers (e.g. slightly higher stage and grade of disease). As a result, it is important to be mindful of these differences (and the analyses should attempt to adjust for them) when comparing EBRT to other therapies. Brachytherapy patients, in contrast, generally have a demographic and disease profile similar to radical prostatectomy patients.

Many of the initial comparisons of treatment-specific HRQOL were based on cross-sectional studies from single institutions. In the first study to employ the UCLA PCI, Litwin et al[10] evaluated HRQOL outcomes among 214 patients with localized prostate cancer, as well as among 273 age-matched control patients. In this

Table 6.1 Studies demonstrating differences in HRQOL across therapies.*

Author/reference	Study design	n	HRQOL instrument	Follow-up	Mean HRQOL scores by therapy			Statistically significant
					RP	EBRT	BT	
Lee et al[82]	Longitudinal	90	FACT P	1 month	117.7	129.5	120.5	Yes (RP vs EBRT and BT vs EBRT)
Davis et al[81]	Cross-sectional	528	AUASI	5 years	17.2	13.8	20.8	NR
			SF-36 domains:					
			Physical function		83.3	74.3	80.8	Yes (BT vs EBRT)
			Role limitation		74.6	58.6	69.1	Yes (RP vs EBRT)
			Bodily pain		82.9	78.0	78.8	NS
			General health		70.9	63.9	66.3	NS
			Vitality		67.8	65.5	62.5	Yes (RP vs EBRT)
			PCI domains:					
			Bowel function		85.5	76.8	82.5	Yes (RP vs EBRT and BT vs EBRT)
			Bowel bother		83.0	71.8	79.3	Yes (RP vs EBRT)
			Sexual function		17.9	26.0	32.2	Yes (RP vs EBRT and RP vs BT)
			Sexual bother		25.2	40.0	40.4	Yes (RP vs EBRT and RP vs BT)
			Urinary function		68.4	86.4	86.8	Yes (RP vs EBRT and RP vs BT)
			Urinary bother		73.9	82.6	76.8	Yes (RP vs EBRT)
Bacon et al[83]	Cross-sectional	842	SF-36 domains:	5 years				
			Physical function		90	83	90	NR
			Role limitation		86	72	79	NR
			Bodily pain		85	79	81	NR
			General health		80	74	78	NR
			Vitality		71	64	66	NR
			Social function		92	87	92	NR
			Emotional function		90	82	86	NR
			Mental health		84	81	84	NR
			Physical component		52	49	51	NR
			Mental component		55	53	54	NR
		752	CARES domains:					
			Physical		0.20	0.33	0.26	NR
			Psychosocial		0.36	0.43	0.37	NR
			Medical interaction		0.17	0.22	0.22	NR
			Sexual problems		1.04	1.09	0.93	NR
			Marital interaction		0.41	0.43	0.45	NR
			Cancer rehabilitation		0.26	0.31	0.27	NR
		752	PCI domains					
			Bowel function		86	81	80	NR
			Bowel bother		86	78	72	NR
			Sexual function		26	34	36	NR
			Sexual bother		43	51	54	NR
			Urinary function		76	89	87	NR
			Urinary bother		82	83	75	NR
Wei et al[9]	Cross-sectional	1014	EPIC summary measures:	4 years				
			Urinary irritative		89.6	84.2	71.5	Yes (all pairwise comparisons)
			Urinary incontinence		77.5	92.8	82.1	Yes (RP vs EBRT)

(Continued)

Table 6.1 Continued

Author/reference	Study design	n	HRQOL instrument	Follow-up	Mean HRQOL scores by therapy			Statistically significant PCI domains:
					RP	EBRT	BT	
Madalinska et al[84]	Prospective		Bowel	1 year	93.2	85.2	76.0	Yes (all pairwise comparisons)
			Sexual		33.9	38.8	26.9	Yes (EBRT vs BT)
			Hormonal		90.9	87.2	83.7	No
			FACT P		36.9	36.4	32.4	Yes (RP vs BT and BT vs EBRT)
			PCI domains:					
			Bowel function		92	80	—	Yes
			Bowel bother		94	78	—	Yes
			Sexual function		NR	NR	—	–
			Sexual bother		NR	NR	—	–
			Urinary function		70	79	—	Yes
			Urinary bother		81	88	—	Yes
Talcott et al[8]	Prospective	391	Validated, study-specific instrument:	2 years				
			Urinary irritative		18.8	12.1	11.1	NR
			Urinary incontinence		23.9	15.7	15.1	NR
			Bowel		4.8	8.9	7.2	NR
			Sexual		68.5	69.2	45.0	NR
Downs et al[88]	Prospective (CaPSURE)		PCI domains:	2 years				
			Bowel function		88.3	—	89.5	NR
			Bowel bother		90.6	—	87.1	NR
			Sexual function		28.0	—	33.8	NR
			Sexual bother		38.8	—	44.5	NR
			Urinary function		75.5	—	88.1	NR
			Urinary bother		83.6	—	85.6	NR
Litwin et al[89]	Prospective (CaPSURE)	452	SF-36 domains:	2 years				
			Mental health		85	75	—	Yes
			Role limitation		94	81	—	Yes
			Vitality		73	61	—	Yes
			Social function		100	86	—	Yes
Potosky et al[12]	Prospective	1591	PCOS domains:#	2 years				
			Incontinence bother		11.2%	2.3%	—	Yes
			Bowel bother		3.3%	8.4%	—	No
			Sexual bother, ages 55–59		59.4%	25.3%	—	Yes
			Sexual bother, ages 60–74		53.2%	46.1%	—	No

*Higher scores on the PCI, EPIC, SF-36 and FACT P represent better HRQOL, whereas lower scores on the CARES, AUASI, and instrument used by Talcott et al8 represent better HRQOL.
#Percent of patients reporting being bothered for each domain.
BT, brachytherapy; EBRT, external beam radiation therapy; NR, not reported; RP, radical prostectomy.

pioneering study, patients treated with radiation therapy or observation reported significantly better urinary function when compared to men treated with radical prostatectomy. This difference was explained primarily by treatment-specific variations in the frequency and severity of urinary incontinence; notably, patients undergoing radiation therapy were equally bothered by their current urinary function. In contrast to urinary function, Litwin et al[10] observed that radical prostatectomy patients were less likely to have bowel dysfunction when compared with men receiving EBRT. More recently, Davis et al[81] also utilized the UCLA PCI and SF-36 instruments to carry out a single-institution, cross-sectional comparison of HRQOL among men treated with surgery, EBRT, and brachytherapy. This study compared 269 brachytherapy patients with a mean follow-up of 22 months, to 222 men treated with EBRT and 142 men treated with RP. Even after adjustment for patient age, follow-up time, and co-morbidity, EBRT patients tended to have poorer general health function as measured by the SF-36. In terms of disease-specific outcomes, the investigators observed more favorable sexual and urinary HRQOL among brachytherapy and EBRT patients, relative to men treated surgically. In contrast, radical prostatectomy was associated with more favorable bowel function. Using the EPIC instrument, a similar study of men undergoing radical prostatectomy, EBRT, and brachytherapy was conducted at our institution during the same period of time.[9] Relative to radical prostatectomy and EBRT, we observed less favorable urinary HRQOL among brachytherapy patients, primarily due to a greater prevalence of bothersome irritative and obstructive symptomatology. Similarly, bowel HRQOL was lowest among the brachytherapy group. Although these findings may be attributable to differences in patient selection or implantation technique, it seems likely that the observed declines in HRQOL for brachytherapy patients simply reflect the greater sensitivity of the EPIC instrument to irritative urinary and bowel symptoms.[9]

Although critical for hypothesis generation, cross-sectional studies are subject to a number of limitations including a lack of baseline HRQOL data. As a result, investigators are generally unable to control for unmeasured differences in baseline function that may explain the observed variations in HRQOL among the distinct therapy groups. Recognizing this limitation, a number of longitudinal prostate cancer HRQOL studies have been completed or are in progress, and provide valuable insight regarding the differential HRQOL impact of contemporary therapies. In a study with short-term follow-up, Lee et al[82] administered the FACT-P and the AUASI to a cohort of men treated with brachytherapy, EBRT or radical prostatectomy. In this analysis, in which HRQOL data were collected pretreatment and again at 1, 3, and 12 months post-therapy, clinically and statistically significant decreases in HRQOL were observed for all three treatment cohorts. The changes were greatest following prostate brachytherapy and radical prostatectomy, but the observed differences disappeared by 12 months. They also noted that moderate to severe urinary complaints persisted for at least 3 months following brachytherapy. Although the mean score for the AUASI was not statistically different from baseline, it is noteworthy that significantly lower (better) scores were evident for the radical prostatectomy and EBRT groups.

In a separate study based on prospectively collected data from the Health Professionals Follow-up Study, Bacon et al[83] examined the impact of cancer therapy on HRQOL in a sample of 1201 men with localized prostate cancer. General health function as measured by the SF-36 was highest for the surgery group and lowest among EBRT patients, even after adjusting for differences in demographic features. However, surgical patients tended to report worse sexual bother and urinary function, as measured by the UCLA PCI. In

contrast, EBRT patients experienced greater decrements in bowel HRQOL compared to the radical prostatectomy group. Although the brachytherapy group was small, these men did report general health function that was equivalent to surgical patients, but the disease-specific outcomes were more variable. Specifically, brachytherapy patients had less favorable bowel function and greater bowel bother than men treated surgically; moreover, urinary bother was more pronounced among brachytherapy patients than among the radical prostatectomy cohort.

In a more recent report, Talcott et al[8] prospectively assessed short-term, disease-specific HRQOL outcomes among a contemporary cohort of men receiving initial primary therapy with radical prostatectomy (n = 129), EBRT (n = 182) or brachytherapy (n = 80). After adjustment for baseline differences in socio-demographics, cancer severity, and disease-specific HRQOL, greater decrements were observed in urinary incontinence HRQOL in the first 12 months after radical prostatectomy relative to EBRT and brachytherapy. In contrast, brachytherapy and EBRT patients reported less favorable urinary irritative and bowel HRQOL in the first year after therapy. Sexual HRQOL declined substantially for all three treatment groups, although the magnitude was greatest for surgery patients. Moreover, minimal benefit was noted from nerve-sparing techniques with regard to preservation of postsurgical sexual HRQOL.

Another prospective cohort study worth noting is the Rotterdam Trial of the European Randomized Study of Screening for Prostate Cancer (ERSPC). In the framework of the ERSPC, Madalinska et al[84] prospectively compared HRQOL (UCLA PCI) at baseline, as well as at 6 and 12 months post-radical prostatectomy or EBRT among a large cohort of men with either screen-detected or clinically-diagnosed prostate cancers. Treatment-specific variations in HRQOL impairment were noted, with radical prostatectomy patients reporting significantly larger declines in sexual and urinary function versus men treated with EBRT. At the same time, the incidence of post-therapy bowel dysfunction was greater among the EBRT cohort.

To date, most prospective HRQOL studies using validated instruments have evaluated patients with relatively short-term (e.g. 2 years or less) follow-up and there has been limited data that examine patient-report HRQOL changes during the later survivorship phase (4–8 years) after radical prostatectomy, EBRT, and brachytherapy. To address this, we recently prospectively reassessed a large cohort (n=1008) of patients from our institution, at a time when the survivors of prostate cancer treatment were a median of 6.2 years after primary treatment with radical prostatectomy, EBRT or brachytherapy.[78] During the interval between 2.6 and 6.2 years of median follow-up, no significant change in general HRQOL (measured with the SF-12 instrument) was observed for any treatment group. In contrast, treatment-specific changes in disease-specific HRQOL (as measured by the EPIC instrument) were evident during this extended follow-up period. Specifically, as patients transition from early to later stages of survivorship, significant improvement was observed for the urinary irritative–obstructive domain among brachytherapy patients, whereas urinary incontinence HRQOL actually worsened among both brachytherapy and three-dimensional EBRT patients. With longer follow-up, overall sexual HRQOL deteriorated for the EBRT patients. In contrast, bowel HRQOL improved among brachytherapy patients. Among radical prostatectomy patients, urinary, bowel, and sexual HRQOL were similar at long-term (median, 6.2 years) and earlier (median, 2.6 years) follow-up. Taken together, these data suggest that, whereas post-prostatectomy HRQOL remains relatively stable beyond 2 years after treatment, disease-specific HRQOL continues to evolve among men treated with brachytherapy and three-dimensional CRT, with improvements in some domains and deterioration in others.

Although the above prospective studies have furthered understanding of treatment-specific HRQOL outcomes, they often draw subjects exclusively from tertiary care centers and, therefore, may have limited generalizability to the entire population of men treated for localized prostate cancer. Therefore, it is particularly informative to consider HRQOL data gleaned from more population-based samples.

CaPSURE is a nationwide observational cohort comprising more than 10,000 patients with prostate cancer accrued at 31 primarily community-based sites across the US.[85] As part of the CaPSURE protocol, patient-report HRQOL is collected on multiple occasions, including pretreatment or baseline assessments, using the SF-36 and UCLA PCI instruments. Thus, data from CaPSURE have played an important role in advancing understanding, on a national level, of the HRQOL impact of various localized prostate cancer therapies.

In an early study from CaPSURE, Lubeck et al[86] prospectively compared changes in general and disease-specific HRQOL in the first 2 years following radical prostatectomy (n = 351) and EBRT (n = 75). Although immediate post-therapy outcomes were less favorable among surgical patients, men treated with radical prostatectomy generally reported significant improvements in urinary, sexual, and bowel HRQOL during the first year post-treatment. Sexual health recovery continued during the second postoperative year, while slight declines in urinary and bowel HRQOL were concurrently noted. Comparatively, short-term HRQOL changes were less pronounced following EBRT, although sexual function did decline over time. In subsequent studies, Litwin et al[11,87] again compared urinary and sexual HRQOL during the first 2 years after radical prostatectomy (nerve sparing and non-nerve sparing) and EBRT.[11,87] Once again, while short-term declines in sexual and urinary HRQOL were more prominent among surgical patients, subsequent improvements in disease-specific HRQOL among radical prostatectomy patients, combined with deteriorating and/or stable sexual and urinary function following EBRT, resulted in largely convergent HRQOL outcomes by 2 years after treatment.

In a more recent publication from the CaPSURE database, Downs et al[88] prospectively compared general and disease-specific HRQOL changes during the first 24 months following brachytherapy monotherapy and radical prostatectomy. No significant changes (from baseline) were detected in general HRQOL among patients more than 12 to 18 months after radical prostatectomy or brachytherapy. In contrast, using the PCI instrument, treatment-specific changes in disease-specific HRQOL were observed during this interval. Urinary function declined significantly for both treatment cohorts, although brachytherapy patients reported less substantial declines for this domain during the first 2 years post-therapy. Notably, and perhaps reflecting the limited sensitivity of the PCI for irritative and obstructive urinary concerns, post-therapy changes in urinary bother did not differ between treatment groups. In contrast to the stable outcomes for surgical patients, brachytherapy patients also experienced concurrent declines in bowel function during the first 12 months following implantation; by 2 years, however, bowel HRQOL had essentially returned to baseline for both therapy groups. Consistent with prior studies, Downs et al[88] also observed significant (and relatively large magnitude) declines in sexual HRQOL during the follow-up interval. While sexual HRQOL did not return to baseline for either cohort, it is worth noting that the magnitude of the observed declines in sexual function and bother were generally greater for men treated with radical prostatectomy.

In addition to this variation in disease-specific outcomes, the CaPSURE investigators have also observed significant differences in post-therapy mental health among 452 men treated with radical prostatectomy, EBRT, and watchful waiting.[89] Based on the mental health domains of the SF-36 instrument, Litwin et al[89] observed that mental health outcomes varied by therapy group, with surgical patients reporting more favorable mental health, vitality, and social function at 24 months post-therapy.

Like CaPSURE, the PCOS is a rich source of data regarding the HRQOL effects of localized prostate cancer therapy, and is both unique and exemplary in that a population-based sample was used, thereby greatly enhancing the generalizability of the analyses.[12,90] One limitation of the PCOS study design, which should be kept in mind when considering the findings from this study, is that baseline HRQOL was assessed via post-treatment patient recall rather than prospective, pretherapy assessment, and is therefore subject to potential recall bias.

In an early PCOS report, Potosky et al[12] compared the effects of radical prostatectomy and conventional EBRT on urinary, sexual, and bowel function among a population of patients treated in multiple and diverse healthcare settings. With an average of 2 years of follow-up, the PCOS investigators observed that both severe urinary incontinence (9.6% vs 3.5%) and impotence (79.6% vs 61.5%) were more common among radical prostatectomy patients compared to EBRT patients. In contrast, bowel dysfunction, including pain with bowel movements and rectal urgency, was more common for EBRT patients. In a subsequent report, Penson et al[91] examined general HRQOL outcomes (SF-36 instrument) following radical prostatectomy and EBRT and noted that type of therapy (e.g. radical prostatectomy vs EBRT) was not independently associated with general quality of life at 2 years after treatment. However, regardless of treatment, men with greater sexual and urinary dysfunction were noted to have less favorable general HRQOL, suggesting an indirect effect of treatment on long-term physical and emotional function. In future, the PCOS dataset will undoubtedly provide additional insight regarding the long-term HRQOL effects of radical prostatectomy and conventional EBRT.

Summary

The composite results of existing studies suggest that general health-related quality of life is favorable following treatment for localized prostate cancer and does not differ substantially by therapy choice. In contrast, sexual, urinary, and bowel dysfunction are both prevalent and bothersome among men treated with radical prostatectomy, EBRT, and brachytherapy. A number of studies suggest that declines in urinary incontinence and sexual HRQOL are more pronounced in the first 2 years after radical prostatectomy compared with radiotherapeutic techniques, although this finding is not universal and differences in function do not always correlate with levels of bother. In contrast, urinary irritative concerns and lower gastrointestinal dysfunction compromise postradiation HRQOL to a greater extent than those reported by surgical patients. Although limited long-term data are available, there is some evidence that, while post-radical prostatectomy HRQOL remains stable beyond 2 years, post-radiation (brachytherapy and EBRT) HRQOL may continue to evolve and change.

Currently, there is insufficient evidence to support one treatment as superior with regard to preservation of urinary, sexual, and bowel HRQOL. Instead, patients should be counseled about the potential

HRQOL effects of each treatment option and encouraged to choose a therapeutic option based on their own preferences and utilities. In future, urologists and radiation oncologists will undoubtedly continue to refine these therapeutic techniques such that cancer control is preserved, while the degree of collateral damage to surrounding tissues is diminished. In this context, progressive improvements in HRQOL can be anticipated for patients with prostate cancer patients, regardless of choice of therapy.

Conclusion

HRQOL assessment for prostate cancer is a rapidly evolving field. Choice of therapy has been shown to have a significant and measurable effect on a patient's HRQOL after treatment for localized prostate cancer. In spite of recent progress in the evaluation of prostate cancer-related HRQOL, more research is still necessary. Several prospective studies that seek to compare HRQOL between therapies are underway, including a multicenter observational study (PROST-QA) that will provide a detailed examination of HRQOL and satisfaction with cancer care in men who self-selected treatment with radical prostatecomy, EBRT or brachytherapy.

In considering HRQOL as an endpoint, it is important to be cognizant of other factors that affect HRQOL, including disease and sociodemographic factors, as well as technical aspects of the treatment provided (e.g. nerve-sparing radical prostatectomy and urethral-sparing brachytherapy). Such confounding factors may have measurable effects on HRQOL and must be controlled for in the analyses of future comparative studies. Moreover, investigators should select HRQOL tools that are reliable, valid, and meet the needs of their study objectives. In some studies, generic HRQOL would suffice, whereas cancer-specific and prostate cancer-specific HRQOL assessments may be desirable in others. With the proliferation of HRQOL tools, it must be kept in mind that these tools generally only provide summary scores and do not in and of themselves quantify urinary incontinence and sexual impotence. Results from such evaluations must be considered together with the clinical condition of the patient. Assessments of HRQOL are an established component of prostate cancer clinical research and are poised to become a valuable addition to the clinical care of patients with prostate cancer.

References

1. Roehl KA, Han M, Ramos CG, et al. Cancer progression and survival rates following anatomical radical retropubic prostatectomy in 3,478 consecutive patients: long-term results. J Urol 2004;172:910–914.
2. Blasko JC, Mate T, Sylvester JE, et al. Brachytherapy for carcinoma of the prostate: techniques, patient selection, and clinical outcomes. Semin Radiat Oncol 2002;12:81–94.
3. Blasko JC, Wallner K, Grimm PD, et al. Prostate specific antigen based disease control following ultrasound guided ^{125}iodine implantation for stage T1/T2 prostatic carcinoma. J Urol 1995;154:1096–1099.
4. Gerber GS, Thisted RA, Scardino PT, et al. Results of radical prostatectomy in men with clinically localized prostate cancer. JAMA 1996;276:615–619.
5. Pound CR, Partin AW, Eisenberger MA, et al. Natural history of progression after PSA elevation following radical prostatectomy. JAMA 1999;281:1591–1597.
6. Blasko JC, Ragde H, Luse RW, et al. Should brachytherapy be considered a therapeutic option in localized prostate cancer? Urol Clin N Am 1996;23:633–650.
7. Albertsen PC, Hanley JA, Gleason DF, et al. Competing risk analysis of men aged 55 to 74 years at diagnosis managed conservatively for clinically localized prostate cancer. JAMA 1998;280:975–980.
8. Talcott JA, Manola J, Clark JA, et al. Time course and predictors of symptoms after primary prostate cancer therapy. J Clin Oncol 2003;21:3979–3986.
9. Wei JT, Dunn RL, Sandler HM, et al. Comprehensive comparison of health-related quality of life after contemporary therapies for localized prostate cancer. J Clin Oncol 2002;20:557–566.
10. Litwin MS, Hays RD, Fink A, et al. Quality-of-life outcomes in men treated for localized prostate cancer. JAMA 1995;273:129–135.
11. Litwin MS, Pasta DJ, Yu J, et al. Urinary function and bother after radical prostatectomy or radiation for prostate cancer: a longitudinal, multivariate quality of life analysis from the Cancer of the Prostate Strategic Urologic Research Endeavor. J Urol 2000;164:1973–1977.
12. Potosky AL, Legler J, Albertsen PC, et al. Health outcomes after prostatectomy or radiotherapy for prostate cancer: results from the Prostate Cancer Outcomes Study. J Natl Cancer Inst 2000;92:1582–1592.
13. Schapira MM, Lawrence WF, Katz DA, et al. Effect of treatment on quality of life among men with clinically localized prostate cancer. Med Care 2001;39:243–253.
14. Wei JT, Dunn RL, Litwin MS, et al. Development and validation of the expanded prostate cancer index composite (EPIC) for comprehensive assessment of health-related quality of life in men with prostate cancer. Urology 2000;6:899–905.
15. Penson DF, Litwin MS, Aaronson NK. Health related quality of life in men with prostate cancer. J Urol 2003;169:1653–1661.
16. Krupski TL, Saigal CS, Litwin MS. Variation in continence and potency by definition. J Urol 2003;170: 1291–1294.
17. Ware JE Jr, Brook RH, Davies AR, et al. Choosing measures of health status for individuals in general populations. Am J Public Health 1981;71:620–625.
18. Barry MJ. Quality of life and prostate cancer treatment. J Urol 1999;162:407.
19. Moinpour CM, Lovato LC. Ensuring the quality of quality of life data: the Southwest Oncology Group experience. Stat Med 1998;17:641–651.
20. Moinpour CM, Lovato LC, Thompson IM Jr, et al. Profile of men randomized to the prostate cancer prevention trial: baseline health-related quality of life, urinary and sexual functioning, and health behaviors. J Clin Oncol 2000;18:1942–1953.
21. Ganz PA, Moinpour CM, Cella DF, et al. Quality-of-life assessment in cancer clinical trials: a status report. J Natl Cancer Inst 1992;84:994–995.
22. Sloan JA, Varricchio C. Quality of life endpoints in prostate chemoprevention trials. Urology 2001;57(4 Suppl 1):235–240.
23. Sloan JA, Loprinzi CL, Kuross SA, et al. Randomized comparison of four tools measuring overall quality of life in patients with advanced cancer. J Clin Oncol 1998;16:3662–3673.
24. Moinpour CM, Hayden KA, Thompson IM, et al. Quality of life assessment in Southwest Oncology Group trials. Oncology 1990;4:79–84, 89, discussion 104.
25. Testa MA, Simonson DC. Assessment of quality-of-life outcomes. N Engl J Med 1996;334:835–840.
26. Wilson IB, Cleary PD. Linking clinical variables with health-related quality of life. A conceptual model of patient outcomes. JAMA 1995;273:59–65.
27. Kielb S, Dunn RL, Rashid MG, et al. Assessment of early continence recovery after radical prostatectomy: patient reported symptoms and impairment. J Urol 2001;166:958–961.
28. Litwin MS, Melmed GY, Nakazon T. Life after radical prostatectomy: a longitudinal study. J Urol 2001;166:587–592.
29. Melmed GY, Kwan L, Reid K, et al. Quality of life at the end of life: trends in patients with metastatic prostate cancer. Urology 2002;59:103–109.
30. Lubeck DP, Kim H, Grossfeld G, et al. Health related quality of life differences between black and white men with prostate cancer: data from the cancer of the prostate strategic urologic research endeavor. J Urol 2001;166:2281–2285.

31. Penson DF, Stoddard ML, Pasta DJ, et al. The association between socioeconomic status, health insurance coverage, and quality of life in men with prostate cancer. J Clin Epidemiol 2001;54:350–358.

32. Eton DT, Lepore SJ, Helgeson VS. Early quality of life in patients with localized prostate carcinoma: an examination of treatment-related, demographic, and psychosocial factors. Cancer 2001;92:1451–1459.

33. Macdonagh R. Quality of life and its assessment in urology. Br J Urol 1996;78:485–496.

34. Streiner DL, Norman J. Health Measurement Scales. New York: Oxford University Press, 1995.

35. Yarbro CH, Ferrans CE. Quality of life of patients with prostate cancer treated with surgery or radiation therapy. Oncol Nurs Forum 1998;25:685–693.

36. Ellison LM, Heaney JA, Birkmeyer JD. Trends in the use of radical prostatectomy for treatment of prostate cancer. Effective Clin Practice 1999;2:228–233.

37. Mettlin CJ, Murphy GP, Cunningham MP, et al. The National Cancer Data Base report on race, age, and region variations in prostate cancer treatment. Cancer 1997;80:1261–1266.

38. Mettlin C. Changes in patterns of prostate cancer care in the United States: results of American College of Surgeons Commission on Cancer studies, 1974–1993. Prostate 1997;32:221–226.

39. Stanford JL, Feng Z, Hamilton AS, et al. Urinary and sexual function after radical prostatectomy for clinically localized prostate cancer: the Prostate Cancer Outcomes Study. JAMA 2000;283:354–360.

40. Hu JC, Elkin EP, Pasta DJ, et al. Predicting quality of life after radical prostatectomy: results from CaPSURE. J Urol 2004;171:703–707, discussion 707–708.

41. Steineck G, Helgesen F, Adolfsson J, et al. Quality of life after radical prostatectomy or watchful waiting. N Engl J Med 2002;347:790–796.

42. Steiner MS, Morton RA, Walsh PC. Impact of anatomical radical prostatectomy on urinary continence. J Urol 1991;145:512–514.

43. Wei JT, Dunn RL, Marcovich R, et al. Prospective assessment of patient reported urinary continence after radical prostatectomy. J Urol 2000;164:744–748.

44. Eastham JA, Kattan MW, Rogers E, et al. Risk factors for urinary incontinence after radical prostatectomy. J Urol 1996;156:1707–1713.

45. Talcott JA, Rieker P, Propert KJ, et al. Patient-reported impotence and incontinence after nerve-sparing radical prostatectomy. J Natl Cancer Inst 1997;89:1117–1123.

46. Kim ED, Nath R, Slawin KM, et al. Bilateral nerve grafting during radical retropubic prostatectomy: extended follow-up. Urology 2001;58:983–987.

47. Kim ED, Scardino PT, Kadmon D, et al. Interposition sural nerve grafting during radical retropubic prostatectomy. Urology 2001;57:211–216.

48. Scardino PT, Kim ED. Rationale for and results of nerve grafting during radical prostatectomy. Urology 2001;57:1016–1019.

49. Guillonneau B, Cathelineau X, Doublet JD, et al. Laparoscopic radical prostatectomy: assessment after 550 procedures. Crit Rev Oncol Hematol 2002;43:123–133.

50. Guillonneau B, el Fettouh H, Baumert H, et al. Laparoscopic radical prostatectomy: oncological evaluation after 1,000 cases a Montsouris Institute. J Urol 2003;169:1261–1266.

51. Tewari A, Peabody JO, Fischer M, et al. An operative and anatomic study to help in nerve sparing during laparoscopic and robotic radical prostatectomy. Eur Urol 2003;43:444–454.

52. Tewari A, Gamito EJ, Crawford ED, et al. Biochemical recurrence and survival prediction models for the management of clinically localized prostate cancer. Clin Prostate Cancer 2004;2:220–227.

53. Menon M, Shrivastava A, Sarle R, et al. Vattikuti Institute Prostatectomy: a single-team experience of 100 cases. J Endourol 2003;17:785–790.

54. Guillonneau B, Vallancien G. Laparoscopic radical prostatectomy: the Montsouris technique. J Urol 2000;163:1643–1649.

55. Guillonneau B, Vallancien G. Laparoscopic radical prostatectomy: the Montsouris technique. J Urol 2000;163:1643–1649.

56. Olsson LE, Salomon L, Nadu A, et al. Prospective patient-reported continence after laparoscopic radical prostatectomy. Urology 2001;58:570–572.

57. Michalski JM, Winter K, Purdy JA, et al. Trade-off to low-grade toxicity with conformal radiation therapy for prostate cancer on Radiation Therapy Oncology Group 9406. Semin Radiat Oncol 2002;12(Suppl):75–80.

58. Sandler HM, Dunn RL, McLaughlin PW, et al. Overall survival after prostate-specific-antigen-detected recurrence following conformal radiation therapy. Int J Radiat Oncol Biol Phys 2000;48:629–633.

59. Dearnaley DP, Khoo VS, Norman AR, et al. Comparison of radiation side-effects of conformal and conventional radiotherapy in prostate cancer: a randomised trial. Lancet 1999;353:267–72.

60. Hanlon AL, Watkins Bruner D, Peter R, et al. Quality of life study in prostate cancer patients treated with three-dimensional conformal radiation therapy: comparing late bowel and bladder quality of life symptoms to that of the normal population. Int J Radiat Oncol Biol Phys 2001;49:51–59.

61. Nguyen LN, Pollack A, Zagars GK. Late effects after radiotherapy for prostate cancer in a randomized dose-response study: results of a self-assessment questionnaire. Urology 1988;51:991–997.

62. Fransson P, Damber JE, Tomic R, et al. Quality of life and symptoms in a randomized trial of radiotherapy versus deferred treatment of localized prostate carcinoma. Cancer 2001;92:3111–3119.

63. Widmark A, Fransson P, Tavelin B. Self-assessment questionnaire for evaluating urinary and intestinal late side effects after pelvic radiotherapy in patients with prostate cancer compared with an age-matched control population. Cancer 1994;74:2520–2532.

64. Janda M, Gerstner N, Obermair A, et al. Quality of life changes during conformal radiation therapy for prostate carcinoma. Cancer 2000;89:1322–1328.

65. Michalski JM, Purdy JA, Winter K, et al. Preliminary report of toxicity following 3D radiation therapy for prostate cancer on 3DOG/RTOG 9406. Int J Radiat Oncol Biol Phys 2000;46:391–402.

66. Hamilton AS, Stanford JL, Gilliland FD, et al. Health outcomes after external-beam radiation therapy for clinically localized prostate cancer: results from the Prostate Cancer Outcomes Study. J Clin Oncol 2001;19:2517–2526.

67. Caffo O, Fellin G, Graffer U, et al. Assessment of quality of life after radical radiotherapy for prostate cancer. Br J Urol 1996;78:557–563.

68. Mettlin CJ, Murphy GP, McDonald CJ, et al. The National Cancer Database Report on increased use of brachytherapy for the treatment of patients with prostate carcinoma in the U.S. Cancer 1999;86:1877–1882.

69. D'Amico AV, Vogelzang NJ. Prostate brachytherapy: increasing demand for the procedure despite the lack of standardized quality assurance and long term outcome data. Cancer 1999;86:1632–1634.

70. Talcott JA, Clark JA, Stark PC, et al. Long-term treatment related complications of brachytherapy for early prostate cancer: a survey of patients previously treated. J Urol 2001;166:494–499.

71. Merrick GS, Butler WM, Wallner KE, et al. Late rectal function after prostate brachytherapy. Int J Radiat Oncol Biol Phys 2003;57:42–48.

72. Merrick GS, Butler WM, Wallner KE, et al. Long-term urinary quality of life after permanent prostate brachytherapy. Int J Radiat Oncol Biol Phys 2003;56:454–461.

73. Merrick GS, Wallner KE, Butler WM. Management of sexual dysfunction after prostate brachytherapy. Oncology (Huntington) 2003;17:52–62; discussion 62, 67–70, 73.

74. Merrick, GS, Butler, WM, Wallner KE, et al. Dysuria after permanent prostate brachytherapy. Int J Radiat Oncol Biol Phys 2003;55:979–985.

75. Lee WR, McQuellon RP, Harris-Henderson K, et al. A preliminary analysis of health-related quality of life in the first year after permanent source interstitial brachytherapy (PIB) for clinically localized prostate cancer. Int J Radiat Oncol Biol Phys 2000;46:77–81.

76. Al Booz H, Ash D, Bottomley DM, et al. Short-term morbidity and acceptability of ^{125}iodine implantation for localized carcinoma of the prostate. BJU Int 1999;83:53–56.

77. Henderson A, Cahill D, Laing RW, et al. (125)Iodine prostate brachytherapy: outcome from the first 100 consecutive patients and selection strategies incorporating urodynamics. BJU Int 2002;90:567–572.

78. Miller DC, Sanda MG, Dunn RL, et al. Long-term outcomes among localized prostate cancer survivors: health-related quality-of-life

changes 4 to 8 years following brachytherapy, external radiation and radical prostatectomy. J Clin Oncol 2005;23:2772–2780.

79. Merrick GS, Butler WM, Galbreath RW, et al. Erectile function after permanent prostate brachytherapy. Int J Radiat Oncol Biol Phys 2002;52:893–902.

80. Merrick GS, Wallner KE, Butler WM. Minimizing prostate brachytherapy-related morbidity. Urology 2003;62:786–792.

81. Davis JW, Kuban DA, Lynch DF, et al. Quality of life after treatment for localized prostate cancer: differences based on treatment modality. J Urol 200;166:947–952.

82. Lee WR, Hall MC, McQuellon RP, et al. A prospective quality-of-life study in men with clinically localized prostate carcinoma treated with radical prostatectomy, external beam radiotherapy, or interstitial brachytherapy. Int J Radiat Oncol Biol Phys 2001;51:614–623.

83. Bacon CG, Giovannucci E, Testa M, et al. The impact of cancer treatment on quality of life outcomes for patients with localized prostate cancer. J Urol 2001;166:1804–1810.

84. Madalinska JB, Essink-Bot ML, de Koning HJ, et al. Health-related quality-of-life effects of radical prostatectomy and primary radiotherapy for screen-detected or clinically diagnosed localized prostate cancer. J Clin Oncol 2001;19:1619–1628.

85. Cooperberg MR, Broering JM, Litwin MS, et al. The contemporary management of prostate cancer in the United States: lessons from the cancer of the prostate strategic urologic research endeavor (CaPSURE), a national disease registry. J Urol 2004;171:1393–1401.

86. Lubeck DP, Litwin MS, Henning JM, et al. Changes in health-related quality of life in the first year after treatment for prostate cancer: results from CaPSURE. Urology 1999;53:180–186.

87. Litwin MS, Flanders SC, Pasta DJ, et al. Sexual function and bother after radical prostatectomy or radiation for prostate cancer: multivariate quality-of-life analysis from CaPSURE. Cancer of the Prostate Strategic Urologic Research Endeavor. Urology 1999;54:503–508.

88. Downs TM, Sadetsky N, Pasta DJ, et al. Health related quality of life patterns in patients treated with interstitial prostate brachytherapy for localized prostate cancer—data from CaPSURE. J Urol 2003;170:1822–1827.

89. Litwin MS, Lubeck DP, Spitalny GM, et al. Mental health in men treated for early stage prostate carcinoma: a posttreatment, longitudinal quality of life analysis from the Cancer of the Prostate Strategic Urologic Research Endeavor. Cancer 2002;95:54–60.

90. Potosky AL, Harlan LC, Stanford JL, et al. Prostate cancer practice patterns and quality of life: the Prostate Cancer Outcomes Study. J Natl Cancer Inst 1999;91:1719–1724.

91. Penson DF, Feng Z, Kuniyuki A, et al. General quality of life 2 years following treatment for prostate cancer: what influences outcomes? Results from the prostate cancer outcomes study. J Clin Oncol 2003;21:1147–1154.

7

Natural history and expectant management of prostate cancer

Jonathan R Osborn, Gerald W Chodak

Introduction

Adenocarcinoma of the prostate is a growing health problem in the US, and is now the most common solid tumor in adult men. Unlike most malignancies, there is a wide disparity between the prevalence and mortality of this disease; prostate cancer is present in approximately 30% of 50-year-old men, and over 50% of 80-year-old men,[1] yet only a small percentage of men actually die from the disease.[2,3] Although one in every six men living in the US will be diagnosed with prostate cancer during his lifetime,[4] the risk of dying is only 3%.[2] In 2004, the number of prostate cancer-related deaths is predicted to be 30,000.[4]

The advent of the prostate-specific antigen (PSA) blood test, combined with the increased testing of asymptomatic men and the use of more core biopsies in each patient, has increased the chances of finding clinically insignificant cancers. Up to a third of men in PSA-screened populations, diagnosed with nonpalpable prostate cancer and undergoing radical prostatectomy, have small (<0.5 cm^3) low-grade (Gleason 6 or less) tumors.[5,6] Such tumors are associated with a long natural history and are unlikely to affect the lifespan of select older men.[7] The median time from diagnosis to death from prostate cancer for men diagnosed with nonpalpable disease in the pre-PSA era was approximately 17 years.[7] Since the US male life-expectancy at 65 years of age is estimated at 15 years, it is unlikely that aggressive treatment is going to add significantly to the average lifespan of most men.[8] Thus, PSA overdetects prostate cancer and may subject many patients to the morbidity of treatment with only a small, if any, measurable gain. The challenge is to identify those patients who harbor non-life-threatening tumors and those whose tumor is progressing rapidly.

Because of the unusual biology of prostate cancer, *watchful waiting* (also called active surveillance or expectant management) has received increased attention as an option for patients with early-stage disease. Traditionally, this strategy followed patients with small volume low-grade prostate cancer without immediate local treatment. If and when progression occurred, androgen ablation was administered. Clearly, watchful waiting was not a curative therapy; however, the risks from this therapy are more than offset by avoiding the complications that result from definitive therapies.

The advent of PSA, however, has led to a change in watchful waiting. Now patients are followed and monitored to identify those cases with early progression. When that occurs, watchful waiting is abandoned and local therapy often is instituted. Men with slowly progressive disease continue on watchful waiting. To understand why conservative therapy is appropriate for the management of some patients, the outcomes from this approach must be reviewed.

Results of conservative therapy

One of the earliest reports on conservative management was published in 1969 by Barnes.[9] He reviewed the outcomes of patients presenting to his institution between 1930 and 1958 and identified 86 patients who were treated conservatively and who were thought to have localized disease based on digital rectal examination (DRE). Only 50% of these patients survived 10 years and only 30% survived 15 years. Barnes noted that over two-thirds of these patients died from competing medical conditions rather than prostate cancer. He recognized that concurrent medical conditions were equally important as tumor stage and grade when selecting therapy and that prostate cancer often was a slowly progressive disease, which could recur more than 10 years after seemingly curative treatment. Barnes concluded that "conservative therapy" was indicated for patients with an expected survival of 10 years or less.

From 1970 to 1990, several cohort series were published on the outcome from watchful waiting. In 1994, Chodak et al[10] assembled a cohort of 828 patients from six of these reports that included patients from throughout Europe, North America, and Israel.[10] They showed that patients with poorly differentiated carcinomas have a 10-fold greater risk of death from prostate cancer compared to men with well-differentiated disease. Specifically, men with poorly differentiated prostate cancer had a 10-year cause-specific survival of only 34% compared to men with well- or moderately-differentiated disease, who have a cause-specific survival of 87%. These findings demonstrated that for the latter group of men, the outcomes from watchful waiting might not differ significantly from aggressive therapy. At the very least, watchful waiting should be offered to patients at the time a well- or moderately-differentiated prostate cancer is diagnosed.

In 1997, Lu-Yao and Yao[11] evaluated long-term overall survival and cause-specific survival for patients treated with surgery, radiation, and conservative management. Using the Surveillance Epidemiology and End Results database, the outcome of 59,876 patients diagnosed with prostate cancer over a 10-year period was reviewed retrospectively. Patients had been treated according to the preferences of the physicians and patients. The authors concluded that the overall survival for men with well- or moderately-differentiated cancers did not differ substantially from the survival observed for men treated by radiation therapy. Small differences were seen when watchful waiting was compared to radical prostatectomy; however, this could be explained by methodologic differences—the tumor grade for men treated by watchful waiting or radiation therapy was based on the initial biopsy, whereas the tumor grade for the surgery patients was based on the final pathology. Studies have clearly demonstrated that biopsy grade underestimates actual tumor grade.

As a result, some men in the surgery group with a biopsy showing moderately-differentiated cancer would have been moved to the higher grade group, thus making the survival for those with moderately-differentiated cancers appear better.

To date, only one sizeable prospective study has compared the outcomes of patients managed aggressively to those managed by watchful waiting. Holmberg et al[12] performed a prospective randomized trial comparing watchful waiting (followed by palliative therapy) and radical prostatectomy. A total of 675 patients were enrolled in 14 Scandinavian hospitals between 1988 and 1998. Patients had T1B, T1C or T2 disease that was judged to be well- or moderately-differentiated at enrollment. All patients had a PSA less than 50 ng/ml and a negative baseline bone scan. Patients were randomized to radical prostatectomy or watchful waiting. Recommended treatment for local progression was transurethral resection of the prostate in the watchful waiting arm, and androgen ablation in the radical prostatectomy arm. The primary outcome measure was disease-specific mortality, with overall mortality, time to metastasis, and local progression being secondary endpoints. A blinded independent endpoint committee determined cause of death, with prostate cancer deaths being autopsy diagnosed or associated with evidence of progressive metastatic disease, with a mean duration of follow-up of 6.2 years. The authors reported a statistically significant decreased risk of death from prostate cancer in patients treated with radical prostatectomy versus those followed expectantly (4.6% vs 8.9% respectively, $P = 0.02$). Additionally, the risk of metastases was significantly increased in the watchful waiting group. The overall survival, however, was not statistically different between these two groups. A more recent follow-up shows a small but significant difference in overall survival at 10 years and a difference in cancer-specific survival holding at approximately 5%.

One potential problem with this study is the unequal distribution of higher grade tumors with 13 more men in the watchful waiting group having Gleason 7 disease. Given the worse natural history of these men compared with Gleason 5 or 6 cancers, the true difference in survival actually might be smaller. A second problem is that the average PSA at diagnosis was substantially higher than found for patients in the US, where the average PSA is less than 10 ng/ml at diagnosis. Had patients with PSA levels similar to those diagnosed in the US been enrolled, the difference also would have been smaller, at least for the same, relatively short follow-up. A third problem is that the primary endpoint is of some concern, as discussed by Alibhai and Klotz.[13] They argue that determination of cause of death is difficult, even by an independent, blinded committee, and that if the six excess noncancer deaths in the surgery arm are added to the 16 prostate cancer deaths, then the benefit from surgery is attenuated.

The advent of PSA testing appears to have advanced the date of diagnosis of prostate cancer (the "lead time") by 5 years or more, and the onset of secondary treatment by a similar amount.[14–16] Therefore, it is reasonable to suggest that our current knowledge base underestimates rather than overestimates a man's survival, if diagnosed with localized prostate cancer by PSA and managed by watchful waiting.

Impact of competing medical hazards

Albertsen et al[17,18] have written extensively on the impact of concomitant medical conditions on survival. They showed that men with well-differentiated disease managed by watchful waiting

experienced little if any loss of life compared to men with no evidence of prostate cancer. In contrast, men with moderately-differentiated prostate cancer lost an average of 4 to 5 years of life, while men with poorly-differentiated disease lost approximately 6 to 8 years of life, in comparison to age-matched controls. A multiple stepwise regression analysis in men treated conservatively demonstrated that the grade of tumor was the most powerful predictor of survival, followed by co-morbidities. Among all men diagnosed with clinically localized disease, 40% died of competing medical conditions rather than prostate cancer within 10 years of diagnosis.[17,18]

Identifying men for delayed local therapy

Given the variable natural history of prostate cancer, one of the most important questions to answer is, which tumors will progress slowly and which will progress rapidly? One approach is to use changes in PSA and the findings on prostate biopsy. In 1994 Epstein et al[6] retrospectively examined the use of PSA criteria and needle biopsy findings to predict small volume tumors in patients with clinical T1C prostate cancer. Using PSA density and identifying favorable (Gleason 6 or less, fewer than three cores containing cancer, ≤50% of any core involving cancer) and adverse needle biopsy findings (Gleason score 7 or higher, more than two cores containing cancer, >50% cancer involvement in any core), this study correlated the pathologic extent of disease to already existing pretreatment parameters. Seventy-nine percent of patients with a PSA density less than 0.15 ng/ml/cm³ and favorable needle biopsy findings had a tumor of total volume 0.5 cm³ or smaller, which was not of high grade and was organ confined. In contrast, 83% of men with a PSA density of 0.15 ng/ml/cm³ or greater or adverse findings on needle biopsy had tumors of volume 0.5 cm³, or which were high grade or nonorgan confined. A subsequent prospective study validated these parameters as accurate predictors of tumor volume.[19]

Choo et al[20] described PSA doubling time as a useful predictor of progression to guide treatment intervention for patients managed with watchful waiting. While PSA doubling time varies wildly between patients, a doubling time of less than 2 years shows a high risk of local progression, with a doubling time of 3 years being the suggested threshold for initiation of curative treatment. El-Geneidy et al[21] confirmed the predictive power of PSA doubling time, and also found that age and percentage positive biopsy cores were independent predictors of delayed therapy.

The dedifferentiation of prostate cancer grade with time in men undergoing watchful waiting has recently been studied.[22] Almost 13% showed a significant change in grade from Gleason 6 or less to Gleason 7 or more. It is interesting to note that in all but one of the upgraded cases the change occurred within 15 months of the initial biopsy, with no difference in initial PSA level, percent-free PSA or PSA density and velocity between the upgrading and grade-stable groups. Therefore, it is possible that these tumors did not progress, but that the area of higher grade was missed in the initial biopsy. One conclusion from these data is that men with a Gleason 6 cancer who are considering conservative therapy might undergo a repeat biopsy to rule out higher grade disease that might have been missed on the original biopsy.

Taking a delayed approach initially, Choo et al[23] reported that 23% of patients received delayed curative therapy after a median follow-up of 2.4 years. Other investigators reported somewhat lower incidences of such therapy in contemporary watchful-waiting patients,[24–26] although the follow-up was less than 2 years. Zeitman et al[27] reported 57% of such patients receiving curative therapy within 5 years and 74% within 7 years (median follow-up 3.4 years). They also commented that 81% of patients perceived the therapy was initiated by physicians, due to increasing PSA or the presence of a nodule, while physicians believed that they advocated treatment in only 24% of cases. This might be a function of anxiety regarding sequential PSA levels ("PSA-itis").[28] Each of these approaches has some merit, but the optimal approach for selecting men for delayed therapy has not yet been defined.

Counseling patients about watchful waiting

After all the benefits and risks have been presented, a common question asked by patients is, "What would you do if you were in my position?" Not surprisingly urologists would mostly select prostatectomy, and radiation oncologists would select radiation therapy.[29] Both physicians and patients should be aware of this possible bias when they are being counseled about therapy. Ultimately, the patient should make decisions by prioritizing his goals, with help from the physician to ensure he is in possession of accurate information and has no misconceptions.

All patients should understand that watchful waiting is an option that has its own set of risks and benefits, which are different from those for radiation therapy or radical prostatectomy. Clearly, if a patient wishes to maximize his survival and minimize the chance that prostate cancer will cause him pain or suffering, then aggressive therapy should be selected. On the other hand, if the patient views the potential complication rates as too high, or the relative gains from treatment as too low to warrant the risk of the various complications, or if he wants to maximize his immediate quality of life even if it potentially means a shorter survival, then watchful waiting is the best choice.

The two most important factors for a patient to consider when making his decision are the grade of tumor and his anticipated lifespan. Watchful waiting poses the least risk to a man with a well- or moderately-differentiated palpable tumor and a life-expectancy of 10 years or less. For a man whose cancer was detected by PSA (stage T1C) and is nonpalpable, watchful waiting may be equally reasonable, even if his life-expectancy approaches 15 years due to the lead time (the time between screen detection and predicted clinical detection) of diagnosis associated with this test. Essentially, watchful waiting represents a throw of the dice with the degree of risk dependent on the growth rate of the tumor and the lifespan of the patient, neither of which can be reliably predicted for an individual. In the end, the decision for the patient is about balancing risk versus benefit.

The future for watchful waiting with delayed therapy

As the average age of the population gradually increases, it is likely that watchful waiting with delayed curative therapy will become an increasingly important option for patients. It is generally assumed that the rate of PSA increase remains stable over time in men with prostate cancer; however, it has been clearly documented that some patients have sudden and rapid increases in PSA after long periods

of stability (PSA acceleration). It is unknown at which stage in the natural history of prostate cancer these accelerations occur. Perhaps acceleration is related either to a change in tumor grade or the growth of tumor beyond the prostate. Studying the long-term outcome of patients after delayed therapy and the value of periodic repeat biopsies will be important in furthering our understanding of prostate cancer.

Conclusion

With the recent dramatic increase in the detection of prostate cancer, there has been the enormous challenge to recommend the best treatment for patients with localized prostate cancer. This challenge has been difficult because of the absence of well-conducted comparative trials. Since the primary goal of the urologist is to "cure" prostate cancer and prolong life, the concept of watchful waiting seems somewhat inappropriate. However, few other diseases have treatments that can so negatively impact on a man's daily quality of life. In addition, the natural history of this cancer, in contrast to many others, does not invariably lead to metastasis or death during the normal lifespan of most patients. Therefore, many patients may wish to maximize their quality of life rather than their duration of survival. This choice depends on the probability of the good and bad outcomes that are possible with each treatment option. Watchful waiting is a reasonable option for many patients. The key is to determine when cancers are becoming life-threatening, and to intervene in these, while observing the remainder. Physicians would do well to be mindful of Hippocrates' maxim, *primum non nocere* (first, do no harm). Ultimately, it is the patient's choice to make, with help and unbiased guidance from his physician.

References

1. Scardino PT. Early detection of prostate cancer. Urol Clin North Am 1989;16:635–655.
2. Sakr WA, Grignon DJ. Prostate cancer: indicators of aggressiveness. Eur Urol 1997;32(Suppl 3):15–23.
3. Franks LM. Proceedings: etiology, epidemiology, and pathology of prostatic cancer. Cancer 1973;32:1092–1095.
4. Jemal A, Murray T, Samuels A, et al. Cancer statistics, 2003. CA Cancer J Clin 2003;53:5–26.
5. Humphrey PA, Keetch DW, Smith DS, et al. Prospective characterization of pathological features of prostatic carcinomas detected via serum prostate specific antigen based screening. J Urol 1996;155:816–820.
6. Epstein JI, Walsh PC, Carmichael M, et al. Pathologic and clinical findings to predict tumor extent of nonpalpable (stage T1c) prostate cancer. JAMA 1994;271:368–374.
7. Horan AH, McGehee M. Mean time to cancer-specific death of apparently clinically localized prostate cancer: policy implications for threshold ages in prostate-specific antigen screening and ablative therapy. BJU Int 2000;85:1063–1066.
8. Minino AM, Arias E, Kochanek KD, et al. Deaths: final data for 2000. Natl Vital Stat Rep 2002;50:1–119.
9. Barnes RW. Survival with conservative therapy. JAMA 1969;210:331–332.
10. Chodak GW, Thisted RA, Gerber GS, et al. Results of conservative management of clinically localized prostate cancer. N Engl J Med 1994;330:242–248.
11. Lu-Yao GL, Yao SL. Population-based study of long-term survival in patients with clinically localised prostate cancer. Lancet 1997;349:906–910.

12. Holmberg L, Bill-Axelson A, Helgesen F, et al. A randomized trial comparing radical prostatectomy with watchful waiting in early prostate cancer. N Engl J Med 2002;347:781–789.
13. Alibhai SM, Klotz LH. A systematic review of randomized trials in localized prostate cancer. Can J Urol 2004;11:2110–2117.
14. Draisma G, Boer R, Otto SJ, et al. Lead times and overdetection due to prostate-specific antigen screening: estimates from the European Randomized Study of Screening for Prostate Cancer. J Natl Cancer Inst 2003;95:868–878.
15. Gann PH, Hennekens CH, Stampfer MJ. A prospective evaluation of plasma prostate-specific antigen for detection of prostatic cancer. JAMA 1995;273:289–294.
16. Tornblom M, Eriksson H, Franzen S, et al. Lead time associated with screening for prostate cancer. Int J Cancer 2004;108:122–129.
17. Albertsen PC, Fryback DG, Storer BE, et al. Long-term survival among men with conservatively treated localized prostate cancer. JAMA 1995;274:626–631.
18. Albertsen PC, Fryback DG, Storer BE, et al. The impact of co-morbidity on life expectancy among men with localized prostate cancer. J Urol 1996;156:127–132.
19. Carter HB, Sauvageot J, Walsh PC, et al. Prospective evaluation of men with stage T1C adenocarcinoma of the prostate. J Urol 1997;157:2206–2209.
20. Choo R, DeBoer G, Klotz L, et al. PSA doubling time of prostate carcinoma managed with watchful observation alone. Int J Radiat Oncol Biol Phys 2001;50:615–620.
21. El-Geneidy M, Garzotto M, Panagiotou I, et al. Delayed therapy with curative intent in a contemporary prostate cancer watchful-waiting cohort. BJU Int 2004;93:510–515.
22. Epstein JI, Walsh PC, Carter HB. Dedifferentiation of prostate cancer grade with time in men followed expectantly for stage T1c disease. J Urol 2001;166:1688–1691.
23. Choo R, Klotz L, Danjoux C, et al. Feasibility study: watchful waiting for localized low to intermediate grade prostate carcinoma with selective delayed intervention based on prostate specific antigen, histological and/or clinical progression. J Urol 2002;167:1664–1669.
24. Carter HB, Walsh PC, Landis P, et al. Expectant management of nonpalpable prostate cancer with curative intent: preliminary results. J Urol 2002;167:1231–1234.
25. Koppie TM, Grossfeld GD, Miller D, et al. Patterns of treatment of patients with prostate cancer initially managed with surveillance: results from The CaPSURE database. Cancer of the Prostate Strategic Urological Research Endeavor. J Urol 2000;164:81–88.
26. McLaren DB, McKenzie M, Duncan G, et al. Watchful waiting or watchful progression?: Prostate specific antigen doubling times and clinical behavior in patients with early untreated prostate carcinoma. Cancer 1998;82:342–348.
27. Zeitman AL, Thakral H, Wilson L, et al P. Conservative management of prostate cancer in the prostate specific antigen era: the incidence and time course of subsequent therapy. J Urol 2001;166:1702–1706.
28. Lofters A, Juffs HG, Pond GR, Tannock IF. "PSA-itis": knowledge of serum prostate specific antigen and other causes of anxiety in men with metastatic prostate cancer. J Urol 2002;168:2516–2520.
29. Moore MJ, O'Sullivan B, Tannock IF. How expert physicians would wish to be treated if they had genitourinary cancer. J Clin Oncol 1988;6:1736–1745.

Clinical trials comparing expectant management to definitive treatment of prostate cancer

Chris Parker

Introduction

For cancers of other primary sites, it would be unethical to even contemplate the idea of clinical trials comparing expectant manage-ment with definitive treatment. Expectant management of most cancers would lead to certain disease progression, disfigurement, and death. Prostate cancer is different. While prostate cancer *can* follow an aggressive and ultimately fatal course, similar to that of other cancers, a significant proportion of cases will behave in an indolent fashion, and have no effect either on health or longevity. For these patients, definitive treatment is both unnecessary and potentially harmful. Furthermore, there has been much uncertainty as to whether definitive treatment of the more aggressive, potentially lethal, prostate cancers does in fact prolong survival.

It is for these reasons that, in the case of prostate cancer, comparison between expectant management and definitive treatment is a vitally important issue. Given that it is so important, it is unfortunate that there is such a paucity of quality data comparing the outcome of expectant management with that of definitive treatment. Furthermore, almost all available data relate to cases typical of the pre-prostate-specific antigen (PSA) era, and such data may not be generalizable to contemporary, PSA screen-detected disease.

Retrospective comparisons of expectant management and definitive treatment

Retrospective comparisons between expectant manage-ment and definitive treatment are of very limited value, given the possibility (indeed the likelihood) of significant confounding variables. That said, two retrospective comparisons merit consideration, not least because they generate the hypothesis that the magnitude of any ben-efit for definitive treatment will vary with tumor grade.

The population-based study of outcome from the SEER database was based on data for 59,876 cancer-registry patients aged between 50 and 79 years who had clinically localized prostate cancer diagnosed between 1982 and 1992.[1] Overall and disease-specific survival were analyzed by grade and by type of treatment (Table 8.1). By the intention-to-treat approach, 10-year prostate cancer-specific survival for grade 1 cancer was 94% (95% CI, 91–95) after prostatectomy, 90% (87–92) after radiotherapy, and 93% (91–94) after conservative management. The corresponding survival figures for grade 2 cancers were

87% (85–89), 76% (72–79), and 77% (74–80); those for grade 3 cancer were 67% (62–71), 53% (47–58), and 45% (40–51).

It is no surprise that disease-specific mortality increases with tumor grade. Nor is it any surprise, given the likely differences in co-morbidities, quite apart from anything else, that survival following definitive treatment appears better than that for watchful waiting. It is, however, interesting to note that the apparent benefit of radical treatment varies markedly with tumor grade. The absolute difference in 10-year disease-specific survival between radical prostatectomy and watchful waiting was 1%, 10%, and 22% for grade 1, 2 and 3 disease, respectively. Although the watchful waiting patients no doubt differ markedly from the radical prostatectomy patients in terms of co-morbidity as well as in other important respects, it is at least arguable that such differences would be similar regardless of cancer grade. Thus, this study generates the hypothesis that the magnitude of any benefit for definitive treatment will vary with tumor grade.

This possibility is supported by another retrospective comparison of expectant management and definitive treatment. Albertsen et al[2] reported a watchful waiting series that has been held in high regard on account of its size, the maturity of the outcome data, and the use of centralized pathology review with the Gleason scoring system. The Albertsen series included men aged 55 to 74 years, diagnosed with prostate cancer between 1971 and 1984, who were identified from the Connecticut Tumor Registry. Cases were excluded if they were known to have metastatic disease at presentation, or if they had undergone radical treatment. Of 767 evaluable cases, 610 were known to have died at the time of analysis. Mean follow-up for the remaining 157 patients was 15 years. Outcome, expressed in terms of 15-year mortality from prostate cancer, was derived from a regression-based competing risks model. Subsequently, an analysis from the Mayo Clinic of long-term outcome following radical prostatectomy was designed to be as comparable as possible to the Albertsen data set.[3] This surgical series was based on 751 men with clinically localized disease, also aged between 55 and 74, who underwent radical prostatectomy during the same time period (1971–1984). The outcome in terms of 15-year mortality from prostate cancer was derived using the same competing risks methodology. Figure 8.1 shows the results of the two studies for men aged between 60 and 64 at diagnosis. It must be remembered that these are two different series, from two very different healthcare settings, and that any comparison between them should be interpreted with great caution. With that strong proviso, it is interesting to note that the apparent benefit of radical treatment over watchful waiting is modest for Gleason scores less than or equal to 6, and becomes larger for the more poorly-differentiated cancers. Specifically, the absolute difference in 15-year disease-specific mortality between radical

Table 8.1 Actuarial 10-year disease-specific mortality (DSM) in men with localized prostate cancer by type of treatment according to the SEER population-based retrospective study[1]

	Radical prostatectomy		Watchful waiting	
	n	*10-year DSM (%)*	*n*	*10-year DSM (%)*
Grade 1	3854	6 (5–9)	9804	7 (6–9)
Grade 2	14,287	13 (11–15)	6198	23 (20–26)
Grade 3	5133	33 (29–38)	2236	55 (49–60)

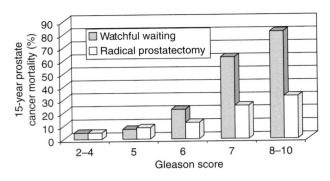

Figure 8.1

Fifteen-year prostate cancer mortality for men aged 60–64 at diagnosis: comparison of Mayo Clinic radical prostatectomy series[3] with Albertsen et al watchful waiting data.[2]

prostatectomy and watchful waiting was 0% for Gleason scores 2 to 4, –1% for Gleason score 5, 10% for Gleason score 6, 37% for Gleason score 7, and 49% for Gleason scores 8 to 10.

These retrospective comparisons suggest that subgroup analysis by tumor grade should be an important part of randomized trials which compare expectant management and definitive treatment.

Randomized comparisons of expectant management and definitive treatment

There are just two published randomized controlled trials comparing expectant management and definitive treatment of prostate cancer. Of these, one, which included just 142 patients, is too small for meaningful analysis.[4] The other, the Scandinavian Prostatic Cancer Group Study, randomized almost 700 men with localized disease between radical prostatectomy and watchful waiting, and the first results were published in 2002.[5] Interpretation of these results has varied widely. According to Patrick Walsh, "for the first time we have clear evidence that surgical treatment reduces the risk of death from prostate cancer."[6] In contrast, the British Medical Journal's account of the same data appeared under the heading, "Watchful waiting as good as surgery for prostate cancer." While interpretations may differ, there is wide agreement that this trial provides the best available data comparing expectant management and definitive treatment.

The Scandinavian trial was designed in 1988, with the main aim of comparing prostate cancer mortality following radical prostatectomy and watchful waiting. Eligible patients were younger than 75 years, with newly diagnosed, clinically localized prostate cancer, with a negative bone scan, a PSA of less than 50 ng/ml, and a life-expectancy of at least 10 years. Cases were graded according to the World Health Organization (WHO) classification, and those with either well- or moderately (but not poorly)-differentiated tumors were included. Gleason scoring was also used, and eligibility was restricted to patients in whom less than 25% of the tumor tissue examined was Gleason grade 4 and less than 5% was Gleason grade 5. Patients were randomized between watchful waiting and radical prostatectomy. Following surgery, adjuvant treatment was not used. For patients on watchful waiting, transurethral resection was recommended for local progression. Patients were followed up with PSA levels and annual bone scans. The study accrued 695 patients from 14 centers between 1989 and 1999. Thirty of 348 patients (9%) randomized to watchful waiting received treatment with curative

intent, and 25 of 347 patients (7%) randomized to surgery were in fact managed by watchful waiting (in addition to 23 patients who were found to be node positive at the time of surgery and did not proceed to radical prostatectomy). All analyses were performed according to intention to treat, rather than treatment received.

Results were obtained at a median follow-up of 6.2 years, and so must be regarded as preliminary, with just 115 (17%) of the 695 patients having died. Forty-seven (41%) of the deaths were attributed to prostate cancer, and 68 (59%) to other causes. Randomization to radical prostatectomy was associated with improved disease-specific mortality, with a hazard ratio of 0.50 (95% CI, 0.27–0.9; $P = 0.02$), which translated into an absolute benefit of 6.6% (95% CI, 2.1–11.1) at 8 years. While this is an important endpoint, it is not beyond criticism, because ascertainment of cause of death in patients with prostate cancer can be problematic. In terms of overall mortality, a statistically nonsignificant trend was seen in favor of radical prostatectomy with a hazard ratio of 0.83 (95% CI, 0.57–1.20). It seems likely that a significant overall survival advantage will emerge with longer follow-up, given that radical prostatectomy was associated with a reduction in the risk of metastatic disease (hazard ratio 0.63; 95% CI, 0.41–0.96). The main outcomes are shown in Figures 8.2 to 8.4.

Although the Scandinavian trial provides the best available data comparing expectant management and definitive treatment, there are obvious, major differences between Scandinavian practice during the early 1990s and contemporary, state-of-the-art clinical practice. First, the case-mix is certainly not representative of screen-detected prostate cancer—only 11% of patients in the trial had stage T1C disease, and the mean initial PSA level was as high as 13 ng/ml, with 18% of patients having a PSA greater than 20 ng/ml. Second, traditional watchful waiting as practiced in the trial, with palliative treatment for symptomatic progression, is very different from expectant management as it is now widely practiced, with radical treatment for those patients with biochemical or histologic progression. Third, radical prostatectomy in the trial was used as a sole modality of treatment, rather than with adjuvant or early salvage radiation and/or hormonal therapy.

The differences in outcome between the two arms of the trial are usually attributed to the effects of surgery. However, an alternative, and apparently plausible, explanation is that the benefits in the surgical arm were due, at least in part, to the earlier use of hormone therapy. Data on the timing of hormone therapy are not publicly available. However, it seems likely that the 23 patients (7%) randomized to radical prostatectomy but found to be node positive at

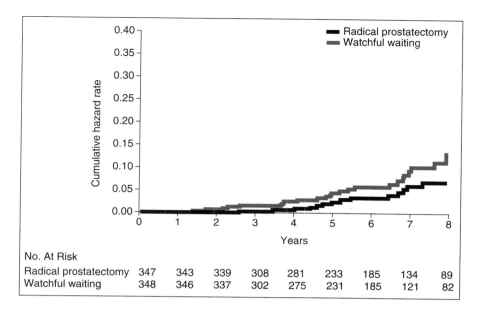

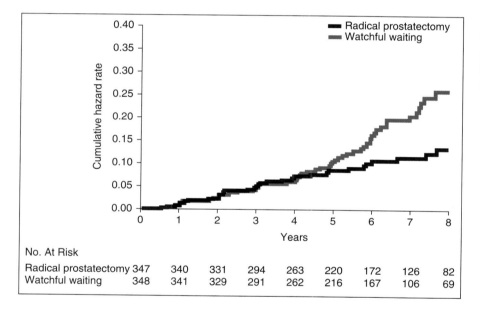

the time of surgery, commenced hormone therapy at that time. Furthermore, hormonal therapy was recommended for patients with local recurrence after radical prostatectomy, but not for patients with local progression on watchful waiting. It is conceivable that differences in the timing of hormone therapy between the two arms of the trial could have introduced a bias, delaying the development of metastatic disease in patients randomized to radical prostatectomy.

Notwithstanding these limitations, the Scandinavian trial remains a very important study. It is now known that treating localized prostate cancer is not always a waste of time and effort. It is now hard to argue that traditional watchful waiting is as effective as surgery for all patients with localized disease. The reduction in the risk of metastatic prostate cancer, even in the absence of an overall survival benefit, is a clinically meaningful benefit of treatment. The challenge now is to identify *which* patients stand to benefit from curative treatment.

In addition to the efficacy data described above, the Scandinavian trial also provides the only randomized comparison of quality of life following expectant management and definitive intervention.[7] Of the 695 patients in the main trial, those who were recruited either in Finland or after February 1996, were excluded from the quality-of-life comparison, leaving 376 eligible patients. Self-reported data were obtained using a study-specific 77-item questionnaire that was mailed to patients following an introductory letter and telephone call. The response rate was impressive, with 87% of questionnaires returned, suggesting that the findings are likely to be representative of the entire cohort. It is important to note that, as in the main trial, a minority (6%) of the patients randomized to watchful waiting actually received radical prostatectomy, and 20% of patients randomized to surgery did not in fact undergo radical prostatectomy. The data reported were analysed by intention to treat.

Radical prostatectomy was associated with increased sexual dysfunction. For example, erectile function "seldom or never sufficient for intercourse" was reported by 80% in the surgical arm, versus 45% of those randomized to watchful waiting (relative risk 1.8; 95% CI, 1.5–2.2). Distress caused by decline in sexual function was also greater among patients randomized to radical prostatectomy (56% vs 40%). A contrasting pattern of urinary dysfunction was

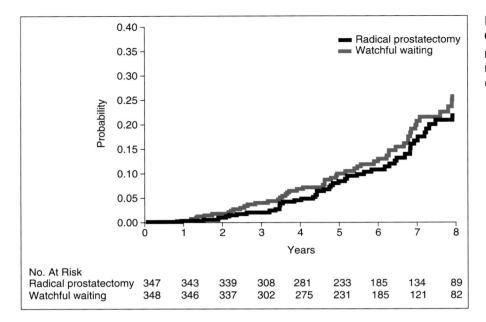

No. At Risk

	0	1	2	3	4	5	6	7	8
Radical prostatectomy	347	343	339	308	281	233	185	134	89
Watchful waiting	348	346	337	302	275	231	185	121	82

Figure 8.4
Overall mortality.

From Holmberg et al,[5] with permission from Massachusetts Medical Society. All rights reserved.

seen in the two groups, with bladder emptying problems more common in the watchful waiting group, and urinary leakage more common in the radical prostatectomy group. For example, bladder emptying difficulty, defined as an American Urological Association symptom index score of greater than 7, was reported by 35% in the radical prostatectomy group versus 49% in the watchful waiting group (relative risk 0.7; 95% CI, 0.5–0.9). Whereas moderate or severe urinary leakage was reported by 18% of patients assigned to radical prostatectomy and 2% of those assigned to watchful waiting (relative risk 9.3; 95% CI, 2.9–29.9). No significant differences were seen between the two groups in terms of either bowel function or psychological symptoms.

These are extremely important data since they are patient- rather than physician-reported, collected prospectively in the context of a randomized trial, and with an excellent compliance rate. The risks of impotence and incontinence associated with radical prostatectomy are much higher than those quoted in series from individual surgeons at academic institutions in the US.[8] It is not clear to what extent this difference reflects disparities in case selection and methods of data collection, and to what extent the morbidity of radical prostatectomy is operator-dependent. However, the data from the Scandinavian trial likely provide a better indication of surgical morbidity for most patients managed in routine clinical practice. That being the case, it is even more important to determine which patients stand to benefit from definitive treatment, and which patients can safely avoid the associated risks of impotence and incontinence.

Ongoing randomized comparisons of expectant management and definitive treatment

There are two ongoing randomized trials which aim to compare definitive treatment with expectant management in PSA screen-detected

disease. The Prostate Cancer Intervention versus Observation Trial (PIVOT) compares radical prostatectomy versus watchful waiting, and has completed enrolment with 731 patients.[9] The Prostate testing for cancer and Treatment (ProtecT) study compares radical prostatectomy, external beam radiotherapy, and active monitoring, and aims to recruit over 2000 patients.[10] The results of these trials will be critically important in helping to determine the relative merits of definitive treatment and expectant management of early prostate cancer.

PIVOT opened to recruitment in 1994 under the auspices of the Department of Veterans Affairs and the National Cancer Institute. Eligible patients were younger than 75 years, with biopsy-proven localized prostate cancer of any grade, a serum PSA less than 50 ng/ml, and a life-expectancy of 10 years or more. Strengths of the trial design include the collection of baseline co-morbidity data and the use of a centralized pathology review. The trial compares two different general approaches to management, rather than two specific interventions. Patients randomized to radical prostatectomy were therefore able to receive adjuvant or salvage postoperative radiation and/or hormone therapy as clinically indicated. Patients randomized to expectant management were managed according to the general principle of using palliative therapies with low morbidity for symptomatic or metastatic progression. Radical prostatectomy, "definitive" radiation, early hormone therapy or treatment for an asymptomatic rising PSA were proscribed for patients in this arm of the trial. Interestingly, patients on expectant management and their physicians were blinded to PSA results in order to minimize intervention for asymptomatic biochemical progression. The main endpoint is overall mortality, and the initial accrual target was 2000 cases. Unfortunately, this target proved unattainable, and the trial closed to recruitment with 731 patients entered, with the plan to analyse the outcome data after 15 years of follow-up.

PIVOT is in many ways similar to the Scandinavian trial of radical prostatectomy versus watchful waiting, but involves a different patient population. On the one hand, PIVOT will likely include a greater proportion of men with PSA screen-detected cancers with a more favorable natural history and less potential to benefit from definitive treatment. On the other, patients with high grade disease for whom the opposite is true were eligible for PIVOT, but not for the Scandinavian trial. The results of exploratory subgroup analyses by tumor grade will be of interest, although the final accrual of just

731 patients will be a limiting factor in such analyses. One important limitation of PIVOT, which it shares with the Scandinavian trial, is that the approach to expectant management, with palliative treatment for symptomatic progression, is very different from expectant management as it is now widely practiced, with radical treatment for those patients with biochemical or histologic progression. If radical treatment for all patients turns out to improve survival compared with radical treatment for none, it will beg the question as to whether radical treatment for some, selected for example according to PSA kinetics, would have been as effective, but less morbid.

It is not surprising that PIVOT failed to reach its target accrual. It is recognized that patients and clinicians may find it difficult to accept the concept of randomization between two such different approaches to treatment. The ProtecT study opened in 1999, supported by the UK Department of Health, with an unusual recruitment methodology designed to address this problem. Individuals are invited, by letter from their general practitioner, to attend a prostate check clinic. Those who agree to attend the clinic are informed about the significance of prostate cancer, and about the randomized trial of treatment options. At this stage men who wish to participate are asked to give informed consent, and have a PSA test. Transrectal ultrasound biopsy is performed in those with a PSA level greater than 3 ng/ml, and those found to have clinically localized prostate cancer are potentially eligible for the treatment randomization, for which a separate informed consent is required. By informing the subjects about the uncertainties of prostate cancer management, and about the treatment trial before, rather than after, diagnosis, it is hoped that randomization between the different treatments will be easier. This approach has been successful in that approximately 70% of eligible patients have agreed to three-way randomization between active monitoring, radical prostatectomy, and radical radiotherapy.[11] However, just as in the Holmberg et al trial,[5] among those who have been randomized, not all patients accept their allocated treatment. One concern is that this approach to recruitment could lead to an increased rate of "crossover" from the allocated treatment, since this could significantly reduce the power of the trial to detect differences in outcome using an intention-to-treat analysis.

Patients randomized to active monitoring are being followed with PSA tests every 3 months in the first year and then at 3- to 6-monthly intervals. Repeat prostate biopsies are not routinely performed. PSA progression is suspected if there is a 50% increase in PSA level within any 12-month period. Suspected progression will prompt restaging investigations, and the decision whether to proceed to curative treatment will be "based on full participant information and joint decision-making." It will be interesting to see what proportion of patients in the active monitoring arm do proceed to curative treatment. A 50% increase in PSA within 12 months is the equivalent of a PSA doubling time of less than 20 months. Only a very small proportion of patients with localized prostate cancer will have such a rapid rate of rise of PSA level,[12] suggesting that this active monitoring policy may be similar in effect to traditional watchful waiting. While there is no evidence-based definition of the criteria that should be used to define disease progression requiring radical treatment, this approach differs from published series of active monitoring in which 25% to 33% of patients receive radical treatment.[13,14]

ProtecT is on course to recruit over 2000 patients by 2006, which will be an outstanding achievement. It promises to be the single most important trial comparing expectant management and definitive treatment of PSA screen-detected prostate cancer. In addition, since the participating general practices represent a random sample of practices within a defined area, and since background rates of PSA screening in nonparticipating general practices remains relatively low, this program will also provide data on the value of PSA screening. Put another way, ProtecT represents the intervention arm of a randomized trial of PSA screening, with those practices not invited to take part acting as the control arm.

The long-term mortality outcomes from PIVOT and the ProtecT trial will provide the best data comparing expectant management and definitive treatment, but will not be available for several years. In the meantime, it is tempting to speculate as to what those results will be. If it is assumed that the 15-year survival for early prostate cancer in the PSA era managed by watchful waiting is that predicted by Nicholson and Harland,[15] and that the improvement in prostate cancer mortality with radical treatment matches the improvement

Table 8.2 Estimated 15-year outcome for PSA screen-detected early prostate cancer managed by watchful waiting (WW) versus radical treatment (RRx)

Age at diagnosis	Alive		Dead from prostate cancer		Dead from other causes	
	WW (%)	RRx (%)	WW (%)	RRx (%)	WW (%)	RRx (%)
50	72.1	75.9 (72.5–78.2)	12.2	7.7 (5.0–11.7)	15.7	16.4 (15.8–16.8)
55	65.2	68.5 (65.6–70.5)	11.6	7.3 (4.8–11.1)	23.2	24.2 (23.3–24.8)
60	56.3	59.1 (56.6–60.7)	11.1	7.0 (4.6–10.7)	32.6	33.9 (32.7–34.7)
65	44.7	47.0 (44.9–48.4)	11.1	7.0 (4.6–10.7)	44.2	46.0 (44.4–47.1)
70	31.4	33.0 (31.5–34.0)	10.5	6.6 (4.3–10.1)	58.1	60.4 (58.3–61.7)
75	7.9	8.3 (7.9–8.6)	7.4	4.7 (3.0–7.1)	84.7	87.0 (85.0–88.4)
80	2.2	2.3 (2.2–2.3)	4.0	2.5 (1.6–3.8)	93.8	95.2 (94.0–96.0)

The estimate for outcome of watchful waiting is taken from Nicholson and Harland.[15] The ranges shown correspond to a range of hazard ratios for effect of RRx on prostate cancer mortality of 0.41–0.96.

seen in the 8-year risk of metastasis observed in the Scandinavian Prostatic Cancer Group study (hazard ratio, 0.63; confidence interval, 0.41–0.96),[5] then the size of the survival benefit of radical treatment can be guesstimated (Table 8.2). These estimates of the potential survival benefit of radical treatment must be regarded with some caution. There is uncertainty with regard to both the predicted natural history of PSA-detected early prostate cancer, and the impact of radical treatment on prostate cancer mortality. However, based on the assumptions stated above, the potential 15-year survival benefit of radical treatment for PSA-detected early prostate cancer appears modest. For example, for men aged 70 at diagnosis, radical treatment is estimated to result in a 1.6% absolute benefit in 15-year survival (number needed to treat [NNT], 62.5), and for men aged 60, the estimated absolute benefit is 2.8% (NNT, 35.7). These results serve as a reminder that, in the absence of good data from randomized trials, the decision whether or not to have radical treatment is a value judgement, comparing the known morbidity of treatment with the unknown, but potential, survival benefit. Faced with a 50% risk of treatment-related impotence and a 2% potential survival benefit, a significant proportion of men will likely elect for expectant management in preference to definitive treatment.

The future for trials of expectant management versus definitive treatment

This chapter has focused on trials of watchful waiting versus definitive treatment with either surgery or radiotherapy. Such trials will leave other important questions to be addressed. First, newer definitive treatments such as brachytherapy, cryotherapy, and high intensity focussed ultrasound (HIFU) offer the promise of less morbidity and greater convenience than either surgery or radiotherapy. Such modalities have the potential to shift the balance of risks and benefits further in favor of definitive treatment. After all, if definitive treatment were effective and had no morbidity, then there would be no case for expectant management.

Second, just as there are advances in definitive treatment techniques over time, so the approach to expectant management is also evolving. At present, there is no consensus on the optimum approach to expectant management. Uncertainties include the frequency of PSA testing, the need for repeat biopsies, the role of imaging investigations, and the criteria used to define disease progression requiring radical treatment. As the approach to active surveillance is optimized, so the ability to target treatment to those who stand to benefit should improve. In future, it can be envisaged that active surveillance could be combined with low-toxicity interventions designed, not to eradicate the disease, but to alter its natural history. This is an attractive possibility, not least because "incidental" prostate cancer is an extremely common postmortem finding even in countries with the lowest rates of clinically significant disease,[16] suggesting that environmental factors, such as diet, may influence prostate cancer progression, rather than initiation. Nutritional interventions require further study, but could become a middle way between definitive treatment and traditional approaches to expectant management.

The long-standing debate concerning the relative merits of expectant management and definitive intervention rests to a large extent on the extraordinary degree of interpatient variation in prostate cancer behavior, together with the inability to predict that behavior in individual cases. While it is known beyond reasonable doubt that half the men diagnosed with early prostate cancer do not need treatment, it is not known which these patients are. As understanding of the molecular pathology of prostate cancer advances, it is likely that new and better predictors of prostate cancer behavior will be identified. In the long-term, the use of such biologic predictors could revolutionize the ability to select patients for definitive treatment on the one hand, or expectant management on the other.

References

1. Lu-Yao G, Yao S. Population-based study of long-term survival in patients with clinically localised prostate cancer. Lancet 1997;349:906–910.
2. Albertsen, P, Gleason D, Barry M. Competing risk analysis of men aged 55 to 74 years at diagnosis managed conservatively for clinically localized prostate cancer. JAMA 1998;280:975–980.
3. Sweat SD, Bergstralh EJ, Slezak J, et al. Competing risk analysis after radical prostatectomy for clinically nonmetastatic prostate adenocarcinoma according to clinical Gleason score and patient age. J Urol 2002;168:525–529.
4. Iversen P, Madsen PO, Corle DK. Radical prostatectomy versus expectant treatment for early carcinoma of the prostate. Twenty-three year follow-up of a prospective randomized study. Scand J Urol Nephrol 1995;172(Suppl):65–72.
5. Holmberg L, Bill-Axelson A, Helgesen F, et al. A randomized trial comparing radical prostatectomy with watchful waiting in early prostate cancer. N Engl J Med 2002;347:781–789.
6. Walsh PC. A randomized trial comparing radical prostatectomy with watchful waiting in early prostate cancer. J Urol 2003;169:1588–1589.
7. Steineck G, Helgesen F, Adolfsson J, et al. Quality of life after radical prostatectomy or watchful waiting. N Engl J Med 2002;347:790–796.
8. Walsh P. Radical prostatectomy for localized prostate cancer provides durable cancer control with excellent quality of life: a structured debate. J Urol 2000;163:1802–1807.
9. Wilt TJ, Brawer MK. The Prostate Cancer Intervention Versus Observation Trial (PIVOT): A randomized trial comparing radical prostatectomy versus expectant management for the treatment of clinically localised prostate cancer. Cancer 1995;75(Suppl7):1963–1968.
10. Donovan J, Hamdy F, Neal D, et al. Prostate testing for cancer and treatment (ProtecT) feasibility study. Health Technol Assess 2003;7:1–88.
11. Donovan J, Mills M, Smith M, et al. Quality improvement report: Improving design and conduct of randomised trials by embedding them in qualitative research: ProtecT (prostate testing for cancer and treatment) study. Commentary: presenting unbiased information to patients can be difficult. BMJ 2002;325:766–770.
12. Choo R, DeBoer G, Klotz L, et al. PSA doubling time of prostate carcinoma managed with watchful observation alone. Int J Radiat Oncol Biol Phys 2001;50:615–620.
13. Choo R, Klotz L, Danjoux C, et al. Feasibility study: watchful waiting for localized low to intermediate grade prostate carcinoma with selective delayed intervention based on prostate specific antigen, histological and/or clinical progression. J Urol 2002;167:1664–1669.
14. Carter HB, Walsh PC, Landis P, et al. Expectant management of nonpalpable prostate cancer with curative intent: preliminary results. J Urol 2002;167:1231–1234.
15. Nicholson PW, Harland SJ. Survival prospects after screen-detection of prostate cancer. BJU Int 2002;90:686–693.
16. Yatani R, et al. Trends in frequency of latent prostate carcinoma in Japan from 1965–1979 to 1982–1986. J Natl Cancer Inst 1988;80:683–687.

9

Anatomic considerations in radical prostatectomy

Robert P Myers, Arnauld Villers

This chapter covers what we believe to be the most important anatomic points for successful radical prostatectomy by whatever method, retropubic or perineal. Illustrations have been fastidiously created by using of specimens from fresh autopsy material, magnetic resonance images of pelvic floor anatomy before radical prostatectomy, and intraoperative photography. On the basis of anatomy, practical observations related to the conduct of surgery are also described.

Pelvic fascia, parietal and visceral, and its surgical importance

Radical prostatectomy must be performed with a clear understanding of the fascia that helps to identify the correct planes of surgical dissection. The pelvic fascia is either *parietal* or *visceral* (fascia pelvis parietalis, fascia pelvis visceralis, *TA**).[1] The parietal component (also commonly called endopelvic fascia) covers the levator ani laterally, and the visceral component covers the bladder, prostate, seminal vesicles, rectum, and pudendal vasculature, the latter coursing anteriorly and superiorly from the dorsal vascular (veins and arteries) complex of the penis. The surgical removal of prostate cancer and the adjacent fasciae in an en-bloc package lessens the risk of local recurrence due to residual tumor.

When the abdominal wall entry is made en route to the prostate in the retropubic approach, the first layer of fascia encountered is the transversalis fascia, extending distally from the posterior rectus abdominis sheath as a prominent thin sheet, which must be incised or penetrated bluntly. Once this is accomplished, there is then an amorphous fascia of loose connective tissue encountered in developing the retropubic and paravesical spaces, the latter space for pelvic lymphadenectomy. This amorphous tissue has no more substance than thin cotton candy.

For a full view of the pelvic fascia, all the retropubic adipose tissue must be teased away. The parietal and visceral components of the pelvic fascia meet in a thickened, curvilinear white line, the fascial tendinous arch of the pelvis (arcus tendineus fasciae pelvis, TA), which stretches from the pubovesical (puboprostatic) ligaments to the ischial spine. The whiteness is due to the thickened nature of the fascia along this line. When the levator ani (parietal or endopelvic) fascia is incised just lateral to the fascial tendinous arch of the pelvis, the bare levator ani muscle that overlies the obturator internus above and the ischioanal fossa below appears laterally.

As the levator muscle is displaced laterally to expose the lateral surfaces of the prostate, its fascia remains abandoned and adherent to the

outer lateral surfaces of the prostate. This remnant levator fascia overlying the outer surface of the prostate (Walsh's lateral pelvic fascia)[2] extends in a posterior direction continuously over the neurovascular bundle (NVB) and the rectum, and distally over the prostatourethral junction and its surrounding vessels. In the retropubic operation, this remnant levator fascia, which is transferred to a visceral location on the lateral surface of the prostate at this point, must be incised anterior and parallel to the NVB in order to preserve it. For wide resection to include the NVBs and the prostatoseminal vesicular (Denonvilliers') fascia (see below) together with the specimen, this fascia must be incised posterior and parallel to the nerve bundle.

Underneath the remnant levator fascia on the lateral surfaces of the prostate, the prostate visceral fascia, where multilayered, contains fat, smooth muscle, and collagen fibers. It is easier to identify grossly when nerves and vessels run among its layers. It consists of three subdivisions (according to its location): 1) anterior prostate visceral fascia, associated with the isthmus or anterior commissure of the prostate; 2) lateral prostate visceral fascia, which covers the lateral glandular prostate; and 3) posterior prostate visceral fascia, known eponymically as Denonvilliers' fascia (septum rectovesicale, *TA*).

The current terminology used above does not capture the continuous sweep of the fascia from the posterior surface of the prostate superiorly over the posterior surfaces of the seminal vesicles. In keeping with the policy of most medical schools currently not to teach eponyms, we propose herein "*prostatoseminal vesicular fascia*" (PSVF) to describe anatomically this posterior fascia, which is neither rectal nor a septum. The PSVF is separated from the rectal fascia propria by a prerectal cleavage plane, which trails distally from the variable distal endpoint of the peritoneal cul-de-sac (rectovesical pouch) (Figure 9.1). This cleavage plane is a remnant of the two peritoneal layers that fused and disappeared before birth. On the posterior surface of the prostate, the PSVF has no macroscopically discernible layers.[3,4] Distally, the PSVF thickens and is demonstrably multilayered just distal to the prostatourethral junction. The PSVF extends posterior to the prostate apex and sphincteric (membranous) urethra and, as a terminal plate,[5] has direct continuity with the midline raphe ending in the perineal body or central tendon of the perineum.

In contrast to the posterior surface of the prostate, the PSVF is frequently multilayered over the seminal vesicles (predominance of smooth muscle fibers), but is, with only very rare exception, a single layer of fascia over the immediate posterior surface of the prostate.[3,6–8] It has been suggested to distinguish a fascial leaf anterior to the seminal vesicles and a fascial leaf posterior to the seminal vesicles and prostate.[9]

Posterolaterally, the NVB is bounded by PSVF, which splits to pass above and below the bundle, and the levator fascia, which passes lateral to the bundle (Figure 9.1B). Thus, in axial or transverse histologic section, the NVB is bounded by a triangle of fascia.[10]

---

* TA = Terminologia Anatomica, New York: Thieme Stuttgart, 1998.

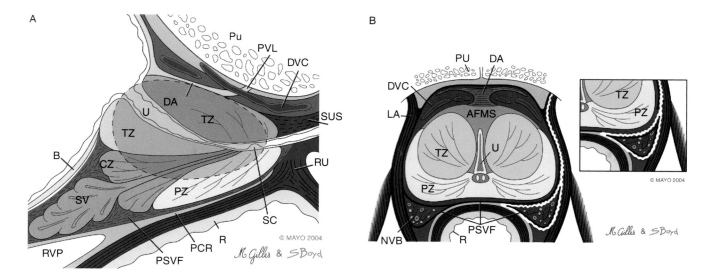

Figure 9.1

Fascial anatomy. *A*, Sagittal and *B*, transverse section of interfascial dissection of neurovascular bundle (NVB). Extrafascial dissection (not shown) would encompass all layers of the periprostatic fascia. AFMS, anterior fibromuscular stroma of McNeal; B, urinary bladder; CZ, central zone; DA, detrusor apron; DVC, dorsal vascular complex; LA, levator ani; PCP, prerectal cleavage plane; PSVF, prostatoseminal vesicular (Denonvilliers') fascia; Pu, pubis; PVL, pubovesical (puboprostatic) ligament; PZ, peripheral zone; R, rectum; RU, rectourethralis; RVP, rectovesical pouch; SC, seminal colliculus; SUS, striated urethral sphincter; SV, seminal vesicle; TZ, transition zone benign prostatic hyperplasia; U, urethra.

Courtesy of Mayo Foundation for Medical Education and Research.

On the basis of these observations, we propose, from an anatomic standpoint with respect to surgical dissection of the prostate, that an *extrafascial plane of dissection* would define the prostate removed with all layers of visceral fascia present on the specimen (wide resection).

Furthermore, an *intrafascial plane of dissection* would define some portion of the visceral fascia being absent from the specimen with prostate capsular and glandular tissue at the margin. In this type of dissection, as the prostate is excised, a triangular layer of PSVF will remain on the posterior surface of the prostate, but the posterolateral surfaces of the prostate where the NVBs resided will be bare of PSVF. Because the PSVF abuts the NVBs laterally and cavernous nerves run in the lateral PSVF, NVB-preserving surgery may injure the nerves associated with the PSVF. Fascia then will be left covering the medial aspect of the NVB as the NVB is dissected away from the posterolateral prostate (Figure 9.1B, inset).

Finally, an *interfascial plane of dissection* would define PSVF covering the entire posterior prostate but not the medial aspect of the NVB (Figure 9.1B). In this case, a safety zone of complete visceral fascial covering will be present on the specimen, thereby reducing the risk of positive posterolateral surgical margins. This is important because perineural tumor extension has been shown to involve microscopic posterolateral nerves to the prostate in the area of the NVB; this is the main mechanism of extraprostatic extension and an important factor for positive margins.[5,8,11]

Dorsal vascular complex (dorsal vein complex, Santorini's plexus, pudendal plexus)

The corpus spongiosum and flanking corpora cavernosa of the penis (corpora) have a rich blood supply that, in part, intimately invests the prostate. Prostate removal cannot be accomplished without some disruption of this blood supply, which is less with the properly performed perineal operation and more with the open retropubic operation. More than veins are involved; the pudendal arteries are multiple and of variable caliber and approach the corpora from below or above the pelvic diaphragm. In some cases, the main arterial supply is found exclusively above the pelvic diaphragm with main, large (e.g. 4 mm in diameter), aberrant pudendal arteries coursing along the pelvic sidewall and diving, immediately posterior to the symphysis pubis, into tissue that sits anterior to the prostatourethral junction. In a cadaveric preparation, Benoit et al[12] illustrated the corpora being subserved by a single, large, aberrant pudendal artery with division into two branches just anterior to the prostatourethral junction. Sacrifice of some arterial blood supply during dorsal vascular complex (DVC) control could contribute directly to postoperative erectile dysfunction.

The pudendal veins course from the DVC in three ways: 1) anterior to the prostate in a hyperbolic path along the lateral edges of the detrusor apron (see below) to enter the vascular pedicle at the junction of the bladder and prostate laterally; 2) posterolateral to the prostate in conjunction with the NVBs; and 3) below the pelvic diaphragm, as the pudendal vein runoff within each ischioanal fossa. Anastomosis between these three main groups is common and variable with respect to quantity, size, and distribution. The unpredictable nature in individual cases can make surgical control of the DVC in the retropubic operation a formidable challenge because failure to understand the nature of the DVC in any one patient and to control bleeding could be rapidly life-threatening. In the perineal operation, the prostate, with care, is shelled away from the overlying DVC when the plane of dissection from the prostatourethral junction to the bladder neck is taken posterior to the visceral preprostatic fascia and the detrusor apron (see below). Serious bleeding in the perineal operation should be very rare if the DVC is not violated.

Relation of the urinary bladder to the prostate

Detrusor apron

From the bladder neck to approximately the mid-anterior commissure of the prostate, the anterior surface of the prostate is covered by outer longitudinal smooth muscle of the bladder in a layer, the detrusor apron, that extends distally to end as two pubovesical (officially "puboprostatic") ligaments on either side of the pubic symphysis (Figure 9.2).[13] Because the core of each ligament contains smooth muscle from the detrusor apron, the ligaments are essentially pubovesical in men, just as they are in women. However, because the smooth muscle stroma of the prostate merges imperceptibly with the inferior surface of the detrusor apron at the vesicoprostatic junction, the ligaments also have a puboprostatic basis. The detrusor apron is just one component of McNeal's anterior fibromuscular stroma.[14,15] In radical prostatectomy, it is useful anatomically to separate the detrusor apron component from McNeal's anterior fibromuscular stroma, as originally illustrated,[14] because it is so intimately involved in control of the DVC. Pubourethral association of the ligaments (pubourethral ligaments) is recognized;[16] this concept has much to do with the continuity of these ligaments and the periurethral levator fascia.

The detrusor apron can serve as a buttress to compress and tamponade with clamp or suture the large flanking, often multiple, anterolateral pudendal veins that emanate from the DVC (Figures 9.1B and 9.2).[17] These veins, bulging and situated in loose connective tissue (fascia), are decompressed when bunched together. This bunching maneuver over the anterior commissure of the prostate allows hemostasis of the anterolateral pudendal plexus and significantly increases visibility of the adjacent anterolateral surfaces of the prostate for the purpose of subsequent NVB preservation. Furthermore, the bunching facilitates control of any anastomotic veins (and there is pronounced variability) traversing the lateral surface of the prostate from NVBs to the anterolateral plexus.

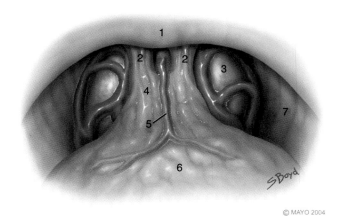

© MAYO 2004

Figure 9.2
Retropubic view after endopelvic fascia is incised and levator fascia (lateral pelvic fascia of Walsh) is removed from lateral surfaces of prostate to allow bulging of pudendal veins emanating from dorsal vascular complex. 1, pubis; 2, pubovesical (puboprostatic) ligaments; 3, prostate; 4, detrusor apron; 5, superficial vein; 6, urinary bladder; 7, levator ani.
Courtesy of Mayo Foundation for Medical Education and Research.

Bundle of Heiss

Relatively thick bundles of the outer longitudinal smooth muscle sweep distally from the lateral surfaces of the bladder and then pass anterolaterally in a loop across the vesicoprostatic junction. This loop was described by Heiss in 1916,[18] illustrated by Wesson in 1920,[19] and emphasized by Woodburne in 1968.[20] It is separate and posterior in relation to the anterior longitudinal muscle that courses off the anterior surface of the bladder to form the detrusor apron. The wall of the bladder is typically much thinner superior to the bundle of Heiss. Anatomically, the bundle of Heiss adheres closely to the prostate and is easily sacrificed in radical prostatectomy when the bladder is entered anteriorly in the process of resecting the prostate. If the bundle of Heiss is preserved, it then can be incorporated in racquet plication and, because of its relative thickness, some passive continence often may be observed if the caliber of the reconstructed bladder neck is no larger than 24 to 26 Charrière and the bladder mucosa is everted (personal observation, RPM).

Proximal bladder neck sphincter at the internal urethral meatus

The inner circular smooth muscle of the bladder neck forms a sphincteric ring of smooth muscle that may extend distally to the veru as the preprostatic sphincter in the absence of benign prostatic hyperplasia (BPH). When nodules of BPH begin within the wall of the preprostatic sphincter distal to the bladder neck as well as outside the preprostatic sphincter, the sphincteric function from the bladder neck to the veru progressively disappears. Whether there are one or two sphincters at the bladder neck has been a matter of controversy. Grossly, during radical prostatectomy, it is our observation that there is only one sphincter at the bladder neck and its function must be very much dependent on circular smooth muscle integrity. Loss of anatomic integrity and compromised neural innervation must then contribute to the observation that the bladder neck never regains normal sphincteric function postoperatively. After healing takes place, the bladder neck is always fixed and open.

Prostate shape

Variation in prostate appearance includes 1) size; 2) presence or absence of BPH; 3) degree of prostate urethral angulation at the veru (verumontanum, seminal colliculus); 4) size of the anterior commissure (isthmus); and 5) apical configuration. We ascribe McNeal's prostate components as peripheral zone, central zone, transition zone, and anterior fibromuscular stroma.[21] We include also the anterior commissure or isthmus and the detrusor apron.

Size

Radical prostatectomy specimens may vary in weight from as little as 10 g to as much as 200 g (personal experience, RPM).

The primary contributor to this considerable range is BPH, but there is variation in size and configuration without BPH, and a phenotypic difference can be appreciated in teenagers.[22]

Prostate urethral angulation

McNeal[23] emphasized a 35° bend at the verumontanum (veru, seminal colliculus) in the prostatic urethra. Rarely, it is 0°, and on occasion it may subtend at a 90° angle even in young men.[24] It is in the latter case that "rigid cystoscopy" is difficult, and the introduction of "flexible cystoscopy" has brought peace and comfort to awake patients.

Variable anterior commissure

The anterior commissure (isthmus) is the bridge of prostate tissue anterior to the urethra that connects the left and right sides of the prostate. It varies from narrow to broad, which means the distance from the bladder to the prostatourethral junction may be very short or relatively long, especially in the presence of BPH. *The practical application of this concept is that the sphincter and neurovascular tissue may be damaged if the technique to secure the DVC is the use of a large right-angle forceps in the presence of a narrow anterior commissure.* The narrow anterior commissure is most often associated with small prostates.

Apical configuration

Variations in apical configuration of the prostate affect the exit of the sphincteric (membranous) urethra from the prostate. Many variations manifest (Figure 9.3). Variations in apical configuration will be completely overlooked by surgeons who blindly transect the urethra at the apex without allowing for the phenomenon of overlap of the sphincter by prostate at the prostatourethral junction. Overlap was emphasized by Turner Warwick[25] and has been confirmed in coronal section in phosphotungstic acid-hematoxylin stain.[26] Overlap varies from 1) circumferential; 2) symmetrically bilateral; 3) asymmetrically unilateral; 4) anterior only; 5) posterior only in the not uncommon posterior lip configuration;[27] and 6) absent. Whatever the apical configuration, the net result of urethral transection should be the delivery of a cylindrical urethral stump that protrudes proximally from the surrounding NVBs (Figure 9.3). If overlap is present but not appreciated and not dealt with properly, urethral transection may leave the patient with a urethral stump far too short for urinary control. In the perineal operation, in order to obtain a more proximal point for urethral transection, Hudson[28] used a scalpel handle to retract proximally the posterior apex. In the retropubic operation, a vein retractor can be used effectively to hold the parenchyma slightly cephalad and thereby to expose precisely the point where the striated sphincter ends and the smooth muscle of the urethral wall begins at the apex.[27] After transection of the anterior half of the urethra, the veru can be appreciated in relation to the point of transection. Also, if the urethra is transected just distal to the veru, the same boundary will be respected as in transurethral resection of the

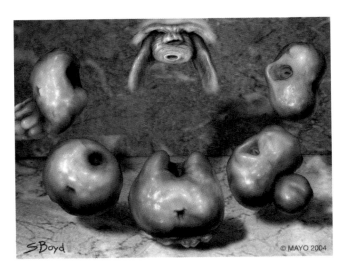

Figure 9.3
Diversity of prostate shape, including apices. Regardless of shape, the prostate has to be removed so that the intact cylindrical urethral stump protrudes proximally with intact flanking neurovascular bundles (NVB) (*center top*) in the NVB-preserving operation.
Courtesy of Mayo Foundation for Medical Education and Research.

prostate, wherein resection distal to the veru often results in urinary incontinence. *This principle is no different in radical prostatectomy.*

Although the urethra can be separated from the adjacent prostate apex, it must be emphasized that the prostate apex is the most treacherous and common site for the occurrence of positive resection margins. Ukimura et al[29] recently recommended the use of realtime ultrasonography during laparoscopic radical prostatectomy to assess apical configuration, including the important posterior lip variant mentioned above.

Urethral stump (sphincteric urethra, membranous urethra) preservation

Urethral support

As a column of tissue, the membranous urethra with its striated sphincter is supported by its attachment to the prostate proximally and corpus spongiosum of the penis distally. Anteriorly and distally, the transverse ligament of the perineum fixes the base of the striated sphincter. Laterally, thickened fascial band components of the DVC (Walsh's pillars,[30] Müller's ischioprostatic ligaments[31]) provide insertion for the anterior layer of the striated sphincter (Figure 9.4). Posteriorly, there is a variably thick fibrous tissue raphe into which is inserted the circular component fibers of the striated sphincter (Figure 9.5). The degree of circumferentiality of the striated sphincter is variable depending on the thickness of the raphe. Even when the sphincter appears to be circumferential grossly during transection, a raphe will be identifiable histologically

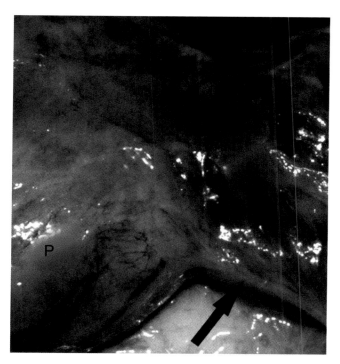

Figure 9.4
Prostatosphincteric urethral junction (gross cadaveric dissection). P, prostate; S, striated urethral sphincter with its superficial layer inserting into lateral fascial band (Walsh's pillar, Müller's ischioprostatic ligament) (*arrow*).

in axial section, should one be obtained. This then gives rise to the concept that the striated sphincter is essentially horseshoe-shaped in axial section.[27,32] However, the actual transverse or axial shape is difficult to describe because the striated sphincter changes configuration in serial axial section from the apex of the prostate to the bulb of the penis. *The lateral bands and posterior raphe, however, are constant anatomic features that contribute to support of the residual urethral stump in the male adult age group that undergoes radical prostatectomy.*

Urogenital hiatus versus urogenital diaphragm

In coronal sections of the pelvis, the sphincteric (membranous) urethra is flanked by the anterior levator (urogenital) hiatus proximally (Figure 9.6). Between the levator hiatus and the corpus spongiosum, the urethra is flanked by the fibrofatty and vascular recesses of the ischioanal fossae. By magnetic resonance imaging (MRI) in coronal section, it is the combination of the perineal membrane and penile corporal body complex bridging the ischiopubic rami that forms an irregular, thick urogenital diaphragm. Importantly, the urethral stump after urethral transection will not be part of a urogenital diaphragm, as illustrated by Netter.[33] Netter illustrated, at the apex of the prostate, a mythical plate of muscle spanning the ischiopubic rami, containing the striated sphincter. He sandwiched his muscle plate between a superior and inferior fascia (of a urogenital diaphragm) from which he suspended the corpora cavernosa and corpus

spongiosum. There is no evidence from gross dissection, histologic section, or MRI to support Netter's illustrated urogenital diaphragm.

Urethral stump function from an anatomic standpoint

When the prostate is removed, only the sphincter of the urethral stump functions to provide urinary control. As described above, the proximal or bladder neck smooth muscle urethral sphincter at the internal meatus is destroyed. As readily confirmed endo-scopically in the postoperative period and reiterated here, the bladder neck always becomes fixed and open regardless of what is done to preserve, plicate, or intussuscept it.[34]

Turner Warwick[25] used "distal sphincter mechanism" to describe the functional system of the residual urethra and periurethral tissue. In this "mechanism," urinary continence depends on six anatomic elements. From urethral stump lumen outward, these six elements consist of 1) the mucosal seal; 2) urethral wall smooth muscle and elastic tissue; 3) striated urethral sphincter; 4) puboperineal portion of the levator ani; 5) associated autonomic and somatic nerves, and 6) blood vessels.

Mucosal seal

A delicate mucosa with numerous luminal invaginations is apparent in cross-sections of the membranous urethra. The mucosa is thus subject to injury from prolonged flattening from an indwelling Foley catheter and disruption from rotations of a grooved sound. To protect the mucosal seal, surgeons should use only a small-caliber smooth sound for anastomotic suture placement and the smallest diameter catheter that can function properly.

Urethral wall smooth muscle and elastic tissue (lissosphincter, intrinsic sphincter)

This element is the single most important component of the distal sphincter mechanism. If this element is not intact, the patient will be rendered incontinent. It extends the entire length of the urethral stump and from the verumontanum (veru, seminal colliculus) to the penile bulb or corpus spongiosum when the prostate is intact. Injury occurs if its full functioning length is shortened by surgical transection that sacrifices the length necessary for urinary control. How much residual urethral length is necessary? The normal membranous urethra is of variable length and, in one MRI study, was measured in a range of 1.5 to 2.4 cm, with 2 cm on average.[35] Study by endorectal coil MRI before surgery has shown that the longer the membranous portion of the urethra before surgery, the more rapid the return of urinary continence.[36] Although not fully established, patients probably need at least 1 cm of functioning residual membranous urethral length to be continent. Thus, a patient with a 1.5-cm membranous urethra before transection cannot tolerate sacrifice of as much length as a patient with a 2.4-cm membranous urethra. Because the prostate gland may overlap the membranous urethra up to approximately 1 cm, urethral transection made

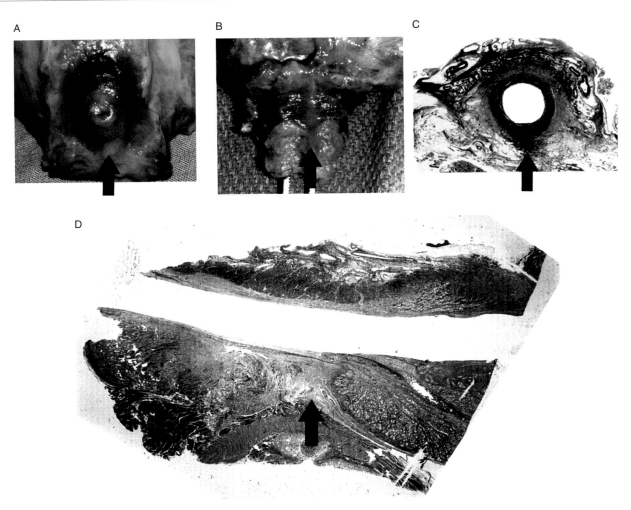

Figure 9.5
Posterior urethral raphe (*arrows*) to confirm horseshoe configuration of striated urethral sphincter. *A*, Cadaveric specimen, gross axial section through mid-membranous urethra. *B*, Cadaveric specimen, posterior view of raphe from apex of prostate above to paired bulbourethral glands below. *C*, Histologic section through mid-membranous urethra. (Masson-trichrome.) *D*, Histologic sagittal section from penile bulb on left to prostate on right to anorectal junction at bottom (Masson-trichrome).

without knowledge of the placement of the veru may result in serious risk of subsequent urinary leakage.

Another variable factor is the placement of the veru with respect to the posterior apical extent of the prostate. The veru may sit exactly at the posterior apex or as much as 1 cm proximal to the apex with prostate posterior to the membranous urethra. If the veru is situated right at the apex, it will have no urethral crest distal to it. In this case, transection of the posterior apex will not sacrifice the membranous urethral stump length. If the veru is proximal to the posterior apex margin and urethral transection is made at the apex, variable urethral stump length will be lost. Technique to optimize residual urethral stump length then might involve preoperative retrograde urethrography to measure the distance from veru to corpus spongiosum to determine whether it is unduly short. Additionally, midline sagittal T_2-weighted MRI can be used to assess urethral stump length and the presence or absence of posterior lip of prostate beneath the membranous urethra. Such studies allow preoperative assessment of prostate apical and urethral stump variability and potentially can help in planning the operation. If patients have positive results of apical biopsy, this assessment could prove to be particularly worthwhile and preoperatively allow the patient to be informed of a pending challenging dissection.

Striated urethral sphincter (rhabdosphincter, sphincter urethrae, ta)

Composed of unique striated fibers (smaller with primarily slow-twitch capacity), the striated urethral sphincter most probably functions to assist passive continence during bladder filling or in the absence of micturition. The striated urethral sphincter covers the critical smooth muscle urethral wall and functions in the male from the apex of the prostate to the bulb. In Caine and Edwards' classic study,[37] when the pelvic floor musculature was paralyzed, subjects maintained urinary continence. Krahn and Morales[38] found the same phenomenon after transurethral resection of the prostate when proximal bladder neck sphincter function had been destroyed.

The striated urethral sphincter is much bulkier in young men undergoing the retropubic operation; older patients often have visible age-related sphincter atrophy. Older patients often also have BPH with detrusor hypertrophy, as evidenced by trabeculation, cellule, and diverticula formation, and this produces detrusor instability. If the prostate is removed, the combination of sphincter

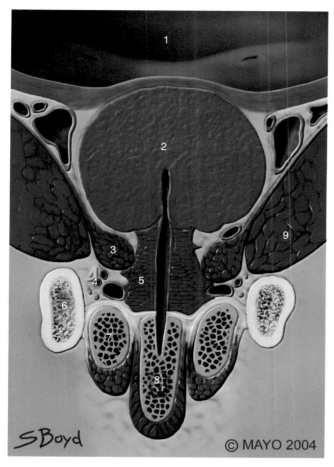

Figure 9.6
Anatomy of radical prostatectomy, coronal section through midprostate (2) and striated urethral sphincter (5), adapted from magnetic resonance image of a 52-year-old man. 1, urinary bladder; 3, levator ani; 4, anterior recess of ischioanal fossa; 6, ischiopubic ramus; 7, corpus cavernosum; 8, corpus spongiosum; 9, obturator internus.
Courtesy of Mayo Foundation for Medical Education and Research.

atrophy plus detrusor instability makes the older patient more vulnerable to pad usage despite meticulous preservation of all the continence components of the urethral stump. Preoperative older patients should be counseled accordingly.

Puboperineal portion of the levator ani (pubourethralis, levator urethrae, "quick stop muscle" of Gosling)

As mentioned above, the striated sphincter is flanked by the thickened anteromedial edges of the anterior levator ani, or what Oelrich called the urogenital hiatus (Figure 9.6).[39] This anterior levator hiatus begins posterior to the urethra at the level of and anteriorly adjacent to the anorectal junction and perineal body. As the

puboperineal portion of the levatores ani,[40] the medial fibers of the puborectalis sling do not follow its outer fibers around the anorectal junction; they descend diagonally downward on either side of the sphincteric (membranous) urethra to insert in the midline perineal body anterior to the anorectal junction. Thus, they form an incomplete sling behind the urethra. On contraction, they forcefully propel the prostate, prostatourethral junction, and striated sphincter upward and forward toward the posterior pubis. Santorini[41] called these thickenings "projectors," and their action has been confirmed in dynamic MRI.[42] This action then allows the quick stop of urination.[43] The upward, forward movement is countered by the horseshoe-shaped striated sphincter, which contracts downward and backward toward the perineal body. This counter-contraction of the striated sphincter has been corroborated by transluminal urethral ultrasonography during pelvic floor contraction.[44] Thus, there is an opposing active loop system: outer levator ani loop upward and forward, and striated sphincter loop backward and downward. The bladder neck is thought to function similarly, but the opposing loops, outer longitudinal detrusor (bundle of Heiss) and inner circular detrusor, are both smooth muscle loops, whereas the distal sphincter mechanism is essentially opposing striated muscle loops.

Intact blood vessels and nerves

Urethral length and integrity of the urinary continence tissue components of mucosa, urethral wall, smooth muscle, elastic tissue, and striated sphincter are moot if the blood vessels and nerves are significantly injured during dissection. How can this occur? Somatic branches of the pudendal nerve innervate the levator ani muscle superiorly and inferiorly. Practically speaking, this means that there are significant branches on the inner surface of the levator ani during lateral mobilization of the levator ani in the retropubic operation and on the undersurface of the levator ani in the perineal operation. Branches from above and below the pelvic diaphragm also supply the striated sphincter. Autonomic innervation is also thought to be dual. Whether above or below the pelvic diaphragm, somatic and autonomic fibers predominate at the 5- and 7-o'clock positions in relationship to the striated sphincter. Some fibers travel in the NVBs. Not all autonomic fibers are destined for the cavernous bodies of the penis. In 1982, Walsh and Donker[45] elucidated the nature of the cavernous nerve supply to the penis with respect to the prostate and clarified why men subject to radical prostatectomy were virtually always rendered impotent. Walsh et al[2] then showed how the cavernous nerves in the NVB could be saved and the patient rendered potent on a consistent basis. Walsh's monumental work paved the way for significant evolution in surgical technique. Of interest, in 1975, Finkle et al[46] reported potency preservation in four of five patients undergoing the perineal operation, but did not explain why. Cavernous nerves are multiple in each bundle and originally were characterized as major and minor.[31] In a study of one NVB, the nerves varied in diameter from approximately 0.04 to 0.37 mm, averaging 0.12 mm.[47]

Takenaka et al[48] recently performed cadaveric dissections and showed the "spray-like" entry of pelvic splanchnic nerve components as they join hypogastric nerve components to the nerve bundle distal to the vesicoprostatic junction. Their findings may be of significance with respect to sural nerve graft interposition in replacing a resected NVB.

In radical prostatectomy, it is possible to find a plane between the NVB and periprostatic "visceral" fascia overlying the capsule (interfascial dissection). Of anatomic importance, the nerves may travel very close to the medial surface of the NVB; when they also travel in close proximity to small arteries and veins that bleed, hemostasis by metal clip or suture may damage these tiny nerve fibers. The nerve bundles in cross-section subtend a crescentic shape as they hug the posterolateral aspect of the prostate. Autonomic nerves, some of which are destined for the cavernous bodies, are distributed throughout the NVB, and those situated at the tips of the crescent are particularly vulnerable to injury. The anterior tip of the crescent often contains veins and associated small arteries, as mentioned above, and the posterior tip of the crescent runs along the lateral aspect of the line of division of the PSVF. More recent studies[10,49] corroborate significant numbers of autonomic nerves in the lateral aspects of the PSVF. These PSVF-associated nerve fibers then are vulnerable to injury and sacrifice as a result of freeing the NVB from the adjacent prostate.

The NVB is delicate and tolerates little shear without breaking. It is tethered along the posterolateral prostate by fine capsular vessels that may angulate the NVB at the prostatourethral junction.[50] From an anatomic and surgical standpoint, release of these vessels from the adjacent prostate fascia then allows release of the NVB. The result of release at the apex of the prostate is the creation of an anatomic triangle formed by the NVB laterally and the prostate and urethra medially as the two additional legs of the triangle immediately adjacent to the prostatourethral junction. This relationship does not become apparent until the fibrous bands (ischioprostatic ligaments, Walsh's pillar tissue) are severed at their prostate junction, as mentioned above.

In the region of the vascular pedicle to the prostate at the vesicoprostatic junction laterally, the NVB is relatively thick.[50] The reason for this is that the pedicle contains, in addition to the inferior vessels to the bladder, numerous ganglia and branch points for autonomic nerves supplying the seminal vesicles, vasa deferentia, and bladder.[31,48,49,51] From the pedicle running distally toward the apex of the prostate, there is notable narrowing of the bundle.

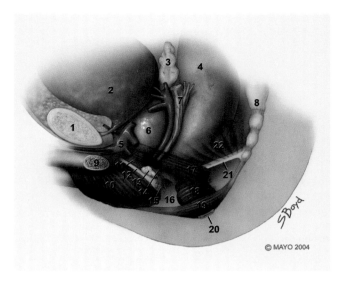

Figure 9.7

Anatomy of radical prostatectomy, three-dimensional side view of male pelvis, developed from sagittal magnetic resonance image. 1, pubis; 2, urinary bladder with pubovesical (puboprostatic) ligament; 3, seminal vesicle; 4, rectum; 5, dorsal vein complex with venous sinus; 6, prostate; 7, neurovascular bundle; 8, coccyx; 9, corpus cavernosum; 10, bulbospongiosus; 11, striated urethral sphincter; 12, perineal membrane; 13, bulbourethral gland; 14, "rectourethralis;" 15, transverse superficial perinei; 16, retrobulbar "space;" 17, puboanalis (puborectalis); 18, deep external anal sphincter; 19, superficial external anal sphincter; 20, anus; 21, anococcygeal ligament; 22, pubococcygeus, iliococcygeus, and coccygeus components of pelvic diaphragm (from anterior to posterior).

Courtesy of Mayo Foundation for Medical Education and Research.

Levatores ani and anal sphincters

Radical prostatectomy by any route is impossible without mobilization of the levator ani, whose muscle fibers embrace the lateral surfaces of the prostate, urethra, and anorectal junction. Fecal soiling after radical prostatectomy is a serious health-related quality-of-life issue. Determination of its frequency requires a validated prospective questionnaire like the UCLA prostate cancer index, which measures both bowel function (dysfunction) and bother (distress).[52] If a surgeon denies that it happens in his practice, he simply may not have asked his patients about an embarrassing subject. Reduced anal manometry pressures and fecal soiling have been reported after both perineal and retropubic operations.[53] The cause is very likely damage to the levator ani and its nerve supply.

Retropubic operation

The levatores ani, which form a conical pelvic diaphragm,[54] are first encountered after the endopelvic fascia is incised 3 to 5 mm lateral to the fascial tendinous arch (arcus tendineus fasciae pelvis, *TA*). This muscle bulges medially on each side because it overlies the inner convex surface of the underlying obturator internus superiorly and adipose tissue to the underlying ischioanal fossae inferiorly

(Figure 9.6). (The obturator internus is covered and usually not seen in this maneuver unless there is the rare convergence of the fascial and muscular tendinous arches of the pelvis.[55]) Fibers of the levator ani that comprise its puborectalis (puboanalis) portion pass posteriorly toward the anorectal junction where the anal canal, situated below the pelvic diaphragm, meets the rectum above the pelvic diaphragm (Figure 9.7).

During dissection of the prostate, the first fibers of the levator ani laterally to be disturbed are those of the pubococcygeus, which tightly embrace the lateral surface of the prostate in a very thin sheet. In the retropubic operation, these fibers are displaced laterally with an instrument or index finger in order to see the lateral surfaces of the prostate; it is this maneuver that may disrupt muscle fiber integrity as well as pelvic nerve innervation along the superior surface of the pelvic diaphragm.[56]

As the prostatourethral junction is exposed, the thickened anteromedial edges of the anterior levator hiatus are evident immediately adjacent to the insertion of the pubovesical (puboprostatic) ligaments. The pubic insertion points of the levator ani are tiny but serve as the take-off for the sling (puborectalis, puboanalis[35]) around the anorectal junction that is so important to fecal control. The deep external anal sphincter fuses to the puborectalis posteriorly, and together they are primarily responsible for fecal continence (Figure 9.7). The tiny tendinous insertion points of the puborectalis sling are situated only 1.3 cm lateral to the midline.[57] *Because these points of insertion are immediately adjacent to the insertion points of the pubovesical (puboprostatic) ligaments, they are subject to inadvertent transection if the pubovesical ligaments are transected at their pubic attachment. If this happens, the patient might experience compromised fecal control.*

Perineal operation

Once the perineal skin incision is made, the first sphincter to be encountered is the superficial external anal sphincter (superficial sphincter). It has prominent bow-shaped extensions (bows) on either side of the anus. Anteriorly, the bows converge in the midline tendinous insertion into the midline raphe of the bulb along its inferior surface. *The insertion point of this muscle is not into the perineal body, as commonly illustrated.* It is the anterior insertion point into the bottom of the bulb of the penis that allows the creation of a retrobulbar space with an index finger (Figure 9.8). With the finger so placed, the sphincter can be taken down at its bulbar insertion point, or divided transversely anterior to the anus in what is known as the Young technique of dividing the "central tendon."[58] It is not commonly appreciated that the anterior bowlike extensions of the superficial sphincter may be transected along with the midline fibrous tissue. Alternatively, the superficial sphincter is so situated that entry into the retrobulbar space can be achieved by retraction of the bows anterolaterally in what is known as the Belt technique.[59] The superficial sphincter has perianal subcutaneous attachment as the bows pass the anus, and this is sometimes illustrated as a separate cutaneous sphincter. However, in gross dissection, the cutaneous fibers are not separate but an integral part of the superficial sphincter. Posteriorly, the bows converge into tendinous attachment to the tip of the coccyx. Importantly, the superficial sphincter is not essential to anal continence. Some of its anterior fibers have been diagrammed converging with the bulbospongiosus and the superficial transverse perinei muscles.[60]

Just superior to the superficial sphincter is the deep external anal sphincter (Figure 9.7), which is closely bound to the anterior wall of the anal canal. In the perineal operation, it should be passed over without disturbance in progressing from the retrobulbar space to the rectourethralis attachment at the anorectal junction. As noted above, the deep sphincter fuses posteriorly with the puborectalis and is absolutely essential for anal continence. In the perineal operation, the recto-urethralis attachment to the perineal body, which centers on the midline posterior aspect of the perineal membrane at the superior backside of the bulb, is transected. Transecting the rectourethralis allows the anorectal junction to lose its sharp anterior angulation and to drop away posteriorly. The anal canal (3–4-cm long in the adult male) has a thick wall due to the presence of the smooth muscle internal anal sphincter. The wall of the rectum superior to the rectourethralis is much thinner. It is at this junction of thick anal canal wall to thin rectal wall that provides the opportunity for inadvertent rectotomy.

After takedown of the rectourethralis, the posterior prostatourethral junction is first exposed. The levator ani muscle that must be retracted laterally to expose the prostate is first the puborectalis sling and more deeply the pubococcygeus. The puborectalis is a misnomer in the sense that its sling passes behind the anococcygeal ligament; it is literally more puboanalis than puborectalis. Some of its inferior fibers insert directly into the wall of the anal canal intercalating with fibers of the smooth muscle internal sphincter, the conjoined longitudinal fibers.[61]

Rectourethralis

The rectourethralis is a fibromuscular complex that produces anterior angulation of the anorectal junction, as noted above. It consists primarily of a dominant (more substantial) midline component of smooth muscle from the anterior wall of the anal canal coming from below (anoperinealis, *TA*) and a less dominant midline component of smooth muscle from the anterior wall of the rectum coming from above (rectoperinealis, *TA*). These two components then converge from below and above, respectively, and insert into the perineal body (central tendon of the perineum). There is no direct urethral attachment. Importantly, the attachment anteriorly is distal to the posterior apex of the prostate, and therefore *the rectourethralis is not part of the retropubic operation as it is in the perineal operation.* Descriptions of the retropubic operation often mistakenly describe transection of the rectourethralis after urethral transection, when what is being described is actually transection of the termination of the PSVF as it joins the midline fibrous tissue raphe of the perineal body. The rectourethralis attachment varies considerably in bulk from thick to thin.

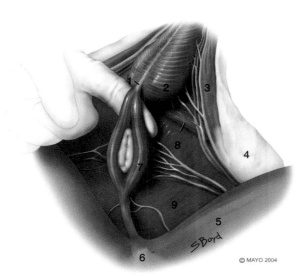

© MAYO 2004

Figure 9.8
Anatomy of radical perineal prostatectomy, initial index finger development of retrobulbar space beneath anterior extension of the superficial external anal sphincter (7). 1, central tendon; 2, bulbospongiosus; 3, ischiocavernosus; 4, ischial tuberosity; 5, gluteus maximus; 6, coccyx; 8, superficial transverse perinei; 9, levator ani.

Courtesy of Mayo Foundation for Medical Education and Research.

References

1. Federative Committee on Anatomical Terminology. Terminologia Anatomica: International Anatomical Terminology/FCAT. Stuttgart: Thieme, 1998.
2. Walsh PC, Lepor H, Eggleston JC. Radical prostatectomy with preservation of sexual function: anatomical and pathological considerations. Prostate 1983;4:473–485.

3. Silver PH. The role of the peritoneum in the formation of the septum recto-vesicale. J Anat 1956;90:538–546.

4. Lindsey I, Guy RJ, Warren BF, et al. Anatomy of Denonvilliers' fascia and pelvic nerves, impotence, and implications for the colorectal surgeon. Br J Surg 2000;87:1288–1299.

5. Villers A, Stamey TA, Yemoto C, et al. Modified extrafascial radical retropubic prostatectomy technique decreases frequency of positive surgical margins in T2 cancers <2 cm³. Eur Urol 2000;38:64–73.

6. Benoit G, Delmas V, Quillard J, et al. Surgical significance of Denonvilliers' aponeurosis [French]. Ann Urol (Paris) 1984;18:284–287.

7. van Ophoven A, Roth S. The anatomy and embryological origins of the fascia of Denonvilliers: a medico-historical debate. J Urol 1997;157:3–9.

8. Villers A, McNeal JE, Freiha FS, et al. Invasion of Denonvilliers' fascia in radical prostatectomy specimens. J Urol 1993;149:793–798.

9. Vordos D, Delmas V, Hermieu JF, et al. Can a precise vesiculectomy be performed during radical prostatectomy? [French]. Prog Urol 2001;11:1259–1263.

10. Kourambas J, Angus DG, Hosking P, et al. A histological study of Denonvilliers' fascia and its relationship to the neurovascular bundle. Br J Urol 1998;82:408–410.

11. Stamey TA, Villers AA, McNeal JE, et al. Positive surgical margins at radical prostatectomy: importance of the apical dissection. J Urol 1990;143:1166–1172.

12. Benoit G, Droupy S, Quillard J, et al. Supra and infralevator neurovascular pathways to the penile corpora cavernosa. J Anat 1999;195:605–615.

13. Myers RP. Detrusor apron, associated vascular plexus, and avascular plane: relevance to radical retropubic prostatectomy: anatomic and surgical commentary. Urology 2002;59:472–479.

14. McNeal JE. The prostate and prostatic urethra: a morphologic synthesis. J Urol 1972;107:1008–1016.

15. McNeal JE. New morphologic findings relevant to the origin and evolution of carcinoma of the prostate and BPH. UICC Technical Rep Series 1979;48:24–37.

16. Steiner MS. The puboprostatic ligament and the male urethral suspensory mechanism: an anatomic study. Urology 1994;44:530–534.

17. Myers RP. The surgical management of prostate cancer: radical retropubic and radical perineal prostatectomy. In Lepor H (ed): Prostatic Diseases. Philadelphia: WB Saunders, 2000, pp 410–443.

18. Heiss R. Über den Sphincter vesicae internus. Archiv Anat Physiol 1916;24:367–384.

19. Wesson MB. Anatomical, embryological and physiological studies of the trigone and neck of the bladder. J Urol 1920;4:279–315.

20. Woodburne RT. Anatomy of the bladder and bladder outlet. J Urol 1968;100:474–487.

21. McNeal JE. Normal histology of the prostate. Am J Surg Pathol 1988;12:619–633.

22. Myers RP. An anatomic approach to the pelvis in the male. In Crawford ED, Das S (eds): Current Genitourinary Cancer Surgery, 2nd ed. Baltimore: Williams & Wilkins, 1997, pp 155–169.

23. McNeal JE. The zonal anatomy of the prostate. Prostate 1981;2:35–49.

24. Glenister TW. The development of the utricle and of the so-called 'middle' or 'median' lobe of the human prostate. J Anat 1962;96:443–455.

25. Turner Warwick R. The sphincter mechanisms: their relation to prostatic enlargement and its treatment. In Hinman F Jr (ed): Benign Prostatic Hypertrophy. New York: Springer-Verlag, 1983, pp 809–828.

26. Blacklock NJ. Surgical anatomy of the prostate. In Williams DI, Chisholm GD (eds): Scientific Foundations of Urology, vol 2. London: William Heinemann Medical Books, 1976, pp 113–125.

27. Myers RP. Male urethral sphincteric anatomy and radical prostatectomy. Urol Clin North Am 1991;18:211–227.

28. Hudson PB. Perineal prostatectomy. In Campbell MF, Harrison JH (eds): Urology, vol 3, 3rd edn. Philadelphia: WB Saunders, 1970, p 2436.

29. Ukimura O, Gill IS, Desai MM, et al. Real-time transrectal ultrasonography during laparoscopic radical prostatectomy. J Urol 2004;172:112–118.

30. Walsh PC. Radical prostatectomy, preservation of sexual function, cancer control: the controversy. Urol Clin North Am 1987;14:663–673.

31. Müller J. Ueber die organischen Nerven der erectilen männlichen Geschlectsorgane des Menschen und der Säugethiere. Berlin: F Dümmler, 1836.

32. Yucel S, Baskin LS. An anatomical description of the male and female urethral sphincter complex. J Urol 2004;171:1890–1897.

33. Netter FH. Atlas of Human Anatomy, Pelvis and Perineum. Summit, NJ: Ciba-Geigy, 1989, Plate 361.

34. Walsh PC, Marschke PL. Intussusception of the reconstructed bladder neck leads to earlier continence after radical prostatectomy. Urology 2002;59:934–938.

35. Myers RP, Cahill DR, Devine RM, et al. Anatomy of radical prostatectomy as defined by magnetic resonance imaging, J Urol 1998;159:2148–2158.

36. Coakley FV, Eberhardt S, Kattan MW, et al. Urinary continence after radical retropubic prostatectomy: relationship with membranous urethral length on preoperative endorectal magnetic resonance imaging. J Urol 2002;168:1032–1035.

37. Caine M, Edwards D. The peripheral control of micturition: a cineradiographic study. Br J Urol 1958;30:34–42.

38. Krahn MD, Mahoney JE, Eckman MH, et al. Screening for prostate cancer: a decision analytic view. JAMA 1994;272:773–780.

39. Oelrich TM. The urethral sphincter muscle in the male. Am J Anat 1980;158:229–246.

40. Myers RP, Cahill DR, Kay PA, et al. Puboperineales: muscular boundaries of the male urogenital hiatus in 3D from magnetic resonance imaging. J Urol 2000;164:1412–1415.

41. Santorini GD. Observationes Anatomicae. Venetiis: JB Recurti, 1724, pp173–205.

42. Mikuma N, Tamagawa M, Morita K, et al. Magnetic resonance imaging of the male pelvic floor: the anatomical configuration and dynamic movement in healthy men. Neurourol Urodyn 1998;17:591–597.

43. Gosling JA, Dixon JS, Critchley HO, et al. A comparative study of the human external sphincter and periurethral levator ani muscles. Br J Urol 1981;53:35–41.

44. Strasser H, Poisel S, Stenzl A, et al. Anatomy and innervation of the male urethra, the rhabdosphincter, and the corpora cavernosa (Lesson 16). AUA Update Series 2001;20:122–127.

45. Walsh PC, Donker PJ. Impotence following radical prostatectomy: insight into etiology and prevention. J Urol 1982;128:492–497.

46. Finkle JE, Finkle PS, Finkle AL. Encouraging preservation of sexual function postprostatectomy. Urology 1975;6:697–702.

47. Myers RP. Gross and applied anatomy of the prostate. In Kantoff PW, Carroll PR, D'Amico AV (eds): Prostate Cancer: Principles and Practice. Philadelphia: Lippincott Williams & Wilkins, 2002, pp 3–15.

48. Takenaka A, Murakami G, Soga H, et al. Anatomical analysis of the neurovascular bundle supplying penile cavernous tissue to ensure a reliable nerve graft after radical prostatectomy. J Urol 2004;172:1032–1035.

49. Costello A, Brooks M, Cole OJ. Anatomical studies of the neurovascular bundle and cavernous nerves. BJU Int 2004;94:1071–1076.

50. Walsh PC. Anatomic radical retropubic prostatectomy. In Walsh PC, Retik AB, Vaughan ED Jr, Wein AJ (eds): Campbell's Urology, 8th edn. Philadelphia: WB Saunders, 2002, pp 3107–3129.

51. Lepor H, Gregerman M, Crosby R, et al. Precise localization of the autonomic nerves from the pelvic plexus to the corpora cavernosa: a detailed anatomical study of the adult male pelvis. J Urol 1985;133:207–212.

52. Litwin MS, Sadetsky N, Pasta DJ, et al. Bowel function and bother after treatment for early stage prostate cancer: a longitudinal quality of life analysis from CaPSURE. J Urol 2004;172:515–519.

53. Bishoff JT, Motley G, Optenberg SA, et al. Incidence of fecal and urinary incontinence following radical perineal and retropubic prostatectomy in a national population. J Urol 1998;160:454–458.

54. Brooks JD, Chao WM, Kerr J. Male pelvic anatomy reconstructed from the visible human data set. J Urol 1998;159:868–872.

55. Thompson P. On the arrangement of the fasciae of the pelvis and their relationship to the levator ani. J Anat Physiol 1901;35:127–141.
56. Hollabaugh RS Jr, Dmochowski RR, Steiner MS. Neuroanatomy of the male rhabdosphincter. Urology 1997;49:426–434.
57. Uhlenhuth ECA. Problems in the Anatomy of the Pelvis. Philadelphia: Lippincott, 1953.
58. Young HH, Davis DM. Young's Practice of Urology: Based on a Study of 12,500 Cases, vol 2. Philadelphia: WB Saunders, 1926, pp 414–512.
59. Belt E, Ebert CE, Surber AC Jr. New anatomic approach in perineal prostatectomy. J Urol 1939;41:482–497.
60. Roux C. Beiträge zur Kenntniss der Aftermuskulatur des Menschen [German]. Archiv Mikr Anat 1880–1881;19:721–733.
61. Lawson JO. Pelvic anatomy: I: pelvic floor muscles. Ann R Coll Surg Engl 1974;54:244–252.

10

Anatomic radical retropubic prostatectomy

J Kellogg Parsons, Alan W Partin, Patrick C Walsh

Introduction

Since its initial description by Walsh, anatomic radical retropubic prostatectomy (RRP) has become the gold standard to which all other therapies for localized prostate cancer are compared. The first surgical procedure to provide definitive therapy with acceptably low rates of morbidity, RRP has transformed prostate cancer treatment paradigms and galvanized basic science research by making available for study previously unprecedented amounts of prostate tissue. In this chapter, the evolution, preoperative evaluation, surgical technique, and postoperative management of RRP for treatment of clinically localized prostate cancer are discussed.

Evolution of radical retropubic prostatectomy

The modern RRP developed from two distinct but complementary insights: first, that prostate removal is technically feasible; second, that prostate removal may potentially benefit patients with prostate cancer. Kuchler[1] reported the earliest documented prostatectomy in 1858 via a perineal approach. Forty years later, Young[2] both refined the technical performance of the radical perineal prostatectomy and conceived of its application to prostate cancer. In 1947, Millin[3] first described the retropubic approach for radical prostatectomy and the removal of benign adenomas. Over the next decade, a number of investigators modified Millin's technique.[4–8] The radical retropubic approach, however, failed to gain widespread acceptance due to its associations with severe intraoperative hemorrhage and inappropriately high rates of postoperative urinary incontinence and impotence.

During the late 1970s and early 1980s, a series of seminal observations provided three key insights into periprostatic anatomy that vastly improved the surgeon's ability to radically excise the prostate with substantially reduced morbidity. First, detailed anatomic characterization of the dorsal vein improved intraoperative hemostasis and permitted more precise dissection in a relatively bloodless field,[9,10] which in turn resulted in fewer transfusions, shorter hospital stays, substantially improved postoperative urinary continence,[11–13] and superior cancer control. Second, elucidation of the anatomy of the pelvic nerve plexus and its structural relationship to sexual function led to precise modifications in surgical technique that, for the first time, made it possible to systematically preserve this plexus and thereby maintain potency in appropriately selected men.[10] Third, Oelrich's descriptions[14] of striated urethral sphincter structure allowed for greater preservation of urinary continence.

Thereafter, RRP was widely adopted as a primary therapy for localized prostate cancer.

Preoperative evaluation

Preoperative evaluation should include clinical staging when indicated (see Chapter 43) and discussion of the risks, complications, and expected benefits of the procedure. Surgery should be deferred for a minimum of 4 to 6 weeks following prostate biopsy or transurethral resection of the prostate. This delay, which will not compromise long-term cancer control,[15] allows for resolution of inflammatory adhesions or hematomas that may obscure visualization of the anatomic relationships between the prostate and adjacent structures.

During the preoperative period, patients may elect to donate 2 or 3 units of blood to decrease the risk of receiving a perioperative homologous transfusion. The relative costs and benefits of preoperative autologous transfusion, however, remain a focus of debate. Although some investigators have observed significantly lower rates of homologous transfusion among preoperative autologous blood donors,[16,17] others have not,[18] while still others have noted that a majority of autologous units are either discarded[19] or inappropriately given to patients with low cardiac risk.[20] In counseling these patients, therefore, the surgeon may wish to consider two pieces of information. First, the probability of receiving a perioperative homologous blood transfusion among those who do not donate blood appears to be low: 2.4% to 3.8% at three high-volume university hospitals.[18,21,22] Second, the following variables have been associated with increased risk of homologous transfusion: a low-volume surgeon (defined as <15 RRPs performed annually) (OR, 8.63; 95% CI, 3.95–18.86), neoadjuvant hormonal therapy (OR, 3.35; 95% CI, 1.51–7.44), general anesthesia (OR, 2.22; 95% CI, 1.12–4.41), and prostate volume greater than 50 g (OR, 1.74; 95% CI, 1.33–2.29).[22]

Another potential option to lower the risk of homologous transfusion is preoperative administration of erythropoietin (Epoetin alfa). Lepor et al[23–25] have observed that preoperative erythropoietin increases serum hemoglobin concentration and is associated with rates of perioperative homologous transfusion comparable to patients who donate autologous blood. However, it is unclear if preoperative erythropoietin decreases the risk of homologous transfusion among men who do not donate autologous blood.

Regardless of preoperative transfusion status, patients should be counseled to avoid medications with potential antiplatelet effects—including vitamin E greater than 400 IU/day, aspirin, clopidogrel (Plavix®), and nonaspirin nonsteroidal anti-inflammatory drugs—for at least 1 week prior to donating blood or having surgery.

We recommend restriction to a clear liquid diet on the day before surgery, oral ingestion of magnesium citrate 250 ml the evening before surgery, and administration of a Fleets® enema early in the morning on the day of surgery. We also recommend administration of standard preoperative antibiotic prophylaxis and application of thromboembolic deterrent stockings and sequential compression devices to the lower extremities prior to beginning the procedure.

Surgical technique

Instruments and positioning

RRP requires few special instruments. We recommend use of a fiberoptic headlight, which facilitates illumination of the retropubic space; a Balfour retractor with narrow and standard wide malleable blades for retraction of the peritoneum; coagulating forceps; and 2.5 to 4.5 power loupes to enhance visualization of the neurovascular bundles (NVBs).

Preexisting medical conditions and anesthesiologist and patient preferences should dictate choice of anesthesia. General, spinal or epidural anesthetics are all acceptable alternatives. Data suggest that regional (spinal or epidural) anesthesia may be associated with less operative blood loss,[17,22,26,27] but not with decreased postoperative morbidity.[28]

The patient is placed supine and flat on the operative table. After skin preparation and sterile draping, a 16-Fr Foley catheter is passed into the bladder, the balloon inflated with 20 ml of saline, and the catheter connected to sterile, closed, continuous drainage.

Incision and pelvic lymph node dissection

A midline, infraumbilical incision is extended from the pubis to the umbilicus. The rectus muscles are separated along the midline and the transversalis fascia is opened sharply without violation of the peritoneal cavity. The anterior fascia is incised inferiorly to the pubis, while the posterior fascia is left intact. The space of Retzius is developed manually, and the peritoneum is mobilized off the external iliac vessels—with care taken not to disturb the tissue overlying the external iliac artery—just caudal to the vas deferens to allow for placement of the narrow retractor blade. We do not recommend isolation and/or division of the vasa, nor development of the retroperitoneal space, as these maneuvers do not facilitate subsequent performance of the operation.

Next, after the Balfour retractor is placed, a narrow malleable blade is used to expose the iliac vessels and provide visualization of the lateral pelvis for staging pelvic lymph node dissection. If necessary, a deep Deaver retractor may provide additional medial retraction of the bladder. Lymph node dissection is initiated on the side of the dominant tumor. Careful division of the adventitia over the external iliac vein with Metzenbaum scissors facilitates access to the obturator fossa and allows for development of the space immediately posterior to the external iliac vein (Figure 10.1). A Gil-Vernet or similar retractor is placed under the external iliac vein to provide gentle anterior retraction. The dissection then moves inferiorly toward the femoral canal, with the surgeon bluntly sweeping the nodal package away from the pelvic sidewall while simultaneously

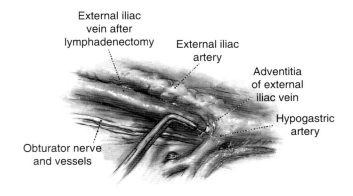

Figure 10.1
View of the right pelvis after completion of the staging lymph node dissection. Note that the fibroadipose tissue around the obturator nerve and vessels—but not that overlying the external iliac artery—has been removed.

Courtesy of the Brady Urological Institute.

identifying the obturator nerve. The nodal tissue should be ligated distal to Cloquet's node, with care taken not to injure the obturator nerve.

The dissection then proceeds superiorly along the pelvic side wall to the bifurcation of the common iliac artery, where the lymph nodes lying in the angle between the external iliac and hypogastric arteries are removed. Posteriorly, the dissection is carried down to the hypogastric veins.[29] The adventitia overlying the external iliac artery should be preserved to maintain lymphatic drainage from the lower extremities. Next, the obturator lymph nodes are removed with care taken to avoid injury to the obturator nerve, artery, and vein. The narrow retractor blade is then removed and the dissection is repeated on the contralateral side. We do not routinely perform frozen-section analyses unless there are palpable nodal abnormalities.

Incision of the endopelvic fascia

Once the nodal dissection is completed, we recommend that the surgeon utilizes 2.5 to 4.5 power loupes for the remainder of the operation. To expose the anterior surface of the prostate, the peritoneum is gently retracted superiorly with the wide malleable Balfour blade.

The fibroadipose tissue covering the anterior and anterolateral surfaces of the prostate is cleared with forceps to expose the pelvic fascia, puboprostatic ligaments, and superficial branches of the dorsal vein. The superficial branch of the dorsal vein complex medial to the puboprostatic ligaments is coagulated and divided. The endopelvic fascia is entered sharply with Metzenbaum scissors at its reflection over the pelvic sidewall, well away from the attachments to the bladder and prostate (Figure 10.2). Here, the endopelvic fascia fibers are translucent and should allow for visualization of the underlying levator ani musculature. After entering the endopelvic fascia, care should be taken not to injure the lateral aspect of the venous plexus of Santorini, which may be appreciated medially. The incision in the endopelvic fascia is extended anteromedially toward the puboprostatic ligaments. During this step, small arterial and

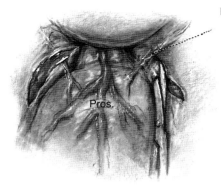

Internal pudendal
vessel branches
divided

Incising endopelvic
fascia

Pros.

Figure 10.2
Incision in the endopelvic fascia is made at the junction with the pelvic sidewall, well away from the bladder and prostate. Small anterior branches from the internal pudendal vessels are often encountered, and should be clipped and divided. Pros, prostate.

Courtesy of the Brady Urological Institute.

venous branches of the pudendal vessels may be encountered as they emerge from the pelvic musculature to supply the prostate. To avoid coagulation injury to the pudendal artery and nerve, located just deep to the muscle along the pubic ramus, these vessels should be ligated with clips.

After division of the endopelvic fascia bilaterally, a sponge stick is used to displace the prostate posteriorly, and the puboprostatic ligaments are sharply divided bilaterally with Metzenbaum scissors (Figure 10.3A). We suggest only dividing the ligaments enough to expose the apical surface of the prostate. The pubourethral component of the complex should remain intact to preserve the anterior fixation of the striated urethral sphincter to the pubis.[30]

Division of the dorsal complex and urethra

While displacing the prostate posteriorly with a sponge stick, a 3-0 monofilament suture on a 5/8 circle needle is passed anterior to the urethra through the dorsal vein complex just distal to the apex of the prostate (Figure 10.3B and C). Next, the needle is reversed in the needle driver and placed through the perichondrium of the pubic symphysis. This maneuver is repeated as a figure-of-eight suture and tied (Figure 10.3D and E), which accomplishes two objectives: first, because it elevates the distal complex, it enables the surgeon to visualize the plane on the anterior apex of the prostate during division of the dorsal vein complex; and second, it provides superior hemostasis (Figure 10.3F).

While again displacing the prostate posteriorly with a sponge stick, Metzenbaum scissors or a No 15 blade on a long handle are used to completely divide the dorsal vein complex (Figure 10.3G). Absolute hemostatic control of the complex is mandatory to provide a bloodless field for the remainder of the procedure. To achieve hemostasis, the same 3-0 monofilament suture placed through the pubic perichondrium during the previous step is used to oversew the superficial edges of the complex (Figure 10.4). In addition, clips may be used to control bleeding from circumflex veins often present at the posterior edges of the complex at 5 and 7 o'clock.

The proximal dorsal vein on the anterior surface of the prostate is oversewn with a 2-0 absorbable suture (Figure 10.4).

Once the vein is oversewn, attention is turned toward urethral division. Gentle posterior displacement of the prostate with a sponge stick should provide excellent visualization of the prostatourethral junction. A right-angle clamp should be passed immediately posterior to the urethral smooth muscle near the apex of the prostate to ensure that the urethra is transected as close to the apex as possible. The anterior urethra is then sharply divided with care taken to avoid entering the Foley catheter (Figure 10.4C). This should provide excellent exposure for urethral suture placement. If additional exposure is necessary, however, the anterior surface of the lateral bands of the striated urethral sphincter may be divided at their midpoint beyond the apex of the prostate.

Five 3-0 monofilament sutures on 5/8 circle tapered needles are then placed, from outside to inside, through the urethra at the following positions: 12, 2, 5, 7, and 10 o'clock. Each suture should incorporate the urethral mucosa and submucosa but exclude the smooth muscle of the sphincter (Figure 10.5). The 2 o'clock suture should be placed first, as it will elevate the urethral mucosa and submucosa, and thus facilitate placement of the remaining sutures. After placement, the sutures are tagged and covered with towels to avoid inadvertent traction or displacement. The Foley catheter is removed. A single suture is then placed through the urethra at the 6 o'clock position in the same manner as the previous five (Figure 10.6A), and the posterior wall of the urethra sharply divided (Figure 10.6B).

To divide the posterior portion of the sphincter complex and develop the plane between the prostate and rectum, the right-angle clamp is placed immediately posterior to the left edge of the complex at a point midway between the prostatic apex and the distal urethra (Figure 10.7). At this midway point, the NVBs are relatively posterior and thus should lie deep to the clamp.[31] Placement of the clamp too close to the prostatic apex may result in NVB damage.

The left border of the complex exposed by the clamp is sharply divided. Next, the right-angle clamp is placed immediately posterior to the right edge of the complex at the midway point (Figure 10.8, top) and the remaining complex is sharply divided (Figure 10.8, bottom). Division of the complex in this manner—lateral to medial on each side—minimizes the potential for inadvertent injury to the NVBs or rectum.

Incision of the superficial lateral pelvic fascia and apical dissection of the neurovascular bundle

During initial dissection of the NVBs, there should be no upward traction placed on the prostate; exposure should instead be accomplished by rolling the prostate from side to side with the sponge stick. The superficial layers of the lateral pelvic fascia are first released with the right-angle clamp at the bladder neck where the fibers coalesce into a thick band (Figure 10.9). Division of this band should immediately increase prostate mobility. The remainder of the superficial lateral pelvic fascia is then divided from the bladder neck to the apex (Figure 10.10). This maneuver, performed on each side, releases the NVBs laterally, which in turn facilitates performance of the next step—posterior release of the NVBs at the apex.

Division of the superficial lateral pelvic fascia should reveal the subtle groove on the posterolateral edge of the prostate that

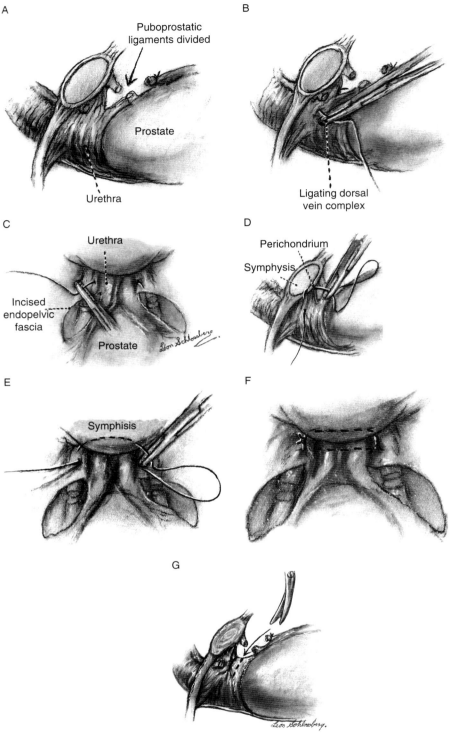

A
Puboprostatic
ligaments divided

Prostate

Urethra

B

Ligating dorsal
vein complex

C
Urethra

Incised
endopelvic
fascia

Prostate

D
Perichondrium

Symphysis

E
Symphisis

F

G

Figure 10.3

Steps in division of the dorsal vein complex. *A*, Superficial puboprostatic ligaments are sharply divided, exposing the junction between the apex of the prostate and the anterior surface of the dorsal vein complex. The pubourethral component of the complex should remain intact. *B* and *C*, 3-0 Monofilament suture is passed superficially through the dorsal vein complex just distal to the apex of the prostate. *D* and *E*, Needle is then reversed, and the same suture is placed through the perichondrium of the pubic symphysis. *F*, This horizontal suture is tied. *G*, Striated sphincter dorsal vein complex is then divided using Metzenbaum sutures.

Courtesy of the Brady Urological Institute.

marks the location of the NVB. Beginning at the apex, each bundle is released by gently rolling the prostate to the contralateral side and spreading with the right angle (Figure 10.11). Initial release of the bundles at the apex mitigates two potential difficulties that may be encountered. First, in patients in whom the bundle lies more anterior, apical release reduces the likelihood of confusing the groove with the potential space lying between the prostate and rectum. Second, in most patients, it facilitates identification and management of veins on the lateral surface of the prostate that run between Santorini's plexus anteriorly and the NVBs posteriorly. The dissection should proceed toward the base along the plane that leaves Denonvilliers' fascia and the prostatic fascia intact on the prostate but releases the residual fragments of the levator fascia laterally. If the NVBs do not fall easily from the prostate, there may be small apical vessels tethering it in place (Figures 10.12 and 10.13). These are best controlled with small clips placed parallel to the bundle followed by sharp division with fine scissors. Due to the potential for nerve injury, electrocoagulation should never be used on the bundle or its branches.[32] If fixation of a bundle to the prostate cannot be explained by vascular tethering, then tumor-induced desmoplasia should be suspected and the bundle excised.

A

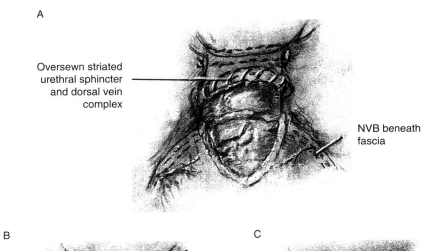

Oversewn striated urethral sphincter and dorsal vein complex

NVB beneath fascia

B

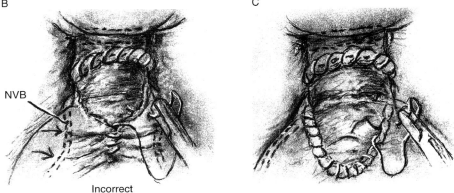

NVB

Incorrect

C

Figure 10.4
Ligation of the dorsal vein complex. *A*, Superficial edges of the distal striated urethral sphincter–dorsal vein complex have been oversewn utilizing the same 3-0 monofilament suture illustrated in Figures 10.3B and C. The edges of the proximal dorsal vein over the prostate are oversewn. If they are pulled together in the midline (*B*), the neurovascular bundles (NVBs) may be advanced too far anteriorly on the prostate, and thus may be in harm's way. Instead, the edges are oversewn in the shape of a "V" using a running 2-0 absorbable suture (*C*).

Courtesy of the Brady Urological Institute.

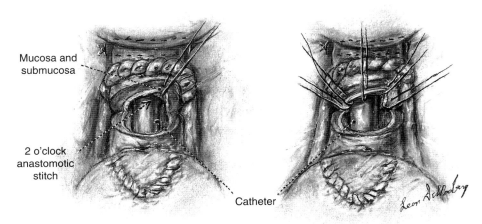

Mucosa and submucosa

2 o'clock anastomotic stitch

Catheter

Figure 10.5
Placement of urethral anastomotic sutures and division of the posterior urethra. 3-0 Monofilament sutures on 5/8 circle tapered needles are placed in the distal urethral segment, from outside to inside, at 12, 2, 5, 7, and 10 o'clock. The suture should incorporate only the mucosa and submucosa of the urethra. Placement of the 2 o'clock suture first facilitates placement of the other four.

Courtesy of the Brady Urological Institute.

A

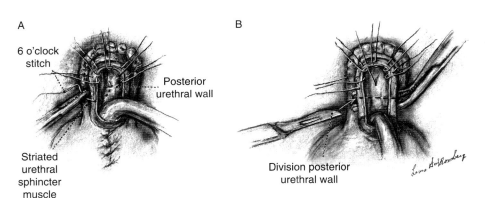

6 o'clock stitch

Posterior urethral wall

Striated urethral sphincter muscle

B

Division posterior urethral wall

Figure 10.6
A, After Foley catheter removal, a single 3-0 monofilament suture on a 5/8 circle tapered needle is placed at 6 o'clock in the same manner as the previous five. *B*, Posterior wall of the urethra is divided.

Courtesy of the Brady Urological Institute.

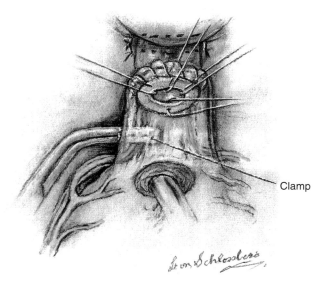

Figure 10.7
Right-angle clamp is passed immediately posterior to the left edge of the striated urethral sphincter complex, anterior to the neurovascular bundle (NVB), midway between the prostatic apex and the distal urethra.

Courtesy of the Brady Urological Institute.

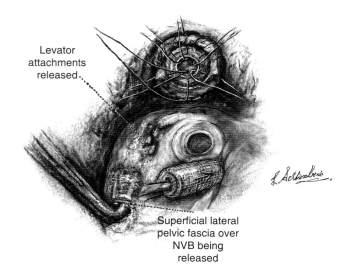

Figure 10.9
Incision of the superficial lateral pelvic fascia and exposure of the neurovascular bundle (NVB) grooves. The superficial layers of the lateral pelvic fascia are released with a right-angle clamp where the fibers coalesce into a thick broad surface.

Courtesy of the Brady Urological Institute.

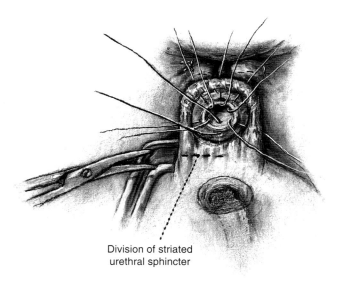

Figure 10.8
Division of the remaining striated urethral sphincter complex. A right-angle clamp is passed posterior to the right edge of the striated urethral sphincter complex midway between the prostatic apex and the distal urethra, and the complex is sharply divided.

Courtesy of the Brady Urological Institute.

Excision of the lateral pelvic fascia and the neurovascular bundle

Excision of the lateral pelvic fascia and NVBs on one or both sides may be necessary. The decision to excise should be based on preoperative evaluation and intraoperative findings. It is important to note that the bundle should not always be excised on the side of the positive biopsy or palpable lesion.[33,34]

Preoperative evaluation should include assessment of sexual function, lesion location (apex versus base), Partin Table probability of capsular extension, and presence of perineural invasion. These criteria should not be used as absolute indications. For example, when considering NVB excision in impotent men, it should be remembered that innervation from the NVBs to the smooth musculature of the urethra may play a role in the recovery of urinary control.[11,35]

There are three intraoperative findings which favor wide excision of the NVB: induration in the lateral pelvic fascia, adherence of the NVB to the prostate during release, and inadequate tissue covering the posterolateral surface of the prostate after prostate removal. This last point is important—the decision to excise or preserve the NVB may be made after prostate removal, and if there is insufficient soft tissue covering the prostate, secondary wide excision of the NVB may be performed.

It is almost never necessary to excise both NVBs.[34,36] Before performing unilateral NVB excision, the contralateral NVB should be freed from the prostate starting at the apex to avoid traction injury. The NVB to be excised is identified at the apex and isolated with a right-angle clamp, which is passed from medial to lateral immediately on the anterior surface of the rectum (Figure 10.14). To maximize the amount of soft tissue excised, the bundle is divided without ligation; if necessary, the distal end may be clipped later for hemostasis.

The dissection is then continued by dividing the fascia on the lateral surface of the rectum from the apex to the base; this allows for the NVB and abundant fascial tissue to be included in the specimen. This procedure is performed under direct vision, with the dissection terminating at the tip of the seminal vesicle, where the NVB is ligated and divided (Figure 10.15).

A

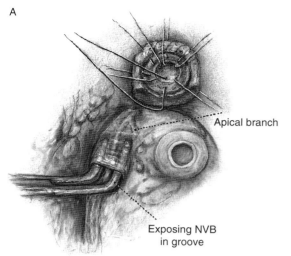

Apical branch

Exposing NVB
in groove

B

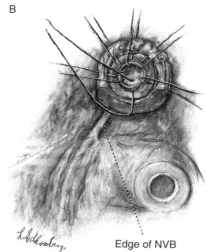

Edge of NVB

Figure 10.10
A and B, Remainder of the superficial lateral pelvic fascia is
divided from the bladder neck to
the apex. NVB, neurovascular
bundle.

Courtesy of the Brady Urological
Institute.

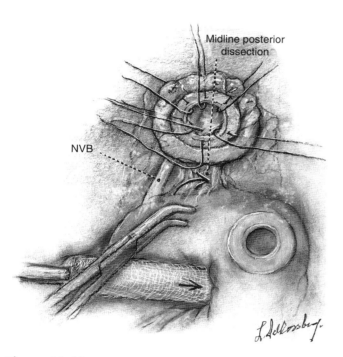

Midline posterior
dissection

NVB

Figure 10.11
Apical dissection of the neurovascular bundle (NVB). Each bundle
is released by gently rolling the prostate to the contralateral side
and spreading with the right angle.

Courtesy of the Brady Urological Institute.

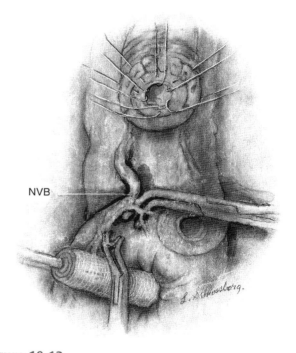

NVB

Figure 10.12
Using the plane that was established posteriorly, the vessels
should be released beginning at the apex. There is often an apical
vessel near the midline that tethers the neurovascular bundle
(NVB), causing it to kink as the prostate is pushed on its side.
Once these apical vessels are released, the bundle straightens out,
and the plane along the posterolateral surface of the prostate
becomes clearer.

Courtesy of the Brady Urological Institute.

Posterior dissection and division of the lateral pedicles

Once the NVBs have been released from the apex to the midpoint of
the prostate or widely excised, the catheter is replaced. Because the
NVBs have been released from the caudal aspect of the prostate,
cephalad-directed traction may now be applied to the catheter to
maximize exposure of the prostatic base and seminal vesicles. While
holding cephalad-directed traction on the catheter, the attachment
of Denonvilliers' fascia to the rectum is sharply divided in the

midline posteriorly. Denonvilliers' fascia overlying the seminal vesicles should be left intact (Figure 10.16A). Next, a prominent arterial branch arising from the NVB and running over the seminal
vesicles to supply the base of the prostate should be identified. This
vessel should be ligated on each side and divided (Figure 10.16B).
Division should cause each bundle to fall away posteriorly from the

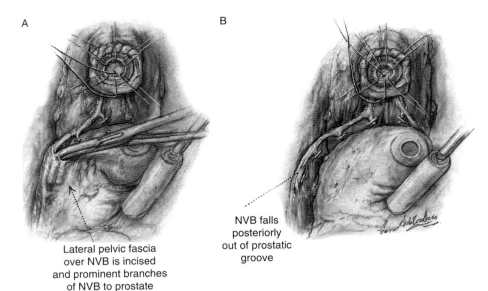

Figure 10.13

A, Small arterial and venous branches at the apex are divided using clips. *B*, Once the bundle has been identified and released at the apex, it should be released up to the mid-portion of the prostate.

Courtesy of the Brady Urological Institute.

Lateral pelvic fascia over NVB is incised and prominent branches of NVB to prostate are divided

NVB falls posteriorly out of prostatic groove

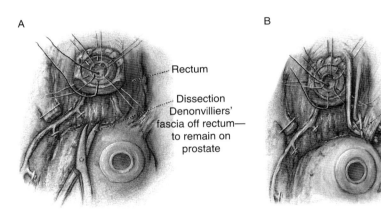

Figure 10.14

A, Residual attachments of the apex of the prostate in the midline are sharply released in preparation for wide excision of the right neurovascular bundle (NVB). *B*, Right-angle clamp is passed directly on the anterior surface of the rectum from medial to lateral, which minimizes the potential for rectal injury.

Courtesy of the Brady Urological Institute.

Rectum

Dissection Denonvilliers' fascia off rectum— to remain on prostate

NVB to be divided

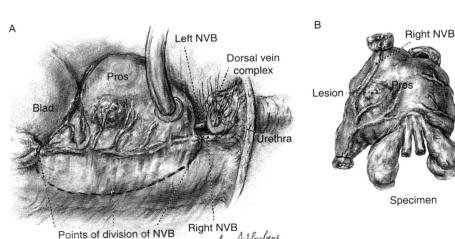

Figure 10.15

A, Lateral extent of neurovascular bundle (NVB) excision from the apex to the tip of the seminal vesicle, where the neurovascular bundle is ligated. *B*, Neurovascular bundle excision provides extensive soft tissue covering the primary lesion.

Courtesy of the Brady Urological Institute.

Left NVB

Dorsal vein complex

Pros

Blad

Urethra

Points of division of NVB   Right NVB

Right NVB

Lesion   Pros

Specimen

prostate and thus allow for safe division of the lateral pedicle on the lateral surface of the seminal vesicles without bundle injury (Figure 10.17).

The plane between the lateral edge of the seminal vesicles and the overlying lateral pelvic fascia is developed, and then each of the lateral pedicles is divided without ligation: superficial layers first,

followed by the deeper layers. Arterial bleeders are controlled with clips. In this manner, the dissection proceeds superiorly onto the anterolateral surface at the junction between the bladder and prostate. Denonvilliers' fascia is then divided over the tips of the seminal vesicles. If preferred, division of the vasa deferentia and mobilization of the seminal vesicles may be performed at this point.

A

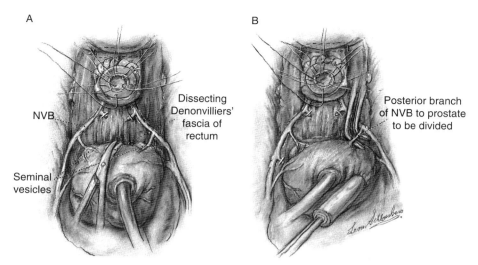

NVB

Dissecting Denonvilliers' fascia of rectum

Seminal vesicles

B

Posterior branch of NVB to prostate to be divided

Figure 10.16

Posterior dissection. *A,* Attachment of Denonvilliers' fascia to the rectum is released. Denonvilliers' fascia overlying the posterior surface of the seminal vesicles should be left intact. *B,* Arterial branch arising from the neurovascular bundle and running over the seminal vesicles to supply the base of the prostate is identified, ligated, and divided.

Courtesy of the Brady Urological Institute.

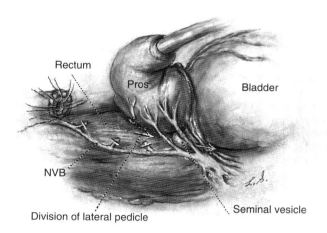

Rectum

Pros

Bladder

NVB

Division of lateral pedicle

Seminal vesicle

Figure 10.17

Lateral view demonstrating location of the neurovascular bundle (NVB) following ligation of the posterior branch to the prostate. Division of this posterior branch should free the NVB and allow it to fall away. Pros, prostate.

Courtesy of the Brady Urological Institute.

Prostatic bladder junction

Pros

Division of anterior bladder wall

Figure 10.18

Anterior bladder neck is incised along the anterior prostatovesicular junction.

Courtesy of the Brady Urological Institute.

Division of the bladder neck and excision of the seminal vesicles

Now that the prostate is nearly completely mobilized, the bladder neck is incised along the anterior prostatovesicular junction (Figure 10.18). The incision is carried through the mucosa. The Foley balloon is deflated, and the two ends of the catheter are clamped together to provide traction. As the incision in the bladder neck is widened, vessels running from the inferior vesical pedicle to the prostate will be encountered at 5 and 7 o'clock (Figure 10.19). Division of these vessels should reveal the plane lying between the anterior surface of the seminal vesicles and the posterior wall of the bladder. The posterior bladder neck is safely divided by using scissor dissection that hugs the anterior surface of the seminal vesicles, with attention paid to the location of the ureteral orifices (Figure 10.20).

After dividing the posterior bladder wall, the bladder neck is retracted with an Allis clamp. If not performed prior to division of the bladder neck, the vasa deferentia are now ligated with clips and divided, and the seminal vesicles are dissected free from surrounding structures (Figure 10.21). Since the pelvic plexus is located on the lateral surface of the seminal vesicles, as the tips of the seminal vesicles are freed, small arterial branches should be identified, ligated, and divided with care to avoid pelvic plexus injury. Any residual attachments of Denonvilliers' fascia are then divided, and the specimen is removed. The specimen is inspected carefully to identify any areas where the margin of resection is uncertain. If there is any concern about either of the margins on the posterolateral surfaces of the prostate, the NVB on that side should be excised.

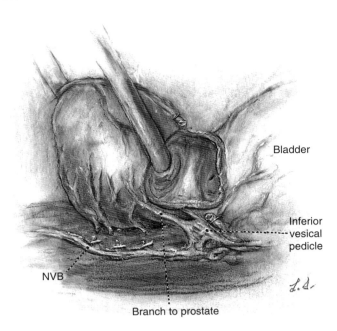

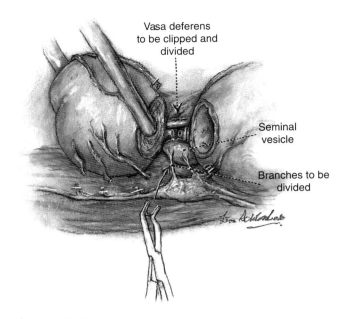

Figure 10.19

As the incision in the anterior bladder neck is extended, vessels running from the inferior vesical pedicle to the prostate will be encountered at 5 and 7 o'clock. Division of these vessels should reveal the plane lying between the anterior surface of the seminal vesicles and the posterior wall of the bladder.

Courtesy of the Brady Urological Institute.

Figure 10.21

Vasa deferentia are ligated and divided, and the seminal vesicles dissected free from the pelvic plexus with direct visualization and ligation of the small arterial branches.

Courtesy of the Brady Urological Institute.

The operative site is inspected carefully for bleeding. Small bleeding vessels near the NVB should be clipped—not cauterized—in order to avoid nerve injury.[32] Hemostatic control of these vessels is important for preventing hematoma development between the bladder and rectum.

Bladder neck closure and urethral anastomosis

The bladder neck is reconstructed using a running suture or interrupted sutures of 3-0 monofilament incorporating full-thickness muscularis and mucosa. A tennis-racket configuration is formed by initiating the closure in the posterior midline and proceeding anterior until the bladder neck is narrowed to the approximate the diameter of the urethra. To facilitate construction of a mucosa-to-mucosa urethrovesical anastomosis, three interrupted 4-0 monofilament sutures should be used to advance the mucosa over the raw musculature of the bladder neck (Figure 10.22). One of these sutures should be placed at the 6 o'clock position and left long to facilitate later placement of the urethral sutures.

To hasten the recovery of urinary control, Walsh has suggested the use of two additional buttressing sutures that intussuscept the bladder neck and prevent it from pulling open as the bladder fills.[37] These sutures are placed in three steps (Figure 10.23). First, a 2-0 monofilamanet suture is placed through the edges of the posterior bladder wall, approximately 2 cm posterior to the reconstructed bladder neck, where the bladder was previously attached to the prostate. This suture is tied in the midline.

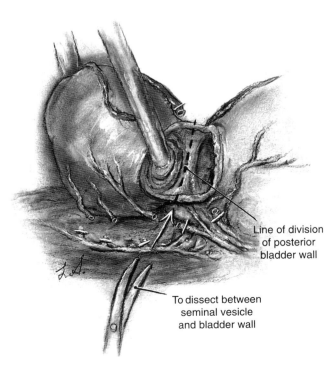

Figure 10.20

Posterior bladder neck is divided with careful scissor dissection.

Courtesy of the Brady Urological Institute.

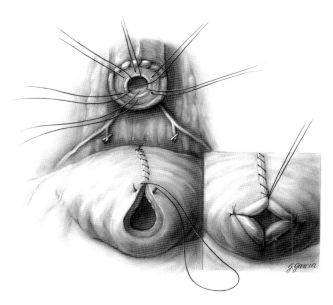

Figure 10.22
Tennis-racket closure of bladder neck using running 2-0 monofilament suture incorporating all layers of the bladder wall. The suture is tied and left long. *Inset,* Three interrupted 4-0 monofilament sutures are used to advance the mucosa over the raw musculature of the bladder neck.

Courtesy of the Brady Urological Institute.

A

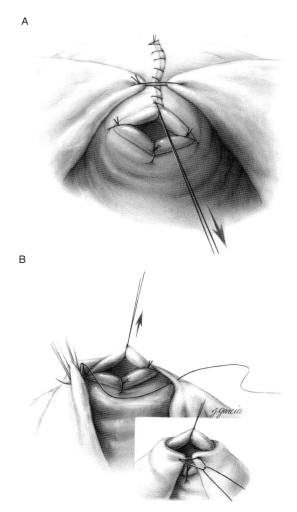

B

Figure 10.23
Intussusception of the bladder neck. *A,* 2-0 Chromic catgut suture is placed in the edges of the posterior bladder wall, about 2 cm from the reconstructed bladder neck, and is tied loosely in the midline. *B,* A second 2-0 monofilament suture is placed as a figure-of-eight approximately 2 cm lateral to the bladder neck on each side and is tied (*inset*).

Courtesy of the Brady Urological Institute.

Second, tension on the anterior bladder wall is released by loosening the malleable blade. This maneuver helps identify the loose perivesical tissue that should be incorporated in the next stitch. Third, another 2-0 monofilament suture is placed as a figure-of-eight approximately 2 cm lateral to the bladder neck on each side and tied loosely. The bladder neck should now lie beneath the anterior hood of tissue created by the anterior stitch, resembling a turtle that has pulled its head inside its shell.

The operative site is inspected carefully for bleeding. A new silicone Foley catheter (16-Fr, 5-ml balloon) is placed through the urethra and into the pelvis. Traction on the long ends of the mucosal advancement suture at the 6 o'clock position may now be used to expose the bladder neck. The six 3-0 monofilament sutures that were previously placed in the distal urethra are now placed in their corresponding positions through the bladder neck, from inside to outside and incorporating only the mucosa and submucosa (Figure 10.24). The catheter is irrigated free of clots, the balloon is tested, and the catheter is placed through the bladder neck and inflated with 15 ml of saline.

To ensure that the bladder neck remains in close approximation to the urethra during tying of the sutures, the bladder should be pushed down to the urethra with a Babcock positioned on its anterior surface and held there while the sutures are tied. The anterior suture is initially tied without tension. If tension is present, the bladder should be released from the peritoneum prior to tying the remaining sutures. The sutures are then tied in the following sequence: 2, 5, 10, 7, and 6 o'clock. To ensure that no sutures have entrapped the catheter, the catheter should be rotated through 360° after tying each suture.

The catheter is then irrigated with saline to eliminate clots. A small suction drain is placed through the anterior rectus sheath on one side of the midline. The drain should run between (not through) the rectus muscles with the tip sited in the operative bed in the midline. The incision is closed with a running number 2 nylon suture and skin clips. The catheter is carefully fixed to the thigh with tape or a catheter strap.

Postoperative management

The postoperative recovery of men who undergo radical retropubic prostatectomy is usually uneventful. Patients should ambulate the morning after the procedure. For the first 12 h, pain control is

A

B

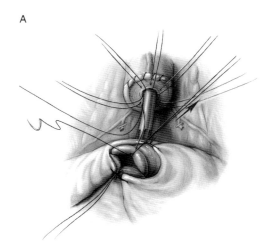

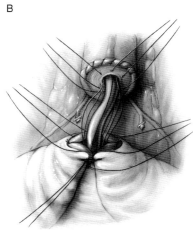

Figure 10.24

A and *B*, Final anastomosis is performed by placing the six 3-0 monofilament sutures previously placed in the distal urethra through their corresponding positions in the bladder neck, from inside to outside and incorporating only the mucosa and submucosa. The anterior sutures are tied first.

Courtesy of the Brady Urological Institute.

achieved with intravenous patient-controlled narcotic analgesia. Thereafter, nonaspirin nonsteroidal anti-inflammatory drugs—intravenous ketorolac or oral agents—may reduce narcotic analgesic requirements, postoperative nausea, and ileus. Patients are fed a regular diet on the evening of the first postoperative day. Closed-suction drains are left in place until output is minimal. Patients are discharged from hospital on the second postoperative day with a Foley catheter in place and return 10 to 14 days after surgery for catheter removal. Management of postoperative complications is discussed in detail in Chapter 19.

Summary

The development and dissemination of anatomic RRP has had a major impact on the treatment of localized prostate cancer. Its operative principles have proven durable: novel, minimally invasive techniques for radical prostatectomy utilizing laparoscopy and robot-assistance are firmly grounded in the same fundamental anatomic and surgical techniques. More than that, though, RRP remains an ideal form of treatment for younger men with localized disease, offering a standard of durable cancer-free survival with acceptably low morbidity to which other primary treatments for prostate cancer—both surgical and nonsurgical—are compared. It will likely continue as such for some time.

References

1. Kuchler H. Uber prostatavergrosserungh. Deutsch Klin 1866;18:458.
2. Young HH. The early diagnosis and radical cure of carcinoma of the prostate: a study of 40 cases and presentation of a radical operation which was carried out in four cases. Johns Hopkins Hosp Bull 1905;16:315–321.
3. Millin T. Retropubic Urinary Surgery. Baltimore: Williams and Wilkins, 1947.
4. Ansell JS. Radical transvesical prostatectomy: preliminary report on an approach to surgical excision of localized prostate malignancy. J Urol 1959;82:373–374.
5. Campbell EW. Total prostatectomy with preliminary ligation of the vascular pedicle. J Urol 1959;81:464–467.
6. Chute R. Radical retropubic prostatectomy for cancer. J Urol 1954;71: 347–372.
7. Lich R, Grant O, Maurer JE. Extravesical prostatectomy: a comparison of retropubic and perineal prostatectomy. J Urol 1949;61:930.
8. Memmelaar J. Total prostatovesiculectomy: retropubic approach. J Urol 1949;62:349.
9. Reiner WG, Walsh PC. An anatomical approach to the surgical management of the dorsal vein and Santorini's plexus during radical retropubic surgery. J Urol 1979;121:198–200.
10. Walsh PC. Anatomic radical prostatectomy: evolution of the surgical technique. J Urol 1998;160:2418–2424.
11. Steiner MS, Morton RA, Walsh PC. Impact of anatomical radical prostatectomy on urinary continence. J Urol 1991;145:512–514; discussion 514–515.
12. Walsh PC, Quinlan DM, Morton RA, et al. Radical retropubic prostatectomy. Improved anastomosis and urinary continence. Urol Clin North Am 1990;17:679–684.
13. Walsh PC, Marschke P, Ricker D, et al. Patient-reported urinary continence and sexual function after anatomic radical prostatectomy. Urology 2000;55:58–61.
14. Oelrich TM. The urethral sphincter muscle in the male. Am J Anat 1980;158:229–246.
15. Khan MA, Mangold LA, Epstein JI, et al. Impact of surgical delay on long-term cancer control for clinically localized prostate cancer. J Urol 2004;172:1835–1839.
16. Nash PA, Schrepferman CG, Rowland RG, et al. The impact of pre-donated autologous blood and intra-operative isovolaemic haemodilution on the outcome of transfusion in patients undergoing radical retropubic prostatectomy. Br J Urol 1996;77:856–860.
17. Peters CA, Walsh PC. Blood transfusion and anesthetic practices in radical retropubic prostatectomy. J Urol 1985;134:81–83.
18. Goldschlag B, Afzal N, Carter HB, et al. Is preoperative donation of autologous blood rational for radical retropubic prostatectomy? J Urol 2000;164:1968–1972.
19. Goh M, Kleer CG, Kielczewski P, et al. Autologous blood donation prior to anatomical radical retropubic prostatectomy: is it necessary? Urology 1997;49:569–573, discussion 574.
20. O'Hara JF Jr, Sprung J, Klein EA, et al. Use of preoperative autologous blood donation in patients undergoing radical retropubic prostatectomy. Urology 1999;54:130–134.
21. Koch MO, Smith JA Jr. Blood loss during radical retropubic prostatectomy: is preoperative autologous blood donation indicated? J Urol 1996;156:1077–1079; discussion 1079–1080.
22. Dash A, Dunn RL, Resh J, et al. Patient, surgeon, and treatment characteristics associated with homologous blood transfusion requirement during radical retropubic prostatectomy: multivariate nomogram to assist patient counseling. Urology 2004;64:117–122.
23. Chun TY, Martin S, Lepor H. Preoperative recombinant human erythropoietin injection versus preoperative autologous blood donation in patients undergoing radical retropubic prostatectomy. Urology 1997;50:727–732.

24. Nieder AM, Rosenblum N, et al. Comparison of two different doses of preoperative recombinant erythropoietin in men undergoing radical retropubic prostatectomy. Urology 2001;57:737–741.

25. Rosenblum N, Levine MA, Handler T, et al. The role of preoperative epoetin alfa in men undergoing radical retropubic prostatectomy. J Urol 2000;163:829–833.

26. Salonia A, Crescenti A, Suardi N, et al. General versus spinal anesthesia in patients undergoing radical retropubic prostatectomy: results of a prospective, randomized study. Urology 2004;64:95–100.

27. Shir Y, Raja SN, Frank SM, et al. Intraoperative blood loss during radical retropubic prostatectomy: epidural versus general anesthesia. Urology 1995;45:993–999.

28. Shir Y, Frank SM, Brendler CB, et al. Postoperative morbidity is similar in patients anesthetized with epidural and general anesthesia for radical prostatectomy. Urology 1994;44:232–236.

29. Allaf ME, Palapattu GS, Trock BJ, et al. Anatomical extent of lymph node dissection: impact on men with clinically localized prostate cancer. J Urol 2004;172:1840–1844.

30. Burnett AL, Mostwin JL. In situ anatomical study of the male urethral sphincteric complex: relevance to continence preservation following major pelvic surgery. J Urol 1998;160:1301–1306.

31. Walsh PC, Marschke P, Ricker D, et al. Use of intraoperative video documentation to improve sexual function after radical retropubic prostatectomy. Urology 2000;55:62–67.

32. Ong AM, Su LM, Varkarakis I, et al. Nerve sparing radical prostatectomy: effects of hemostatic energy sources on the recovery of cavernous nerve function in a canine model. J Urol 2004;172:1318–1322.

33. Rogatsch H, Horninger W, Volgger H, et al. Radical prostatectomy: the value of preoperative, individually labeled apical biopsies. J Urol 2000;164:754–757; discussion 757–758.

34. Walsh PC. Re: Radical prostatectomy: the value of preoperative, individually labeled apical biopsies. J Urol 2001;165:915.

35. Wei JT, Dunn RL, Marcovich R, et al. Prospective assessment of patient reported urinary continence after radical prostatectomy. J Urol 2000;164:744–748.

36. Walsh PC. Nerve grafts are rarely necessary and are unlikely to improve sexual function in men undergoing anatomic radical prostatectomy. Urology 2001;57:1020–1024.

37. Walsh PC, Marschke PL. Intussusception of the reconstructed bladder neck leads to earlier continence after radical prostatectomy. Urology 2002;59:934–938.

11

Radical retropubic prostatectomy: contemporary modifications

Murugesan Manoharan, Mark Soloway

Introduction

Retropubic radical prostatectomy (RRP) was first described by Millin in 1947,[1] but never gained popularity because of significant morbidity and mortality. This trend changed following the description of the anatomic retropubic prostatectomy by Walsh.[2] In the past two decades, it has become one of the most common oncologic procedures performed in the US.[3] Better understanding of the structural and functional anatomy of the pelvic floor, including the cavernosal nerves, dorsal venous complex, sphincter muscles, and puboprostatic ligaments has led to several modifications which result in better oncologic and functional outcome with a dramatic reduction in perioperative morbidity. This chapter summarizes various contemporary modifications to RRP.

Modified Pfannenstiel approach

RRP is traditionally performed using a vertical midline incision. However, a transverse Pfannenstiel incision[4] is commonly used by gynecologists for a variety of pelvic procedures. We have modified this incision,[5] and over the past 2 years vhave performed every RRPs using a modified Pfannenstiel approach that provides excellent exposure and better cosmetic results than a vertical incision.

Surgical technique

The patient is placed in a supine position with the anterosuperior iliac spine at the level of the kidney bridge. The bridge is raised and the operating table flexed to provide better access to the pelvis. A transverse curvilinear incision, approximately 8- to 10-cm long, is made along the pubic hairline centered over the pubic symphysis (Figure 11.1A). The superficial and deep fasciae are divided along the line of the skin incision to the level of the rectus sheath.

A V-shaped incision is initially made in the rectus sheath, with the midpoint of the V situated 2 cm above the symphysis pubis (Figure 11.1B). The limbs of the V are directed superiorly and laterally at a 30° angle to the skin incision. This avoids entering the inguinal canal inadvertently. The rectus sheath is opened on either side up to the lateral border of the rectus muscle.

The superior leaflet of the rectus sheath is reflected off the rectus muscle for a distance of 3 to 4 cm. To achieve this, two Allis clamps are applied to the superior leaflet of the rectus sheath on either side of the midline, and gentle traction is exerted. The rectus sheath is connected to the rectus muscle only by loose areolar tissue laterally and fibrous tissue along the midline. This is separated easily by a combination of blunt dissection and electrocautery (Figure 11.1C). A few small branches of the inferior epigastric artery pierce the rectus muscle and supply the rectus sheath. These should be identified and cauterized, because they may be avulsed easily and retract into the rectus muscle, possibly leading to a rectus hematoma.

The V incision is converted to a Y incision by making a vertical incision on the inferior leaflet of the rectus sheath along the midline up to the pubic symphysis (Figure 11.1D). It is not necessary to reflect the inferior leaflet of the rectus sheath off the rectus muscle.

The rectus and pyramidalis muscles are then exposed and are separated in the midline. The transversalis fascia is incised close to the pubis, and the retropubic space of Retzius is entered. By gentle blunt dissection, the peritoneum is mobilized superiorly from the pelvis. A Buckwalter self-retaining retractor is used to expose the wound. Two lateral blades are applied over the rectus muscle to retract the wound laterally. A small Richardson retractor is placed inferiorly to retract the skin and fatty tissue. A 16-F Foley catheter is inserted into the bladder, and the balloon inflated with 30 ml of water. The grooved Holtgrewe-Yu retractor is applied over the balloon, and the bladder neck is retracted superiorly (Figure 11.2A). This provides excellent exposure of the prostate. A standard RRP is performed. The transverse incision provides excellent exposure for a pelvic lymph node dissection. A malleable retractor is fitted to the Buckwalter frame to retract the bladder and facilitate exposure of the external iliac vessels and pelvic lymph nodes.

After completion of the RRP, the rectus muscle is approximated with absorbable suture. The rectus sheath is closed with a 0 Vicryl suture. The subcutaneous layers are closed with 3-0 chromic catgut. The skin is closed with a 4-0 Monocryl subcuticular technique (Figure 11.2B).

This incision is well accepted by patients because of the better cosmetic results and wound healing. We have performed more than 200 consecutive RRPs using this approach. The exposure is not dependent on the patient's body habitus. This incision provides excellent access to the inguinal canal. Five to 10% of patients with clinically localized prostate cancer have a detectable inguinal hernia. The modified Pfannenstiel approach allows for concurrent mesh repair of the inguinal hernia without the need for a separate incision.[6]

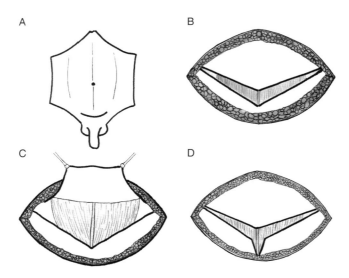

Figure 11.1

A, Skin incision. *B*, V-shaped incision of rectus sheath. *C*, Reflection of superior leaflet of rectus sheath. *D*, V to Y conversion of rectus sheath incision.

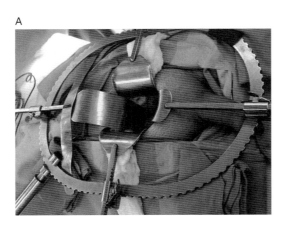

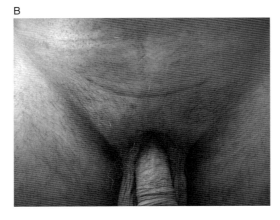

Figure 11.2

A, Wound exposure with self-retaining Buckwalter retractor. *B*, Healed incision.

Anesthesia and analgesics

The administration of analgesia prior to a painful stimulus reduces short- and long-term analgesic requirements and permits earlier resumption of normal activities.[7] Such "preemptive" analgesia may

act via a reduction in central nervous system sensitization before the nocioceptive input.

In a prospective randomized trial, Gottschalk et al[8] showed that preoperative epidural analgesia significantly decreased postoperative pain during hospitalization and long after discharge in patients undergoing radical prostatectomy. RRP has been successfully performed under epidural anesthesia in many centers. However, intrathecal administration of the anesthetic has some advantages over epidural anesthesia.[7,9] It allows faster onset of action and is technically easier than epidural anesthesia.[9] Failure rates of 2% to 5% have been reported for epidural administration of analgesia due to misplacement of the epidural catheter. In addition, intrathecal administration of opioids is less expensive than epidural analgesia when drug costs, delivery tubing, and administration trays are considered.[7,10]

In a retrospective analysis of factors affecting length of stay after radical prostatectomy, Gardner et al[11] showed that patients receiving epidural analgesia combined with general anesthesia had longer hospital stays compared to those not receiving epidural analgesia. This was believed to be the result of delayed ambulation and prolonged administration of epidural analgesia. Such factors are eliminated with a single preoperative dose of intrathecal opioid.

The safety of intrathecal opioids has been confirmed by Gwirtz et al,[10] who reported a series of approximately 6000 patients who received intrathecal morphine immediately following a variety of operative procedures. The efficacy of preoperative intrathecal morphine for reducing pain after radical prostatectomy has been evaluated by Eandi et al.[7] In a retrospective study of 62 patients who received a single dose of intrathecal morphine sulfate prior to RRP, 45% did not require postoperative narcotics and 95% were satisfied with their postoperative pain control. Mean hospital stay was 2.3 ± 0.3 days and patients resumed normal activities by a mean of 5.3 weeks after surgery.

In a prospective study involving 103 patients, Sved et al[12] demonstrated that RRP can be performed safely with spinal anesthesia and a single dose of intrathecal long-acting morphine. In their series, the mean times to tolerate oral fluids and unassisted ambulation were 11 and 20 h, respectively. Forty-three percent of patients were discharged on the first postoperative day and mean length of stay was 37.5 ± 11.8 h. The average narcotic requirements were 7.4 morphine equivalents (ME) prior to discharge and 28.1 ME in the first week after discharge. Mean visual analog pain score was 4.47 at the time of discharge and fell significantly to 1.6 by the time of catheter removal on postoperative day 7 to 8.

It is recommended that, whenever feasible, the RRP be performed under spinal anesthesia and intrathecal opioids. This provides better pain control and early ambulation of the patient.

Surgical techniques for improved continence

Continence rates following RRP range from 85% to 100% depending on subtle differences in surgical technique.[13–16] In 1982, Walsh and Donker[17] described the anatomic or nerve-sparing RRP with early control of the dorsal vein complex, careful apical dissection, precise urethral–vesical anastomosis, and preservation of the neurovascular bundles. Since then, many modifications have been described to improve post-prostatectomy continence further, including bladder neck preservation, meticulous dissection of the rhabdosphincter, puboprostatic ligament preservation, and maximal urethral preservation with dissection within the prostate to maintain the integrity of the proximal continence mechanism (posterior urethral segment sparing technique).

The puboprostatic "complex" consists of three components. The *pyramidal portion* (also called the puboprostatic ligament) lies between the base of the prostate and the pubic symphysis, and extends laterally into the endopelvic fascia that covers the lateral pelvic muscles (levator ani, internal obturator) constituting the dense medial part of the endopelvic fascia. The *dorsal vein complex* (Santorini plexus) lies below the first portion and behind the pubic symphysis in the retropubic fat, and is separated from the prostate by fibromuscular and soft connective tissue. The *fibromuscular and soft connective tissue* attach the prostate to the pubic arch in the median plane, forming the intermediate pubourethral ligament that inserts at the anterior commissure of the prostate, the isthmus prostate. The anterior urethral ligament and the urethra lie at the distal margin of this third portion.

Preservation of the distal striated sphincter is the most critical aspect for maintaining urinary continence following RRP.[18,19] In addition, supporting structures of the external striated urethral sphincter, such as the puboprostatic ligaments, may play a role in normal continence by maintaining the normal position of the urethra in the pelvic floor.[15,20] This is the anatomic principle underlying the placement of the suture that ligates the dorsal vein to the symphysis pubis[21] or the preservation of the supporting puboprostatic ligaments.[15]

Complete cancer removal remains the goal of RRP and modifications in the surgical technique should not compromise the pathologic outcome. It is conceivable that by preserving the bladder neck, cancer at the base of the prostate may be left behind with increased incidence of positive margin rates. On a similar note, puboprostatic ligament sparing not only makes the ligation of the Santorini venous plexus difficult, but might also leave the apical prostatic tissue behind with a high incidence of positive apical surgical margin rate. Myers et al[19] demonstrated that the posterior lip of the prostate extends more caudally and an inappropriate urethral dissection might result in dissection through the posterior prostatic tissue at the level of the prostatic apex. In addition, the risk of positive margins exists anteriorly during the dissection between the dorsal vein complex and the prostate.[14]

Maintenance of the integrity of the external striated muscle urethral sphincter and its attachments is of paramount importance for continence. Presti et al[22] demonstrated that continence rates correlate with the mean functional urethral length and maximal urethral closure pressure following RRP. Sphincteric integrity of the pelvic floor has been found to be more important for continence than retubularization of the bladder neck.[19] It is, therefore, very important to preserve, as far as possible, the integrity of the periurethral tissues that form the posterior urethral plate.

Bladder neck preservation

The so-called "bladder neck preservation" technique involves careful sharp and blunt dissection between the circular fibers of the bladder neck and base of the prostate.[13,23] Deliveliotis et al,[18] Braslis et al,[24] Lowe,[25] Gaker et al,[26] and Klein[27] reported improved early (3–6 months) continence rates following bladder neck preservation, and suggested that the early return of continence is the result of the added passive outlet resistance from the unaltered bladder neck. The reported continence rates are variable and may be due to the differing definitions of continence.[4,13] Following the initial period, the external sphincter becomes stronger and recovers from the surgery, playing a more important role in continence and, therefore, masking the effect of the bladder neck preservation. At 9 and 12 months

most patients have similar excellent continence rates whether the bladder neck has been preserved or not.

Deliveliotis et al[18] reported similar cancer control rates in terms of positive margins following bladder neck preservation (21%), puboprostatic ligament sparing (18%), and both (22%) in patients with a final Gleason score of greater than 7, similar to the rates reported by Braslis et al[24] in patients with a prostate-specific antigen (PSA) level of less than 10 ng/ml. Bladder neck dissection could have avoided positive margins in 5 of 149 (3%) patients. In contrast, Srougi et al[16] demonstrated in a randomized, prospective study that, although the positive margin rates were similar following bladder neck preservation or wide bladder neck resection, margins were positive only at the bladder neck in 10% of the preservation group, whereas no patients in the bladder neck resection group had a positive bladder neck margin.

Bladder neck preservation avoids the need for bladder neck reconstruction and mucosal eversion, and in our experience reduces the incidence of vesicourethral anastomotic strictures.[13] However, care should be exercised in using this modification in patients with high volume, high-grade cancers at the base of the prostate. Bianco et al[28] found positive margins at the apex and bladder neck in 104 (19%) and 13 (2%) patients, respectively, of 555 patients. Of those with a positive bladder neck margin, eight had a Gleason score of 7 or greater, three had seminal vesicle invasion, and two had nodal disease. Only two patients had a positive bladder neck margin as the sole adverse pathologic feature. Significant independent predictors of survival in their study included Gleason score, PSA, pathologic stage, and presence of positive margins in more than one location. Marcovich et al[29] reported that bladder neck preservation can be associated with an increased rate of positive surgical margins in a pT3A cancer subset with focal penetration through the prostatic capsule, with an associated trend toward decreased PSA-free survival.

Puboprostatic ligament preservation

Puboprostatic ligament (PL) preservation during RRP entails division of the ligaments adjacent to the prostate rather than the pubis, and is believed to preserve the tissues that provide support to the proximal urethra and striated sphincter complex.[14,15]

Poore et al[14] reported earlier return of continence following PL-sparing prostatectomy. However, final outcome was similar to non–PL-sparing techniques. Deliveliotis et al[18] did not find any advantage with the PL-sparing prostatectomy, and the discrepancies can be attributed to the definition of continence (no need for pads[14] vs use of one pad daily[17]). Noh et al[3] demonstrated that mean time to recovery of continence was similar for bladder reconstruction (2.3 months) and bladder neck preservation (2.9 months) but was significantly longer ($P \leq 0.05$) for bladder neck and PL preservation (4.3 months). None of their patients had "bladder neck-only positive margins," although 9% had positive margins.

It remains unclear whether PL preservation improves the continence both in the short- and long-term.

Posterior urethral sparing technique

Urethral length at the time of anastomosis has been shown to correlate with continence rates.[30,31] The modified technique of RRP with urethral preservation entails preservation of the 1.5 cm of the posterior urethra, which should be circumferentially intact.

Proximal urethral dissection is performed at the time of bladder neck preservation. The tissue plane between the bladder base and prostate is identified, and the proximal urethra is carefully separated from the prostate by blunt dissection. Exposure to the area of dissection is the primary challenge, as the surrounding prostate limits visualization. The preserved urethra includes mucosa and immediate periurethral tissue for 1 to 1.5 cm distal to the bladder neck. Splitting of the anterior fibromuscular septum of the prostate allows direct visualization of the prostatic urethra with an improved angle of dissection. Using this technique, Tongco et al[32] demonstrated positive margins in 5 of 12 (41.66%) patients with a PSA greater than 10 ng/ml and/or a Gleason score of greater than 7. They found residual prostate adenoma on the dissected urethral specimens. Gaker et al[26] performed true urethra-urethrostomy in 24 patients, sparing the distal urethra to the level of the verumontanum by blunt dissection of the apical urethra from the surrounding prostatic tissue. Proximal urethral dissection was performed to the proximal verumontanum (average length, 2.0 cm), sparing the prostatic and periurethral musculature. Two of the 24 patients had positive margins, but none of the urethral biopsies had benign or malignant prostatic tissue. Eight-three percent of patients were continent by 7 weeks following prostatectomy. There were no anastomotic complications.

There is no unequivocal evidence that this technique improves continence rates significantly. There are no large series to confirm the long-term benefits and oncologic safety of this technique and hence this technique is not recommended at present.

In conclusion, 1-year continence rates after bladder neck preservation and/or PL sparing do not differ. Using strict continence definition criteria, bladder neck preservation achieves earlier return to continence. PL preservation has been found to be associated with slower recovery of continence and does not alter the long-term continence rates. Bladder neck sparing can safely be performed to obtain earlier return to continence without compromising cancer control. Bladder neck preservation further improves morbidity with fewer incidences of anastomotic strictures.

Other modifications

Role of pelvic drain

Though it is a common practice to drain the pelvis following a RRP, Savoie et al[33] reported that routine drainage of the pelvis is not required in all cases. In their series, after the RRP was performed and the anastomotic sutures were tied, the bladder was filled with saline through the urethral catheter. If there was no significant leakage, a drain was not placed (73% of 116 consecutive patients who underwent RRP). None had clinical evidence of lymphocele, hematoma or infection. One patient developed an urinoma that required percutaneous drainage without any sequelae. We have performed 397 consecutive radical prostatectomies in the past 3 years and have not placed a drain in 76% of these, with excellent outcome.

If the bladder neck is preserved or meticulously reconstructed, there may be little or no extravasation and, thus, routine drainage may be unnecessary. Moreover, studies from other specialties have demonstrated several disadvantages associated with wound drains, including drain site pain, retained drains, infection, and cost.[34] In properly selected cases, morbidity is not increased by omitting a drain from the pelvic cavity after RRP.

Blood transfusion and cell saver

Transfusion rates during RRP have decreased steadily over the past several years as increasing surgeon skill and familiarity with the operation have reduced estimated blood loss (EBL). An analysis of the Department of Defense Center for Prostate Disease Research Multicenter National Research Database of 2918 patients undergoing radical prostatectomy showed statistically significant decreases in the median EBL (from 1800 to 800 ml), rates of preoperative blood donation (from 81.7% to 10.9%), and transfusion rates (from 93.2% to 13.7%) from 1985 to 2000.[35] Other recent studies have reported homologous blood transfusion rates of 4.6%, 7.1%, and 9.7%.[36–38] Thus, although the likelihood of a patient receiving blood is relatively low, the risk is still present.

Different means of managing blood loss include preoperative donation of autologous blood, preoperative recombinant erythropoeitin injection, intraoperative hemodilution, allogenic blood transfusion, and intraoperative cell salvage (IOCS). IOCS, commonly referred to as "cell saver," is an attractive blood management strategy since it is relatively inexpensive, obviates a trip to the blood bank, and prevents the risks associated with allogeneic blood transfusion, such as viral infection.

Many oncologic surgeons have been reluctant to utilize IOCS because of the theoretical risk of tumor dissemination. Davis et al[39] published our institutional experience with IOCS between 1992 and 1998 and reported no short-term increased risk of biochemical recurrence among 408 patients. We further evaluated 1038 patients from our database and there was no significant difference in the biochemical recurrence rate between those who did and those who did not receive cell salvaged blood. Further stratification of our patients according to low, intermediate, and high risk did not demonstrate any significant differences in the biochemical recurrence rate between the cohorts.[40]

The use of IOCS is a safe and valuable technique of blood management for patients undergoing RRP and decreases the need for allogenic transfusion.

Table 11.1 "University of Miami approach" to retropubic radical prostatectomy

- Spinal anesthesia and intrathecal long-acting morphine ± laryngeal mask
- Intermittent compression device prior to induction, no routine use of heparin or heparinoid prophylaxis
- Intraoperative cell salvage (IOCS) system and salvaged red cells transfused as required
- Supine position, bridge elevated at the level of the anterior superior iliac spine and the table is flexed to provide better exposure to the pelvis
- Modified Pfannenstiel incision, Buckwalter retractor to expose the wound
- Bilateral pelvic lymph node dissection performed routinely, but not obligatory
- Standard retropubic prostatectomy, preservation of neurovascular bundles, bladder neck preservation, no routine mucosal eversion
- Pelvic drain not routinely used
- Early mobilization and routine discharge from the hospital within 36–48 h
- Foley catheter for 7 days, no routine cystogram prior to removal of the catheter

Instrumentation

Various advances in the field of medical instrumentation have facilitated the ease of performing RRP and improved outcome. Several surgeons routinely use magnifying optical loupes and headlight to improve the visualization and dissection of the apex of the prostate and neurovascular bundle.[41] We use 2.5X loupes but do not routinely use headlights.

Devices such as Ligasure and vascular staplers have been reported to facilitate the dorsal venous complex control.[42] These devices, however, have not gained widespread acceptance as most surgeons are comfortable with suture ligation of the dorsal venous complex. The harmonic scalpel is another useful device that can be used to secure the vascular pedicles of the prostate. We routinely use this device and find it reliable.

Conclusion

With the perceived benefits of reduced postoperative morbidity, earlier return to normal activity, and improved cosmesis, minimally invasive surgical options for localized prostate cancer, such as laparoscopic radical prostatectomy (LRP) and robot-assisted prostatectomy (RAP) have gained popularity in recent years. However, these procedures are expensive and technically difficult, with a steep learning curve. The total operating time is usually longer than with a standard RRP. Moreover, these technologies are not available universally and many centers cannot afford them.

On the other hand, simple modifications to the standard RRP (Table 11.1) have resulted in dramatic improvement in patient outcome without any significant increase in cost. These modifications can be easily adapted by urologists, both in the community and in referral centers.

The contemporary RRP offers a viable alternative treatment option to the expensive and technically challenging minimally invasive procedures.

References

1. Millin T. Retropubic Urinary Surgery. London: Livingstone, 1947.
2. Walsh PC. Radical prostatectomy for the treatment of localized prostatic carcinoma. Urol Clin North Am 1980;3:583–591.
3. Noh C, Kshirsagar A, Mohler JL. Outcome after radical retropubic prostatectomy. Urology 2003;61:412–416.
4. Griffiths DA. A reappraisal of the Pfannenstiel incision. BJU Int 1976; 48: 469–474.
5. Manoharan M, Gomez P, Sved P, Soloway MS. Modified Pfannenstiel approach for radical retropubic prostatectomy. Urology 2004;64:369–371.
6. Manoharan M, Gomez P, Soloway MS. Concurrent radical retropubic prostatectomy and inguinal hernia repair through a modified Pfannenstiel incision. BJU Int 2004;93:1203–1206.
7. Eandi JA, de Vere White RW, Tunuguntla HS, et al. Can single dose preoperative intrathecal morphine sulfate provide cost-effective postoperative analgesia and patient satisfaction during radical prostatectomy in the current era of cost containment. Pros Can Pros Dis 2002;5:226–230.
8. Gottschalk A, Smith DS, Jobes DR, et al. Preemptive epidural analgesia and recovery from radical prostatectomy. JAMA 1998;279:1076–1082.
9. Stoelting RK. Intrathecal morphine: an understood combination for postoperative pain management. Anesth Analg 1989;68:707–709.
10. Gwirtz KH, Young JV, Byers RS, et al. The safety and efficacy of intrathecal opioid analgesia for acute postoperative pain: Seven years' experience with 5969 surgical patients at Indiana University Hospital. Anesth Analg 1999;88:599–604.
11. Gardner TA, Bissonette EA, Petroni GR, et al. Surgical and postoperative factors affecting length of stay after radical prostatectomy. Cancer 2000;89:424–430.
12. Sved PD, Nieder AM, Manoharan M, et al. Evaluation of analgesic requirements and postoperative recovery after radical retropubic prostatectomy using long-acting spinal anesthesia. Uroloy 2005;65:509–512.
13. Shelfo SW, Obek C, Soloway M. Update on bladder neck preservation during radical retropubic prostatectomy: impact on pathologic outcome, anastomotic strictures, and continence. Urology 1998;51:73–78.
14. Poore RE, McCullough DL, Jarow JP. Puboprostatic ligament sparing improves urinary continence after radical retropubic prostatectomy. Urology 1998;51:67–72.
15. Jarow JP. Puboprostatic ligament sparing radical retropubic prostatectomy. Semin Urol Oncol 2000;18:28–32.
16. Srougi M, Nesrallah LJ, Kauffmann JR, et al. Urinary continence and pathological outcome after bladder neck preservation during radical retropubic prostatectomy: a randomized prospective trial. J Urol 2001;165:815–818.
17. Walsh PC, Donker PJ. Impotence following radical prostatectomy: insight into etiology and prevention. J Urol 1982;128:492–497.
18. Deliveliotis C, Protogerou V, Alargof E, Varkarakis J. Radical prostatectomy: bladder neck preservation and puboprostatic ligament sparing-effects on continence and positive margins. Urology 2002;60:855–858.
19. Myers RP. Male urethral sphincgteric anatomy and radical prostatectomy. Urol Clin North Am 1991;18:211–227.
20. Steiner MS. Anatomic basis for the continence-preserving radical retropubic prostatectomy. Semin Urol Oncol 2000;18:9–18.
21. Eastham JA, Kattan MW, Rogers E, et al. Risk factors for urinary incontinence after radical prostatectomy. J Urol 1996;156:1707–1713.
22. Presti JC Jr, Schmidt RA, Narayan PA, et al. Pathophysiology of urinary incontinence after radical prostatectomy. J Urol 1990;143:975–978.
23. Soloway MS, Neulander E. Bladder-neck preservation during radical retropubic prostatectomy. Semin Urol Oncol 2000;18:51–56.
24. Braslis KG, Petsch M, Lim A, et al. Bladder neck preservation following radical prostatectomy: continence and margins. Eur Urol 1995;28:202–208.
25. Lowe BA. Comparison of bladder neck preservation to bladder neck resection in maintaining postprostatectomy urinary incontinence. Urology 1996;48:889–893.
26. Gaker DL, Gaker LB, Stewart JF, et al. Radical prostatectomy with preservation of urinary continence. J Urol 1996;156:445–449.
27. Klein EA. Early continence after radical prostatectomy. J Urol 1992;148:92–95.
28. Bianco FJ Jr, Grignon DJ, Sakr WA, et al. Radical prostatectomy with bladder neck preservation: impact on positive margins. Eur Urol 2003;43:461–466.
29. Marcovich R, Wojno KJ, Wei JT, Rubin MA, Montie JE, Sanda MG. Bladder neck-sparing modification of radical prostatectomy adversely affects surgical margins in pathologic T3a prostate cancer. Urology 2000;55:904–908.
30. Levy JB, Seay TM, Wein AJ. Postprostatectomy incontinence. In Ball TP (ed): AUA Update Series, vol XV, Lesson 8. Houston: American Urologic Association, 1996.
31. McGuire EJ. Urethral sphincter mechanisms. Urol Clin North Am 1979;6:39–49.
32. Tongco WP, Wehner MS, Basler JW. Does urethral-sparing prostatectomy risk residual prostate cancer? Urology 2001;57:495–498.
33. Savoie M, Soloway MS, Kim SS, Monoharan M. A pelvic drain may be avoided after radical retropubic prostatectomy. J Urol 2003;170:112–114.
34. Scott H, Brown AC. Is routine drainage of pelvic anastomosis necessary? Am Surg 1996;62:452–457.
35. Moul JW, Sun L, Wu H, et al. Factors associated with blood loss during radical prostatectomy for localized prostate cancer in the prostate-specific antigen (PSA)-era: an overview of the Department of Defence

(DOD) Center for Prostate Disease Research (CPDR) national database. Urol Oncol 2003;21:447–455.

36. Lepor H, Kaci L. Contemporary evaluation of operative parameters and complications related to open radical retropubic prostatectomy. Urology 2003;62:702–706.

37. Nuttall GA, Cragum MD, Hill DL, et al. Radical retropubic prostatectomy and blood transfusion. Mayo Clin Proc 2002;77:1301–1305.

38. Lepor H, Nieder AM, Ferrandino MN. Intraoperative and postoperative complications of radical retropubic prostatectomy in a conservative series of 1,000 cases. J Urol 2001;166:1729–1733.

39. Davis M, Sofer M, Gomez-Marin O, Bruck D, Soloway MS. The use of cell salvage during radical retropubic prostatectomy: does it influence cancer recurrence? BJU Int 2003;91:474–476.

40. Nieder AM, Manoharan M, Soloway MS, et al. Intraoperative cell salvage during radical prostatectomy is not associated with greater biochemical recurrence. Urology 2005;65:730–734.

41. Altwein JE. Enhancing the efficacy of radical prostatectomy in locally advanced prostate cancer. Urol Int 1998;60(Suppl):2–10.

42. Daskalopoulos G, Karyotis I, Heretis I, Delakas D. Electrothermal bipolar coagulation for radical prostatectomies and cystectomies: a preliminary case-controlled study. Int Urol Nephrol 2004;36:181-185.

12

Role of lymphadenectomy in prostate cancer

Fiona C Burkhard, Martin Schumacher, Natalie Tschan, Urs E Studer

Introduction

When and to what extent lymphadenectomy should be performed in patients undergoing radical prostatectomy remains a matter of intense debate. Lymphadenectomy provides important information for prognosis (number of nodes involved, tumor volume, capsular perforation) that is not matched by any other procedures. Whether, in addition, a potential therapeutic effect of extended lymph node dissection with removal of all diseased nodes can be expected has still not been fully documented, due to the relatively benign course of this disease. In contrast, in other malignancies such as gastric, breast, colorectal, and cervical cancer, and in recent years also bladder cancer, it has become apparent that survival and accuracy of staging improve with the number of nodes removed and therefore the extent of lymph node dissection.[1–6]

Pelvic lymphadenectomy as a staging procedure

Precise tumor staging is the basis for optimal therapeutic management. In prostate cancer the availability of biochemical markers and preoperative biopsies allows a differentiated staging. Based on these, nomograms have been developed to help decide which patients will benefit from pelvic lymphadeonectomy and in which it can be avoided.[7] To date all nomograms are based on standard lymph node dissection and with the increasing awareness of possible lymph node metastasis outside the region of standard dissection, these nomograms may prove increasingly inadequate.

Classic imaging modalities, such as computerized tomography (CT) and magnetic resonance imaging (MRI), are relatively insensitive for the detection of lymph node metastasis in the pelvis and are of no value in deciding therapeutic strategies.[8–10] Newer developments such as sentinel node lymphoscintigraphy with gamma probe detection and high-resolution MRI with magnetic nanoparticles are emerging. If these are only a slight improvement over available methods or are truly of advantage with high sensitivity and specificity remains to be determined. For the time being, a meticulous pelvic lymph node dissection remains the most accurate and cost-efficient solution, requiring only minor additional surgical time.

Lymphatic drainage from the prostate shows large variability, with sentinel nodes found mainly along the external iliac vein, in the obturator fossa, or along the internal iliac vessels.[11] Single sentinel nodes have not been identified. For this reason, dissection should include all primary drainage areas from the diseased organ (Figures 12.1 and 12.2). Accordingly, the boundaries for extended lymphadenectomy are: laterally, the upper limit of the external iliac vein (leaving the periarteric tissue untouched); distally, the femoral canal; proximally, the bifurcation of the common iliac artery; medially, the side wall of the bladder; and inferiorly, the floor of the obturator fossa and the internal iliac (hypogastric) vessels. Tissue medial to the internal iliac artery should be included, which some may describe as the presacral/pararectal area.

With these templates in our series at the University of Bern a median of 21 (range 6–50) nodes were removed in 365 patients with prostate cancer.[12] The number of removed nodes corresponds well with the results of an anatomic study by Weingaertner et al,[13] who determined that approximately 20 removed lymph nodes can be considered a representative pelvic lymphadenectomy. Stone et al[14] compared 150 patients with modified and 39 with extended laparoscopic lymph node dissection; not only did they find, as to be expected, a significant difference in the number of nodes removed (9.3 vs 17.8 [P $\leq$0.05]), but also three times as many patients with lymph node metastasis (7.3% versus 23.1% [P = 0.02]). This was confirmed by Heidenreich et al[15] in a study comparing a historical control group with standard lymph node dissection (external iliac vein and obturator fossa) and a contemporary group with extended lymph node dissection (external iliac vein, obturator fossa, internal iliac artery, common iliac vessels, and presacral). A median of 11 (6–19) and 28 (21–46) nodes were removed for standard and extended lymph node dissection, respectively. At the same time, the number of patients with diseased nodes increased from 12 of 100 to 27 of 103. The authors concluded that as only three of all the positive nodes were found along the common iliac vessels and in the presacral area, removing lymphatic tissue from these regions could be neglected. In our prospective study of 365 patients undergoing extended lymph node dissection, we detected positive nodes in 24%.[12]

These percentages are significantly higher than the 5% to 10% positive nodes described in other, albeit not necessarily comparable, series without extended lymph node dissection.[16–18] One explanation for the noticeably higher percentage of positive nodes in our series may be that a significant number of nodes were found outside the standard area of dissection and the importance of removing nodes along the internal iliac vessels is becoming increasingly clear. Indeed, when performing extended lymphadenectomy, almost two-thirds of all patients with lymph node metastasis have positive nodes along the internal iliac vessels and approximately one-fifth of these patients have them solely at this location.[12,19] The proportion of patients with positive nodes either exclusively in this area or in combination with another location was 59% in our series and 67% in a series by Tenaglia and Ianucci.[20] Not only would a significant number of patients be understaged if the internal iliac nodes were not removed, but many would also be left with diseased nodes.

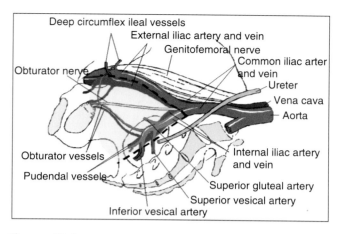

Figure 12.1
Boundaries of extended lymph node dissection and
subdivision into three different locations, including the
external iliac vein, obturator fossa, and internal iliac artery.
Note that tissue medial to the internal iliac artery is also
removed.

Considering the fact that many urologists do not remove nodes in
this region, this may seem quite astonishing. Despite support from
evolving highly sensitive detection techniques for the existence
of lymph node metastasis outside the standard area of dissection,
controversy still persists concerning the extent of dissection.

A study by Clark et al[21] appears to support those who consider
standard dissection to be adequate. They performed a randomized
prospective evaluation of extended versus limited lymph node dissection in 100 patients with clinically localized prostate cancer and
found no difference between these two groups concerning metastatic disease. However, they did describe a significantly higher rate of
complications after extended versus lymph node dissection in 123.
This study, although addressing an important subject, does have
some limitations, which may explain why the findings are in contrast
to most other studies. The number of patients is too small to test for
equivalence. In the low-risk patient groups, the majority would not
have required lymph node dissection, which further limits the power
of the trial. In addition, the researchers randomly assigned patients
to extended lymph-adenectomy on one side only, independent of
tumor localization, thus introducing a large risk of lymph node dissection on the non–tumor-bearing side. They also did not define the
pathologic work-up or the number of nodes removed.

Complications of lymph node dissection

The typical complications associated with lymph node dissection
are lymphoceles, lymphedema, venous thrombosis, and pulmonary
embolism. Reported complication rates for patients with prostate
cancer range from 4% to 50%.[22] Clark et al[21] described a total complication rate of 13 of 123 (10.5%) patients, with 75% of complications occurring on the side of extended pelvic lymphadenectomy.
Heidenreich et al,[19] however, found no statistical difference concerning intraoperative complications, postoperative complications,
blood loss, and lymphocele formation. In our series of 463 patients,

the incidence of prolonged hospitalization or rehospitalization
attributable to extended lymph node dissection was as low as 2%
and only one patient developed persisting lymphedema. We ascribe
this low rate of complications to a meticulous surgical technique: 1)
ligation, instead of clipping, of all the lymphatics from the lower
extremities—hemoclips have a tendency to be torn away during
subsequent surgery; 2) placement of two drains instead of one, with
one on each side of the pelvis where lymphadenectomy was performed—these are not removed until the total amount drained is
less than 50 ml/24 h; and 3) injection of low molecular heparin into
the upper arm instead of the thigh.

Indication for extended lymphadenectomy

Is extended lymph node dissection necessary in all patients? In general, we feel that all patients requiring lymph node dissection need
extended dissection, including nodes along the internal iliac artery.
Many urologists now consider patients with a clinically localized
tumor, a prostate-specific antigen (PSA) level of less than 10 ng/ml to
be at low risk for metastatic disease. In our series, we found positive
nodes in 11% of patients in this low-risk group. Only patients with a
PSA of less then 10 ng/ml and a Gleason score less than 6 have a minimal chance of node metastasis.[23] However, as approximately 30% of
preoperative biopsies are understaged, it is difficult to recognize this
low-risk group with certainty preoperatively. Therefore, we feel that
extended lymphadenectomy should be performed in all patients.

Possible advantage of extended lymphadenectomy in prostate cancer

Prostate cancer generally has quite a benign course. In contemporary series, the 10-year cancer-specific survival rates are approximately 85% for watchful waiting and 90% to 94% for radical
retropubic prostatectomy in patients with clinically localized
prostate cancer (Table 12.1). A high rate of biochemical failure has
been reported after radical prostatectomy, but the interpretation of
biochemical failure remains controversial and may not have an
impact on survival in the majority of patients.[24]

Lymph node metastasis, however, does have a negative impact on
prognosis. This is not as obvious after 5 years (Table 12.1 vs Table
12.2) as after 10 years, when recurrence/metastasis-free rates (without immediate hormonal therapy) range from 10% to 68%,[25–29] and
cancer-specific survival rates from 56% to 62% (Table 12.2).[26,28,30–32]
For this reason it is often stated that once patients have node-
positive disease, this should be considered systemic and treated
accordingly, and that removal of further nodes shows no benefit for
the patient. However, there are findings suggesting that in certain
patients treatment can be curative even in lymph node-positive
prostate cancer. In Catalona et al's[33] relatively small series of
12 patients with minimal lymph node involvement (micrometasta-
sis and only one positive node) and no adjuvant therapy, no tumor
was detectable at 5 and 10 years in 75% and 58% of patients, respectively. In Pound et al's[34] in patients with lymph node metastasis
found in a 10-year metastasis-free survival rate of 68%, again

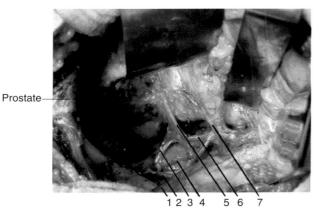

Prostate

1. External iliac vein
2. Obturator vein
3. Pudendal vessels
4. Obturator artery
5. Inferior vesical artery
6. Internal iliac artery
7. Superior vesical artery

1 2 3 4   5 6   7

Figure 12.2
Intraoperative photograph after extended lymph node dissection. The pubis is on the left and the bladder on the right. All tissue has been removed from the external iliac vein, the obturator fossa, and along the internal iliac artery.

Table 12.1 Survival rates following radical retropubic prostatectomy (RRP) for prostate cancer, including patients with positive nodes

	Number of patients	Median follow-up (years)	Treatment	Projected metastasis-free survival (%)		Projected cancer-specific survival (%)	
				5 years	10 years	5 years	10 years
Jhaveri et al[24]	1132	2.8	RRP	–	–	–	90[†]
Pound et al[34]	1997	5.3	RRP	–	87	99	94
Han et al[25]	2404	6.3	RRP	84[‡]	74[‡]	–	–

˙8-year follow-up.
[†]Overall survival.
[‡]Recurrence free

Table 12.2 Survival rates in node-positive patients without immediate hormonal therapy

	Number of patients	Median follow-up (years)	Treatment	Metastasis-free survival (%)		Cancer-specific survival (%)	
				5 years	10 years	5 years	10 years
Han et al[25]	135	6.3	RRP	26[‡]	10[‡]	–	–
Bader et al[26]	92	3.75	RRP	~50	~25	74	~62
Catalona et al[35]	12	7	RRP	75	58§	–	–
Steinberg et al[28]	64	3.75	RRP	83	68	97	62
Caddedu et al[33]	19*	5.5	RRP	–	–	93	56
Messing et al[34]	51	10	RRP	–	–	–	57

[‡]Recurrence free.
§7-year follow-up.
˙33% with hormonal therapy, 3% with radiation therapy

without adjuvant therapy. After a 60- and 80-month follow-up, 83% and 68% of patients were free of detectable tumor in Steinberg et al's[28] series of 64 patients. Golimbu et al[35] reported on 42 patients with lymph node metastasis with a mean follow-up of 5 years. Their patients with microscopic metastatic disease or fewer than one positive node had an 85% 5-year and a 50% 10-year survival free of disease. In a more recent series by Bader et al,[26] 74% of patients with only one positive node remained free of tumor progression and only

14% have died to date. Daneshmand et al[37] observed a clinical recurrence-free survival rate of 70% and 73% in patients with one or two positive nodes versus 49% in those with more than five positive nodes. In Steinberg et al's[30] study, the number of positive nodes did not have a significant prognostic value. However, in Frazier et al's[30] series patients with two or fewer positive nodes showed improved cancer-specific survival compared to patients with more than two positive nodes. In our series of 92 patients with lymph node metastasis, time to progression was significantly correlated with the number of positive nodes.26 Allaf et al[38] reported a survival difference in men with less than 15% of positive nodes, the 5-year PSA-free survival rate was 43% versus 10% for extended versus limited lymph node dissection, respectively.

In contrast, Dimarco et al[39] detected no survival advantage after extended lymphadenectomy for prostate cancer. In their study, the median number of nodes removed decreased from 14 between 1987 and 1989 to 5 between 1999 and 2000. Interestingly, removing more nodes in the earlier period led to similar results for disease progression and survival as removing fewer nodes in the later period. As T-stage migration is an accepted phenomenon these results may imply that, thanks to the more extended lymphadenectomy, patients with a higher T-stage had comparable survival chances to the more recent population with earlier stage disease.

The need for extended lymphadenectomy is further supported by Di Blasio et al's[40] analysis showing that the number of nodes removed is associated with progression. Removal of 13 nodes had the lowest risk of disease progression, regardless of nodal disease status. Bader et al[38] reported similar findings, with 16%, 12%, 8%, and 8% of patients showing disease progression after removing 0 to 4, 5 to 9, 10 to 14 and more than 14 nodes for pT1/pT2N0 prostate cancer, respectively.

There are few reports concerning the percentage of positive nodes in prostate cancer. In a univariate and multivariate analysis, Steinberg et al[28] found the percentage of positive nodes to have a significant prognostic value. In a series from the John Hopkins Universtiy, 52% of patients with less then 15% positive nodes, Gleason score less than 7, and negative seminal vesicle invasion remained free of progression at 5 years.[38,41] In agreement with this, Daneshmand et al[37] reported that patients with a lymph node density (number of positive nodes removed/total number of removed nodes) of 20% or greater were at higher risk for progression than those with a density of less than 20%.

Overall, there does seem to be a subset of patients with a good chance of asymptomatic long-term survival in the presence of minimal lymph node metastasis (two or fewer positive nodes, low metastatic volume), most likely as a consequence of having the diseased nodes removed.

Conclusion

Lymph node dissection remains the only reliable method for exact staging. Extended lymphadenectomy, including tissue along the external iliac vein, obturator fossa, and internal iliac vessels, should be performed in all patients undergoing radical prostatectomy. There is an increasing amount of data suggesting that removal of all diseased nodes that contain minimal metastatic disease may have a positive impact on disease-free and, perhaps, overall survival. Due to the relatively benign course of prostate cancer, longer follow-up is still necessary before a definitive statement can be made.

References

1. Mathiesen O, Carl J, Bonderup O, et al. Axillary sampling and the risk of erroneous staging of breast cancer. An analysis of 960 consecutive patients. Acta Oncol 1990;29:721–725.
2. Siewert JR, Böttcher K, Stein HJ, et al. Relevant prognostic factors in gastric cancer. Ann Surg 1998;228:449–461.
3. Friedberg V. Results of 108 exenteration operations in advanced gynecologic cancers [German]. Geburtshilfe Frauenheilkd1989;49:423–427.
4. Caplin S, Cerottini JP, Bosman FT, et al. For patients with Duke's B (TNM Stage II) colorectal carcinoma, examination of six or fewer lymph nodes is related to poor prognosis. Cancer 1998;83:666–672.
5. Mills RD, Turner WH, Fleischmann A, et al. Pelvic lymph node metastases from bladder cancer: outcome in 83 patients after radical cystectomy and pelvic lymphadenectomy. J Urol 2001;166:19–23.
6. Leissner J, Hohenfellner R, Thüroff JW, et al. Lymphadenectomy in patients with transitional cell carcinoma of the urinary bladder; significance for staging and prognosis. Br J Urol 2000;85:817–823.
7. Partin AW, Mangold LA, Lamm DM, et al. Contemporary update of prostate cancer staging nomograms (Partin Tables) for the new millennium. Urology 2001;58:843–848.
8. Wolf JS Jr, Cher M, Dall'era M, et al. The use and accuracy of cross-sectional imaging and fine needle aspiration cytology for detection of pelvic lymph node metastases before radical prostatectomy. J Urol 1995;153:993–999.
9. Paik ML, Scolieri MJ, Brown SL, et al. Limitations of computerized tomography in staging invasive bladder cancer before radical cystectomy. J Urol 2000;163:1693–1696.
10. Tempany CM, McNeil BJ. Advances in biomedical imaging. JAMA 2001;285:562–567.
11. Wawroschek F, Vogt H, Wengenmair H, et al. Prostate lymphoscintigraphy and radio-guided surgery for sentinel lymph node identification in prostate cancer. Technique and results of the first 350 cases. Urol Int 2003;70:303–310.
12. Bader P, Burkhard FC, Markwalder R, et al. Is a limited lymph node dissection an adequate staging procedure for prostate cancer? J Urol 2002;168:514–518, discussion 518.
13. Weingaertner K, Ramaswamy A, Bittinger A, et al. Anatomical basis for pelvic lymphadenectomy in prostate cancer: results of an autopsy study and implications for the clinic. J Urol 1996;156:1969–1971.
14. Stone NN, Stock RG, Unger P. Laparoscopic pelvic lymph nodes dissection for prostate cancer: comparison of the extended and modified techniques. J Urol 1997;158:1891–1894.
15. Heidenreich A, Varga Z, Von Knobloch R. Extended pelvic lymphadenectomy in patients undergoing radical prostatectomy: high incidence of lymph node metastasis. J Urol 2002;167:1681–1686.
16. Bluestein DL, Bostwick DG, Bergstralh EJ, et al. Eliminating the need for bilateral pelvic lymphadenectomy in select patients with prostate cancer. J Urol 1994;151:1315–1320.
17. Petros JA, Catalona WJ. Lower incidence of unsuspected lymph node metastases in 521 consecutive patients with clinically localized prostate cancer. J Urol 1992;147:1574–1575.
18. Bishoff JT, Reyes A, Thompson IM, et al. Pelvic lymphadenectomy can be omitted in selected patients with carcinoma of the prostate: development of a system of patient selection. Urology 1995;45:270–274.
19. Heidenreich A, Von Knobloch R, Varga Z, et al. Extended pelvic lymphadenectomy in men undergoing radical retropubic prostatectomy (RRP) — an update on >300 cases. J Urol 2004;171:312 (A1183).
20. Tenaglia JL, Iannucci M. Extended pelvic lymphadenectomy for the treatment of localized prostate carcinoma. Eur Urol Today 2004;15.
21. Clark T, Parekh DJ, Cookson MS, et al. Randomized prospective evaluation of extended versus limited lymph node dissection in patients with clinically localized prostate cancer. J Urol 2003;169:145–147, discussion 147–148.
22. Link RE, Morton RA: Indications for pelvic lymphadenectomy in prostate cancer. Urol Clin North Am 2001;28:491–498.
23. Burkhard FC, Schumacher M, Thalmann GN, et al. Is pelvic lymphadenectomy really necessary in patients with a serum prostate-specific antigen level of <10 ng/ml undergoing radical prostatectomy for prostate cancer? BJU Int 2005;95:275–278.
24. Jhaveri FM, Zippe CD, Klein EA, et al. Biochemical failure does not predict overall survival after radical prostatectomy for localized prostate cancer: 10-year results. Urology 1999;54:884–890.
25. Han M, Partin AW, Pound CR, et al. Long-term biochemical disease-free and cancer-specific survival following anatomic radical retropubic prostatectomy. The 15-year Johns Hopkins experience. Urol Clin North Am 2001;28:555–565.

26. Bader P, Burkhard FC, Markwalder R, et al. Disease progression and survival of patients with positive lymph nodes after radical prostatectomy. Is there a chance of cure? J Urol 2003;169:849–854.

27. Roehl KA, Han M, Ramos CG, et al. Cancer progression and survival rates following anatomical radical retropubic prostatectomy in 3,478 consecutive patients: long-term results. J Urol 2004;172:910–914.

28. Steinberg GD, Epstein JI, Piantadosi S, et al. Management of stage D1 adenocarcinoma of the prostate: the Johns Hopkins experience 1974 to 1987. J Urol 1990;144:1425–1432.

29. Zwergel U, Lehmann J, Wullich B, et al. Lymph node positive prostate cancer: long-term survival data after radical prostatectomy. J Urol 2004;171:1128–1131.

30. Frazier HA, 2nd, Robertson JE, Paulson DF. Does radical prostatectomy in the presence of positive pelvic lymph nodes enhance survival? World J Urol 1994;12:308–312.

31. Cadeddu JA, Partin AW, Epstein JI, et al: Stage D1 (T1–3, N1–3, M0) prostate cancer: a case-controlled comparison of conservative treatment versus radical prostatectomy. Urology 1997;50:251–255.

32. Messing E, Manola J, Sarosdy M, et al. Immediate hormonal therapy compared with observation after radical prostatectomy and pelvic lymphadenectomy in men with node positive prostate cancer; Results at 10 years of EST 3886. J Urol 2003;169:396.

33. Catalona WJ, Miller DR, Kavoussi LR. Intermediate-term survival results in clinically understaged prostate cancer patients following radical prostatectomy. J Urol 1988;140:540–543.

34. Pound CR, Partin AW, Eisenberger MA, et al. Natural history of progression after PSA elevation following radical prostatectomy. JAMA 1999;281:1591–1597.

35. Golimbu M, Provet J, Al-Askari S. Radical prostatectomy for stage D1 prostate cancer. Urology 1987;30:427–435.

36. Bader P, Spahn M, Huber R, et al. Limited lymph node dissection in prostate cancer may miss lymph node metastasis and determines outcome of apparently pN0 prostate cancer. Eur Urol 2004;3:16 (A55).

37. Daneshmand S, Quek ML, Stein JP, et al. Prognosis of patients with lymph node positive prostate cancer following radical prostatectomy: long-term results. J Urol 2004;172:2252–2255.

38. Allaf ME, Palapattu GS, Trock BJ, et al. Anatomical extent of lymph node dissection: impact on men with clinically localized prostate cancer. J Urol 2004;172:1840–1844.

39. Dimarco DS, Zincke H, Slezak JM, et al. Does the extent of lymphadenectomy impact disease free survival in prostate cancer? J Urol 2003;169:295 (A1145).

40. Di Blasio CJ, Fearn P, Seo HS, et al. Association between number of lymph nodes removed and freedom from disease progression in patients receiving pelvic lymph node dissection during radical prostatectomy. J Urol 2003;169:456 (A1708).

41. Palapattu GS, Allaf ME, Trock BJ, et al. Prostate specific antigen progression in men with lymph node metastases following radical prostatectomy: results of long-term followup. J Urol 2004;172:1860–1864.

13

Clinical management of rising prostate-specific antigen after radical retropubic prostatectomy

J Kellogg Parsons, Alan W Partin

Introduction

Approximately 40% of men diagnosed with prostate cancer will undergo radical prostatectomy.[1] Of these, 15% to 46% will manifest an isolated, asymptomatic rise in postoperative PSA within 15 years. This phenomenon is referred to as biochemical recurrence. Since an estimated 75,000 radical prostatectomies are performed annually in the US, biochemical recurrence after prostatectomy represents a healthcare issue of considerable magnitude, affecting several thousand men each year.[2]

This chapter reviews the definition, natural history, diagnosis, and treatment of biochemical recurrence after radical prostatectomy, emphasizing practical considerations in the management of these patients.

Definition of biochemical recurrence

Appropriate prostate-specific antigen assays

The gold standard for detecting biochemical recurrence after surgery is measurement of total prostate-specific antigen (PSA). Subsequent statements regarding PSA in this chapter are in reference only to total PSA.

Ultrasensitive assays for total PSA, capable of detection thresholds of 0.001 to 0.01 ng/ml, are not recommended for routine surveillance since they are of unproven clinical value,[3] may detect minute amounts of PSA originating from nonmalignant extraprostatic sources,[4] and may generate problems with false-positive results.[5]

Timing of postoperative prostate-specific antigen surveillance

The oncologic goal of radical prostatectomy is removal of all prostatic tissue. Since the half-life of PSA is 3.15 days,[6] serum PSA should fall to undetectable levels within 21 to 30 days after successful surgery.[7]

There are no uniform standards for the timing of postoperative PSA surveillance. Practice patterns vary considerably. Typically, PSA is drawn every 3 months during the first year, every 6 months during the second through fifth years, and every 12 months thereafter, unless there is clinical or laboratory evidence of recurrent disease.[8]

There are also no uniform standards for the required duration of follow-up for patients with a persistently undetectable PSA. Although some investigators have observed that biochemical recurrence after 7 years is rare,[9] other data suggest that it may occur in a substantial number of patients up to 10 years after surgery.[10,11]

Definition of recurrence: prostate-specific antigen level

There has been considerable debate as to what level of PSA constitutes true biochemical failure. Recommendations for cut-off values range from 0.2 to 0.5 ng/ml.[3,9–16] If postoperative PSA never falls below 0.2 to 0.4 ng/ml, the presence of systemic disease should be strongly considered. If postoperative PSA is initially undetectable but then rises above 0.2 to 0.4 ng/ml, the presence of local recurrence and/or systemic disease should be strongly considered. In 2004, the Group on Clinical Trials in the State of a Rising PSA defined a cut-off of 0.4 ng/ml for eligibility for enrollment in clinical trials.[17]

Rarely, PSA will fail to reach undetectable levels after surgery but remains stable at levels less than 0.4 ng/ml.[16] Should this occur, it is reasonable to consider retained benign tissue as a potential etiology,[15] and expectant management with serial PSAs is an acceptable treatment option. If a persistently detectable PSA rises above 0.4 ng/ml within 3 years of surgery, the presence of recurrent local or systemic disease should be considered.[16]

Natural history of biochemical recurrence

Incidence

Among patients who undergo radical retropubic prostatectomy (RRP), biochemical failure will eventually occur in about one-third, with 15-year PSA-free actuarial survival ranging from 54% to 85%.[5,9,10,13,18–20] PSA-free survival varies depending upon pathologic stage of tumor, grade, margin status, and institutional series.

Data on the incidence of biochemical failure after perineal prostatectomy are considerably less extensive but appear to be similar when compared by equivalent stage, grade, and margin status.[21,22]

Data from laparoscopic radical prostatectomy are not yet mature, but at least one institution has observed 3-year recurrence rates comparable to some retropubic series.[23]

Prediction of biochemical recurrence

A number of equations, graphs, and tables have been developed to predict which patients are most likely to develop biochemical recurrence.[24] The clinical goal of these prediction instruments is to improve the delivery of care by providing clinicians and patients with additional information on which to base treatment decisions.

In the case of biochemical recurrence, stratifying patients by risk identifies those who would potentially benefit from adjuvant treatment *before* biochemical recurrence occurs. The rationale is to delay or prevent biochemical recurrence in those patients most likely to develop it.

There are at least 16 models for predicting the likelihood of biochemical recurrence after radical prostatectomy (Table 13.1). Consistently, the most important variables in these models are preoperative PSA, Gleason score, specimen confinement status, and seminal vesicle or lymph node involvement.[15] Although a number of other variables independently predict biochemical recurrence,[25,26] it is not yet clear whether these individual markers add anything to existing predictive models.[27]

There is no consensus as to how these nomograms should be applied to clinical practice, nor any data to support the hypothesis that adjuvant treatment of patients likely to experience biochemical recurrence improves cancer-specific survival. Nevertheless, our institution and others[9,15] recommend the use of validated nomograms to direct at-risk patients into appropriate clinical trials or more rigorous surveillance programs.

Prediction of time to metastases and death

The natural history of progression to frank metastases and death after biochemical recurrence is variable but is generally prolonged.[10,28,29] Among 304 patients with biochemical recurrence followed for up to 15 years, 34% progressed to metastases over a median period of 8 years. Of those who progressed, median time to cancer-specific death after documented metastases was 5 years.[10]

The challenge in clinical practice has been to identify the minority of men who will progress rapidly after the onset of biochemical recurrence. PSA kinetics, the study of changes in PSA over time, has been useful in this regard. Three measures are associated with rapid clinical progression after biochemical recurrence: time to biochemical recurrence (time between surgery and onset of biochemical recurrence), PSA velocity (PSAV; change in PSA/unit time), and PSA doubling time (PSADT; time it takes for serum PSA levels to double).

Shorter time to recurrence is associated with faster progression. Men who recur within 1 to 3 years of surgery will progress more quickly to metastases and death.[10,16,30,31] Larger PSAV is associated with faster progression. A PSAV greater than or equal to 0.75 ng/ml/year at 1 year after surgery is associated with an increased likelihood of early metastatic disease.[6]

PSADT is calculated by: 1) log-transforming longitudinal PSA levels to create a linear relationship between serum PSA level and time; 2) determining the slope of this log-transformed curve; and 3) multiplying the slope of the log-transformed curve by the inverse of the natural log of 2.[32] Shorter PSADT is associated with decreased time to metastases[10,31–33] and increased prostate cancer-specific mortality.[28,34] The advantage of PSADT over time to recurrence or PSAV at 1 year is that it predicts metastatic progression independently of the number of years since surgery.[11,32] PSADT cut-off values for stratifying patients into low and high-risk groups for metastatic progression and death range from 3[28] to 6[32,33] to 12 months.[34]

Diagnosis of biochemical recurrence

Local versus systemic disease

One of the most problematic aspects of evaluating patients with biochemical recurrence is determining whether the source of the PSA is localized or metastatic disease. Ideally, identifying isolated localized disease allows for therapy to be directed towards the prostatic fossa. Estimates for the incidence of isolated local recurrence vary from 4% to 53%, reflecting the difficulty in establishing this diagnosis.[5,35–38]

Current diagnostic modalities for distinguishing between local and systemic disease remain limited. Available options (Tables 13.2 and 13.3) are described below.

Prostate-specific antigen kinetics and tumor pathology

PSA kinetics and tumor pathology are the most useful parameters for estimating the likelihood that systemic disease is present.[3] With respect to the three PSA kinetic measurements mentioned above, the following criteria suggest the presence of systemic disease: 1) time to biochemical recurrence of less than 1 to 2 years,[6,31,32,39] 2) a PSAV at 1 year greater than or equal to 0.75 ng/ml/year,[6] and 3) a PSADT less than 3 to 12 months.[10,28,32–34]

Higher tumor grade and advanced stage also suggest the presence of systemic disease.[30] Table 13.3 summarizes the PSA and pathologic criteria associated with an increased likelihood of distant disease. Table 13.4 presents data for predicting the probability of metastasis-free survival at 3, 5, and 7 years with Gleason score, time to biochemical recurrence, and PSADT.[5,10]

Digital rectal examination

Digital rectal examination should be performed with the recognition that its diagnostic utility is limited. The postoperative contour of the prostatic fossa is highly variable and is not consistently associated with the presence of local recurrence.[36,40–42] Management decisions, therefore, should not be based on examination findings alone.

Table 13.1 Models for prediction of biochemical recurrence after radical retropubic prostatectomy

Reference	Year	Number of patients	Prediction instrument	Prediction variables	Validated?
Partin et al[66]	1995	216	Equation categorizing men into low-, intermediate-, and high-risk groups	PSA, specimen Gleason score, specimen confinement status	Yes
Bauer et al[67]	1997	132	Equation categorizing men into low-, intermediate-, and high-risk groups	BCL2 status, p53 status, PSA, race, specimen confinement status	No
Bauer et al[68]	1998	378	Equation categorizing men into low-, intermediate-, and high-risk groups	PSA, race, specimen confinement status, specimen Gleason score	Yes
D'Amico et al[69]	1998	862	Probability graph	Pathologic stage, PSA specimen Gleason score, surgical margin status	No
Kattan et al[70]	1998	983	Probability nomogram	Biopsy Gleason score, clinical stage, PSA	Yes
D'Amico et al[71]	1999	892	Probability nomogram	Biopsy Gleason score clinical stage, PSA	Yes
Graefen et al[72]	1999	318	Quantitative analysis of high-grade cancer categorizing men into low- and high- risk groups	Biopsy Gleason score, number of positive biopsy cores, pathologic stage, PSA, specimen Gleason score	No
Kattan et al[9]	1999	996	Probability nomogram	Lymph node invasion, PSA, seminal vesicle invasion, specimen confinement status, specimen Gleason score	Yes
Potter et al[73]	1999	214	Neural network	DNA ploidy, patient age, quantified nuclear grade, specimen confinement status, specimen Gleason score	Yes
D'Amico et al[74]	2000	823	Percent of positive biopsy cores categorizing men into risk groups	Biopsy Gleason grade, Clinical stage, Percentage of positive biopsy cores, PSA	Yes
Stamey et al[75]	2000	326	Equation for probability of biochemical failure	Gleason score, lymph node invasion, percent of intraductal cancer, prostate weight, PSA, tumor volume, vascular invasion	Yes
Blute et al[76]	2001	2518	Equation categorizing men into low- and high-risk groups	Adjuvant therapy, Gleason score, PSA, seminal vesicle invasion, surgical margin status	Yes
Moul et al[25]	2001	1012	Equation categorizing men into four different risk groups	PSA, race, specimen confinement status, specimen Gleason score	Yes
Roberts et al[77]	2001	904	Equation categorizing men into low- and high-risk groups	Gleason score, lymph node invasion, seminal vesicle invasion, surgical margin status	Yes
Khan et al[78]	2003	1955	Probability nomogram	Gleason score, pathologic stage, surgical margin status	No
Freedland et al[79]	2004	459	Model categorizing men into low-, intermediate-, high-, and very high-risk groups	Gleason score, percent of positive biopsy cores, PSA	No

Ultrasound-guided biopsy

We do not recommend routine biopsy of the prostatic fossa or vesicourethral anastomosis. Despite some favorable initial reports,[36] there are at least four substantial problems with biopsy as a diagnostic tool for guiding therapy in this setting. First, the true sensitivity of ultrasound in detecting local recurrence is not known. Second, since the true false-negative rate is not known,[2,3] negative biopsy does not preclude the presence of local disease. Third, distant disease may exist concomitantly with local disease.[3,39] Fourth, post-biopsy salvage radiation therapy to the prostatic bed has produced similar results regardless of whether the biopsy was positive or negative.[43,44]

Computed tomography

Computed tomography (CT) of the abdomen and pelvis has poor yield for identifying either local or metastatic disease after prostatectomy.[45–49] Its clinical usefulness is particularly limited in asymptomatic patients with a PSA of less than 10 ng/ml. It may hold limited value in patients with a PSADT of less than 6 months.[49]

Magnetic resonance imaging

The primary role for endorectal magnetic resonance imaging (MRI) is to rule out osseous metastases after an equivocal bone scan.[3] The efficacy of MRI in identifying soft-tissue and nodal disease is unclear and is under study.[50]

Bone scan

Bone scan also possesses limited clinical usefulness in asymptomatic men with biochemical recurrence and low PSA.[3,15,49,51] For asymptomatic patients, most investigators recommend bone scan only for select patients with a serum PSA of greater than 10 to 50 ng/ml and/or a PSADT of less than 6 months.[3,15,49,51]

Table 13.2 Prostate-specific antigen (PSA) and pathologic variables for distinguishing between local and systemic disease in patients with biochemical recurrence after radical prostatectomy

Variable	Local recurrence	Systemic recurrence
Gleason score[30]	≤7	>7
Lymph node invasion[30]	No	Yes
PSA doubling time (PSADT)[10,28,32–34]	≥3–12 months	<3–12 months
PSA velocity at 1 year[6,30]	<0.75 ng/ml/year	0.75 ng/ml/year
Seminal vesicle invasion[30]	No	Yes
Time to PSA recurrence[6,31,32,39]	>1–2 years	<1–2 years

Table 13.3 Diagnostic modalities for distinguishing between local and systemic disease in patients with biochemical recurrence after radical prostatectomy

Diagnostic modality	Clinical usefulness
Digital rectal examination	None
Ultrasound-guided biopsy	None
Computed tomography	Marginal. May consider if PSA >10 ng/ml or PSA doubling time (PSADT) <6 months
Magnetic resonance imaging	Under investigation
Bone scan	Marginal. May consider if PSA >10–50 ng/ml or PSADT <6 months
Radiolabeled antibody to PSMA	Potentially useful. Further trials needed in setting of biochemical recurrence
Positron emission tomography	Under investigation

PSMA, prostate-specific membrane antigen.

Radiolabeled antibody to prostate-specific antigen (Prostascint)

Prostate-specific membrane antigen (PSMA) is a prostate-restricted cell-surface antigen expressed by all prostate cancers. Expression tends to be increased in poorly differentiated, metastatic, and hormone refractory tumors. Capromab pendetide (ProstaScint, Cytogen Corporation, Princeton, NJ) is a monoclonal, radiolabeled anti-PSMA antibody that is FDA-approved for imaging of soft-tissue metastases. Sensitivities for capromab pendetide for the detection of metastatic prostate cancer range from 62% to 75%.[52,53] Although it may potentially distinguish local from systemic disease in patients with a PSA as low as 0.5 ng/ml,[54] more prospective trials are needed to evaluate its usefulness in post-prostatectomy patients.

Positron emission tomography

Positron emission tomography (PET) scanning, which utilizes a radiolabeled glucose analog to identify areas of increased tumor activity, has only a limited role in the evaluation of biochemical recurrence.[55,56] Studies of newer radiotracers are ongoing.[57]

Treatment of biochemical recurrence

Discussion of the management of biochemical recurrence after prostatectomy merits contemplation of one important caveat: currently, there are no prospective data as to whether treatment of biochemical recurrence, at any time point or with any modality, improves cancer specific survival. While many current treatment modalities are effective at returning serum PSA to undetectable levels, it is unclear as to whether or not this alters the natural history of the disease.

Expectant management

Since there is no definitive evidence that treatment of biochemical recurrence will improve cancer-specific mortality, and since the median time for the onset of metastases in untreated patients after an initial rise in PSA is 8 years,[10] expectant management may be an appropriate treatment option in older patients with significant co-morbidity and/or a lower probability of disease progression. These patients may be followed closely, with treatment reserved for those with a PSADT of less than 3 to 12 months or clinical symptoms.

Salvage radiotherapy

Salvage radiotherapy is radiotherapy applied to the prostatic bed with curative intent for postoperative biochemical recurrence.[58] It should be considered if PSA kinetics, pathologic variables, and/or radiologic imaging suggest an isolated local recurrence.

The efficacy of salvage radiotherapy at improving cancer-specific survival remains unproven. In most studies, the primary outcome is a PSA response to treatment. Although 60% to 90% of patients may initially achieve an undetectable PSA after radiation, only 10% to 45% remain free of PSA recurrence 5 years later.[58–60]

The single most important prognostic factor in predicting objective PSA response to salvage radiotherapy is pretreatment PSA. A lower PSA is associated with increased likelihood of response.[60–63] Accordingly, in 1999 the American Society for Therapeutic Radiology and Oncology (ASTRO) consensus panel recommended that treatment be initiated at a PSA of less than 1.5 ng/ml with a minimum dose of 64 to 65 Gy.[58]

The benefit of adjuvant hormonal therapy with salvage radiotherapy is also unproven. Although retrospective data suggest that hormonal therapy may improve PSA response,[64] there are no prospective data. The Radiation Therapy Oncology Group is conducting a study (RTOG 96-01) randomizing patients with biochemical recurrence after radical prostatectomy to radiotherapy alone versus radiotherapy plus bicalutamide 150 mg/day.[60]

Table 13.4 Estimation of metastasis-free survival following biochemical recurrence after radical prostatectomy

| | | | Percent with metastasis-free survival (95% CI) | | |
			3 years	*5 years*	*7 years*
All patients			78 (73–84)	63 (56–70)	52 (44–60)
Gleason score 5–7	Recurrence >2 years	PSADT >10 months	95 (83–96)	86 (74–92)	82 (69–90)
		PSADT ≤10 years	82 (54–94)	69 (40–86)	60 (32–80)
	Recurrence ≤2 years	PSADT >10 months	79 (65–88)	76 (61–86)	59 (40–73)
		PSADT ≤10 years	81 (57–93)	35 (16–56)	15 (4–33)
Gleason score 8–10	Recurrence >2 years		77 (55–89)	60 (33–79)	47 (17–72)
	Recurrence ≤2 years		53 (39–66)	31 (17–45)	21 (9–35)

Data adapted from Pound et al[5] and Laufer et al.[10]
PSADT, PSA doubling time.

In summary, salvage radiotherapy is effective at lowering PSA. It should be considered in patients in whom isolated local recurrence is suspected. Treatment when PSA is less than 1.5 ng/ml maximizes the potential response. Studies are ongoing as to whether adjuvant hormonal therapy will improve response.

Hormonal therapy

The rationale for treating biochemical recurrence with androgen ablation is that, in the absence of isolated local recurrence, biochemical recurrence represents systemic disease. The appropriate timing of androgen ablation in the treatment of advanced prostate cancer—early versus late—is disputed. In the post-prostatectomy patient, androgen ablation for asymptomatic biochemical recurrence represents early therapy, while ablation for symptomatic metastases represents late therapy.

Regardless of timing, androgen ablation will reduce serum PSA levels in men with biochemical recurrence after radical prostatectomy.[65] Retrospective data suggest that select men with aggressive disease who receive early hormonal therapy for biochemical recurrence have improved PSA progression-free survival and increased time to the onset of metastases.[65] However, there is no evidence that either early or late androgen ablation improves cancer-specific survival.

Other means by which the androgen axis may be manipulated include maximum androgen blockade, oral androgen antagonists, and 5-alpha reductase inhibitors. There are no conclusive data on the benefits of any of these modalities for the treatment of biochemical recurrence.

Summary

The most appropriate assay for diagnosing biochemical recurrence is serum total PSA, which should be checked every 3 months for the first year after surgery and at least every 12 months thereafter for a minimum of 10 years. Definitions for the diagnosis of biochemical recurrence after radical prostatectomy range from 0.2 to 0.4 ng/ml. A multidisciplinary group has recommended a cut-off of 0.4 ng/ml as a criterion for inclusion in clinical trials. Persistent, stable levels below 0.4 ng/ml for up to 3 years following surgery may be followed expectantly.

Fifteen-year PSA-free actuarial survival rates vary from 54% to 85%. Several validated prediction models exist for predicting biochemical recurrence. Disease progression following biochemical recurrence is generally indolent. Time to recurrence, PSAV, PSADT, and tumor pathology are all associated with the risk of progression to metastases and death.

In distinguishing between patients with local and systemic recurrence, PSA kinetics and tumor features remain the most valuable clinical parameters. Digital rectal examination should be performed, but its usefulness at planning therapy is limited. Ultrasound-guided biopsy of the prostatic fossa is not recommended. CT and bone scan have marginal clinical utility. MRI, ProstaScint, and PET scanning are investigational modalities at this time.

Expectant management should be considered in patients with an onset of recurrence more than 2 years after surgery, a PSADT of greater than 3 to 12 months, and no evidence of clinical disease. Salvage radiotherapy is efficacious at lowering serum PSA in men suspected of having isolated local recurrence, particularly with a PSA of less than 1.5 ng/ml. However, it is unclear whether it improves survival. Early hormonal therapy will lower PSA and, in men with aggressive disease, potentially increase time to metastases. However, there is no evidence that either early or delayed hormonal therapy will improve cancer-specific survival.

References

1. Burkhardt JH, Litwin MS, Rose CM, et al. Comparing the costs of radiation therapy and radical prostatectomy for the initial treatment of early-stage prostate cancer. J Clin Oncol 2002;20:2869–2875.
2. Moul JW. Prostate specific antigen only progression of prostate cancer. J Urol 2000;163:1632–1642.
3. Swindle PW, Kattan MW, Scardino PT. Markers and meaning of primary treatment failure. Urol Clin North Am 2003;30:377–401.
4. Diamandis EP, Yu H. Nonprostatic sources of prostate-specific antigen. Urol Clin North Am 1997;24:275–282.
5. Laufer M, Pound CR, Carducci MA, et al. Management of patients with rising prostate-specific antigen after radical prostatectomy. Urology 2000;55:309–315.
6. Partin AW, Oesterling JE. The clinical usefulness of prostate specific antigen: update 1994. J Urol 1994;152:1358–1368.
7. Oesterling JE, Chan DW, Epstein JI, et al. Prostate specific antigen in the preoperative and postoperative evaluation of localized prostatic cancer treated with radical prostatectomy. J Urol 1988;139:766–772.
8. Oh J, Colberg JW, Ornstein DK, et al. Current followup strategies after radical prostatectomy: a survey of American Urological Association urologists. J Urol 1999;161:520–523.
9. Kattan MW, Wheeler TM, Scardino PT. Postoperative nomogram for disease recurrence after radical prostatectomy for prostate cancer. J Clin Oncol 1999;17:1499–1507.

10. Pound CR, Partin AW, Eisenberger MA, et al. Natural history of progression after PSA elevation following radical prostatectomy. JAMA 1999;281:1591–1597.

11. Ward JF, Blute ML, Slezak J, et al. The long-term clinical impact of biochemical recurrence of prostate cancer 5 or more years after radical prostatectomy. J Urol 2003;170:1872–1876.

12. Moul JW, Douglas TH, McCarthy WF, et al. Black race is an adverse prognostic factor for prostate cancer recurrence following radical prostatectomy in an equal access health care setting. J Urol 1996;155:1667–1673.

13. Zincke H, Oesterling JE, Blute ML, et al. Long-term (15 years) results after radical prostatectomy for clinically localized (stage T2c or lower) prostate cancer. J Urol 1994;152:1850–1857.

14. Freedland SJ, Sutter ME, Dorey F, et al. Defining the ideal cutpoint for determining PSA recurrence after radical prostatectomy. Prostate-specific antigen. Urology 2003;61:365–369.

15. Moul JW. Variables in predicting survival based on treating "PSA-only" relapse. Urol Oncol 2003;21:292–304.

16. Amling CL, Bergstralh EJ, Blute ML, et al. Defining prostate specific antigen progression after radical prostatectomy: what is the most appropriate cut point? J Urol 2001;165:1146–1151.

17. Scher HI, Eisenberger M, D'Amico AV, et al. Eligibility and outcomes reporting guidelines for clinical trials for patients in the state of a rising prostate-specific antigen: recommendations from the Prostate-Specific Antigen Working Group. J Clin Oncol 2004;22:537–556.

18. Catalona WJ, Smith DS. 5-year tumor recurrence rates after anatomical radical retropubic prostatectomy for prostate cancer. J Urol 1994;152:1837–1842.

19. Khan MA, Han M, Partin AW, et al. Long-term cancer control of radical prostatectomy in men younger than 50 years of age: update 2003. Urology 2003;62:86–91, discussion 91–92.

20. Trapasso JG, deKernion JB, Smith RB, et al. The incidence and significance of detectable levels of serum prostate specific antigen after radical prostatectomy. J Urol 1994;152:1821–1825.

21. Iselin CE, Robertson JE, Paulson DF. Radical perineal prostatectomy: oncological outcome during a 20-year period. J Urol 1999;161:163–168.

22. Harris MJ. Radical perineal prostatectomy: cost efficient, outcome effective, minimally invasive prostate cancer management. Eur Urol 2003;44:303–308, discussion 308.

23. Guillonneau B, el-Fettouh H, Baumert H, et al. Laparoscopic radical prostatectomy: oncological evaluation after 1,000 cases a Montsouris Institute. J Urol 2003;169:1261–1266.

24. Ross PL, Scardino PT, Kattan MW. A catalog of prostate cancer nomograms. J Urol 2001;165:1562–1568.

25. Moul JW, Connelly RR, Lubeck DP, et al. Predicting risk of prostate specific antigen recurrence after radical prostatectomy with the Center for Prostate Disease Research and Cancer of the Prostate Strategic Urologic Research Endeavor databases. J Urol 2001;166:1322–1327.

26. Rhodes DR, Sanda MG, Otte AP, et al. Multiplex biomarker approach for determining risk of prostate-specific antigen-defined recurrence of prostate cancer. J Natl Cancer Inst 2003;95:661–668.

27. Kattan MW. Judging new markers by their ability to improve predictive accuracy. J Natl Cancer Inst 2003;95:634–635.

28. D'Amico AV, Moul JW, Carroll PR, et al. Surrogate end point for prostate cancer-specific mortality after radical prostatectomy or radiation therapy. J Natl Cancer Inst 2003;95:1376–1383.

29. Jhaveri FM, Zippe CD, Klein EA, Kupelian PA. Biochemical failure does not predict overall survival after radical prostatectomy for localized prostate cancer: 10-year results. Urology 1999;54:884–890.

30. Partin AW, Pearson JD, Landis PK, et al. Evaluation of serum prostate-specific antigen velocity after radical prostatectomy to distinguish local recurrence from distant metastases. Urology 1994;43:649–659.

31. Amling CL, Blute ML, Bergstralh EJ, et al. TM, Slezak J, Zincke H. Long-term hazard of progression after radical prostatectomy for clinically localized prostate cancer: continued risk of biochemical failure after 5 years. J Urol 2000;164:101–105.

32. Patel A, Dorey F, Franklin J, et al. Recurrence patterns after radical retropubic prostatectomy: clinical usefulness of prostate specific antigen doubling times and log slope prostate specific antigen. J Urol 1997;158:1441–1445.

33. Roberts SG, Blute ML, Bergstralh EJ, et al. PSA doubling time as a predictor of clinical progression after biochemical failure following radical prostatectomy for prostate cancer. Mayo Clin Proc 2001;76:576–581.

34. Albertsen PC, Hanley JA, Penson DF, et al. Validation of increasing prostate specific antigen as a predictor of prostate cancer death after treatment of localized prostate cancer with surgery or radiation. J Urol 2004;171:2221–2225.

35. Han M, Partin AW, Pound CR, et al. Long-term biochemical disease-free and cancer-specific survival following anatomic radical retropubic prostatectomy. The 15-year Johns Hopkins experience. Urol Clin North Am 2001;28:555–565.

36. Foster LS, Jajodia P, Fournier G Jr, et al. The value of prostate specific antigen and transrectal ultrasound guided biopsy in detecting prostatic fossa recurrences following radical prostatectomy. J Urol 1993;149:1024–1028.

37. Connolly JA, Shinohara K, Presti JC Jr, et al. Local recurrence after radical prostatectomy: characteristics in size, location, and relationship to prostate-specific antigen and surgical margins. Urology 1996;47:225–231.

38. Zietman AL, Shipley WU, Willett CG. Residual disease after radical surgery or radiation therapy for prostate cancer. Clinical significance and therapeutic implications. Cancer 1993;71(3 Suppl):959–969.

39. Pound CR, Partin AW, Epstein JI, et al. Prostate-specific antigen after anatomic radical retropubic prostatectomy. Patterns of recurrence and cancer control. Urol Clin North Am 1997;24:395–406.

40. Saleem MD, Sanders H, Abu El Naser M, et al. Factors predicting cancer detection in biopsy of the prostatic fossa after radical prostatectomy. Urology 1998;51:283–286.

41. Fowler JE, Jr., Brooks J, Pandey P, et al. Variable histology of anastomotic biopsies with detectable prostate specific antigen after radical prostatectomy. J Urol 1995;153:1011–1014.

42. Lightner DJ, Lange PH, Reddy PK, et al. Prostate specific antigen and local recurrence after radical prostatectomy. J Urol 1990;144:921–926.

43. Cadeddu JA, Partin AW, DeWeese TL, et al. Long-term results of radiation therapy for prostate cancer recurrence following radical prostatectomy. J Urol 1998;159:173–177, discussion 177–178.

44. Koppie TM, Grossfeld GD, Nudell DM, et al. Is anastomotic biopsy necessary before radiotherapy after radical prostatectomy? J Urol 2001;166:111–115.

45. Seltzer MA, Barbaric Z, Belldegrun A, et al. Comparison of helical computerized tomography, positron emission tomography and monoclonal antibody scans for evaluation of lymph node metastases in patients with prostate specific antigen relapse after treatment for localized prostate cancer. J Urol 1999;162:1322–1328.

46. Kramer S, Gorich J, Gottfried HW, et al. Sensitivity of computed tomography in detecting local recurrence of prostatic carcinoma following radical prostatectomy. Br J Radiol 1997;70:995–999.

47. Johnson PAS. Yield of imaging and scintigraphy assessing bNED failure in prostate cancer patients. Urol Oncol 1997;70:995.

48. Kane CJ, Amling CL, Johnstone PA, et al. Limited value of bone scintigraphy and computed tomography in assessing biochemical failure after radical prostatectomy. Urology 2003;61:607–611.

49. Okotie OT, Aronson WJ, Wieder JA, et al. Predictors of metastatic disease in men with biochemical failure following radical prostatectomy. J Urol 2004;171:2260–2264.

50. Harisinghani MG, Barentsz J, Hahn PF, et al. Noninvasive detection of clinically occult lymph–node metastases in prostate cancer. N Engl J Med 2003;348:2491–2499.

51. Cher ML, Bianco FJ Jr, Lam JS, et al. Limited role of radionuclide bone scintigraphy in patients with prostate specific antigen elevations after radical prostatectomy. J Urol 1998;160:1387–1391.

52. Quintana JC, Blend MJ. The dual-isotope ProstaScint imaging procedure: clinical experience and staging results in 145 patients. Clin Nucl Med 2000;25:33–40.

53. Hinkle GH, Burgers JK, Neal CE, et al. Multicenter radioimmunoscintigraphic evaluation of patients with prostate carcinoma using indium-111 capromab pendetide. Cancer 1998;83:739–747.

54. Raj GV, Partin AW, Polascik TJ. Clinical utility of indium 111-capromab pendetide immunoscintigraphy in the detection of early, recurrent prostate carcinoma after radical prostatectomy. Cancer 2002;94:987–996.

55. Hofer C, Laubenbacher C, Block T, et al. Fluorine-18-fluorodeoxyglucose positron emission tomography is useless for the detection of local recurrence after radical prostatectomy. Eur Urol 1999;36:31–35.

56. Effert PJ, Bares R, Handt S, et al. Metabolic imaging of untreated prostate cancer by positron emission tomography with 18fluorine-labeled deoxyglucose. J Urol 1996;155:994–998.

57. Hricak H, Schoder H, Pucar D, et al. Advances in imaging in the postoperative patient with a rising prostate-specific antigen level. Semin Oncol 2003;30:616–634.

58. Cox JD, Gallagher MJ, Hammond EH, et al. Consensus statements on radiation therapy of prostate cancer: guidelines for prostate re-biopsy after radiation and for radiation therapy with rising prostate-specific antigen levels after radical prostatectomy. American Society for Therapeutic Radiology and Oncology Consensus Panel. J Clin Oncol 1999;17:1155.

59. Forman JD, Velasco J. Therapeutic radiation in patients with a rising post-prostatectomy PSA level. Oncology (Huntingt) 1998;12:33–39, discussion 39, 43–44, 47.

60. Macdonald OK, Schild SE, Vora SA, et al. Radiotherapy for men with isolated increase in serum prostate specific antigen after radical prostatectomy. J Urol 2003;170:1833–1837.

61. Anscher MS, Clough R, Dodge R. Radiotherapy for a rising prostate-specific antigen after radical prostatectomy: the first 10 years. Int J Radiat Oncol Biol Phys 2000;48:369–375.

62. Song DY, Thompson TL, Ramakrishnan V, et al. Salvage radiotherapy for rising or persistent PSA after radical prostatectomy. Urology 2002;60:281–287.

63. Liauw SL, Webster WS, Pistenmaa DA, et al. Salvage radiotherapy for biochemical failure of radical prostatectomy: a single-institution experience. Urology 2003;61:1204–1210.

64. Eulau SM, Tate DJ, Stamey TA, et al. Effect of combined transient androgen deprivation and irradiation following radical prostatectomy for prostatic cancer. Int J Radiat Oncol Biol Phys 1998;41:735–740.

65. Moul JW, Wu H, Sun L, et al. Early versus delayed hormonal therapy for prostate specific antigen only recurrence of prostate cancer after radical prostatectomy. J Urol 2004;171:1141–1147.

66. Partin AW, Piantadosi S, Sanda MG, et al. Selection of men at high risk for disease recurrence for experimental adjuvant therapy following radical prostatectomy. Urology 1995;45:831–838.

67. Bauer JJ, Connelly RR, Sesterhenn IA, et al. Biostatistical modeling using traditional variables and genetic biomarkers for predicting the risk of prostate carcinoma recurrence after radical prostatectomy. Cancer 1997;79:952–962.

68. Bauer JJ, Connelly RR, Seterhenn IA, et al. Biostatistical modeling using traditional preoperative and pathological prognostic variables in the selection of men at high risk for disease recurrence after radical prostatectomy for prostate cancer. J Urol 1998;159:929–933.

69. D'Amico AV, Whittington R, Malkowicz SB, et al. The combination of preoperative prostate specific antigen and postoperative pathological findings to predict prostate specific antigen outcome in clinically localized prostate cancer. J Urol 1998;160:2096–2101.

70. Kattan MW, Eastham JA, Stapleton AM, et al. A preoperative nomogram for disease recurrence following radical prostatectomy for prostate cancer. J Natl Cancer Inst 1998;90:766–771.

71. D'Amico AV, Whittington R, Malkowicz SB, et al. Pretreatment nomogram for prostate-specific antigen recurrence after radical prostatectomy or external-beam radiation therapy for clinically localized prostate cancer. J Clin Oncol 1999;17:168–172.

72. Graefen M, Noldus J, Pichlmeier U, et al. Early prostate-specific antigen relapse after radical retropubic prostatectomy: prediction on the basis of preoperative and postoperative tumor characteristics. Eur Urol 1999;36:21–30.

73. Potter SR, Miller MC, Mangold LA, et al. Genetically engineered neural networks for predicting prostate cancer progression after radical prostatectomy. Urology 1999;54:791–795.

74. D'Amico AV, Whittington R, Malkowicz SB, et al. Clinical utility of the percentage of positive prostate biopsies in defining biochemical outcome after radical prostatectomy for patients with clinically localized prostate cancer. J Clin Oncol 2000;18:1164–1172.

75. Stamey TA, Yemoto CM, McNeal JE, et al. Prostate cancer is highly predictable: a prognostic equation based on all morphological variables in radical prostatectomy specimens. J Urol 2000;163:1155–1160.

76. Blute ML, Bergstralh EJ, Iocca A, et al. Use of Gleason score, prostate specific antigen, seminal vesicle and margin status to predict biochemical failure after radical prostatectomy. J Urol 2001;165:119–125.

77. Roberts WW, Bergstralh EJ, Blute ML, et al. Contemporary identification of patients at high risk of early prostate cancer recurrence after radical retropubic prostatectomy. Urology 2001;57:1033–1037.

78. Khan MA, Partin AW, Mangold LA, et al. Probability of biochemical recurrence by analysis of pathologic stage, Gleason score, and margin status for localized prostate cancer. Urology 2003;62:866–871.

79. Freedland SJ, Terris MK, Csathy GS, et al. Preoperative model for predicting prostate specific antigen recurrence after radical prostatectomy using percent of biopsy tissue with cancer, biopsy Gleason grade and serum prostate specific antigen. J Urol 2004;171:2215–2220.

14

Radical perineal prostatectomy

David M Hartke, Martin I Resnick

Introduction

Prostate cancer is the most frequently diagnosed noncutaneous cancer in American men and the second leading cause of cancer death. Fortunately, we are in an era of early detection and men are diagnosed with and present for treatment of adenocarcinoma of the prostate at earlier stages. Though various methods of therapy are available, over the last century, surgical cure has been a mainstay of prostate cancer therapy. Hugh Hampton Young, the first Chairman of Urology at Johns Hopkins School of Medicine, is credited with performing the first radical perineal prostatectomy for treatment of cancer.[1] In 1939, Belt modified the procedure by introducing a subsphincteric dissection as a means of improving exposure of the prostate.[2] For years, many surgeons adopted this approach, which was the principle method for treating those patients with localized prostate malignancies. In 1945, the retropubic prostatectomy was first introduced by Dr Terrence Millin, however, due to the large intra-operative blood loss and high morbidity, the perineal approach remained the accepted method of treatment.[3] In the late 1970s, the importance of pelvic lymphadenectomy for accurate disease staging was understood and the retropubic approach and concomitant pelvic lymph node dissection through the same incision replaced the perineal prostatectomy as the more popular approach. Furthermore, the works of Dr Patrick Walsh improved upon Millin's technique, demonstrating functional anatomic relationships that reduced the intraoperative blood loss and improved outcomes of impotence and urinary incontinence.[4,5,6] Thus, the radical retropubic prostatectomy has been the most common surgical approach over the last two decades.

Recently, there has been a resurgence of interest in the radical perineal prostatectomy. The reason for increased popularity is multifactorial. First, the work of Partin et al. has allowed for a relatively accurate prediction of disease stage and pelvic lymph node involvement through analysis of PSA level, clinical stage, and Gleason pathologic score.[7] This work has allowed for a more selective use of staging lymphadenectomy.[8] Moreover, the advancement of laparoscopy has allowed for a combined laparoscopic pelvic lymphadenectomy and standard radical perineal prostatectomy in those patients who require staging lymph node analysis.[8,9,10] Thus, with the need for an abdominal incision obviated, and due to advancements in technique,[11] the perineal prostatectomy offers patients a cost-effective operation, with shorter hospital stays, shorter time to reconvalescence, low morbidity, and cancer control as effective as with the retropubic approach. Moreover, the perineal prostatectomy may have an easier learning curve than the retropubic approach.[12]

Patient selection

Radical curative surgery is offered to those patients with an expected non-cancer survival of greater than 15 years who demonstrate a high likelihood of organ-confined disease. Those with a biopsy Gleason score of 8 or less, a PSA level below 20 ng/ml and are without palpable bilateral disease are eligible candidates; patients with higher values tend to have more advanced disease and are not eligible for the procedure. Laparoscopic pelvic lymphadenectomy is deemed unnecessary because of the low likelihood of nodal disease if the biopsy Gleason score is less than 7 in the presence of unilateral disease and the serum PSA level is less than 10 ng/ml. When required, the laparoscopic lymphadenectomy is usually carried out immediately prior to prostatectomy.[10] While the lymph nodes specimens are processed as frozen sections, the patient is repositioned. RPP is aborted if the lymph nodes are positive for metastatic disease.

In patients with localized prostate cancer, there are few contraindications to this procedure. Patients with severe ankylosis of the hips or spine and those with unstable artificial hip replacements may not tolerate the exaggerated lithotomy position. However, common degenerative disc disease is not a contra-indication to positioning. Furthermore, patients with extreme obesity may not be eligible secondary to the restrictive force upon ventilation generated by excessive weight on the diaphragm. These extremely obese patients are poor candidates for the retropubic approach as well and are often offered non-surgical treatment. Some patients, such as those having a renal transplant or those with severe inflammation secondary to placement of synthetic mesh for repair of a hernia may not be amenable to a retropubic approach but typically can have the prostate removed perineally without incident.

Preoperative care

A full bowel preparation is administered the day prior to surgery. Although the patient may consume a regular diet, he is instructed to consume 4 L of polyethylene glycol in the afternoon prior to the surgery. Also, 1.0 g of neomycin is administered orally at 12:00, 2:00, 4:00, 6:00, 8:00 and 10:00 pm. This bowel prep allows for primary closure of any inadvertent rectal injury at the time of surgery.

A blood type and antibody screen is obtained from all patients in the days or hours prior to surgery. Because blood loss is minimal and transfusions rarely required, a cross-match is unnecessary.

In the preoperative holding area, knee-high antithromboembolic surgical stockings are placed without the need for sequential compression devices. The patient is given 1.0 g of intravenous cefazolin in the operating room. Patients with cephalosporin allergy are administered intravenous gentamicin at a dose of 2 to 5 mg/kg body weight.

Anesthesia

Anesthetic options are discussed with the patient pre-operatively. Although regional anesthetics such as spinal or epidural anesthesia are possible, they are somewhat limited by the exaggerated lithotomy positioning of the patient. Thus, most patients elect to receive a general anesthetic.

Position

After the induction of anesthesia, the patient is positioned supine so that when the leg portion of the operating table is lowered, the buttocks are extended beyond the table edge. Allen® stirrups are stationed 2 inches cranially on the rail so that there is ample room for the attachment of the self-retaining retractor. The patient's feet are placed in the Allen® stirrups with the stirrups at the level of his legs. The stirrups are then simultaneously elevated into a modified exaggerated dorsal lithotomy position such that the upper thigh is at a 75° angle with the spine. The perineum is at a right angle to the floor (Figure 14.1). The perineum, anus, and scrotum are shaved and the anterior abdomen inferior to the umbilicus, penis, scrotum, perineum, anus, and both thighs are painted with povidone-iodine in the standard sterile fashion. After gowning, a sterile towel is sewn from the 9 o'clock to the 3 o'clock position around the anus at the mucocutaneous pigmentation line with silk suture. Leg and perineal drapes are placed. The upright of the self-retaining retractor is secured to the table rail on the patient's left while maintaining the sterility of the upright. A headlight is adorned to supplement the overhead lighting.

Exposure of the prostate

A curved Lowsley tractor is placed transurethrally into the bladder and its wings are opened. A curvilinear incision is made from a position just medial to the right ischial tuberosity to a position just medial to the left ischial tuberosity. The incision should not extend posteriorly beyond the 3 and 9 o'clock positions relative to the anus (Figure 14.2). Subcutaneous tissues and Colle's fascia are then sharply incised along the same direction as the incision. Electrocautery and blunt dissection are employed to open and develop each ischiorectal fossa lateral to the central tendon. The central tendon is then divided using electrocautery. The fibers of the superficial external anal sphincter are dissected and retracted anteriorly using an appendiceal retractor (Belt modification).[2] The longitudinal muscle fibers of the rectum are identified and gentle traction is placed dorsally on the rectum using a dampened sponge. The plane is developed leading to the rectourethralis muscle, which is formed by fascicles of the rectal muscle, connecting the rectum to the perineal body. It appears as a strap of muscle tenting the rectum ventrally (Figure 14.3). For the next step, traction should not be placed on the Lowsley tractor to avoid rectal injury. The rectourethralis muscle is divided close to the apex of the prostate using vertically oriented scissors or electrocautery, allowing the rectum to fall dorsally; caution must be exercised to prevent rectal injury at this point of the procedure. Gentle pressure is applied on the Lowsley tractor toward the anterior abdominal wall. This maneuver delivers the prostate well into the field of view and allows the blunt, digital dissection of the prostate from the rectum in a cephalad direction until the base of the prostate is identified at the vesicoprostatic junction. The proper plane is between the anterior and posterior leafs of Denonvillier's fascia.[35]

Nerve-sparing dissecton

Resumed traction on the Lowsley tractor toward the anterior abdominal wall again brings the prostate into the incision. If preservation of the neurovascular bundles is intended, the exposed anterior layer of Denonvillier's fascia is incised vertically in the midline from the vesicoprostatic junction to the apex of the prostate using a number 15-blade scalpel. Careful lateral dissection with gentle lateral traction preserves the neurovascular bundles as they course between the leaves of Denonvillier's fascia at the posterolateral edge of the prostate. The fascia and enclosed nerves must be mobilized sufficiently to allow for eventual extraction of the prostate without stretching or damaging the bundles.

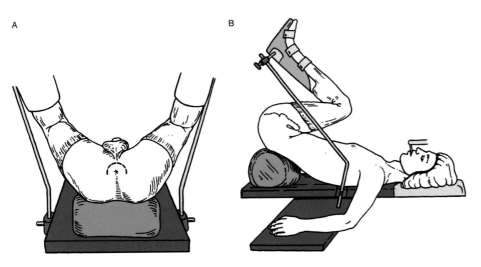

A

B

Figure 14.1
The exaggerated lithotomy position.

Attention is then directed toward the prostatic apex and urethra. The Lowsley tractor can be palpated within the urethra and a right-angle clamp is placed with the open points facing cephalad on either side of the urethra to dissect the neurovascular bundles off of the urethra as they course distally. The number 15 blade scalpel is again used to incise the posterior aspect of the urethra over the Lowsley tractor. The curved Lowsley tractor is then replaced by a straight Lowsley tractor and the wings opened. With moderate traction on the Lowsley tractor, and the right-angle clamp beneath the remaining intact urethra, the anterior aspect of the membranous urethra is transected from the prostatic apex using scissors.

The self-retaining retractor is attached to the previously placed upright and blades are placed in the 6, 9, 12, and 3 o'clock positions. Dissection is then directed over the anterior prostate from the apex toward the bladder neck. Traction on the Lowsley tractor aids in this portion by bringing the prostate into the incision. The surgeon must be mindful not to dissect too far ventrally and come upon the dorsal venous complex. The puboprostatic ligaments are encountered during this dissection and are divided with scissors, not avulsed.

The junction of the bladder neck and prostate base is then identified by palpating the wings of the Lowsley tractor. This junction is then further developed with blunt and sharp dissections, preserving the bladder neck. This dissection is continued and the bladder entered anteriorly using a scalpel (Figure 14.4). The Lowsley tractor is removed from the urethra and a long right-angle clamp is passed retrograde through the prostatic urethra and bladder neck. A 14-French red rubber catheter is then fed into the open right angle clamp and pulled through the prostatic urethra; the ends are clamped together with a Kelly clamp. Traction on the catheter further delivers the prostate into the incision and dissection of the anterior bladder neck is continued circumferentially around the prostate base. Identification of the ureteral orifices is generally unnecessary unless the dissection inadvertently involves the trigone posteriorly. The lateral attachments and vascular pedicles are found coursing

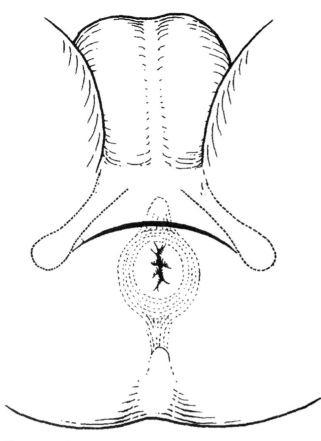

Figure 14.2
The curvilinear skin incision is made approximately 1 to 2 cm above anal verge.[35]

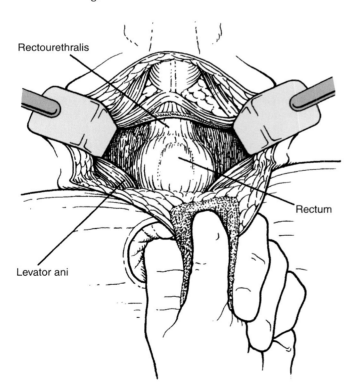

Figure 14.3
Dissection along the longitudinal fibers of the rectal wall exposes the rectourethralis muscle.[35]

Rectourethralis

Rectum

Levator ani

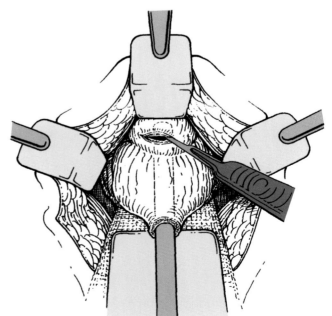

Figure 14.4
The incision of the anterior bladder with a straight Lowsley retractor in place.[35]

toward the base of the prostate and are dissected, sharply divided between right-angle clamps, and secured using 3-0 absorbable ties. To preserve the neurovascular bundles, the lateral pedicles should be divided close to the prostate, taking care not to compromise the surgical margin. Electrocautery is avoided during this phase.

The dissection is continued posteriorly at the bladder neck to separate it completely from the prostate. The red-rubber catheter is then removed and a right-angle clamp is passed along the midline posterior surface of the prostate with tips directed toward the base. The 14-French red-rubber is passed through the open tips of the right-angle clamp, pulled through, and ends secured together with a Kelly clamp. Traction can then be applied around the entirety of the prostate toward the incision, exposing the vasa deferentia and seminal vesicles (Figure 14.5). Each vas deferens is grasped with a right-angle clamp, bluntly dissected, and divided with electrocautery. Each seminal vesicle is similarly grasped with a right-angle clamp, bluntly dissected and divided, ligating the seminal vesicle artery with 3-0 absorbable ties. The complete surgical specimen is removed and passed-off for pathologic examination.

Vesicourethral anastomosis

Occasionally, it may be necessary to reconstruct the bladder neck using simple interrupted absorbable suture placed posteriorly in a tennis racquet fashion. The ureteral orifices should be identified and care should be taken to prevent harm.

The retractor placed at the 12 o'clock position is removed and a 12-French red-rubber catheter is placed retrograde through the penile urethra and grasped at the glans with a Kelly clamp. This

catheter aids in the ability to identify the membranous urethra and prevents risk of damage to a catheter balloon. A 3-0 polyglycolic acid suture is placed from outside the anterior bladder neck at the 12 o'clock position and from inside to outside the membranous urethra at the same position and tied. While the assistant places traction on the red-rubber catheter toward the contralateral side, the surgeon places sutures at the 2 and 10 o'clock positions. The red-rubber catheter is removed and a 22-French silastic Foley catheter is carefully passed retrograde from the penile urethra and into the bladder. The 5-ml balloon is inflated with 15-mL of sterile water. Sutures are then placed at the 4, 6, and 8 o'clock positions and tied, completing the anastomosis.

Closure

The field is inspected for hemostasis and again for rectal injury. A penrose drain is positioned near the vesicourethral anastomosis and brought through the incision. The levator ani are reapproximated using 2-0 absorbable sutures, avoiding damage to the neurovascular bundles and penrose drain. The central tendon and Colles' fascia is reapproximated respectively with 2-0 absorbable sutures. The skin is closed with 4-0 caprosyn suture interrupted in a vertical mattress fashion. The penrose drain is sutured to the skin with a simple stitch. The wound is dressed with a fluffed gauze dressing.

Postoperative care

Regardless of whether the patient underwent a laparoscopic lymph node dissection at the time of prostatectomy, the postoperative care remains the same. Patients are started on a clear liquid diet on the day of surgery and are advanced to a regular diet by the first postoperative day. Patients are encouraged to ambulate routinely beginning the evening of surgery and at least 4 times per day thereafter. Lower-extremity sequential compression devices are used while in bed. Likewise, incentive spirometry is encouraged every hour while in bed to prevent atelectasis. Rectal stimulation, instrumentation, and medication insertion is pro-hibited. Furthermore, gentle irrigation of the catheter is performed only when absolutely necessary and only by a physician. The patients are provided oral narcotic analgesia; intravenous narcotics are given only for breakthrough pain. Docusate is prescribed until the patient no longer requires the oral narcotic. All patients are maintained on a prophylactic oral antibiotic until the catheter is removed. The Penrose drain is typically removed on postoperative day 1 and the urethral catheter is removed in the office 2 to 3 weeks after the day of surgery. The majority of patients are discharged on post-operative day number 2; however, nearly one-third are discharged on the first postoperative day.

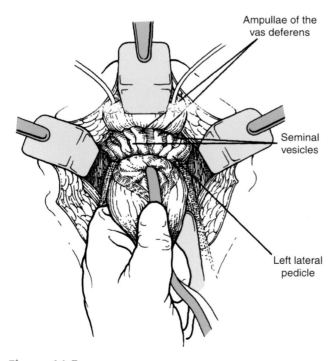

Ampullae of the vas deferens

Seminal vesicles

Left lateral pedicle

Figure 14.5
Dissection of the posterolateral prostate reveals the lateral vascular pedicles, seminal vesicles, and ampullae of the vas deferens. All figures from Haas and Resnick[35]

Perioperative morbidity

Without the need for an abdominal incision and as a result of relatively short operative times,[13] perioperative morbidity is low. Weldon and colleagues reported that 18% of their perineal prostatectomies experienced adverse events. However, most events were not serious and no deaths were reported.[14] Patients are typically administered general anesthetic and may have comorbidities such as hypertension, atherosclerosis, and diabetes; they are at risk of perioperative myocardial infarction, stroke, and death. Given a relatively low operative blood loss and short operative time, these serious risks are small.[10,14,15] Anastomotic strictures which can usually be managed with urethral dilatations under local anesthetic or direct vision urethrotomy occur from 1% to 8% and often occur within the first 4 months of surgery.[10,14,16,17] The incidence of transient lower extremity neurapraxia increases with increased operative time in the extended lithotomy position as reported by Price, noting a 21% incidence with a mean operative time of 188 min.[18] Keller reported a 0% incidence of neurapraxia in 284 prostatectomies with a mean operative time of 99 minutes.[13] Other series note a neurapraxia incidence rate of less than 2%.[14,15,16] Keller postulates that operative times with a patient in the exaggerated lithotomy position of less than 180 minutes is paramount to prevention of neurapraxia.[13]

Blood loss

Blood loss incurred during a radical perineal prostatectomy is less than that during a radical retropubic prostatectomy.[17,19] This is attributed to the fact the dorsal venous complex is merely reflected from the specimen during the perineal approach whereas it is transected during a retropubic prostatectomy. A review of the literature supports an average blood loss from perineal prostatectomy between 400 and 800 ml and the need for red blood cell transfusions is found to vary from 1–11%.[10,14–17,19–21] Ruiz-Deya et al. report that, over time, their transfusion rates improved from 11% to 5%.[15]

Rectal injury

Rectal injuries have been reported to occur during 0.6–11% of perineal prostatectomies.[10,14,16,19,22,23] When recognized at the time of surgery and repaired primarily with a two layer closure, clinical sequelae are typically avoided. If unrecognized, or when occurring in concert with postoperative urinary extravasation, a rectocutaneous or rectourethral fistula may develop. These fistulas can usually be managed conservatively with a short period of bowel rest followed by a low-residue diet. If spontaneous closure does not occur, the fistula must be explored and excised. In rare cases, a temporary diverting colostomy is required.

Fecal incontinence

As with rectal injury, fecal incontinence occurs at a higher rate following a radical perineal prostatectomy than retropubic prostatectomy. Bishoff et al. surveyed 227 patients 12 months following radical prostatectomy and report 18% of perineal patients had new onset of fecal incontinence compared with only 5% in the retropubic group.[24] In a prospective longitudinal assessment by Dahm and colleagues, rectal urgency was the most common complaint and symptoms resolved over time; only 2.9% of patients reported involuntary stool leakage by 12 months after radical perineal prostatectomy.[25] Of note, less than 50% of incontinent patients in the Bishoff study had mentioned this problem to their surgeon.[24] Thus, surgeons may be underestimating this problem in their practices.

Outcomes

Urinary continence

Postoperative urinary continence is an outcome that has garnered much attention due to its impact on quality of life. As a result of the excellent exposure of the bladder neck and prostatic apex enjoyed through the perineal approach, it is generally believed to offer a higher percentage of urinary continence to patients. In a survey by Bishoff, a higher rate of urinary continence and a faster time to continence postoperatively were supported.[24] Unfortunately, controlled studies are lacking. Furthermore, the different definitions of incontinence employed among the various studies make comparisons difficult. It is of the authors' opinion that the 2 procedures are comparable in this regard and that has been shown in several studies.[19,26]

Based on a number of series, the rate of incontinence following radical perineal prostatectomy is reported to range from 4 to 8%.[14,17,20] In Weldon's experience of 220 consecutive perineal cases where incontinence was described as the use of daily pads, continence returned in 23% of patients by 1 month, in 56% by 3 months, in 90% by 6 months and in 95% by 10 months. The only variable significantly related to continence status was age greater than 69; all men in the incontinent group after 10 months were older than 69 years of age.[14] Thus, patients are counseled that final continence status may not be achieved until 1 year after surgery and evaluation for treatment is limited only to those patients who remain incontinent at that time.

Potency

In 1988, Weldon applied the nerve-sparing technique previously unique to the retropubic approach to the radical perineal prostatectomy.[11] In the time since, it has been established that potency is preserved at rates similar to those achieved using a retropubic approach. Patients are instructed that potency may be regained up to 24 months after nerve-sparing surgery and that, although they may have an erection sufficient for vaginal penetration, the overall quality is likely to be diminished. Potent men following radical retropubic prostatectomy were reported by Walsh and colleagues to have erection quality at 60% to 95% of their preoperative state.[27] Moreover, patients who were impotent prior to surgery will remain so post-operatively and those with decreased sexual function preoperatively are at a higher risk for impotence. Investigations are currently under way to assess the benefit of early, regimented use of phosphodiesterase inhibitors in the post-prostatectomy patients. It has been shown that regimented use of sildenafil may help to preserve and increase intrcorporeal smooth muscle content, maintaining the pro-erectile ultrastructure of post-prostatectomy patients.[28] Improved nocturnal erections were demonstrated in post-prostatectomy patients who were administered nightly sildenafil compared to those given placebo.[29] As our understanding of pharmacotherapy improves, so may potency outcomes.

In the series by Weldon and colleagues, post-operative potency was reported in 70% of the 50 patients who met preoperative criteria for nerve-sparing dissection (preoperative potency, unlikely compromise of posterolateral margins) and had follow-up for a minimum of 18 months.[14] 50% of Weldon's patients achieved potency at 1 year and 70% at 2 years. Preservation of only a unilateral neurovascular bundle did not produce significantly different results from a bilateral nerve-sparing operation (68% versus 73%).[14] These results are similar to the 68% potency rates following radical retropubic prostatectomy reported by Walsh et al.[27] However, it is reported that, with older patients, bilateral nerve preservation may afford improved potency compared to only unilateral nerve-sparing operation.[30]

Cancer control

Although outcomes of potency and urinary continence are exceedingly important for patient satisfaction, radical perineal prostatectomy is foremost an operation to treat cancer. Lance et al. reviewed 1382 men treated by radical retropubic prostatectomy and 316 by radical perineal prostatectomy.[19] To eliminate the selection bias of men with higher preoperative PSA and Gleason score in the retropubic group, patients were matched by race, preoperative PSA level, and Gleason sum. Results did not show any differences among the numbers of organ confined, specimen confined and margin positive disease. As expected by the different exposures afforded, there were higher instances of posterior margin-positive disease in the radical retropubic group, while the perineal group revealed a higher incidence of positive margins at the bladder neck and anterior surface.[19] In Weldon's series of patients with T1 and T2 disease, the rate of positive margins was 44%.[31] The rate of positive margins was 7%, 16%, and 25% for the apex, posterolateral, and anterior prostate respectively. Korman and colleagues reviewed the pathology specimens from 60 radical retropubic and 40 perineal prostatectomies and did not find a statistically significant difference in the 2 groups: positive margins were apparent in 16% of the retropubic patients and 22% of the perineal patients (p = 0.53) and the capsular incision rate was 4% in each group.[32] Likewise, Frazier and coworkers did not find a difference in the positive margins between retropubic and perineal approaches.[17] In the experience of 508 consecutive radical perineal prostatectomies in the PSA-era, Harris reported 36% of patients had extracapsular disease, but only 18% of cases had margin-positive disease.[33] Clearly, the literature supports radical perineal prostatectomy as an excellent operation for cancer control.

In general, cancer outcomes following surgery are favorable. In the 20-year experience of Paulson whereby radical perineal prostatectomy was performed on 1,242 men with clinically confined adenocarcinoma of the prostate the median time to non-cancer death was 19.3 years.[34] Median cancer-associated death was not reached for patients with organ and specimen confined disease, but it was 12.7% in those with positive margins at time of excision. After 5 years, PSA failure (defined by PSA > 0.5 ng/ml) occurred in 8%, 35%, and 65% of men with organ confined, specimen confined, and margin positive disease respectively. In patients with positive margins, the median time to PSA failure was 2.4 years. Approximately 20% of patients with positive margins did not have biochemical failure. Cancer-associated death occurred approximately 10 years following the time of PSA failure.[34]

Summary

The resurgence of the radical perineal prostatectomy for the treatment of localized prostate cancer has been facilitated by the current emphasis on reducing medical costs, the identification of prostate cancer at earlier stages, and the selected use of laparoscopic lymph node sampling. This technique offers cancer control for localized prostate cancer as efficacious as the radical retropubic prostatectomy in a manner that is cost-effective, and with low morbidity.

References

1. Young HH. The early diagnosis and radical cure of carcinoma of the prostate: being a study of 40 cases and presentation of a radical operation which was carried out in 4 cases. Bull Johns Hopkins 1905;16:315.
2. Belt E, Ebert CE, Surber AC. A new anatomic approach in perineal prostatectomy. J Urol 1939;41:482.
3. Millen T. Retropubic Prostatectomy. A new extravesical technique: report of 20 cases. Lancet 1945;2:693–6.
4. Reiner WJ, Walsh PC. An anatomic approach to the surgical management of the dorsal vein and Santorini's plexus during radical retropubic surgery. J Urol 1979;147:1574.
5. Walsh PC, Donker PJ. Impotence following radical prostatectomy: insight into etiology and prevention. J Urol 1982;128:492–494.
6. Walsh PC, Lepor H, Eggleston JC. Radical prostatectomy with preservation of sexual function: anatomical and pathological considerations. Prostate 1983;4:473.
7. Partin AW, Kattan MW, Subong EN, et al. Combination of prostate-specific antigen, clinical stage, and Gleason score to predict pathological stage of localized prostate cancer. J Am Med Assoc 1997;277:1445–1451.
8. Parra RO, Isorna S, Perez MG, et al. Radical perineal prostatectomy without pelvic lymphadenectomy: selection criteria and early results. J Urol 1996;155:612–615.
9. Lerner SE, Fleischmann J, Taub HC, et al. Combined laparoscopic lymph node dissection and modified Belt radical perineal prostatectomy for localized prostate adenocarcinoma. Urology 1994;43:493–498.
10. Levy DA, Resnick MI. Laparoscopic Pelvic Lymphadenectomy and radical perineal prostatectomy: a viable alternative to radical retropubic prostatectomy. J Urol 1994;151:905–908.
11. Weldon VE, Tavel FR. Potency-sparing radical perineal prostatectomy: anatomy, surgical technique, and initial results. J Urol 1988;140:559–562.
12. Mokulis J, Thompson I. Radical prostatectomy: is the perineal approach more difficult to learn? J Urol 1997;157:230–232.
13. Keller H. Comment: Re: Transient lower extremity neurapraxia associated with radical perineal prostatectomy. A complication of exaggerated lithotomy position. J Urol 1999;162:171.
14. Weldon VE, Tavel FR, Neuwirth H. Continence, potency and morbidity after radical perineal prostatectomy. J Urol 1997;158:1470–1475.
15. Ruiz-Deya G, Davis R, Srivastav SK, et al. Outpatient radical prostatectomy: impact of standard perineal approach on patient outcome. J Urol 2001;166:581–586.
16. Gillitzer R, Thuroff JW. Relative advantages and disadvantages of radical perineal prostatectomy versus radical retropubic prostatectomy. Crit Rev Oncol Hematol 2002;43:167–190.
17. Frazier HA, Robertson JE, Paulson DF. Radical prostatectomy: the pros and cons of the perineal versus retropubic approach. J Urol 1992;147:888–890.
18. Price DT, Vieweg J, Roland F, et al. Transient lower extremity neurapraxia associated with perineal prostatectomy. A complication of the exaggerated lithotomy position. J Urol 1998;160:1376–1378.
19. Lance RS, Freidrichs PA, Kane C, et al. A comparison of radical retropubic with perineal prostatectomy for localized prostate cancer within the Uniformed Services Urology Research Group. BJU 2001;87:61–65.
20. Boczko J, Melman A. Radical perineal prostatectomy in obese patients. Urology 2003;62:467–469.
21. Parra RO, Boullier JA, Rauscher JA, et al. The value of laparoscopic lymphadenectomy in conjunction with radical perineal or retropubic prostatectomy. J Urol 1994;151:1599–1602.

22. Lassen PM, Kearse WS. Rectal injuries during radical perineal prostatectomy. Urology 1995;45:266–269.

23. Zincke H, Oesterling JE, Blute ML, et al. Long-term (15 years) results after radical prostatectomy for clinically localized (stage T2c or lower) prostate cancer. J Urol 1994;152:1850–1857.

24. Bishoff JT, Motley G, Optenberg SA, et al. Incidence of fecal and urinary incontinence following radical perineal and retropubic prostatectomy in a national population. J Urol 1998;160:454–458.

25. Dahm P, Silverstein AD, Weizer AZ, et al. A longitudinal assessment of bowel related symptoms and fecal incontinence following radical perineal prostatectomy. J Urol 203;169:2220–2224.

26. Gray M, Petroni GR, Theodorescu D. Urinary function after radical prostatectomy: a comparison of the retropubic and perineal approaches. Urology 1999;53:881–891.

27. Walsh PC, Partin AW, Epstein JI. Cancer control and quality of life following anatomical radical retropubic prostatectomy: results at 10 years. J Urol 1994;152:1831–1836.

28. Schwartz EJ, Wong P, Graydon RJ. Sildenafil preserves intracorporeal smooth muscle after radical retropubic prostatectomy. J Urol 2004;171:771–774.

29. Levine LA, McCullough AR, Padma-Nathan H. Longitudinal randomized placebo-controlled study of the return of nocturnal erections after nerve-sparing radical prostatectomy in men treated with nightly sildenafil citrate. J Urol Abstracts 2004;171:231 (Abstract)

30. Quinlan DM, Epstein JI, Carter BS, et al. Sexual function following radical prostatectomy: influence of preservation of neurovascular bundles. J Urol 1991;145:998–1002.

31. Weldon VE, Travel FR, Neuwirth H, et al. Patterns of positive specimen margins and detectable prostate-specific antigen after radical perineal prostatectomy. J Urol 1995;153:1565–1569.

32. Korman HJ, Leu PB, Huang RR, et al. A centralized comparison of radical perineal and retropubic prostatectomy specimens: Is there a difference according to the surgical approach? J Urol 2002;168:991–994.

33. Harris MJ. Radical perineal prostatectomy: cost efficient, outcome effective, minimally invasive prostate cancer management. European Urology 2003;44:303–308.

34. Iselin CE, Robertson JE, Paulson DF. Radical perineal prostatectomy: oncological outcome during a 20-year period. J Urol 1999;161:163–168.

35. Haas CA, Resnick MI. Radical perineal prostatectomy: late division of seminal vesicles. In: Resnick MI, Thompson IM, Eds. Surgery of the Prostate. New York: Churchill Livingstone, 1998:131–148.

15

Laparoscopic and robotic radical prostatectomy

Xavier Cathelineau, Carlos Arroyo, Marc Galiano, Francois Rozet, Eric Barret, Guy Vallancien

Introduction

Laparoscopic surgery dates back to 1901 when Kelling performed a "celioscopic procedure" by inserting a cystoscope into an air insufflated abdomen of a dog to inspect the abdominal viscera. However, it was not until the 1940s, that laparoscopic surgery was actually developed in the field of gynecology, and afterwards in gastrointestinal surgery from 1986 onwards. There was a significant delay in its use in urologic procedures if we consider that it was not until 1990 that the first laparoscopic nephrectomy was performed by Ralph Clayman, and 2 years later Schuessler et al reported the first attempt to perform a laparoscopic prostatectomy; then, in 1997, they published 9 cases of laparoscopic radical prostatectomy finding it a difficult procedure with no advantages over open surgery.[1] During that same year, Raboy published a case of an extraperitoneal radical prostatectomy.[2] By December that same year, Richard Gaston (Bordeaux, France), in a personal communication, indicated that he had performed a transperitoneal radical prostatectomy in less than 6 hours. Six weeks later, Bertrand Guillonneau and Guy Vallancien started to perform their first radical prostatectomies;[3,4] followed 5 months later by Claude Abbou.[5] Nowadays, virtually all of the urologic oncologic surgeries can be performed by a laparoscopic approach.[6]

Current progress in robotic manipulators is encouraging for laparoscopic surgery because it could make the procedures easier. The first group includes robots that assist the surgeon by actively positioning the laparoscope, such as the robotic arm AESOP™ that uses speech recognition to maneuver the endoscope to place the camera where it is required. The second group involves what we consider robotic-assisted surgery—this involves a computer-enhanced master–slave telemanipulator, which allows a remote manipulation of the instruments in the operative field; however, they are not really robots.

In the last few years, laparoscopic radical prostatectomy has gained popularity, with a significant increase in the number of procedures performed worldwide.[7] Part of this increase can be explained because minimally invasive surgery is appealing to patients[8] and surgeons, because by maintaining the oncologic results of open surgery it offers the benefit of a minimally invasive technique that should reduce the postoperative pain, shorten the convalescence time, and improve the quality of the procedure by perfecting the urethrovesical anastomosis and preservation of neurovascular bundles.

Currently our experience in the Institut Montsouris adds up to over 2000 laparoscopic radical prostatectomies, performed from 1998 to 2004, distributed as follows: 1400 transperitoneal and 600 extraperitoneal, including over 120 have been robot assisted (70 transperitoneal and 50 extraperitoneal). In this chapter we will discuss the indications, techniques, complications, and results of laparoscopic and robotic radical prostatectomy.

Indications and contraindications

Concerning the indications of laparoscopic or robotic radical prostatectomy, there is no debate because they are exactly the same as in open radical prostatectomy. However, as in open surgery, the adequate selection of the patients who are candidates for a surgical treatment will impact on the results obtained with either approach. The best indication for a radical prostatectomy would be a young patient, without any serious co-morbidity, a PSA lower than 15 ng/mL, clinical stage T1, with less than 50% of biopsies positive and a Gleason score of less than 8.

However, just as in open surgery, laparoscopic radical prostatectomy can be performed in selected T3N0M0 stages, without neurovascular bundle preservation, but always cautioning the patient of the risk of residual disease that may require complementary treatment. Also, salvage laparoscopic radical prostatectomy after radiotherapy or brachytherapy can be done; however, it is important to keep in mind that this surgery involves a high risk of damage to the rectum whether it is performed by open surgery or a laparoscopic approach.

There are some absolute anesthetic contraindications that are shared with any laparoscopic approach, involving high intracranial pressure of whatever etiology. Abdominal laparoscopic surgery, especially in an extraperitoneal approach, causes an increased partial pressure of carbon dioxide (Pco_2), that requires an increased minute ventilation, in order to maintain a Pco_2 between 30 and 35 mmHg (data to be published). This explains additional relative anesthetic contraindications that include, severe emphysema, cardiac insufficiency, atrioventricular defects, chronic respiratory disease, and severe glaucoma.

As in open radical prostatectomy, there are no anatomic contraindications for laparoscopic approach. However, there are some cases considered as potentially challenging, especially those circumstances in which tissues around the prostate are more difficult to dissect. These include a large volume prostate (over 100 g), neoadjuvant hormonotherapy, previous prostatic surgery (transurethral resection of the prostate [TURP] or adenomectomy), history of prostatitis, radiotherapy, brachytherapy, thermal ablation of the prostate (Ablatherm™) or previous major abdominopelvic surgery because of the formation of adhesions.[9–11] Finally, for an extraperitoneal approach the history of previous bilateral mesh hernia repair can make this approach difficult because of the formation of adhesions that can make the Retzius space dissection difficult.[12]

An important consideration for surgeons at the beginning of their learning curve is to carefully select their cases, because it has been shown that the surgeon's experience is inversely related to in-hospital complications and length of stay for open radical prostatectomy.[13] Importantly, always keep in mind that in laparoscopic surgery, conversion to open surgery is not a shame but a sign of wisdom.

Preoperative preparation

The patient is admitted to the hospital the night before the surgery to start prophylactic anticoagulation with an injection of low-molecular-weight heparin, which is continued for at least 7 days postoperatively. Another measure to prevent thromboembolic complications is the systematic use of varicose vein stockings. We do not do any gastrointestinal or skin preparation (shaving), nor do we prescribe any antibiotic prophylaxis.

Patient installation and trocar placement

Patient installation

Laparoscopic radical prostatectomies by the transperitoneal or extraperitoneal approach are performed under general anesthesia, with the patient placed in a dorsal supine position. During the transperitoneal technique an exaggerated Trendelenburg position is preferred compared with a moderate position in the extraperitoneal approach. The lower limbs are in abduction for intraoperative access to the rectum. The upper limbs are positioned alongside the body to avoid the risk of stretch injuries to the brachial plexus. Two security belts are placed across the thorax in an "X" pattern, to ensure that there is no patient movement during surgery, and yet ensuring there is no risk of pressure injury in using shoulder rests.

The surgeon stands on the left side of the patient with the operating room nurse and instrument table, and the assistant stands on the right side of the operating table. The video column with the insufflator and light source are placed between the legs of the patient and the electrocautery and aspirator behind the assistant.

In the case of a robot-assisted technique, before the entry of the patient in the operative room the "robot" is set up. The system is started and performs a self-testing procedure, during which it recognizes its own spatial position and various components. The cameras are black and white, balanced, and calibrated. The patient positioning is the same except for a slight flexion of the lower limbs to allow the robot to approach as close as possible to the surgical table. The surgeon remains in the console for the entire procedure, and a scrub nurse and assistant remain on the left side of the patient.

Trocar placement

In case of laparoscopic radical prostatectomy, we routinely use five trocars, and they are the same with either approach, except for a

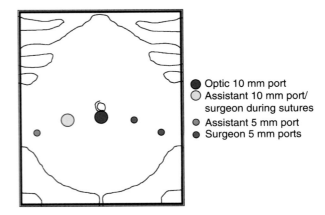

- ● Optic 10 mm port
- ○ Assistant 10 mm port/ surgeon during sutures
- ◉ Assistant 5 mm port
- ● Surgeon 5 mm ports

Figure 15.1
The first trocar position variation involves placement of all the ports as high as possible with respect to the umbilicus; the left side ports are used by the surgeon and the right side for the assistant.

slight displacement in the extraperitoneal approach, in which the trocars tend to be slightly lower than for the transperitoneal approach. They depend on the surgeons preferences and include:

The linear distribution, in which a 10 mm trocar is introduced in the umbilicus for the camera, the surgeon will work with two 5 mm trocars that are introduced—one above and medial to the iliac spine and another one lower and lateral to the umbilical port. The assistant will work with a 5 mm trocar that is placed above and medial to the right iliac spine, and a second 10 mm trocar between the umbilical and lateral ports on the right (Figure 15.1).

The triangular trocar variation involves placement of the surgeon's ports on the left side between the umbilical port and the left iliac spine and the other one two thirds of the distance between the umbilical port and the suprapubic rim along the midline (Figure 15.2).

In the case of a robot-assisted procedure, no matter if it is extra- or transperitoneal, the trocar distribution is as follows: a 12 mm trocar is introduced in the umbilicus for the camera, and two 8 mm trocars for the robot arms are placed on both sides five fingerbreadths lateral to the optic and slightly lower. Finally, for the assistant, a 5 mm trocar is introduced above and medial to the left iliac spine and a 10 mm trocar for the suture introduction is placed slightly higher between the optic and right robot trocar (Figure 15.3).

Techniques

Transperitoneal approach

This approach was the first one to be described for laparoscopic radical prostatectomy,[14,15] and it has been divided into the following six critical steps:

1. Incision of the posterior vesical peritoneum with dissection of the vasa deferens and seminal vesicles. Denonvilliers' fascia is also incised.
2. Dissection of the Retzius space. The intrapelvic fascia is incised with selective suture ligation of the Santorini's plexus.
3. Bladder neck is identified and dissected, with the seminal vesicles delivered.

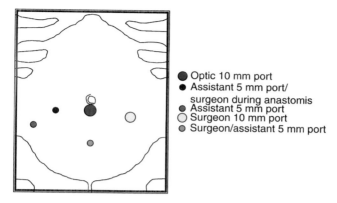

● Optic 10 mm port
● Assistant 5 mm port/
　surgeon during anastomis
● Assistant 5 mm port
○ Surgeon 10 mm port
● Surgeon/assistant 5 mm port

Figure 15.2
The triangular trocar variation involves placement of the surgeon ports on the left side between the umbilical port and the left iliac spine and the other two thirds of the distance between the umbilical port and the suprapubic rim along the midline.

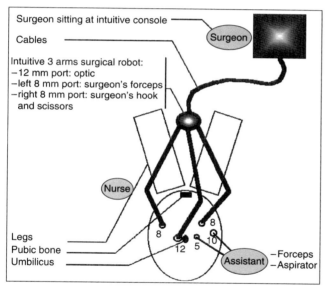

Surgeon sitting at intuitive console

Cables

Intuitive 3 arms surgical robot:
−12 mm port: optic
−left 8 mm port: surgeon's forceps
−right 8 mm port: surgeon's hook
　and scissors

Surgeon

Nurse

Legs
Pubic bone
Umbilicus

8
8
12　5　10
Assistant
−Forceps
−Aspirator

Figure 15.3
Telerobotic system.

4. The lateral surfaces of the prostate are dissected in the intrafascial plane in order to preserve the neurovascular bundles (when indicated).
5. Selective dissection of the urethra with the aid of a metal Béniqué dilator.
6. A urethrovesical anastomosis is performed with interupted or running vicryl sutures. Finally, the prostate is extracted using a laparoscopic bag.

There have been some variations described in the literature concerning the technique, such as the one proposed by Abbou et al,[16,17] in which he prefers to divide the Santorini´s plexus after having opened the bladder neck, which is identified by palpation with scissors to distinguish a mobile bladder wall from solid prostatic substance. Another difference is that the urethrovesical anastomosis is performed with two hemicircumferential running sutures.

Rassweiler et al have also proposed the Heilbronn technique in which he places five trocars in a W-shaped distribution and starts the surgery by immediate access to the Retzius space. They recommend a 6th port for an optimal exposure and describe an ascending part as the incision of the endopelvic fascia and trans-section of the puboprostatic ligaments, and the dorsal vein complex with a previously placed suture, in order to gain access to the urethra at the level of the apex. The descending part of the surgery implies the traction of the prostate ventrally for the dissection of the bladder neck to gain access to the seminal vesicle by a retrovesical approach.[18]

These and other modifications only prove that the steps in the laparoscopic radical prostatectomy can be performed according to the surgeon's preferences, but always with the idea of making the technique more effective and to improve the functional results.

Extraperitoneal approach

This approach has been previously described in the literature[19–21] and can be divided into steps similarly:

1. The dissection of the Retzius space is done by blunt dissection with the laparoscope or by the use of a balloon.
2. Opening of the intrapelvic fascia floor with the suture ligature of Santorini's plexus.
3. Bladder neck dissection, which reveals the initial plane of dissection of the seminal vesicles and the Denonvilliers' fascia.
4. The lateral surfaces of the prostate are dissected in the intrafascial plane in order to preserve the neurovascular bundles (when indicated).
5. The prostatic apex is dissected and mobilized for a selective section of the urethra.
6. A urethrovesical anastomosis is performed with interrupted or running vicryl sutures with extraction of the prostate with a laparoscopic bag.

This retropubic approach, described after the experience gained with the transperitoneal prostatectomy, has gained a lot of interest because it is argued that the anatomy is more comparable to the open technique,22 with the added benefit that by avoiding the peritoneum, the danger of gastrointestinal damage is decreased.23,24 What has been learned from experience is that it also allows a better identification of the hypogastric vessels, which is very helpful during the placement of the lateral ports. Also, if there is an anastomotic urinary leak, it can be managed better because there is no contact with the peritoneal organs.

Telerobotic surgical system

The surgical technique varies only in the placement of the trocars and the equipment. The position of the patient is basically the same as in any laparoscopic radical prostatectomy; however, the umbilical port is a 12 mm trocar for the use of the 3D-endocamera that is attached to the medial arm of the robot. Both 8 mm lateral ports are for the introduction of the specially designed instruments for the robot, that feature the Endo-Wrist™ articulations and include the cautery hook, a short-tip grasper, a bipolar hemostatic grasper, and needle holders.[25] The fourth 10 mm port is for the introduction of the needles and instruments by the assistant, and, finally, the fifth 5 mm port will also be used by the assistant for conventional laparoscopic instruments (clip appliers, large grasper, and suction device).

Once all of the attachments and instruments are placed, the surgery is basically done following the steps mentioned in the transperitoneal or extraperitoneal approach. The da Vinci system' is a master–slave type of surgical robot, that consists of a slave or work unit and a master or control unit, which are connected by a computer-based system. The master unit is located in the remote console and transmits the movements that the surgeons is performing to the slave unit, which will move the camera and two instruments. The role of the assistant is limited to exposing the operative field, assisting in hemostasis by suction and irrigation, and the application of clips.[26]

All of the above require a complete knowledge of the performance capabilities and steps in the attachment of the instruments by the assistant and the operating room nurse, in order to facilitate the introduction of the instruments and assist the surgeon to make it efficient.

The role of robotic technology in laparoscopic urologic surgery is becoming more widely accepted because of the advantages provided by this technology, which include: the improved visualization by the InSitte Vision System that provides a 3D-vision and 10-fold magnification; the handling of the laparoscopic tools that is facilitated by the Endo-Wrist instrument technology, which allows the surgeon to use instruments as in open surgery; and finally, the procedure can be undertaken in a relaxed working position at the console.[27]

The above has allowed not only the performance of radical prostatectomy, but other techniques associated with it, such as sural nerve grafting during the same procedure[28] or more complex procedures, including nerve-sparing radical cystoprostatectomy and urinary diversion.[29]

Postoperative management

The bladder catheter is left for 3 to 7 days depending on the quality of the suture evaluated by the surgeon. Postoperative cystogram is not routinely performed. Our analgesia scheme is limited to i.v. paracetamol during the first 24 hours, followed on day 1, by oral paracetamol/dextropropoxyphene if necessary. Major analgesics are administered if necessary. The intravenous perfusion is stopped on day 1, and oral fluids are started on the next morning after the surgery, and a normal diet can generally be resumed on day 2.

Results

Since 1998 we have been performing laparoscopic radical prostatectomy, and our current experience adds up to over 2000 cases, which include: 1400 transperitoneal cases and 600 extraperitoneal cases. Among them we have performed 120 robot assisted laparoscopic radical prostatectomies, 70 transperitoneal and 50 by the extraperitoneal approach.

The patient characteristics are summarized in Table 15.1.

Morbidity

Intraoperative complications

The median blood loss during laparoscopic radical prostatectomy in our experience was 350 mL with a transfusion rate of 3%. Concerning

retropubic radical prostatectomy, Catalona et al,[30] using the technique of hemodilution, reported that most of the patients received autologous transfusion during or after surgery; 9% also needed heterologous postoperative transfusion.

Gastrointestinal injuries are rare and directly related to the operator's experience and to the patient's history (especially previous radiotherapy). The rate of rectal injuries is similar regardless of the technique (retropubic or laparoscopic), ranging from 0.5% to 2%.[30]

Early postoperative complications

Thromboembolic complications constitute the main cause of postoperative mortality in open procedures. Catalona et al[30] reported 2% of thromboembolic accidents, while Rassweiler18 as in our experience[31] reported a thromboembolic accident rate of less than 0.5%. Prophylactic anticoagulation and early mobilization (especially after laparoscopic procedure) decrease the frequency of these complications.

Anastomotic leaks are often missed when minimal and correctly drained, and their incidence is, therefore, often underestimated.

Our complications are summarized in Table 15.2. To date, we have had neither deaths nor any cardiac complications.

Functional results

Continence

The quality of continence after radical prostatectomy is difficult to assess, as reflected by the marked variability of incontinence rates reported in the literature. This variability is related to three main factors: definition of incontinence, modalities of evaluation, and follow-up. In our department, the patient is sent a self questionnaire by regular mail. The median follow-up is at 12 months, and reports the continence rates—if they do not use any protection pads, if they

Table 15.1 Preoperative characteristics for 2000 patients who underwent laparoscopic radical prostatectomy

Median age	61 years
Median PSA	9.2 ng/mL
Gleason score	6.5
Number of positive biopsies	2.2

Table 15.2 Intraoperative and early postoperative complications in patients who underwent laparoscopic radical prostatectomy

Complication	Occurrence (%)
Transfusion rate	3.5
Prolonged urinary leakage	1.8
Rectal injury	0.8
Bowel injury	0.2
Lymphocele	0.2
Hematoma	0.2

are continent but prefer to use a precaution pad; and, finally, if they use one pad on a daily basis because of small urine leaks. Our results are encouraging with a continence rate higher than 84% with either approach (the patients report not using any pad) and only 8% to 14% use 1 pad daily for occasional urine leaks.

Potency

As for continence, objective evaluation of sexual potency encounters a number of difficulties: absence of a consensual definition of sexual potency, various methods of evaluation, and variable follow-up.

Currently, for two years, we have evaluated the erectile function with a self applied questionnaire that is mailed to our patients postoperatively. With a median follow-up of 6 months, in the preoperatively potent patients (IIEF5 >20), the erectile function was recovered for 64% with the bilateral nerve-sparing technique, and 43% with unilateral nerve preserving surgery. Longer follow-up is obviously needed.

Oncologic results

For patients with organ-confined disease treated with the open approach, at 3 years, Catalona et al[30] had a recurrence-free survival of 93%. Similar results are observed by the Johns Hopkins group, where their 5-years recurrence-free rate was 97% for organ-confined cancer. Concerning the positive margins in series using retropubic approach, the rate ranges between 10% and 40% depending on the experience of the team, the pathologic stage, and the preservation or not of the neurovascular bundles.

In our experience of laparoscopy and robotic radical prostatectomy, 92% of the patients with organ-confined disease had a PSA of less than 0.1 ng/mL at 5 years. The overall rate of positive margin was 14%. Up to now, no port seeding has been observed.[31,32]

Discussion

Some of the benefits obtained with laparoscopic over open radical prostatectomy are the result of the excellent view and magnification provided by the laparoscope, which enables a more precise dissection, especially for the neurovascular bundles, and a more detailed suturing during the urethrovesical anastomosis.[33] Another advantage during laparoscopy is lower hemorrhage rate compared with open surgery. This is the result of the careful and inherent selective coagulation that is essential in this technique. Moreover, less postoperative pain induces quicker recovery, and the preliminary functional results are really encouraging.

In relation to the controversy between the transperitoneal and extraperitoneal laparoscopic approach, our experience, which includes over 1400 transperitoneal and 600 extraperitoneal radical prostatectomies, has shown both approaches to be equivalent in terms of operative, postoperative, and pathologic data. This is why we consider that there is no gold standard in terms of a technique or approach, but rather the outcome depends on the surgeon's experience.[33,34]

Finally, the most relevant difficulty in laparoscopic urologic surgery is the steep learning curve that has been described to be of a minimum of 50 surgeries, as well as the frequency issue, because it has to be done in a rather short period of time. However, this issue is still in debate, but it is clear that laparoscopic surgery does require a long and intensive training period in order to obtain the most out of this technique.

Concerning robot-assisted laparoscopic surgery, the robotically assisted prostatectomy has proven to be a feasible technique that is safe, associated with less blood-loss, and could shorten the hospital stay and catheterization time with the same oncologic and functional results as open surgery.[35] These results are in accordance with the over 120 prostatectomies (70 transperitoneal and 50 extraperitoneal) performed in our institute with the assistance of the da Vinci robot,[36] and they could be attributed to a better visualization, anatomical dissection, reduced blood loss, and improved ability to reconstruct the anatomy.[35,37]

Disadvantages of the robotic interface include the extremely high cost of the equipment, the limitations in the surgical instruments that are available, and the time involved with the positioning of the robot. However, we have also seen that if the same surgical team is routinely involved with the placement of the robot then the time for the complete preparation for the surgery can be decreased significantly (it currently takes between 20 and 25 minutes to start the surgery with the different ports in place).

Overall, the robotic assistance is a safe and effective procedure, which could be the result of the increased range of movements at the instrument tip and the 3D visualization that make a more precise anatomical dissection possible,[38] making this a promising technique.

However, today, for a surgeon experienced in laparoscopy, there are no real advantages for the patient in having a radical prostatectomy carried out by robot-assisted surgery compared with the "classical" laparoscopic approach. This technique is still under development, and improvement of the instrumentation and long-term studies are necessary, but it is already showing promise regarding ease of instrument handling, and we think that it is a matter of time for the full benefits to come to light.

Conclusions

The development of laparoscopy in surgery is a natural evolution toward a minimally invasive approach with better quality of surgery. The laparoscopic option, through still in evolution, provides a viable alternative with a steep learning curve. The laparoscopic radical prostatectomy remains one of the most technically demanding laparoscopic procedures in view of the difficulty of surgical access and the need for precise intracorporeal suturing. Today, computer-assisted surgery does not currently provide any significant benefit for the patient compared with laparoscopy, but developments are expected. The surgical and oncologic standards of open surgery are maintained by the minimally invasive techniques. Finally, the benefit of an excellent vision, and potential benefits for the patient provided by a laparoscopic approach, requires the surgeon to keep an open attitude for further improvement of the technique.

References

1. Schuessler WW, Schulam PG, Clayman RV, et al. Laparoscopic ra-dical prostatectomy: initial short-term experience. Urology 1997;50:854–857.
2. Raboy A, Ferzli G, Albert P. Initial experience with extraperitoneal endoscopic radical retropubic prostatectomy. Urology 1997;50:849–853.

3. Guillonneau B, Cathelineau X, Barret E, et al. Prostatectomie radical coelioscopique. Premier evaluation apres 28 interventions. Pess Med 1998;27:1570–1574.

4. Guillonneau B, Cathelineau X, Barret E, et al. Laparoscopic radical prostatectomy: Technical and early oncological assessment of 40 operations. Eur Urol 1999;36:14–20.

5. Abbou CC, Salomon L, Hoznek A, et al. Laparoscopic radical prostatectomy: preliminary results. Urology 2000;55:630–634.

6. Gomella LG. Editorial: Laparoscopy and urologic oncology – I now pronounce you man and wife. J Urol 2003;169:2057–2058.

7. Lu-Yao GL, McLerran D, Wasson J, et al. An assessment of radical prostatectomy: time trends, geographic variation and outcomes. JAMA 1993;269:2633–2636.

8. Hara I, Kawabata G, Miyake H, et al. Comparison of quality of life following laparoscopic and open prostatectomy for prostate cancer. J Urol 2003;169:2045–2048.

9. Seifman BD, Dunn RL, Wolf JS. Transperitoneal laparoscopy into the previously operated abdomen: effect on operative time, length of stay and complications. J Urol 2003;169:36–40.

10. Weibel MA, Majno G. Peritoneal adhesions and their relation to abdominal surgery. A postmortem study. Am J Surg 1973;126:345.

11. Parsons JK, Jarrett TJ, Chow GK, et al. The effect of previous abdominal surgery on urological laparoscopy. J Urol 2002;168:2387–2390.

12. Katz EE, Patel RV, Sokoloff MH, et al. Bilateral laparoscopic inguinal hernia repair can complicate subsequent radical retropubic prostatectomy. J Urol 2002;167:637–638.

13. Hu JC, Gold KF, Pashos CL, et al. Role of surgeon volume in radical prostatectomy outcomes. J Clin Oncol 2003;21:401–405.

14. Guillonneau B, Cathelineau X, Barret E, et al. Prostatectomie radical coelioscopique. Premier evaluation apres 28 interventions. Pess Med 1998;27:1570–1574.

15. Guillonneau B, Vallancien G. Laparoscopic radical prostatectomy: The Montsouris technique. J Urol 2000;163:1643–1649.

16. Hoznek A, Solomon L, Rabii R, et al. Vesicourethral anastomosis during laparoscopic radical prostatectomy: the running suture method. J Endourol 2001;14:749–753.

17. Hoznek A, Salomon L, Olsson LE, et al. Laparoscopic radical prostatectomy. The Creteil experience. Eur Urol 2001;40:38–45.

18. Rassweiler J, Sentker L, Seemann O, et al. Laparoscopic radical prostatectomy with the Heilbronn technique: an analysis of the first 180 cases. J Urol 2001;166:2101–2108.

19. Bollens R, Vanden Bossche M, Roumeguere T, et al. Extraperitoneal laparoscopic radical prostatectomy. Results after 20 cases. Eur Urol 2001;40:65–69.

20. Dubernard P, Enchetrit S, Hamza T, et al. Prostatectomie extra-peritoneale retrograde laparoscopique (P.E.R.L.) avec dissection premiere des bandelettes vasculo-nerveuses erectiles – technique simplifiee – a propos de 100 cas. Prog Urol 2003;13;163.

21. Vallancien G, Guillonneau B, Fournier G, et al. Laparoscopic Radical Prostatectomy, Technical Manual, 21st ed. In Vallancien G, Khoury S (eds): European School of Surgery Collection, 2002.

22. Bollens R, Bossche MV, Roumeguere T, et al. Extraperitoneal laparoscopic radical prostatectomy. Eur Urol 2001;40:65–69.

23. Bollens R, Roumeguere T, Vanden Bossche M, et al. Comparison of laparoscopic radical prostatectomy technique. Curr Urol Rep 2002;3: 148–151.

24. Abreu SC, Gill IS, Kaouk JH, et al. Laparoscopic radical prostatectomy: comparison of transperitoneal laparoscopic radical prostatectomy. Urology 2003;61:617.

25. Guillonneau B, Cappele O, Martinez JB, et al. Robotic assisted laparoscopic pelvic lymph node dissection in humans. J Urol 2001;165: 1078–1081.

26. Abbou CC, Hoznek A, Salomon L, et al. Laparoscopic radical prostatectomy with a remote controlled robot. J Urol 2001;165:1964–1966.

27. Binder J, Kramer W. Robotically-assisted laparoscopic radical prostatectomy. Br J Urol Int 2001;87:408–410.

28. Kaouk JH, Sesai MH, Abreu SC, et al. Robotic assisted laparoscopic sural nerve grafting during radical prostatectomy: initial experience. J Urol 2003;170:909–912.

29. Menon M, Hemal AK, Tewari A, et al. Nerve-sparing robot-assisted radical cystoprostatectomy and urinary diversion. Br J Urol Int 2003;92:232–236.

30. Catalona WJ, Carvalhal GF, Mager DE, et al. Potency, continence and complication rates in 1,870 consecutive radical retropubic prostatectomies. J Urol 1999;162:433–438.

31. Guillonneau B, Rozet F, Cathelineau X, et al. Perioperative complications of laparoscopic radical prostatectomy: the Montsouris 3 year experience. J Urol 2002;167:51–56.

32. Vallancien G, Cathelineau X, Baumert H, et al. Complications of transperitoneal laparoscopic surgery in urology: review of 1,311 procedures at a single center. J Urol 2002;168:23–26.

33. Cathelineau X, Arroyo C, Rozet F, et al. Laparoscopic radical prostatectomy: the new gold standard? Curr Urol Report 2004;5:108–114.

34. Cathelineau X, Cahill D, Widmer H, et al. Transperitoneal or extraperitoneal approach for laparoscopic radical prostatectomy: a false debate for a real challenge. J Urol 2004;171:714–716.

35. Tewari A, Srivasatava A, Menon M. A prospective comparison of radical retropubic and robot-assisted prostatectomy: experience in one institution. Br J Urol Int 2003;92:205–210.

36. Cathelineau X, Widmer H, Rozet F, et al. Telerobotic assisted prostatectomy. In Ballantyne GH, Marescaux J, Giulianotti PC (eds): Primer of Robotic and Telerobotic Surgery. Lippincott Williams Wilkins, 2004.

37. Ahlering TE, Skarecky D, Lee D, et al. Successful transfer of open surgical skills to a laparoscopic environment using a robotic interface: initial experience with laparoscopic radical prostatectomy. J Urol 2003;170:1738–1741.

38. Rassweiler J, Frede T. Robotics, telesurgery and telementoring: their position in modern laparoscopy. Arch Esp Urol 2002;55:610–628.

16

Vattikuti Institute prostatectomy: a robotic technique for the management of localized prostate cancer

James A Brown, Ashok K Hemal, Mani Menon

Introduction

In November 2000, the development of robotic radical prostatectomy using the da Vinci surgical system (Intuitive Surgical, Mountain View, CA) began at Henry Ford Hospital. The da Vinci™ combination of three-dimensional magnified vision and wristed instrumentation provided the rationale for incorporating this technology into radical prostatectomy surgery. A structured program was developed to accomplish this goal.[1] The first step was to gain experience with the laparoscopic radical prostatectomy techniques developed by Guillonneau and Vallencien.[2] Two surgeons from Henry Ford spent a month at L'Institut Mutualiste Montsouris learning laparoscopic skills from a trainer in the animal laboratory and observing 50 laparoscopic radical prostatectomy (LRP) cases performed without robotic assistance. The French surgeons then trained the Henry Ford team in Detroit for 50 additional LRP cases. Our initial robotic prostatectomy procedures closely mimicked the Montsouris laparoscopic procedure. We have, however, made several modifications to our technique over the past 4 years, the most significant being the abandonment of the initial dissection of the seminal vesicles, technique of apical dissection, neurovascular bundle dissection, and vesicourethral anastomosis.[3–5] To date, we have performed about 1200 robotic surgeries at our medical center, of which over 1000 have been Vattikuti Institute prostatectomy (VIP). We describe our current technique and provide insight into the lessons we have learned developing robotic radical prostatectomy.

Robotic technology

The da Vinci robotic system uses a sophisticated master–slave system. It provides three-dimensional stereoscopic vision, movement scaling, and wristed instrumentation with 7° of movement. A mobile control console houses two-finger controlled handles (masters) to control the robotic arms and foot pedals to control camera movement and electrocautery. The bedside tower has three (and an optional fourth) multijoint robotic arms. The first controls the binocular endoscope and the others the articulated instruments.[6] Instrument movement can be scaled from 1:1 to 1:3 and 1:5. The former setting allows exact finger-movement transmission to the instrument tip, while the latter two settings scale down the surgeon's movements; all with tremor filtration.

Patient selection

Any patient meeting the requirements for open or laparoscopic radical prostatectomy is a candidate for robotic radical prostatectomy (VIP). The same factors that exclude a patient from open or laparoscopic surgery apply to robotic prostatectomy patient selection; namely, bleeding diatheses or inability to tolerate general anesthesia. In addition, the patient must be able to tolerate the dorsal lithotomy position placed in steep Trendelenburg. Therefore, patients with lower extremity contractures, severe pulmonary conditions (e.g. chronic obstructive pulmonary disease) or a history of cerebrovascular accident, indwelling ventriculo-peritoneal shunt or cerebral aneurysm should be carefully evaluated or avoided. Previous abdominal surgery, including mesh inguinal herniorrhapy, and obesity up to a body mass index of 40 are not contraindications. However, patients who have had previous pelvic surgery should be evaluated prior to embarking on a robotic prostatectomy, given alternative therapeutic options (perineal prostatectomy and radiation therapy). Large prostate size is not a contraindication, as the wristed instruments and scope mobility of the da Vinci robot make this procedure an ideal surgical treatment option for these patients.

Preoperative management

Anticoagulants, including aspirin, are discontinued 5 to 7 days prior to surgery. Patients with mandatory indications for coumadin are hospitalized for intravenous heparin conversion prior to surgery. Antibiotic prophylaxis, typically with a first-generation cephalosporin, and 5000 IU subcutaneous heparin are provided on call to the operating room. Lower extremity sequential compression devices are placed just prior to induction of general anesthesia and intravenous fluids are restricted at surgery to less than 800 ml, beginning the morning of surgery until the anastomosis is complete during the operation.

Robotic prostatectomy technique

The steps and equipment needed in performing a robot-assisted radical prostatectomy are listed in Table 16.1. Table 16.2 gives tips and solutions to problems that may be encountered during the procedure.

Table 16.1 Surgical steps in performing Vattikuti Institute prostatectomy

Step	Procedure	Lens	Right instrument	Left instrument	Equipment
1	Extraperitoneal space development	30° up	Endowrist® permanent cautery hook	Endowrist® long tip forceps	Monopolar cautery setting 80–120
2	Apical exposure	0°	Endowrist® permanent cautery hook	Endowrist® long tip forceps	Monopolar cautery setting 80–120
3	Dorsal vein complex ligation	0°	Endowrist® needle driver	Endowrist® needle driver	0-Vicryl on CT-1 needle (6–7 inches)
4	Bladder neck transection	30° down	Endowrist® permanent cautery hook	Endowrist® long tip forceps	Monopolar cautery setting 80–120
5	Seminal vesical and initial posterior prostate dissection	30° down	Endowrist® permanent cautery hook (or Endowrist® round tip scissors)	Endowrist® long tip forceps (or Endowrist" precise bipolar)	Monopolar cautery setting 80–120 (or bipolar setting 25)
6	Posterior prostate, pedicle and neurovascular bundle dissection	30° down	Endowrist® round tip scissors	Endowrist® precise bipolar	Bipolar cautery setting 25
7	Apical dissection and urethral transaction	0°	Endowrist® round tip scissors	Endowrist® precise bipolar	Bipolar cautery setting 25
8	Pelvic lymphadenectomy	0°	Endowrist® round tip scissors	Endowrist® precise bipolar	Bipolar cautery setting 25
9	Urethrovesical anastomosis	0°	Endowrist® needle driver	Endowrist® needle driver (± Endowrist" long tip forceps for initial suture placement)	3-0 Monocryl on RB-1 needle (two dyed and undyed 7–8 inch tied together)

Table 16.2 Technical tips and troubleshooting caveats

Problem	Solution
Port placement for tall/short patients	Camera port placed infra- or supra-umbilical if much taller/shorter than 5 foot 10 inches
Port placement for narrow pelvis	Move ports medial to keep robotic port medial to anterior superior iliac spine
Bowel adhesions	Alter order of port placement to allow lysis of adhesions
Localizing bladder neck transection	Pull Foley balloon into and out of bladder neck to define, elevate prostate and keep tension on bladder in midline, angle dissection slightly inferiorly
Large intravesical median lobe	Elevate through bladder neck and incise mucosa at margin approximately 1 cm distal to ureteral orifices, dissect bladder neck of adenoma
Capacious bladder neck opening bleeding along neurovascular bundles or prostatic fossa	Narrow using figure-of-eight 2-0 vicryl on SH needle at inferolateral corners, use 8-inch 3-0 monocryl running suture, consider "tennis-racket" reconstruction of bladder neck
Inability to move robotic arm caudally/ inferiorly in pelvis	Place "cottonoid" Codman surgical strip (Codman & Shurtleff Inc), consider FloSeal (FloSeal matrix hemostatic sealant, Baxter Inc)
Inability to move robotic arm laterally in pelvis	"Lengthen" robotic arm by clutching and further introducing robotic port 1–2 cm
Inability to rotate robotic arm further in a given direction	"Medialize" robotic arm by clutching and rotating arm in medial direction
Dorsal vein complex bleeding after division	Release handle and untwist arm 360°, then grasp master
Anastomotic extravasation	Cauterize with bipolar if ineffective monopolar current or relegate with 2-0 vicryl on RB-1 needle, place interrupted or figure-of-eight 2-0 vicryl sutures, consider redoing anastomosis or tacking bladder or peritoneum to sidewall to "reperitonealize" and take pressure of anastomosis
Postoperative ileus or abdominal pain	Abdominal CT scan to rule out urinary ascites, pelvic hematoma, hernia or ileus

Positioning

The patient is placed in the dorsal lithotomy position on a gel pad operative table, with the arms tucked along the sides. Cotton pads are used to protect the axilla and other pressure points. The elbows and hands are protected with egg crate foam padding. The shoulders and chest are also padded with egg crate foam and 3-inch tape and straps are criss-crossed across the chest to secure the patient to the table prior to placing him in the steep Trendelenburg position with the table fully lowered. The lower extremities are secured in Allen-type stirrups and the thighs abducted 45° and placed in line with the torso (Figure 16.1). The abdomen is prepped from the costal margin to the groin, and an 18-Fr Foley catheter is placed.

Port placement

A 20 mmHg pneumoperitoneum is established through a left lateral umbilical incision using a Veress needle (Ethicon Endo-Surgery, Albuquerque, NM). The pressure is reset to 14 mmHg after initial port placement. Six ports are then placed as configured in Figure 16.2. The periumbilical incision is typically made along the

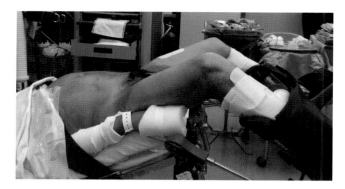

Figure 16.1
Patient positioned in steep Trendelenburg, dorsal lithotomy position.

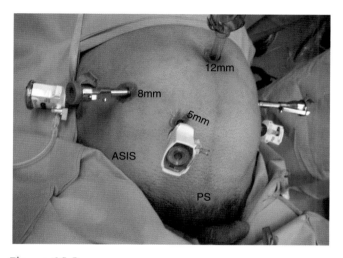

Figure 16.2
Abdominal port locations.

avoidance of leg, hand or abdominal skin contact or injury. It typically takes 15 min from Veress needle insufflation to completion of robot docking.

Development of extraperitoneal space

We have performed several completely extraperitoneal robotic prostatectomies after initially dilating the extraperitoneal space of Retzius with a balloon (Auto Suture, OMS-PDBS2), but we have found port placement to be more challenging than with the transperitoneal approach. Fewer than 50 cases have been done by extraperitoneal VIP technique. The 30° up endoscope is used with the Endowrist® permanent cautery hook (hook cautery) on the right and Endowrist® long tip forceps (long tip forceps) on the left. The cautery (Valley Lab Force FX, Medical Solutions Inc, Minneapolis, MN) power is set as follows: bipolar 25 (standard, medium), cut 50 (pure), and coagulation 80–120 (desiccate, low). Atraumatic graspers (Medtronic Xomed France, LePavillon, France) and the suction/irrigator are used by the assistants. The parietal peritoneum is incised just lateral to the medial umbilical ligament and just medial to the internal inguinal ring over the vas deferens. The latter is grasped and divided, cauterizing the deferential vessel. The dissection is carried anteriorly, 1 cm lateral to the medial umbilical ligament to above the bladder dome (Figure 16.3). The avascular plane of dissection is developed and carried inferiorly through predominantly aereolar tissue until the pubic arch is identified. Care is taken to identify and avoid injuring the iliac vessels just lateral to the plane of dissection. This procedure is repeated on the contralateral side. Subsequently, the medial umbilical ligaments are divided above the bladder, with the assistants providing posterior traction on the ligaments with graspers and anterior traction with suction. The dissection is carried medially, dividing the urachus and then reflecting the bladder posteriorly. Fat is dissected off the pubic arch and endopelvic fascia. The superficial dorsal vein is cauterized and divided and the anterior prostate cleaned of adherent fat.

superior left lateral aspect of the umbilicus for a man 70 inches tall. For shorter men it is moved cephalad and for taller men caudad, approximately 1 to 2 cm. A 12-mm port is placed and the 30° upward lens is introduced. The peritoneum is inspected for injury, abnormalities or bowel adhesions. The right-sided 8-mm robotic port is introduced approximately 3 cm below the level of the umbilicus, 10 to 12 cm off the midline, 2 cm medial to and three finger breadths superomedial to the anterior superior iliac spine. Two right-sided assistant ports are placed for suture introduction/extraction, suction, and tissue grasping. The first is a 12-mm radial dilating port placed two to three finger breadths above the iliac crest as far lateral along the abdominal wall as possible, entering just anterior to the ascending colon. The second is a 5-mm port placed midway between the camera port and the 8-mm right robotic port. It is placed approximately 2 to 3 cm inferior to the robotic port to allow instruments to reach the pelvis. The left-sided ports are then placed; an 8-mm robotic port in the mirror image location of the right and a 5-mm assistant port in a symmetrical position to the 12-mm right lateral assistant port. The robotic tower is then wheeled between the legs and carefully docked into position, with the right- and left-sided bedside assistant surgeons ensuring proper alignment and

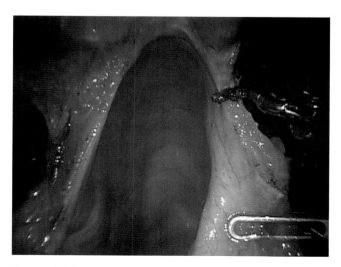

Figure 16.3
Incisions lateral to the medial umbilical ligaments on either side, during development of the extravesical space.

Prostatic apical dissection and control of dorsal venous complex

The 0° endoscope is introduced, and the endopelvic fascia is scored with a hook just lateral to the prostate. Blunt dissection allows exposure of the lateral surface of the prostate as the levator ani muscle fibers are bluntly dissected laterally. Care is taken to minimize use of cautery and avoid inadvertent neurovascular bundle injury. Dissection is carried distally until the urethra with its surrounding puboperinealis muscle is exposed.[7] The wristed action of the instruments allows for precise cephalad retraction of the prostate apex and caudad reflection of adjacent periprostatic levator ani muscle fibers and fascial attachments—a difficult dissection to perform with standard laparoscopic instruments. The puboprostatic ligaments are left intact. The dissection is carried superiorly until a tongue of retroperitoneal fat is identified at the prostatovesical junction. The robotic instruments are exchanged for Endowrist® needle drivers bilaterally and a vertical mattress 7-inch suture of zero polyglactin (0-vicryl) on a CT-1 taper needle is used to secure the dorsal vein complex. We prefer to place the suture without scaling and pass the suture behind the puboprostatic ligaments. The remainder of the suture is used to place a traction suture midway between the prostate apex and base.

Bladder neck transection

The endoscope is changed to 30° down and the hook cautery is replaced on the right and the long tip forceps on the left. We have used Endowrist® round tip scissors (scissors) on the right and Endowrist® precise bipolar (bipolar) on the left, but have found this to be more time consuming and less hemostatic. The assistants sequentially lift the prostate anteriorly with the traction suture, while the surgeon identifies the prostatovesical junction as a shallow groove just cephalad to the prostate, and incises it lateral to the midline approximately 1 cm cephalad to the prostate. The previously identified tongue of retroperitoneal fat is a constant guide to the prostatovesical junction. Laterally, about 2 cm of fatty tissue separates the detrusor muscle from the prostate, and it is quite safe to incise at this location. If fat is not identified when the incision is made, it is likely that the surgeon is too close to the prostate. The transection follows the contour of the prostatovesical junction distally in the midline, where the bladder is entered anteriorly just cephalad to the prostate. The catheter balloon is deflated, grasped by the second assistant and used to provide anterior traction to expose the posterior bladder neck. The latter is incised and the plane between the prostate and bladder is developed inferiorly and laterally. If a prostatic median lobe is present, it is grasped and elevated out of the bladder, and its cephalad margin is incised 1 to 2 cm distal to the visualized ureteral orifices.

Vas deferens, seminal vesicle and posterior prostatic dissection

The posterior lip of the bladder neck is elevated and dissected off the prostate. The anterior layer of Denonvilliers' fascia is identified and incised, exposing the ampullas of the vas deferens and seminal vesicles.

Often the vasa are easily visualized in the midline but may be widely separated with significant prostatic enlargement. Variations in seminal vesicle and vasal anatomy can be recognized more easily if the incision is made wide, before making it deep. Upward traction of the posterior prostate base by the left assistant is applied and the left vas is grasped, cleaned, and divided. The distal and proximal ends are grasped and retracted by the left and right assistants, respectively. The ipsilateral seminal vesicle tip is identified by mobilizing the proximal vas. The seminal vesicle is then skeletonized and freed, avoiding damage to the neurovascular bundle laterally. Subsequently both the left vas and seminal vesicle are grasped by the left assistant, and an identical procedure is performed on the right. The second assistant then grasps and elevates both seminal vesicles and the transected vasa, and the second layer of Denonvilliers' fascia is grasped approximately 1 cm from the prostate and retracted posteriorly. It is divided in the midline and careful blunt dissection allows visualization of the anterior perirectal fat. The plane of dissection between the prostate and rectum is continued with blunt and sharp dissection to the prostatic apex distally and laterally to the medial aspect of the prostatic pedicles. We have recently begun to dissect out the seminal vesicles in select patients using scissors and bipolar cautery in an effort to minimize neurovascular bundle electocautery damage. In addition, we preserve the seminal vesicles (with frozen-section control) in low-risk patients (Gleason score ≤6, clinical T1C, low volume, prostate-specific antigen [PSA] <10 ng/ml) to determine if this modification might improve potency preservation.

Prostatic pedicle control and neurovascular bundle preservation

The scissors are placed on the right and the bipolar instrument on the left (coagulation setting 25). The prostatic pedicles, when discrete and thick, may be controlled with Hem-o-lock MLK clips (Weck Closure Systems, Research Triangle Park, NC) or may be divided sharply with bipolar cauterization of discreet bleeding vessels. The neurovascular bundles run along the posterolateral aspect of the prostate encircled by the inner (prostatic) and outer (levator) layers of periprostatic fascia and anterior layer of Denonvilliers' fascia posteriorly. After dividing the prostatic pedicle, the plane between the prostatic capsule and inner prostatic fascial layer covering the neurovascular bundle is developed at its cranial extent. With the assistants providing superomedial retraction on the prostate and lateral retraction of the neurovascular bundle, careful sharp and blunt dissection of the neurovascular bundle off the prostate is performed until the bundle is mobilized lateral to the prostatic apex. Bipolar cautery is used to coagulate vascular branches or micropedicles that enter the prostate. The wristed instrumentation facilitates this dissection, especially near the prostate apex.

"Veil of Aphrodite" lateral periprostatic fascia dissection

We hypothesize that preservation of the lateral periprostatic fascia along with the posterolateral neurovascular bundle might preserve additional accessory nerves and better preserve the vascular supply to the nerves. We, therefore, in February 2003 initiated preservation of the lateral periprostatic fascia ("veil of Aphrodite") in continuity with the posterolateral "neurovascular bundle" in selected sexually potent patients with low-risk disease (serum PSA <10 ng/ml, clinical T1C, Gleason score ≤ 6, and low-volume tumor) in an effort to determine if this surgical modification would improve erectile potency preservation. The neurovascular bundle is dissected free as described above but, in addition, all periprostatic fascia along the lateral aspect of the prostate up to and including the ipsilateral puboprostatic ligament is preserved in continuity. When performed properly, intact veils of periprostatic tissue, coined "veil of Aphrodite", hang from the puboprostatic ligament(s).

Apical dissection and urethral transection

The 0° endoscope is used for this and the remainder of the operation. Any residual periapical rectal attachments are taken down and the neurovascular bundles are confirmed free. The Foley catheter is inserted and the dorsal vein complex is divided sharply with scissors, with bipolar used to cauterize any bleeders. The periurethral tissues are divided and the prostatic apex and apical notch identified. The anterior and subsequently lateral and posterior urethra is divided sharply, and the rectourethralis and any remaining prostatic attachments are divided (Figure 16.4). Urethral and apical biopsies are typically obtained and sent for frozen-section analysis, and selected biopsies along the neurovascular bundles and rectum are obtained if indicated.[4] The prostate is then entrapped in an Endo-Catch (Auto Suture, Norwalk, CT) bag for later retrieval.

Pelvic lymphadenectomy

The stereoscopic vision and wristed instrumentation of the da Vinci robot make pelvic lymphadenectomy a much easier operation than its standard laparoscopic counterpart. The endoscopic scissors and

bipolar are used to carefully tease the node packet away from the external iliac vein and any accessory vessels. The node packet is cauterized and divided just distal to the node of Cloquet. The obturator nerve is identified and additional distal attachments divided. The packet is mobilized off the obturator nerve and vein and divided proximally. For patients with higher risk disease (Gleason score ≥7, clinical stage T2, PSA 10 ng/ml), we perform an extended node dissection to include all fatty and lymphatic tissues posterior and medial to the obturator nerve up to the bifurcation of the iliac vein.

Urethrovesical anastomosis

We initially performed an interrupted anastomosis but converted to a running anastomosis based on the principles described by Van Velthoven et al[8] for laparoscopic radical prostatectomy. The suture (the MVAC [Menon, Van Velthoven, Ahlering, Clayman] suture) is made by tying a 6 to 8 inch dyed to a similar undyed 3-0 monocryl suture on an RB-1 tapered needle. A needle driver is used on the right and long tip forceps on the left to start the anastomosis. The dyed suture is initially placed out-to-in at the 4 o'clock position of the bladder neck just lateral to the right ureteral orifice. It is run clockwise across the posterior urethra with two to three passes until the suture is just medial to the left ureteral orifice. The suture is cinched down with gentle caudad traction on the bladder (Figure 16.5). The needle driver is placed on the left and the anastomosis continued for two to three passes. It may be intermittently locked or tension may be maintained by the surgeon or assistant. At the 9 o'clock position, the suture is reversed and an additional two passes are performed out-to-in on the urethral and in-to-out on the bladder neck until approximately the 10 o'clock position is reached, where the left assistant holds the suture under tension. The undyed suture is then started by passing it out-to-in at the 4 o'clock position of the urethra and continuing in a counter-clockwise fashion until the anastomosis is complete. If the bladder neck is capacious, it may be closed in a tennis-racket fashion, with the anterior cystotomy closed after completing the anastomosis. A 20-Fr silicone-coated

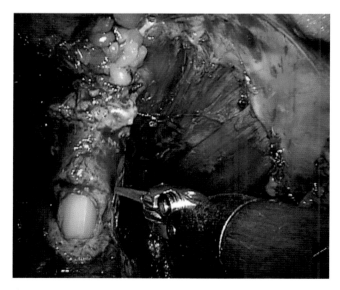

Figure 16.4
Transection of the urethra.

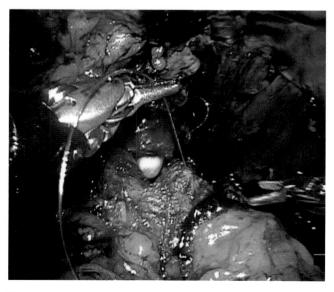

Figure 16.5
Urethrovesical anastomosis.

Foley catheter is positioned in the bladder with 20 ml placed in a 5 ml balloon. The bladder is filled to 120 ml to confirm the anastomosis is water-tight.

Specimen retrieval and completion of surgery

A 15-Fr Jackson-Pratt drain is placed through the left lateral 5-mm port and positioned in the pelvis. The robot is then dedocked and the specimen bag removed through the umbilical port site, enlarging it as necessary. The umbilical port is closed in layers, with 1-0 ethibond on a CTX needle for the fascia. The skin of all port sites is reapproximated with 4-0 vicryl subcuticular sutures and steristrips. Band-Aids or gauze covered with Tegaderm are applied. The drain and Foley catheter are secured, and the patient is transferred to the recovery room.

Postoperative care

The patient is admitted for overnight observation, allowed to ambulate, and given clear liquids the evening of surgery. Pain management is provided with ketorolac and acetaminophen with codeine. He is discharged on postoperative day 1, typically after removal of the drain. A gravity cystogram is obtained on postoperative day 4 to 6, and the Foley catheter is removed if no anastomotic extravasation is noted. The patient resumes full activity 1 to 2 weeks postoperatively.

Results

Technique evolution

Our initial surgical technique included initial posterior dissection of the seminal vesicles,[2] division of the puboprostatic ligaments, use of a urethral sound, and performance of an interrupted anastomosis.[3] We subsequently abandoned initial posterior seminal vesicle dissection, puboprostatic ligament division, and use of a urethral sound, and incorporated use of a running anastomosis into our technique.[9] We have recently initiated preservation of the lateral prostatic fascia ("veil of Aphrodite") and selective preservation of the seminal vesicles in an effort to improve sexual potency preservation. We have completed our first 1000 VIPs and are now compiling and evaluating our results. We have reported results from our initial 100 patients[10] and subsequently our first 200 VIP patients.[11]

Initial experience

We have published the results of our first 100 cases performed between August 2001 and May 2002.[10] Mean patient age was 60 years, and mean body mass index was 27.5. Mean preoperative PSA level was 7.2 ng/ml and follow-up was 5.5 months. Thirty-eight patients had pelvic lymphadenectomy. Mean operative time was

195 $\pm$ 5.0 min. Mean blood loss was 149 ml and no patient required transfusion. Twenty-one, 64, 5, 9, and 1 tumors were pathologic stage pT2a, pT2b, pT3a, pT3b, and pT3BN1, respectively. Positive surgical margin rate was 15%. At 1, 3, and 6 months, the continence rates were 37%, 72%, and 92%, respectively, and the potency rates were 11%, 32%, and 59%. A significant improvement was noted between our initial 40 and subsequent 60 cases. Mean operative time decreased from 274 to 195 min, estimated blood loss (EBL) from 256 to 149 ml, and positive margin rate from 17.5% to 12%.

Interim experience: comparison of VIP and radical retropubic prostatectomy

We subsequently compared the results of our first 200 VIPs to a contemporary series of 100 radical retropubic prostatectomies (RRPs) performed at our institution.[11] No statistically significant difference in patient age, preoperative serum PSA level, body mass index, abdominal or pelvic surgery history, Charlson score or clinical grade or stage was noted. A significant difference favoring VIP was observed in terms of mean EBL (153 vs 910 ml), intraoperative blood transfusion (0% vs 67%), postoperative pain score (3 vs 7), discharge hemoglobin (130 vs 101 g/L), hospital stay (1.2 vs 3.5 days), catheterization time (7 vs 15.8 days), total positive margins (9% vs 23%) and extensive (>1 mm) positive margins (1% vs 15%) in pT2A to pT3A tumors. Analysis of functional outcomes demonstrated faster recovery of continence and potency for the VIP cohort.

Assessment of running urethrovesical anastomosis

We evaluated the results of our first 120 running anastomoses performed by a single surgeon.[4] Mean time was 13 min. Ninety-six (80%) patients had their catheter removed 4 days after surgery after negative cystogram. The remainder had their Foley catheter removed at 7 days. Two patients developed urinary retention requiring recatheterization. Ninety-six percent of patients were continent (no pads) at 3 months follow-up. No patient developed a bladder neck contraction.

Assessment and modification of neurovascular bundle preservation

In an effort to better understand the neurovascular anatomy, we performed a critical analysis of the neurovascular bundles using cadaver dissection.[5] More recently, we have developed the hypothesis that preservation of the lateral periprostatic fascia along with the posterolateral neurovascular bundle might preserve additional accessory nerves and better preserve the vascular supply to the nerves. As described above, we have initiated preservation of the lateral periprostatic fascia ("veil of Aphrodite") in continuity with the posterolateral "neurovascular bundle" in selected patients with low-risk disease in an effort to determine if these surgical modifications would improve erectile potency preservation. A follow-up (conducted by an independent third party) of 33 patients 1 year after surgery with a preoperative sexual function (SHIM) score of 20 or higher was performed. Twenty-two patients had undergone standard nerve preservation and 11 had preservation of the lateral periprostatic fascia ("veil of Aphrodite"). Seven (32%) patients who underwent standard bilateral nerve sparing and 9 (82%) who underwent the "veil of Aphrodite" reported 1-year SHIM scores of 20 or greater (P = <0.05). While the sample size is extremely small, we are encouraged that the return of potency and the quality of erections were superior in the cohort of patients undergoing the "veil of Aphrodite" modification of the VIP.

Our initial postoperative potency preservation results were not improved for patients in whom we spared the tips of the seminal vesicles. We have, therefore, also initiated sparing the entire seminal vesicle in "low-risk" patients. We look forward to analyzing these patients' results to determine if these surgical technique modifications result in improved postoperative outcomes.

Summary

The development of the da Vinci robot has ushered in a new era of surgery.[12] We now have technology that allows us to combine the magnified view and minimally-invasive benefits of laparoscopy with the three-dimensional vision and wristed movements of open surgery. The surgeon is able to operate from a comfortable seated position and provide the patient with outcomes equivalent to or surpassing the best results of open and laparoscopic radical prostatectomy. One can only dream what the future holds for robotic surgery.

References

1. Menon M, Shrivastava A, Tewari A, et al. Laparoscopic and robotic assisted radical prostatectomy: establishment of a structured program and preliminary analysis of outcomes. J Urol 2002;168:945–949.
2. Guillonneau B, Vallancien G. Laparoscopic radical prostatectomy: the Montsouris technique. J Urol 2000;163:1643–2649.
3. Tewari A, Peabody J, Sarle R, et al. Technique of da Vinci robot-assisted anatomic radical prostatectomy. Urology 2002;60:569–572.
4. Menon M, Hemal AK, Tewari A, et al. The technique of apical dissection of the prostate and urethrovesical anastomosis in robotic radical prostatectomy. BJU Int 2004;93:715–719.
5. Tewari A, Peabody JO, Fischer M, et al. An operative and anatomic study to help in nerve sparing during laparoscopic and robotic radical prostatectomy. Eur Urol 2003;43:444–454.
6. Menon M, Hemal AK . Laparoscopic surgery: Where is it going? Prous Science: Timely Topics in Medicine, Oct 10, 2003, ttmed.com (epub), www.prous.com.
7. Myers RP. Detrusor apron, associated vascular plexus, and avascular plane: relevance to radical retropubic prostatectomy—anatomic and surgical commentary. Urology 2002;59:472–9.
8. Van Velthoven RF, Ahlering TE, Peltier A, et al. Technique for laparoscopic running of urethrovesical anastomosis: the single knot method. Urology 2003;61:699–702.
9. Menon M, Tewari A, Peabody J. Vattikuti Institute Prostatectomy: Technique. J Urol 2003;169:2289–2292.
10. Menon M, Shrivastava A, Sarle R, et al. Vattikuti Institute prostatectomy: A single-team experience with 100 cases. J Endourology 2003;17:785–790.
11. Tewari A, Shrivastava A, Menon M. A prospective comparison of radical retropubic and robot-assisted prostatectomy: experience in one institution. BJU Int 2003;92:205–210.
12. Hemal AK, Menon M. Robotics in urology. Curr Opin Urol 2004;14:89–94.

17

Radical prostatectomy: making the transition from open to robotic surgery

Roger S Kirby, Miles A Goldstraw, Prokar Dasgupta, Chris Anderson, Krishna Patil, Peter Amoroso, Jim Peabody

Introduction

Over the past two decades, open nerve-sparing radical retropubic prostatectomy (RRP) has become widely established worldwide as a safe and effective treatment for localized prostate cancer. Recent data from Scandinavia has confirmed that compared with watchful waiting, radical prostatectomy reduces the risk of developing metastases by around 50%, and improves the chances of prostate cancer specific and overall survival.[1] Notwithstanding this, open RRP is still a fairly formidable operation to perform, and even more so to undergo. The lower abdominal incision is associated with significant post-operative discomfort, many patients find the period of up to 3 weeks post-operative catheterization tiresome and convalescence is often slow. Although in expert hands cancer clearance rates (i.e. negative surgical margins and no evidence of biochemical failure) are high, and persistent urinary incontinence is unusual, many patients suffer permanent erectile dysfunction which does not always respond to phosphodiesterase type 5 inhibitors.

The first serious surgical challenge to open RRP came from the laparoscopists in France who discovered that both intraperitoneal[2,3] and extraperitoneal[4] laparoscopic RRP were feasible. Advantages over open RRP in terms of reduced blood loss[5] and diminished post-operative pain[6] soon became apparent and patients were also able to return to normal activities more rapidly. The major problem with laparoscopic RRP relates to the difficulty in learning the procedure. The counter-intuitive movements required to control the laparoscopic instruments, especially when dissecting and suturing deep in the pelvis, take many months to master. This makes the learning curve long and exposes patients to risk of complications while the necessary experience is gained. By contrast, robotically assisted RRP is somewhat easier to master because of the more intuitive way in which the instruments are controlled, and the three-dimensional vision with up to 10× magnification.

In this chapter we describe the way in which our group accomplished the transition from open to robotic RRP. We do not pretend that the journey has been an easy one, but we have recently completed our one-hundredth robotic prostatectomy without any major complications. While we consider this an important milestone, we do not pretend to have mastered this technique. Certainly, others are in a better position to lay claim to this with Dr Mani Menon at the Vattikuti Institute, Henry Ford System, Detroit, USA having reported results from 1100 robotic RRP cases.[7] The learning curve for robotic RRP may differ significantly according to a number of surgeon-related factors. Herrell and Smith[8] reported that more than 150 cases need to be performed before all outcome variables reached parity with the open technique. Furthermore, more than 250 cases needed to be performed before confidence levels of the operating surgeon were similar to the open technique. These figures have important implications for any group intending to set up a robotic prostatectomy program. The median number of radical prostatectomies performed by urologists in the USA is only seven cases per year; clearly, at this rate, many will never overcome the learning curve.

For those considering making the transition, the first step, of course, is the acquisition of a Da Vinci robot, a considerable investment for any institution.[9] Additional funds need to be allocated for the service contract and the ongoing costs of robotic instruments such as scissors, forceps and the diathermy hook. The robotic cart weighs something in the order of 2 tons and the operating department floor has to be sufficiently robust to withstand this weight. The console is light but there has to be sufficient space for both of these bulky pieces of equipment (Figure 17.1A and B).

Once the robot is installed, structured training of the nursing and medical team is required. Careful selection of surgical team members is advisable: we combined a surgeon who was very experienced in open RRP (RSK; more than 1000 cases performed) with an experienced laparoscopic prostatectomist (CA) and the UK's first robotic urologist (PD) who had been using the Da Vinci robot to perform radical cystectomy, colposuspension, live donor nephrectomy and pyeloplasty. We started with so-called "wet lab" training in New York, where we operated robotically on an anesthetized pig and also observed an experienced team undertaking robotic RRP from start to finish. We were then fortunate to have Dr Jim Peabody – who has worked closely with Dr Mani Menon to develop the procedure – come to the UK to mentor the group. It has to be said that the greatest obstacle to this was the rules and regulations imposed by the UK's General Medical Council (GMC) who contrived to make the process of temporary registration as labyrinthine as possible. Eventually the bureaucrats were satisfied and Dr Peabody joined us to guide us through our first six cases. These were accomplished over five consecutive days, informed consent having been achieved from patients who were aware that this was a new undertaking for us. Fortunately, no complications were encountered, in spite of the sometimes prolonged (up to 6 hours) duration of the procedure during this early stage of our experience.

With six cases safely completed, were we ready to "go it alone"? Categorically no; for us, mastering the numerous steps required to perform robotically assisted RRP needed more mentoring support,

A

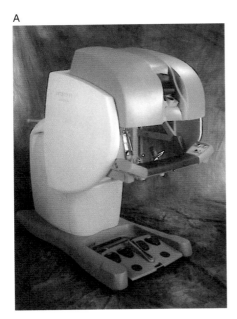

B

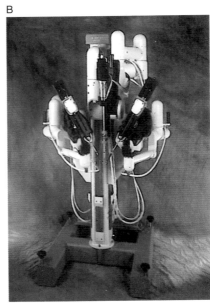

Figure 17.1
A, The Da Vinci console.
B, The Da Vinci surgical cart.

so we persuaded Dr Peabody to return for a further six cases. We also managed to inveigle Dr Ashutosh Tewari from Cornell, New York – who had been in Detroit with Dr Mani Menon while the robotic technique was being developed – to come and help us with a further two cases. Thus, before we went solo we were mentored and supported through a total of 14 robotic RRP. Even then the next few cases were a little nerve-wracking, but as the confidence and skill of the team grew, the operating time diminished and the benefits of the procedure from the patient's viewpoint became increasingly apparent.

Surgical tips for the safe performance of robotic radical retropubic prostatectomy

The goal of RRP is identical to that of open surgery: complete removal of the prostate and seminal vesicles – hopefully with clear margins and a good functional outcome. The role of pelvic lymphadenopathy is controversial and while it is not difficult to perform via the robotic technique we have reserved this for higher grade cancers or those with high prostate-specific antigen (PSA) (>15). Both extraperitoneal[10] and transperitoneal[11] approaches are feasible; however, we adopted the technique of Dr Mani Menon preferring to undertake a transperitoneal approach with antegrade dissection.

Selection criteria are virtually the same for RRP as with open surgery. Whilst obesity is not a particular problem for the operating surgeon (extra-long laparoscopic instruments may be needed), it does appear these patients do worse following this surgery. Ahlering et al[12] noted that baseline sexual and urinary function were significantly worse (versus non-obese comparison) and that there was a strong trend towards delayed recovery time. Obesity may also be a problem for the anesthetist with Trendelenburg tilt and high intra-abdominal pressure making ventilation difficult. The present authors have performed a number of cases with large prostates (>100 cm³),

but we recommend leaving these cases until greater confidence is gained. RP can be an extremely difficult procedure following mesh repair of hernia but with the transperitoneal RRP this has not been a major problem. Any adhesions have to be carefully dissected in the initial phase of the operation but once complete one can proceed as planned. During the first 100 cases we have identified, and treated laparoscopically, a number of undiagnosed inguinal herniae. This takes a matter of a few minutes and involves the insertion of a prolene mesh which is maneuvered around the cord and stapled into position; this would not be possible with the open technique.

After the patient is anesthetized and correctly positioned with all pressure points protected, the abdominal skin is prepared and a urethral catheter passed. Establishing access to the prostate within the pelvis via a transperitoneal route requires safe and careful placement of six laparoscopic ports (two robotic; 2 × 10 mm and 2 × 5 mm). The first key maneuver is the safe establishment of the pneumoperitoneum. This is accomplished through a small vertical incision adjacent to the umbilicus. The fat is dissected down to the level of the rectus sheath, which is elevated using two strong sutures. A 2 mm incision is made in the sheath and a Verres needle cautiously introduced into the peritoneal cavity while an assistant pulls upward on two sutures which have been placed in the rectus sheath. Correct placement of the Verres needle is checked by injection of saline before CO_2 is connected. As the pneumoperitoneum is established, careful checks should be kept on the pressure which should not rise above a few mmHg until several litres is infused, providing that the needle is correctly sited. Incorrect placement of the Verres needle is usually in the extraperitoneal space or within the omentum, but rarely a puncture of the small bowel or other intra-abdominal viscus may occur. Provided this is recognized early in the procedure little harm will ensue. If difficulties are encountered with the insertion of the Verres needle, an open insertion of the midline camera port trocar should be performed. Once the camera port is correctly in place the other five ports can be created under direct vision using a 30°-up lens. Correct port placement is critical and the optimum position of each one is shown in Figure 17.2.[13] It is essential that any pre-existing adhesions, from for example a previous appendicectomy scar, be divided laparoscopically so that safe and secure port placement can be achieved. Care must be taken during

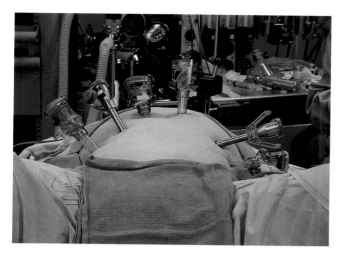

Figure 17.2
Ports in place prior to docking of the Da Vinci robot.

this adhesiolysis as underlying bowel is often extremely close without necessarily being seen; unidentified diathermy injury to bowel has been reported requiring delayed laparotomy.[14] In two of our first 100 cases intra-abdominal adhesions were so extensive that a decision was made after insertion of the camera port to place no further ports and proceed instead with an open extraperitoneal procedure.

The next move is to dock the robot. The machine is advanced between the patient's legs and the camera port connected – ensuring that the robotic cart is central and that the camera arm is correctly positioned. A 30°-up telescope is utilized for the first part of the procedure. The second, third and optional fourth robotic arms are then connected, and each port is inspected in turn to ensure correct positioning and to exclude significant intraperitoneal bleeding. The instruments are then introduced under direct vision and the surgeon at the console then takes over their control.

The bladder is mobilized fully at the time of takedown of the peritoneum. Adhesions to the bladder should be released and the "inverted-U" peritoneal incision should be taken down to the level of the vas on each side. The vasa can be divided laterally at the point they cross the medial umbilical ligament to achieve greater mobility of the bladder, and to allow for easier access to lymph node packets. This additional mobility can allow for easier movement of the bladder to the urethra during anastomosis. An assistant or the fourth robotic arm can grasp the bladder anteriorly to also hold the bladder down. In very overweight patients with large amounts of perivesical fat, the bladder should not be taken down too high on the abdominal wall as this leaves extra weight on the bladder, which can serve to distract the bladder, cranially away from the anastomosis later.

Once the prostate is exposed, scrupulous attention is paid to the removal of the fat that lies on its anterior surface using the 0° telescope. This must be accomplished with care as bleeding may occur from the fragile superficial veins that lie within it, usually in the midline. These can be diathermied with the bipolar forceps. The next move is to divide the lateral pelvic fascia on each side to mobilize the prostate. This plane is usually relatively bloodless, but care does need to be taken as the prostate–urethral junction is approached so as to avoid injury and bleeding from the dorsal venous complex. The muscle of the pelvic floor is gently teased away from the urethra so that the suture to secure the dorsal venous complex can be placed under direct vision. The puboperinealis muscle covers the urethra

and is the most anteromedial component of the levator ani; this appears to have a special role in the urinary continence mechanism.[15] Inferiorly, the incisions are deepened until a characteristic triangle of fat is identified that marks the vesicoprostatic junction. The instruments are then changed to two-needle drivers and a suture is placed through the groove between the dorsal venous complex and the urethra, from right to left, this is then brought back from left to right immediately beneath the puboprostatic ligaments and tied securely on the right-hand side of the urethra. The puboprostatic ligaments fix the prostate to the pubis, maintain support for the striated sphincter[16] and help prevent hypermobility of the penis.[17] Certainly, a number of groups feel that puboprostatic preservation is important in helping gain early continence.[18,19]

The next move is to dissect the prostate away from the bladder neck using the 30°-down telescope. It is important that this incision is made precisely in the correct location to avoid an inadvertent incision into the anterior prostate, which can cause confusion and additional bleeding. Pinching the prostate bilaterally to define the vesicoprostatic junction can be helpful, as can traction applied to the catheter. The relatively thin anterior bladder neck is divided in the midline down to the catheter, which is identified and the balloon deflated. The catheter is then pulled through and held up by the second assistant or the fourth robotic arm to apply anterior traction to the prostate. This maneuver facilitates the incision through the posterior bladder neck which must be beneath any median lobe but well away from the usually easily visualized ureteric orifices. Once the posterior bladder neck is divided, the incision is deepened through Denonvilliers' fascia; at this point, care has to be taken to avoid either button-holing of the bladder neck or inadvertent incision into the prostate itself. Provided the correct plane is located then the vasa and seminal vesicles come into view quite quickly. The right vas is dissected free and divided, and then the first assistant is requested to grasp and lift the proximal end of the vas. This facilitates the dissection of the right seminal vesicle, which is elevated progressively as the vesicular arteries are secured and divided by diathermy. The procedure is then repeated for the left vas and seminal vesicle. Once both seminal vesicles are free, the second assistant or fourth robotic arm are used to elevate the prostate by lifting up on them and the proximal stumps of the divided vasa. A "window" is then apparent just behind the posterior prostate and anterior to the rectum.[20] An incision here soon exposes the pre-rectal fat and the rectum can be pushed gently backwards as the posterior prostatic capsule comes into view. Extending the dissection right and left at this point can facilitate the subsequent dissection of the neurovascular bundles. Sometimes a switch back to the 0° telescope can be helpful. Once the apex is reached, attention is paid to securing each prostatic pedicle which is done using so-called Weck clips and the robotic scissors.

The dissecting scissors are then used to dissect the neurovascular bundles on each side. If a nodule is palpable, a wide excision may be indicated on the side affected in an attempt to achieve a negative surgical margin. Once this maneuver has been accomplished the prostate should be free, apart from its connection to the urethra and ligated dorsal venous complex. These structures are then divided sharply by scissors to avoid diathermy injury to the distal urethral stump. Bleeding from the dorsal venous complex can usually be dealt with by bipolar diathermy and occasionally a suture. The prostate is then bagged and placed in the right iliac fossa.

As in open surgery, the anastomosis can be the most technically challenging part of the procedure; however, the superb vision and 10× magnification facilitate this step considerably. Problems of suture pull-through at the bladder neck can be diminished by proper attention to the posterior bladder neck thickness at the time of division of the bladder off the posterior urethra – don't thin it out too much. At times, with a median lobe, the residual posterior bladder neck can be quite thin. In this case a portion of the thinner tissue can be excised or, preferably, a deeper more secure bite into the bladder can be taken.

Bleeding from the dorsal vein complex and prostatic pedicles should be controlled as necessary to allow for clear vision before division of the urethra. This allows for better visualization to facilitate creation of a good urethral stump. It also allows for improved ability to see the urethra during suturing and makes it more prominent. Perineal pressure can help to demonstrate bleeding points at the dorsal vein which can facilitate precise suture ligature.

Bladder neck tapering: It is important to have a rough concordance (not more than 2–3:1) between the bladder neck and urethra, but a larger bladder neck is easier to anastomose than a smaller one. Sutures can be placed laterally at 3 o'clock and 9 o'clock positions. We typically use interrupted 3 zero vicryl on an RB-1 needle. Care must be taken to avoid the ureteric orifices which can usually be visualized well. Indigo Carmine or Methylene Blue can be injected intravenously for their easier identification but we have not had to do this. If the bladder neck is too small, one or two tapering sutures could be removed, or if no tapering was done an incision could be made at the 12 o'clock position (anterior) on the bladder to improve visualization of the posterior (trigonal) bladder neck. Sometimes we perform an anterior tapering, i.e. we complete the anastomosis leaving a gap anteriorly which is closed separately in a "tennis raquet" fashion.

The pneumoperitoneum causes the urethra to be extruded out of the pelvis which can make it difficult to accurately place the initial sutures. Perineal pressure is used routinely to evert the urethra at the beginning of the anastomosis, and it is used until the bladder is "snugged down" to the urethra, creating the posterior plate.

Use of urethral catheter throughout anastomosis allows for accurate visualization of the urethra, which prevents "backwalling" of the urethra. Prior to each suture being placed through the urethra, the tip of the catheter is passed forward by the assistant to allow visualization of the urethra and a minimal degree of urethral eversion. The catheter must be well lubricated and should be withdrawn a few centimeters by the assistant prior to the bladder bite being taken to ensure that the catheter is not pierced by the needle. The catheter should be changed after completion of the anastomosis.

Sugundh Shetty from William Beaumont Hospital, Detroit, USA described a technique to us whereby a long prolene suture is passed through the bladder neck in the midline. A Foley catheter is then placed through the urethra into the pelvis. The ends of the prolene suture are then passed through the eye of the catheter and the catheter is withdrawn through the urethra, pulling the ends of the prolene suture out through the meatus. Traction on this suture will approximate the bladder neck to the urethra, facilitating the anastomosis.

We use the 0° lens for the anastomosis and the "MVAC" suture exclusively. This was the result of a series of communications between Dr Menon,[18] Professor VanVeltoven,[21] Dr Ahlering and Dr Clayman. A double-armed suture is created by tying two 3 zero monocryl sutures together with a "ten-throw" knot which creates a pledget. The arms are 6–7 inches long; one arm may be dyed and the other left undyed to allow for easier identification of the right and left sides. An RB-1 needle is used on each end with the dyed end used first. At times, the bladder neck can be difficult to identify and in these circumstances we use the needle in the right hand to try to engage the posterior bladder neck and elevate it into view. If this is not successful, the lens could be switched to 30°-down to find the bladder neck. The assistant can also use suction to press the anterior portion of the bladder down and cephalad to further

expose the urethra. Some groups have suggested placing a suture on the posterior bladder neck at the time of division of the bladder from the prostate to facilitate later identification, but we have never found this necessary.

The dyed end is run from the 4 o'clock position in a clockwise fashion to the 11 o'clock position. An outside-in bite is taken at the 4 o'clock position on the bladder neck, just lateral to the right ureteral orifice. This suture must be pulled through until the knot is secure and tight against the bladder muscle. The next bite is taken inside-out in the urethra at the corresponding 4 o'clock position using the perineal pressure and catheter as noted above. The next bite is taken outside-in on the bladder neck, again in the midline. The next bite is inside-out on the urethra in the midline. With these first two urethral bites, an effort is made to include a few millimeters of tissue posterior to the urethra to provide a more secure bite. The next pass of the suture is outside-in on the bladder at the level of the left ureteral orifice. With these five bites placed (three bladder and two urethral) the bladder can be gently pulled down to the urethra by using the left hand to pull on the dyed suture and the right-hand needle-driver to push the bladder neck down. The instrument can be placed behind the trigone to push the bladder forward.

Once the posterior plate is securely together the assistant on the right side will hold traction on the suture while the console surgeon will use both needle-drivers to place the next suture (inside-out on the urethra). Some surgeons will perform a single, double or even triple locking suture at this point. One or two additional bites are taken inside-out on the urethra and outside-in on the bladder. After each bladder bite is secured we have the right-hand side assistant hold tension on the suture. As an alternative, the console surgeon can hold the tension on the suture but this requires a higher degree of skill as the needle must be manipulated with only one instrument; this is not recommended for the novice robotic surgeon. The mucosa should be visualized and taken with each bite on each side. The suture is then "turned around" on the bladder by placing a suture outside-in and then inside-out on the bladder. This serves to both make up some of the difference in size between the bladder and urethra and to allow for easier suturing on the left side anterior urethra. Additional bites are taken outside-in on the urethra and inside-out on the bladder. Suturing continues for one or two more bites until the 11 o'clock position is reached. The suture can then be held by the left-hand side assistant, the fourth robotic arm, or secured to the side wall or bladder.

The right side of the anastomosis is then completed by placing the first pass of the undyed suture outside-in on the urethra, the next bite being inside-out on the bladder. These initial bites are sometimes easier to perform with a right-handed backhand approach. Additional bites are taken in sequence until the anastomosis is complete.

The anastomosis should be inspected to be certain that all sutures are pulled down tight; any gaps should be tightened and then the suture is tied. We generally cut the needle off the dyed suture because this suture end is more easily visualized than the undyed one. We use a single-throw first knot and make an effort to gently pull the sutures horizontally, watching for an indentation in the bladder muscle to indicate that the suture is tight. Six to seven throws are taken and the suture ends are trimmed.

Fluid along the sides of the bladder and anastomosis is suctioned out. A new catheter is advanced into the bladder up to the hub; the balloon is not yet inflated. The bladder is filled with 120–180 cm³ of saline to check for leaks. If none are found, the catheter is inflated and the anastomosis is complete. If a leak is found, the new catheter is removed and the old one replaced to prevent damage to the new catheter during the attempted repair of the leak. We identify the leak with the bladder partially filled. A 3 zero vicryl on an RB-1 needle is used to close the leak, usually with a figure-of-eight suture. After each pass of the needle, the catheter should be advanced into the bladder to assure that the needle has not "backwalled" the urethra or bladder, narrowing the anastomosis. A posterior leak is very difficult to close. A large leak is best treated by prolonged catheterization or takedown and reconstruction of the anastomosis. A leaking anastomosis can be treated by a period of light tension on the Foley catheter.

Before closure, a suction drain is placed under vision on the anterior bladder wall. Some surgeons suture the peritoneum back in place (puboperineoplasty) but this is usually unnecessary. The robot is undocked and the prostate removed through an enlarged paraumbilical incision. The wounds are then closed carefully with particular attention to the larger port entry sites to minimize the risk of hernia formation and subcuticular sutures used to close the skin.

Post-operatively, early mobilization is encouraged and the duration of hospital stay is a matter of only a few days. Catheter removal can be accomplished within a few days but the risk of recatheterization is increased. We usually leave the catheter in place for 1 week and then check hemoglobin and urine culture. We recommend routine performance of a cystogram at the beginning of one's experience, and then as needed for more difficult anastomoses.

If a catheter falls out in the recovery room, or shortly after surgery, we advise using a Coude tip catheter with some rectal pressure to guide the catheter into the bladder. We obtain a cystogram to confirm correct catheter placement. It is extremely unusual to have complete disruption of an anastomosis, which usually happens in the face of a large pelvic hematoma distracting the bladder from the urethra. In this situation it is feasible to laparoscopically re-explore the pelvis and redo the anastomosis. This should be done as soon as possible after the problem is recognized – within a few days of the original operation. The tissues are often edematous and friable and satisfactory completion of the anastomosis can be very difficult.

Functional outcomes

Outcomes following RRP are controversial. Incontinence and erectile dysfunction are the complications with greatest effect on quality of life over the long term. Surgical technique is undoubtedly a contributing factor to the stress incontinence seen after radical prostatectomy. Theoretically, the excellent vision provided by the laparoscopic camera, together with the minimal bleeding, allows precise dissection and limits trauma to the periurethral striated sphincter. This opens the door for the potential for early return of continence with RRP. While results from RRP certainly show very low levels of incontinence,[18,22] none of the currently published studies show a definitive advantage over the open technique.

Since Binder and Kramer[23] performed the first RRP it has been an evolving technique with continual refinements being made. Ong et al[24] used a canine model to study the effects of thermal energy on the cavernous nerve function, and their research supported strict avoidance of thermal energy around the neurovascular bundle. Ahlering et al[25] performed a prospective analysis of 59 potent men (SHIM scores 22–25) looking at short-term potency rates in men undergoing cautery-free robotic prostatectomy and compared them with a closely matched control group undergoing standard bipolar diathermy dissection. Results showed a fivefold improvement (43% versus 8.3%) in 3 month potency with cautery-free prostatectomy

compared to the standard bipolar dissection. Chien et al[26] showed broadly similar potency results of 47% at 3 months using a clipless antegrade nerve preservation approach. Potency rates increased to 69% by 12 months and further long-term improvements may be expected. This study compares favorably with the outcomes for a series on open RRP using the same validated questionnaire (reporting 36.7% and 50%, 3 and 12 month intervals, respectively).[27]

Menon et al[11] have further refined the anatomical nerve-sparing robotic prostatectomy and reported that preservation of the prostatic fascia (the so-called "veil of Aphrodite") is important for the maintenance of erectile function. It is proposed that accessory neural channels exist in this lateral prostatic facia that may supply innervation to the penis. A recent report by this group has shown impressive results: prospective analysis of 76 potent men undergoing RRP with either standard robotic nerve-sparing prostatectomy (control) or the prostatic fascia sparing technique (treatment) was performed. Patients with normal erectile function, low-risk disease – PSA <10 ng/mL, stage T1c, Gleason sum ≤60 – were offered the prostatic fascia preservation technique (n=46), although eight patients were included in this group who did not fit these criteria exactly. Results at 12 months follow-up showed that 51% of treatment patients achieved normal erections compared with 17% of control patients without medication.[28] This percentage increased to 86% and 26%, respectively, with the use of a phosphodiesterase type 5 inhibitor; when the survey included all men able to achieve an erection strong enough for intercourse, the figure reached 97% in the treatment group.

Conclusion

Although RRP is a relatively recent invention it has already become a serious alternative to the open prostatectomy. In the USA, in 2006, there were over 350 robotic systems performing over 35,000 procedures.[29] It is important to not be influenced too greatly by the marketing claims available, but there does appear to be several benefits. While laparoscopic radical prostatectomy results in reduced pain, low blood loss and rapid patient recovery, it is an incredibly difficult operation to learn and one that has counter-intuitive movements with no ergonomic comfort. In contrast, robotic RRP has all of the advantages of minimally invasive surgery but has the benefits of: 10× magnification, tremor reduction, ergonomic design and intuitive movements (seven-degrees of freedom). Theoretically, this may give improvements over the traditional laparoscope. Furthermore, any procedure that minimizes trauma to the periprostatic tissue has the potential to result in improved functional outcomes. This is suggested by recent data showing an improvement in erectile function with robotic RRP compared to the open approach.[28,30] Clearly, data from such small numbers of patients need to be treated with caution, and outcome figures from specialist centers may not always be achievable elsewhere. However, robotic RRP is an evolving technique and outcome figures may be expected to continue to improve. In comparison, open surgery has had two decades of improvements and may have reached a plateau in its development. Perhaps this is the key question which remains to be answered and will be crucial in deciding whether or not to make the transition. The other important factor is the health economics of robotic surgery and cost reduction can be anticipated in the future. However, it does seem possible that robotic RRP may become the new "gold standard" treatment for clinically localized prostate cancer.

References

1. Bill-Axelson A, Holmberg L, Ruutu M et al. Scandinavian prostate cancer group study No 4. Radical prostatectomy versus watchful waiting in early prostate cancer. N Engl J Med 2005;352:1977–1984.

2. Guillonneau B, Vallancien G. Laparoscopic radical prostatectomy: the Montsouris technique. J Urol 2000;163:1643–1649.

3. Schuessler W, Schulam P, Clayman R, Kavoussi L. Laparoscopic radical prostatectomy; initial short-term experience. Urology 1997;50:854.

4. Bollens R, Vanden Bossche M, Roumeguere T et al. Extraperitoneal laparoscopic radical prostatectomy. Results after 50 cases. Eur Urol 2001;40:65–69.

5. Salomon L, Sebe P, De La Taille A et al. Open versus laparoscopic radical prostatectomy: Part II. BJU Int 2004;94:244–250.

6. Bhayani S, Pavlovich C, Strup S et al. Laparoscopic radical prostatectomy: a multi-institutional study of conversion to open surgery. Urology 2004;63:99–102.

7. Menon M, Tewari A, Peabody J et al. Vattikuti Institute prostatectomy, a technique of robotic radical prostatectomy for management of localised carcinoma of the prostate: experience of over 1100 cases. Urol Clin North Am 2004;31:701–717.

8. Herrell S, Smith J Jr. Robotic-assisted laparoscopic prostatectomy: what is the learning curve? Urology 2005;66 (suppl 5A):105–107.

9. Scales C, Jones P, Eisenstein E et al. Local cost structures and the economics of robot assisted radical prostatectomy. J Urol 2005;174:2323–2329.

10. Joseph J, Rosenbaum R, Madeb R, Patel H. Robotic extraperitoneal radical prostatectomy: an alternative approach. J Urol 2006;75:945–950.

11. Menon M, Hemal A, VIP team. Vattikuti Institute prostatectomy: a technique of robotic radical prostatectomy: experience in more than 1000 cases. J Endourol 2004;18:611.

12. Ahlering T, Eichel L, Edwards R, Skarecky D. Impact of obesity on clinical outcomes in robotic prostatectomy. Urology 2005;65:740–744.

13. Hemal A, Eun D, Tewari A, Menon M. Nuances in the optimum placement of ports in pelvic and upper urinary tract surgery using the da Vinci robot. Urol Clin North Am 2004;31:683–692.

14. Menon M. Robotic radical retropubic prostatectomy. BJU Int 2003;91:175–176.

15. Myers R, Cahill D, Kay P et al. Puboperineales: muscular boundaries of the male urogenital hiatus in 3D from magnetic resonance imaging. J Urol 2000;164:1412–1415.

16. Steiner M. The puboprostatic ligament and the male urethral suspensory mechanism: an anatomic study. Urology 1994;44:530–534.

17. Hemal A, Wadhwa S. Repair of the suspensory ligament of the penis: an important step in the transpubic approach. Br J Urol 1994;74:516.

18. Menon M, Hemal A, Tewari A et al. The technique of apical dissection of the prostate and urethrovesical anastamosis in robotic radical prostatectomy. BJU Int 2004;93:715–719.

19. Deliveliotis C, Protogerou V, Alargof E et al. Radical prostatectomy. Bladderneck preservation and puboprostatic ligament sparing-effects on continence and positive margins. Urology 2002;60:855–888.

20. Hemal A, Bhandari A, Tewari A, Menon M. The window sign; an aid in laparoscopic and robotic prostatectomy. Int Urol Nephrol 2005;37:73–77.

21. Van Velthoven R, Ahlering T, Peltier A et al. Technique for laparoscopic running urethrovesical anastomosis: the single knot method. Urology 2003;61:699–702.

22. Smith JJ. Robotically assisted laparoscopic prostatectomy: an assessment of its contemporary role in the surgical management of localised prostate cancer. Am J Surg 2004;188:63S–67S.

23. Binder J, Kramer W. Robotically-assisted laparoscopic radical prostatectomy. BJU Int 2001;87:408–410.

24. Ong A, Su L, Varkarakis L et al. Nerve sparing radical prostatectomy: effects of hemostatic energy sources on the recovery of cavernous nerve function in a canine model. J Urol 2004;172:1318–1322.

25. Ahlering T, Eichel L, Skarecky D. Early potency with cautery-free neurovascular bundle preservation with robotic laparoscopic radical prostatectomy. J Endourol 2005;19:715–718.

26. Chien G, Mikhail A, Orvieto M et al. Modified clipless antegrade nerve preservation in robotic-assisted laparoscopic radical prostatectomy with validated sexual function evaluation. Urology 2005;66:423.

27. Litwin M, Melmed G, Nakazon T. Life after radical prostatectomy: a longitudinal study. J Urol 2001;166:592.

28. Menon M, Kaul S, Bhandari A et al. Potency following robotic prostatectomy: a questionnaire based analysis of outcomes after conventional nerve sparing and prostatic fascia sparing techniques. J Urol 2005;174:2291–2296.

29. Kaul S, Menon M. Robotic radical prostatectomy: evolution from conventional to VIP. World J Urol 2006;24:152–160.

30. Goldstraw MA, Dasgupta P, Anderson C et al. Does robotically assisted radical prostatectomy result in better preservation of erectile function? BJU Int 2006;98:721–722.

18

Role of surgery in the management of high-risk localized prostate cancer

Laurence Klotz, Alessandro Volpe

Introduction

Prostate cancer is a heterogeneous disease with very different phenotypes. Defining the subgroup of patients who are at high risk for developing recurrence after local treatment is a priority.

Historically, initial risk assessment was based on clinical staging and anatomic extent of the disease, assessed by digital rectal examination (DRE) and imaging. However, a large proportion of patients with clinically organ-confined disease are subsequently found to have extracapsular disease at the time of surgery. Such patients are at high risk of recurrence. Partin et al[1] developed a nomogram which improves the ability to clinically predict pathologic stage, taking into account biopsy Gleason grade and prostate-specific antigen (PSA) level along with clinical stage.

Many studies reveal a significant association between an increased biopsy Gleason score and decreased disease-free survival after radical prostatectomy or radiation therapy.[2–4] Superior outcomes occur with a Gleason score of 6 or less, intermediate outcomes with a Gleason score of 7, and poorer outcomes with a Gleason score of 8 or more.[2,4–6] Pretreatment PSA is also a significant predictor of outcome either after surgery[2,3,7] or radiation therapy.[8,9]

Given the independent prognostic significance of pretreatment PSA, Gleason score, and clinical stage, various algorithms have been produced to establish the risk of PSA failure after local therapy of localized prostate cancer. Kattan et al[10] developed a nomogram to predict 5-year prognosis after radical prostatectomy. Similar nomograms have been developed for external beam radiation therapy[11] and brachytherapy.[12] These are widely used in clinical practice.

D'Amico et al[13,14] proposed stratifying patients with localized prostate cancer into categories with low (<25%), moderate (25–50%), and high risk (>50%) of PSA failure at 5 years from definitive local treatment. According to this classification, patients with AJCC clinical stage T2C, a PSA level of more than 20 ng/ml, or a biopsy Gleason score of 8 or more are considered at high risk of recurrence (Table 18.1).

In a recent paper, the same investigators[15] observed that patients presenting with all the characteristics used to define intermediate-risk cancers (Table 18.1) had a time to PSA failure and a prostate cancer-specific mortality after radical prostatectomy significantly shorter than patients whose definition was based on just one or two factors. This observation may support the shift of this group of intermediate-risk patients into the high-risk category.

Blute et al[7] developed a different scoring system called GSPM (Gleason score, Seminal vesicle, PSA, and Margin status) to predict the risk of biochemical failure after radical prostatectomy (Table 18.2).

In their series, 5-year progression-free survival was 94% for a score lower than 5, 60% for a score of 10, and 32% for a score greater than 12.

Several studies have shown that the addition of information about the percentage of prostate biopsy cores involved by cancer can further stratify patients with respect to the probability of PSA failure.[16–20]

Some authors have used results from high-density tissue microarrays to define combinations of biomarkers associated with prostate cancer progression after radical prostatectomy.[21] Neural networks have also been utilized to predict the risk of biochemical failure after surgical treatment.[22]

Role of radical prostatectomy in the management of high-risk localized disease

The first goal in the management of patients diagnosed with localized prostate cancer is the selection of a treatment that can provide the best chance of cure with the least morbidity. Appropriately, high-risk patients who are aware of the life-threatening nature of their disease are more accepting of treatment morbidity. However, the side effects of radical prostatectomy are not increased in patients with high-risk disease.[23–25]

In a randomized trial comparing radical prostatectomy with watchful waiting in clinically localized prostate cancer, Bill-Axelson et al[26] observed a lower cancer-specific mortality in the surgical group at 5 to 10 years from diagnosis (Figure 18.1). According to Pound et al,[27] the median time to death from prostate cancer in men who have had a radical prostatectomy is 16 years.[27] Thus, deaths from prostate cancer at 5 to 10 years from diagnosis reflect high-risk, aggressive disease. This suggests that the survival benefit in the Bill-Axelson et al study is a function of a survival benefit of radical prostatectomy in high-risk patients.

Other than the unique Holmberg et al trial,[26] determining the rational, evidence-based choice of treatment of localized prostate cancer has been hampered by the scarcity of unbiased data on outcome from randomized clinical trials. Few studies have been carried out outside specialized academic centers. However, a population-based approach has provided some convincing evidence for the role of surgery. In 1997, Lu-Yao and Yao[28] analyzed the data for

Table 18.1 Classification of localized prostate cancerin risk groups based on preoperative prognostic factors[13,14]

	Low risk	Intermediate risk	High risk
AJCC clinical stage	T1 – T2a	T2b	T2c
Biopsy Gleason score	≤6	7	≥8
PSA level (ng/ml)	<10	10–20	> 20

Table 18.2 Mayo Clinic GSPM score system[7]

Clinical feature	Score
Gleason score	Gleason score value
PSA 4–10 ng/ml	+1
PSA 10–20 ng/ml	+2
PSA >20 ng/ml	+3
Positive seminal vesicles	+2
Positive surgical margins	+2

High scores are associated with increased risk of biochemical recurrence.

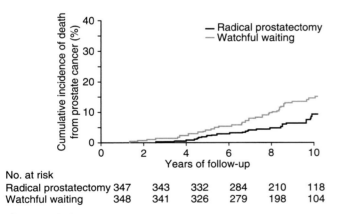

No. at risk						
Radical prostatectomy	347	343	332	284	210	118
Watchful waiting	348	341	326	279	198	104

Figure 18.1

Disease-specific cumulative incidence of death for patients with newly diagnosed, clinically localized prostate cancer who were randomly assigned to watchful waiting or radical prostatectomy.

From Bill-Axelson et al,[26] with permission

59,876 patients included in the Surveillance, Epidemiology and End Results (SEER) program database to establish overall and disease-specific survival in patients treated by surgery, radiotherapy or conservative management for clinically localized prostate cancer in diverse clinical settings. They observed that cancer grade significantly affects overall survival for all treatments, confirming its role as the most important predictor of survival. In each grade group, radical prostatectomy provided higher 10-year cancer-specific survival rates compared to radiation therapy or watchful waiting (Table 18.3). The benefit of surgery when compared to other treatments was greatest in patients with high-grade disease and therefore high risk of mortality; this benefit was apparent within 5 years of diagnosis. Though Lu-Yao and Yao's study[28] was not randomized, these findings support the view that surgical treatment can significantly improve long-term survival in patients with high-risk localized prostate cancer.

Menon et al[29] retrospectively evaluated long-term survival in 3159 men with clinically localized prostate cancer managed conservatively or treated definitively with either radiation therapy or radical prostatectomy. The overall adjusted survival rate was significantly increased in patients with high-grade cancers who underwent surgery when compared to patients treated with radiation therapy ($P = 0.009$), which was superior to conservative treatment ($P = 0.023$). The increase in the duration of survival was 4.6 years with radiation therapy and over 8.6 years with radical prostatectomy.[29]

In another retrospective study, D'Amico et al[13] used a multivariable time-to-PSA-failure analysis to compare PSA outcome after radical prostatectomy, external beam radiation therapy, and interstitial radiation therapy with or without neoadjuvant androgen deprivation for patients stratified by pretreatment risk group of recurrence. The group of patients at low risk for post-therapy PSA failure was estimated to derive equal benefit from the different treatments, while patients at high risk treated with radical prostatectomy had a significantly better 5-year PSA outcome compared to patients treated with seeds implant, and a higher 5-year PSA outcome compared to those treated with external beam radiation therapy, even though this difference was not statistically significant.

The impact on outcome of the improved surgical technique acquired in the PSA era has been reported in more recent series.[2,30,31] Eastham et al[32] identified the surgeon as the single most important independent variable predicting cancer recurrence after radical prostatectomy.

The 10-year postsurgical prostate cancer-specific mortality for high-risk patients in recent studies[2,30,31] is considerably lower than the mortality observed in high-grade cancer after treatment with external beam radiation therapy in the population-based study of Lu-Yao et al,[28] or the mortality observed after radiation therapy in the high-risk patients in the Boston radiotherapy cohort (Table 18.4).[33]

Table 18.3 Ten-year disease-specific survival in patients with clinically localized prostate cancer according to treatment received[28]

Treatment	Gleason 2–4		Gleason 5–7		Gleason 8–10	
	n	% Survival (95% CI)	n	% Survival (95% CI)	n	% Survival (95% CI)
Radical prostatectomy	3402	98 (97–99)	12,922	91 (89–93)	4154	76 (71–80)
Radiation therapy	4188	89 (87–92)	8456	74 (71–77)	2977	52 (46–57)
Watchful waiting	10,133	92 (90–93)	7046	76 (73–78)	2834	43 (38–48)

Table 18.4 Ten-year prostate cancer-specific mortality with different treatment modalities

	Low grade (%)	Intermediate grade (%)	High grade (%)
Population study[28]			
Radical prostectomy	2	9	21
Radiation therapy	11	26	48
Watchful waiting	8	24	57
Baylor College radical prostatectomy cohort[30]			
Radical prostatectomy	2	1	18
Boston radiotherapy cohort[33]			
Radiation therapy	0	6	45

Clearly, current techniques of conformal radiation therapy may also provide better long-term cancer control rates than the radiation therapy modalities used 10 years ago. Other pitfalls exist in comparing the results of surgery to radiation, including different definitions of PSA failure.

Multimodality treatment

Several studies have evaluated whether better outcomes can be achieved in high-risk patients with a multimodality treatment approach. Excellent survival rates with low treatment-related morbidity have been achieved at the Mayo Clinic by performing primary radical prostatectomy with different protocols of adjuvant therapy in a large series of patients with clinical stage T3 prostate cancer. Ten-year crude and cancer-specific survival rates were 70% and 80%, respectively.[24]

Neoadjuvant therapy

Neoadjuvant therapy can provide cytoreduction for locally advanced disease and (in theory) early treatment for micrometastases. Several trials have randomized patients to 3 months of androgen blockade before radical prostatectomy versus surgery alone. A significant decrease in positive surgical margins was observed, but no study was able to show a benefit in term of PSA progression-free survival at 3 to 6 years of follow-up.[34–39] Importantly, none of these studies was enriched for high-risk patients, and none was powered to show a PSA progression difference. The only study to report follow up longer than 5 years found a PSA progression benefit in the patients with a PSA level greater than 20 ng/ml.[39]

Other recent studies suggest that a longer period of androgen deprivation (6–8 months) may be needed to obtain improved pathologic and clinical outcomes.[40,41] Gleave et al[40] randomized 547 patients with clinically localized prostate cancer to 3 versus 8 months of androgen deprivation before radical prostatectomy. They observed ongoing biochemical and pathologic regression of the tumors between 3 and 8 months of neoadjuvant hormonal therapy. These findings suggest that longer androgen blockade in high-risk patients may result in a benefit. A long-term neoadjuvant study in high-risk patients is required to test this hypothesis.

Several groups are studying the role of neoadjuvant chemotherapy in high-risk localized prostate cancer. Most available data come from small phase II trials.[42–45] A randomized phase III study of radical prostatectomy alone versus estramustin and docetaxel before radical prostatectomy has been initiated by the Cancer and Leukemia Group B (CALGB 90203) and will enrol approximately 700 men who will be observed for a follow-up of at least 7 years.[46] The use of more targeted and therefore less toxic drugs (growth factor inhibitors, angiogenesis inhibitors, antioxidants, and inducers of apoptosis) may also have a role in the neoadjuvant setting and have been studied in preliminary trials.[47,48]

Adjuvant radiation therapy

For patients with residual disease after radical prostatectomy, therapy should be more effective shortly after removal of the primary tumor, when the number of malignant cells is low. An advantage of adjuvant therapy is that it does not delay definitive local treatment.

Adjuvant radiation therapy has been widely studied in patients with high risk of recurrence after radical prostatectomy. Retrospective series reported that the 5-year biochemical recurrence rate may be decreased with this approach in patients with positive margins or extracapsular extension,[7,49–54] but the effect on overall and cause-specific mortality is still unclear. Reports of 10-year survival rates range from 52% to 80% in patients without adjuvant radiation, to 60% to 76% in patients receiving adjuvant radiation.[55–58] A survival advantage related to better local control has been often suggested, but has not been confirmed by randomized trials. The Southwest Oncology Group (SWOG) and the European Organization for Research and Treatment of Cancer (EORTC) have completed accrual to two randomized adjuvant radiation studies (SWOG 8794 and EORTC 22911) that will help to clarify this issue. Until these results become available, adjuvant radiation therapy alone should be reserved for patients with positive surgical margins and without Gleason 8 to 10 disease or other poor prognostic features such as seminal vesicles invasion. These latter patients are at high risk for occult distant metastases and are less likely to benefit from further local therapy.

Adjuvant hormonal therapy

Data regarding the use of adjuvant hormonal therapy after radical prostatectomy for high-risk localized disease are limited. Most published studies have enrolled patients with locally advanced or metastatic disease.[59–63] A recent large study by See et al[64] revealed a significant reduction in the risk of PSA progression after radical prostatectomy (hazard ratio, 0.49) with the administration of bicalutamide 150 mg/day in a large cohort of men with early prostate cancer. An obvious concern with this endpoint is that the patients progressing in the bicalutamide arm are not completely hormonally naïve; those in the placebo arm are. The progressing bicalutamide patients may have an increased component of hormone refractory disease. Thus, an improved time to progression may not translate into a disease-specific survival benefit.

Based on a review of their experience, Kupelian et al[65] suggested that patients with localized high-grade disease (Gleason score of 8 or above) but an initial PSA level less than or equal to 10 ng/ml might benefit from only 6 months of adjuvant androgen deprivation following local therapy. A two-fold reduction in mortality with the addition of 6 months of androgen suppression therapy to three-dimensional conformal radiation therapy for high-risk clinically localized prostate cancer has been recently observed by D'Amico et al[66] in a randomized controlled trial. This benefit is comparable to that reported by Bolla et al[67] with 3 years of androgen blockade after radiation therapy for locally advanced disease, and suggests that the benefit of adjuvant hormonal therapy may be achieved with a shorter duration of treatment.

Adjuvant chemotherapy

The identification of chemotherapeutic agents with promising activity in prostate cancer has led to some enthusiasm for the development of adjuvant chemotherapy trials in patients with high-risk disease. Data are still very limited.[68]

Adjuvant radiation and hormonal therapy

The use of hormonal ablation combined with adjuvant radiation therapy soon after surgical treatment has been studied in small cohorts of high-risk patients.

Akakura et al[69] reported a prospective randomized trial comparing the results of radical prostatectomy versus external beam radiation therapy (60–70 Gy) with the combination of endocrine therapy in both modalities in a total of 95 patients with stage B2 and C prostate cancer. The two groups were well balanced in terms of risk factors. The endocrine therapy, consisting in most patients of the daily administration of diethylstilbestrol diphosphate, was initiated approximately 8 weeks before surgery or radiation and continued indefinitely thereafter. The surgery group was associated with a significantly higher 5-year progression-free and cause-specific survival compared to the radiation group (Table 18.5; Figure 18.2). This study demonstrated that radical prostatectomy plus endocrine therapy may contribute to a survival benefit for patients with high-risk clinically localized and locally advanced prostate cancer. This approach is being evaluated in patients with clinically organ-confined prostate cancer in a randomized prospective trial by the Radiation Therapy Oncology Group (RTOG P-0011).

Salvage radiation and hormonal therapy

Another approach is delayed salvage therapy with hormonal and/or radiation treatment at the time of biochemical failure. Androgen deprivation is often recommended in these cases because it is clinically challenging to identify the subgroup of patients who have disease confined to the prostate bed and might therefore receive radiation therapy alone.

Stephenson et al[70] reviewed a multicenter cohort of 501 patients who received radiation therapy for biochemical failure after radical prostatectomy. They observed that patients with a Gleason score of less than 8, positive surgical margins, preradiotherapy PSA level of less than 2 ng/ml, PSA doubling time of greater than 10 months, and absence of seminal vesicle invasion are more likely to have durable

Table 18.5 Five-year survival in patients with stage B2-C prostate cancer treated with radical prostatectomy or radiation therapy plus adjuvant hormonal treatment[69]

	Progression-free survival (%)	Cause-specific survival (%)	Overall survival (%)
Radical prostatectomy	90.5	96.6	85.6
Radiation therapy	81.2	84.6	75.9
Significance	0.044	0.024	NS

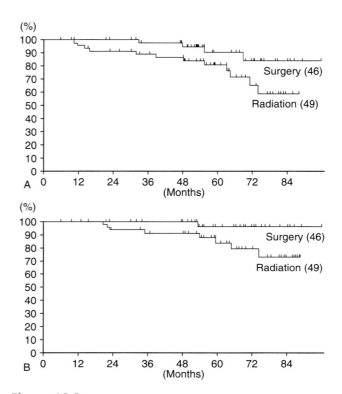

Figure 18.2
A, Progression-free and *B,* cause-specific survival curves by treatment group for patients with clinical stage B2 and C prostate cancer who were randomly treated with radical prostatectomy or external beam radiation therapy with a common endocrine therapy in both modalities.

From Akakura et al,[69] with permission

response with radiation therapy alone. Radiation therapy may prevent metastatic disease progression in patients at high risk if it is delivered early in the course of recurrent disease.

The survival benefit of combined salvage hormonal and radiation therapy is not yet well defined. The RTOG is conducting a phase III trial (RTOG 96-01) that will help to clarify this issue. Meanwhile, the results of several small series provide evidence of durable biochemical control in a significant percentage of patients.

Tiguert et al[71] retrospectively evaluated the benefit of androgen deprivation (3 months of injection of a LH–RH analog) administered before salvage external beam radiation therapy (median, 60 Gy) in 81 patients with biochemical failure following radical prostatectomy. The actuarial biochemical failure-free rate was 50% at 5 years.

Similar results are reported by Katz et al[72] who followed 115 patients treated with salvage three-dimensional conformal radiation therapy with or without neoadjuvant androgen deprivation. The 4-year PSA relapse-free survival rate was 39% for the 70 patients treated with radiation alone and 59% for the 45 patients who also received hormonal therapy. Androgen deprivation significantly improved PSA-free survival in patients with either negative surgical margins, absence of extracapsular extension, or presence of seminal vesicles invasion.

Finally, Eulau et al[73] reviewed the results of 105 consecutive patients treated with pelvic irradiation after radical prostatectomy for locally advanced disease, persistent or rising postoperative PSA or local recurrence. In their experience biochemical relapse-free survival and clinical relapse-free survival were significantly higher in patients who also received 6 months of androgen blockade before and during radiation therapy (56% vs 27% and 100% vs 70% at 5 years, respectively). The short-term use of androgen deprivation was the only significant predictor of biochemical failure at the multivariate analysis.

Conclusion

Randomized studies have shown that radical prostatectomy reduces cancer-specific mortality by 44% compared to watchful waiting.[26] This survival advantage is likely due to benefit in high-risk patients. The use of adjuvant treatments after surgery for high-risk disease can contribute to further decreases in the rate of local and distant failure. In high-risk patients, this likely translates into a survival benefit.

Radical prostatectomy in conjunction with adjuvant radiation and/or androgen deprivation should be considered in the management of young patients who are diagnosed with high-risk localized prostate cancer.

References

1. Partin AW, Kattan MW, Subong EN, et al. Combination of prostate-specific antigen, clinical stage, and Gleason score to predict pathological stage of localized prostate cancer. A multi-institutional update. JAMA 1997;277:1445–1451.
2. Han M, Partin AW, Pound CR, et al. Long-term biochemical disease-free and cancer-specific survival following anatomic radical retropubic prostatectomy. The 15-year Johns Hopkins experience. Urol Clin North Am 2001;28:555–565.
3. Feneley MR, Partin AW. Indicators of pathologic stage of prostate cancer and their use in clinical practice. Urol Clin North Am 2001;28:443–458.
4. Roach M 3rd, Lu J, Pilepich MV, et al. Long-term survival after radiotherapy alone: radiation therapy oncology group prostate cancer trials. J Urol 1999;161:864–868.
5. Roach M, Lu J, Pilepich MV, et al. Four prognostic groups predict long-term survival from prostate cancer following radiotherapy alone on Radiation Therapy Oncology Group clinical trials. Int J Radiat Oncol Biol Phys 2000;47:609–615.
6. Epstein JI, Partin AW, Sauvageot J, et al. Prediction of progression following radical prostatectomy. A multivariate analysis of 721 men with long-term follow-up. Am J Surg Pathol 1996;20:286–292.
7. Blute ML, Bergstralh EJ, Iocca A, et al. Use of Gleason score, prostate specific antigen, seminal vesicle and margin status to predict biochemical failure after radical prostatectomy. J Urol 2001;165:119–125.
8. Shipley WU, Thames HD, Sandler HM, et al. Radiation therapy for clinically localized prostate cancer: a multi-institutional pooled analysis. JAMA 1999;281:1598–1604.
9. Zietman AL, Coen JJ, Shipley WU, et al. Radical radiation therapy in the management of prostatic adenocarcinoma: the initial prostate specific antigen value as a predictor of treatment outcome. J Urol 1994;151:640–645.
10. Kattan MW, Eastham JA, Stapleton AM, et al. A preoperative nomogram for disease recurrence following radical prostatectomy for prostate cancer. J Natl Cancer Inst 1998;90:766–771.
11. Kattan MW, Zelefsky MJ, Kupelian PA, et al. Pretreatment nomogram for predicting the outcome of three-dimensional conformal radiotherapy in prostate cancer. J Clin Oncol 2000;18:3352–3359.
12. Kattan MW, Potters L, Blasko JC, et al. Pretreatment nomogram for predicting freedom from recurrence after permanent prostate brachytherapy in prostate cancer. Urology 2001;58:393–399.
13. D'Amico AV, Whittington R, Malkowicz SB, et al. Biochemical outcome after radical prostatectomy, external beam radiation therapy, or interstitial radiation therapy for clinically localized prostate cancer. JAMA 1998;280:969–974.
14. D'Amico AV, Whittington R, Malkowicz SB, et al. Pretreatment nomogram for prostate-specific antigen recurrence after radical prostatectomy or external-beam radiation therapy for clinically localized prostate cancer. J Clin Oncol 1999;17:168–172.
15. D'Amico AV, Moul J, Carroll PR, et al. Cancer-specific mortality after surgery or radiation for patients with clinically localized prostate cancer managed during the prostate-specific antigen era. J Clin Oncol 2003;21:2163–2172.
16. Freedland SJ, Terris MK, Csathy GS, et al. Preoperative model for predicting prostate specific antigen recurrence after radical prostatectomy using percent of biopsy tissue with cancer, biopsy Gleason grade and serum prostate specific antigen. J Urol 2004;171:2215–2220.
17. D'Amico AV, Whittington R, Malkowicz SB, et al. Clinical utility of the percentage of positive prostate biopsies in defining biochemical outcome after radical prostatectomy for patients with clinically localized prostate cancer. J Clin Oncol 2000;18:1164–1172.
18. Grossfeld GD, Latini DM, Lubeck DP, et al. Predicting disease recurrence in intermediate and high-risk patients undergoing radical prostatectomy using percent positive biopsies: results from CaPSURE. Urology 2002;59:560–565.
19. D'Amico AV, Schultz D, Silver B, et al. The clinical utility of the percent of positive prostate biopsies in predicting biochemical outcome following external-beam radiation therapy for patients with clinically localized prostate cancer. Int J Radiat Oncol Biol Phys 2001;49:679–684.
20. Nelson CP, Dunn RL, Wei JT, et al. Contemporary preoperative parameters predict cancer-free survival after radical prostatectomy: a tool to facilitate treatment decisions. Urol Oncol 2003;21:213–218.
21. Rhodes DR, Sanda MG, Otte AP, et al. Multiplex biomarker approach for determining risk of prostate-specific antigen-defined recurrence of prostate cancer. J Natl Cancer Inst 2003;95:661–668.
22. Ziada AM, Lisle TC, Snow PB, et al. Impact of different variables on the outcome of patients with clinically confined prostate carcinoma: prediction of pathologic stage and biochemical failure using an artificial neural network. Cancer 2001;91(8 Suppl):1653–1660.
23. Fradet Y. Role of radical prostatectomy in high-risk prostate cancer. Can J Urol 2002;9(Suppl 1):8–13.
24. Lerner SE, Blute ML, Zincke H. Extended experience with radical prostatectomy for clinical stage T3 prostate cancer: outcome and contemporary morbidity. J Urol 1995;154:1447–1452.
25. van den Ouden D, Hop WC, Schroder FH. Progression in and survival of patients with locally advanced prostate cancer (T3) treated with radical prostatectomy as monotherapy. J Urol 1998;160:1392–1397.

26. Bill-Axelson A, Holmberg L, Ruutu M et al. Radical prostatectomy versus watchful waiting in early prostate cancer. N Engl J Med 2005 352:1977–1984.

27. Pound CR, Partin AW, Eisenberger MA, et al. Natural history of progression after PSA elevation following radical prostatectomy. JAMA 1999;281:1591–1597.

28. Lu-Yao GL, Yao SL. Population-based study of long-term survival in patients with clinically localised prostate cancer. Lancet 1997;349:906–910.

29. Menon M, Tewari A, Divine G, et al. Comparison of long-term survival in men with clinically localized prostate cancer managed conservatively, with definitive radiation or radical prostatectomy. J Urol 2001;165 (5 suppl):151–152 (abstract 621).

30. Hull GW, Rabbani F, Abbas F, et al. Cancer control with radical prostatectomy alone in 1,000 consecutive patients. J Urol 2002;167:528–534.

31. Roehl KA, Han M, Ramos CG, et al. Cancer progression and survival rates following anatomical radical retropubic prostatectomy in 3,478 consecutive patients: long-term results. J Urol 2004;172:910–914.

32. Eastham JA, Kattan MW, Riedel E, et al. Variations among individual surgeons in the rate of positive surgical margins in radical prostatectomy specimens. J Urol 2003;170:2292–2295.

33. D'Amico AV, Cote K, Loffredo M, et al. Determinants of prostate cancer-specific survival after radiation therapy for patients with clinically localized prostate cancer. J Clin Oncol 2002;20:4567–4573.

34. Soloway MS, Pareek K, Sharifi R, et al. Neoadjuvant androgen ablation before radical prostatectomy in cT2bNxMo prostate cancer: 5-year results. J Urol 2002;167:112–116.

35. Aus G, Abrahamsson PA, Ahlgren G, et al. Three-month neoadjuvant hormonal therapy before radical prostatectomy: a 7-year follow-up of a randomized controlled trial. BJU Int 2002;90:561–566.

36. Witjes WP, Schulman CC, Debruyne FM. Preliminary results of a prospective randomized study comparing radical prostatectomy versus radical prostatectomy associated with neoadjuvant hormonal combination therapy in T2–3 N0 M0 prostatic carcinoma. The European Study Group on Neoadjuvant Treatment of Prostate Cancer. Urology 1997;49(3A Suppl):65–69.

37. Schulman CC, Debruyne FM, Forster G, et al. 4-Year follow-up results of a European prospective randomized study on neoadjuvant hormonal therapy prior to radical prostatectomy in T2–3N0M0 prostate cancer. European Study Group on Neoadjuvant Treatment of Prostate Cancer. Eur Urol 2000;38:706–713.

38. Van Poppel H, De Ridder D, Elgamal AA, et al. Neoadjuvant hormonal therapy before radical prostatectomy decreases the number of positive surgical margins in stage T2 prostate cancer: interim results of a prospective randomized trial. The Belgian Uro-Oncological Study Group. J Urol 1995;154:429–434.

39. Klotz LH, Goldenberg SL, Jewett MA, et al. Long-term followup of a randomized trial of 0 versus 3 months of neoadjuvant androgen ablation before radical prostatectomy. J Urol 2003;170:791–794.

40. Gleave ME, Goldenberg SL, Chin JL, et al. Randomized comparative study of 3 versus 8-month neoadjuvant hormonal therapy before radical prostatectomy: biochemical and pathological effects. J Urol 2001;166:500–506; discussion 506–507.

41. Selli C, Montironi R, Bono A, et al. Effects of complete androgen blockade for 12 and 24 weeks on the pathological stage and resection margin status of prostate cancer. J Clin Pathol 2002;55:508–513.

42. Clark PE, Peereboom DM, Dreicer R, et al. Phase II trial of neoadjuvant estramustine and etoposide plus radical prostatectomy for locally advanced prostate cancer. Urology 2001;57:281–285.

43. Hussain M, Smith DC, El-Rayes BF, et al. Neoadjuvant docetaxel and estramustine chemotherapy in high-risk/locally advanced prostate cancer. Urology 2003;61:774–780.

44. Oh WK, George DJ, Kaufman DS, et al. Neoadjuvant docetaxel followed by radical prostatectomy in patients with high-risk localized prostate cancer: a preliminary report. Semin Oncol 2001;28(4 Suppl 15):40–44.

45. Konety BR, Eastham JA, Reuter VE, et al. Feasibility of radical prostatectomy after neoadjuvant chemohormonal therapy for patients with high risk or locally advanced prostate cancer: results of a phase I/II study. J Urol 2004;171:709–713.

46. Eastham JA, Kelly WK, Grossfeld GD, et al. Cancer and Leukemia Group B (CALGB) 90203: a randomized phase 3 study of radical prostatectomy alone versus estramustine and docetaxel before radical prostatectomy for patients with high-risk localized disease. Urology 2003;62(Suppl 1):55–62.

47. Kucuk O, Sarkar FH, Sakr W, et al. Phase II randomized clinical trial of lycopene supplementation before radical prostatectomy. Cancer Epidemiol Biomarkers Prev 2001;10:861–868.

48. Howe LR, Dannenberg AJ. A role for cyclooxygenase-2 inhibitors in the prevention and treatment of cancer. Semin Oncol 2002;29(3 Suppl 11):111–119.

49. Davis BJ, Pisansky TM, Leibovich BC. Adjuvant external radiation therapy following radical prostatectomy for node-negative prostate cancer. Curr Opin Urol 2003;13:117–122.

50. Leibovich BC, Engen DE, Patterson DE, et al. Benefit of adjuvant radiation therapy for localized prostate cancer with a positive surgical margin. J Urol 2000;163:1178–1182.

51. Do LV, Do TM, Smith R, et al. Postoperative radiotherapy for carcinoma of the prostate: impact on both local control and distant disease-free survival. Am J Clin Oncol 2002;25:1–8.

52. Valicenti RK, Gomella LG, Ismail M, et al. The efficacy of early adjuvant radiation therapy for pT3N0 prostate cancer: a matched-pair analysis. Int J Radiat Oncol Biol Phys 1999;45:53–58.

53. Petrovich Z, Lieskovsky G, Langholz B, et al. Postoperative radiotherapy in 423 patients with pT3N0 prostate cancer. Int J Radiat Oncol Biol Phys 2002;53:600–609.

54. Mayer R, Pummer K, Quehenberger F, et al. Postprostatectomy radiotherapy for high-risk prostate cancer. Urology 2002;59:732–739.

55. Paulson DF, Moul JW, Walther PJ. Radical prostatectomy for clinical stage T1–2N0M0 prostatic adenocarcinoma: long-term results. J Urol 1990;144:1180–1184.

56. Shevlin BE, Mittal BB, Brand WN, et al. The role of adjuvant irradiation following primary prostatectomy, based on histopathologic extent of tumor. Int J Radiat Oncol Biol Phys 1989;16:1425–1430.

57. Thompson IM, Paradelo JC, Crawford ED, et al. An opportunity to determine optimal treatment of pT3 prostate cancer: the window may be closing. Urology 1994;44:804–811.

58. Petrovich Z, Lieskovsky G, Stein JP, et al. Comparison of surgery alone with surgery and adjuvant radiotherapy for pT3N0 prostate cancer. BJU Int 2002;89:604–611.

59. Messing EM, Manola J, Sarosdy M, et al. Immediate hormonal therapy compared with observation after radical prostatectomy and pelvic lymphadenectomy in men with node-positive prostate cancer. N Engl J Med 1999;341:1781–1788.

60. Prayer-Galetti T, Zattoni F, Capizzi A, et al. Disease-free survival in patients with pathological C stage prostate cancer at radical prostatectomy submitted to adjuvant hormonal treatment. Eur Urol 2000;38:48 (abstract).

61. Ghavamian R, Bergstralh EJ, Blute ML, et al. Radical retropubic prostatectomy plus orchiectomy versus orchiectomy alone for pTxN+ prostate cancer: a matched comparison. J Urol 1999;161:1223–1227; discussion 1227–1228.

62. Myers RP, Larson-Keller JJ, Bergstralh EJ, et al. Hormonal treatment at time of radical retropubic prostatectomy for stage D1 prostate cancer: results of long-term followup. J Urol 1992;147:910–915.

63. Schmeller N, Lubos W. Early endocrine therapy versus radical prostatectomy combined with early endocrine therapy for stage D1 prostate cancer. Br J Urol 1997;79:226–234.

64. See W, Iversen P, Wirth M, et al. Immediate treatment with bicalutamide 150 mg as adjuvant therapy significantly reduces the risk of PSA progression in early prostate cancer. Eur Urol 2003;44:512–517; discussion 517–518.

65. Kupelian PA, Buchsbaum JC, Elshaikh M, et al. Factors affecting recurrence rates after prostatectomy or radiotherapy in localized prostate

carcinoma patients with biopsy Gleason score 8 or above. Cancer 2002;95:2302–2307.

66. D'Amico AV, Manola J, Loffredo M, et al. 6-month androgen suppression plus radiation therapy vs radiation therapy alone for patients with clinically localized prostate cancer: a randomized controlled trial. JAMA 2004;292:821–827.

67. Bolla M, Gonzalez D, Warde P, et al. Improved survival in patients with locally advanced prostate cancer treated with radiotherapy and goserelin. N Engl J Med 1997;337:295–300.

68. Wang J, Halford S, Rigg A, et al. Adjuvant mitozantrone chemotherapy in advanced prostate cancer. BJU Int 2000;86:675–680.

69. Akakura K, Isaka S, Akimoto S, et al. Long-term results of a randomized trial for the treatment of Stages B2 and C prostate cancer: radical prostatectomy versus external beam radiation therapy with a common endocrine therapy in both modalities. Urology 1999;54: 313–318.

70. Stephenson AJ, Shariat SF, Zelefsky MJ, et al. Salvage radiotherapy for recurrent prostate cancer after radical prostatectomy. JAMA 2004;291: 1325–1332.

71. Tiguert R, Rigaud J, Lacombe L, et al. Neoadjuvant hormone therapy before salvage radiotherapy for an increasing post-radical prostatectomy serum prostate specific antigen level. Role of radical prostatectomy in high-risk prostate cancer. J Urol 2003;170: 447–450.

72. Katz MS, Zelefsky MJ, Venkatraman ES, et al. Predictors of biochemical outcome with salvage conformal radiotherapy after radical prostatectomy for prostate cancer. J Clin Oncol 2003;21:483–489.

73. Eulau SM, Tate DJ, Stamey TA, et al. Effect of combined transient androgen deprivation and irradiation following radical prostatectomy for prostatic cancer. Int J Radiat Oncol Biol Phys 1998;41:735–740.

19

Prevention and management of complications associated with open radical retropubic prostatectomy

Herbert Lepor

Introduction

An anatomic approach to radical perineal prostatectomy was described by Young in 1905.[1] Forty years later, Millin described the retropubic approach for radical prostatectomy.[2] The primary advantage of the perineal approach was avoidance of the dorsal venous complex, resulting in less bleeding and a quicker recovery. Nevertheless, the radical retropubic prostatectomy (RRP) was preferred by most urologists since they were generally more familiar with retropubic anatomy and this approach provided the opportunity to perform a simultaneous staging pelvic lymphadenectomy through the single lower midline incision.[3]

Historically, radical perineal and radical retropubic prostatectomies were associated with significant morbidity and mortality.[4] In the modern era, radical prostatectomy performed by expert surgeons is associated with exceedingly rare mortality and minimal morbidity.[5] The dramatically lower complication rates in contemporary series can be attributed to greater experience of individual surgeons, improved surgical technique, younger surgical candidates with fewer co-morbidities, better anesthetic agents, and more sophisticated intraoperative monitoring.

Between 1986 and 2004, the author has performed over 2500 RRPs. Two thousand of these were performed between 1994 and 2004 at New York University (NYU) Medical Center. We have reported both a large retrospective and prospective outcomes assessment of 1000[6] and 500[7] cases, respectively. In both of these personal series, complication rates were exceedingly low. The low complication rates may be attributed to high surgical volume, thoughtful patient selection, rigorous preoperative assessment, meticulous surgical technique, and compulsive postoperative management. This chapter focuses on the prevention and management of complications associated with open RRP, and draws on the personal experiences of the author.

Cardiovascular complications

Cardiovascular complications associated with radical prostatectomy include myocardial infarction, cerebral vascular accidents, cardiac arrhythmias, pulmonary embolus, and deep venous thrombosis (DVT). These complications may occur intra- and post-operatively.

In the modern era, these cardiovascular events are the primary cause of rare intra- and post-operative mortalities. For example, our only intra- or post-operative mortality occurred in an individual who experienced a myocardial infarction during his hospitalization and died at home within 30 days of surgery. The rates of DVT (0.2–2.7%), pulmonary embolus (0.3–2.0%), and other cardiovascular complications (myocardial infarction and arrhythmias) (0.1–0.7%) reported by experienced surgeons is exceedingly low (Table 19.1).[6-11]

A detailed preoperative review of systems, social history, and family history should focus on identifying significant cardiovascular disease or associated risk factors. Risk factors include hyperlipidemia, hyper-tension, diabetes, smoking, and a family history of atherosclerotic vascular disease. The presence of erectile dysfunction may represent an early indicator of occult systemic vascular disease. Men with known cardiovascular disease or high-risk factors should undergo a thorough preoperative cardiovascular evaluation, including auscultation for carotid bruits, an echocardiogram to assess ejection fraction and cardiac wall motion, and an exercise stress test to identify cardiac ischemia.

Men with significant functional cardiac compromise or coronary artery disease generally should not be offered radical prostatectomy since their limited life-expectancy and increased surgical risks do not justify surgical attempts to cure the disease. Men with evidence of coronary artery disease who are deemed appropriate candidate for radical prostatectomy should be carefully monitored intraoperatively to avoid sustained hypotension. A lower threshold should be

Table 19.1 Intraoperative technical complications during radical retropubic prostatectomy

Surgeon/ institution	Year	Number of patients	Rectal injury (%)	Ureteral injury (%)
Saint-Jean Cerou, Languedoc[11]	1992	620	0.5	0
Mayo Clinic[8]	1995	1000	0.6	0
Catalona[9]	1999	1870	0.05	0.05
Lepor[6]	2001	1000	0.5	0.10
Lepo[7]	2003	500	0	0.20

established for transfusing blood products if bleeding occurs in order to decrease myocardial ischemia. All men with preexisting coronary artery disease should undergo serial EKGs and cardiac enzyme monitoring immediately postoperatively, independent of their postoperative course. Identifying a myocardial infarction early in its course allows for immediate thrombolytic intervention, which may diminish mortality and damage to the myocardium associated with the event.

Any changes in mental status or extremity weakness should prompt immediate computerized tomography (CT) of the head with contrast in order to identify a cerebrovascular accident. A thromboembolic event arising from a plaque in the carotid or basilar arteries or an intimal dissection of these vessels may represent the etiology for an intra- or post-operative cerebrovascular accident. A thrombus arising from the left atrium in association with atrial fibrillation is another relatively common cause of postoperative cerebrovascular accident. A hypertensive crisis or a right-sided embolus passing to the left side of the heart via a septal defect is a rare etiology for a cerebrovascular accident. An echocardiogram should always be obtained to exclude the heart as the source of the thrombus. In some cases, prompt initiation of anticoagulation may decrease the extent of the final neurologic deficit.

Pulmonary embolus represents the most common life-threatening thromboembolic event associated with radical prostatectomy. The role of prophylaxis for preventing pulmonary embolus and deep venous thrombosis is highly controversial.[12] We do not recommend any routine pharmacologic or mechanical prophylaxis for deep venous thrombosis or pulmonary embolus with the exception of compression stockings. A personal or family history of DVT should trigger a hematology consultation and a more aggressive preventative strategy, including mechanical compression boots and administration of low molecular weight heparin immediately after surgery if there is no evidence of postoperative bleeding. In our recent series of 500 consecutive cases of RRP,[7] only 0.2% of men experienced a DVT and none a pulmonary embolus within 30 days of the surgical procedure. We attribute the extraordinarily low rates of DVT and pulmonary embolus to avoidance of staging a pelvic lymph node dissection in almost 70% of men with a Gleason score of 6 or less, a quick surgical procedure, early ambulation, short hospital stay, and encouragement for early return to activities.

Intraoperative technical complications

Rectal injury

The rate of rectal injury during radical prostatectomy in the modern era ranges between 0.5% and 3% (Table 19.2).[5] Rectal injury, if unrecognized, represents a very serious complication which may lead to sepsis and fistula formation.[13] In the setting where the rectal fistula is identified postoperatively and is associated with an abscess, a diverting colostomy is mandatory with incision and drainage of the associated abscess. The fistula, if persistent, can be closed at a later time and the colostomy taken down. Some smaller fistulas will close spontaneously.[14]

Historically, the standard of practice for all rectal injuries recognized intraoperatively was to primarily close the rectal injury and perform a diverting colostomy. Borland and Walsh[15] reported

Table 19.2 Postoperative complications following radical retropubic prostatectomy

Surgeon/ institution	Percent		
	Deep venous thrombosis	Pulmonary embolism	Cardiovascular (myocardial infarction and arrhythmia)
Saint-Jean Cerou Languedoc[11]	2.3	0.8	0.2
Mayo Clinic[8]	1.3	0.7	0.7
Catalona[9]	–	2.0	0.1
Lepor[6]	0.1	0.1	0.7
Lepor[7]	0.4	0	0.4

excellent outcomes with primary closure of the rectal injury and interposition of omentum between the rectal closure and the vesicourethral anastomosis. Excellent outcomes were achieved in men whose mechanical bowel preparation consisted only of Fleets enemas. It is often advisable to perform a colostomy if the rectal injury occurs in a previously radiated field.

In the recent personal series of 500 RRPs, only one intraoperative rectal injury was identified, which was small and closed primarily in two layers without interposition of omentum. An attempt was made to imbricate the adjacent perirectal soft tissue over the suture line. The wound was copiously irrigated and intravenous ampicillin and gentamicin were administered for 48 h. The anal sphincter was manually dilated and the patient's diet was limited to clear liquids for 48 h. A meticulous effort was made to achieve a water-tight vesicourethral anastomosis. Pelvic drains were removed per routine.

Rectal injury usually occurs while dissecting the apex of the prostate posteriorly. The injury is most likely to occur in men with small prostates since the apex may not be easily discernible. Prior radiation therapy, underlying bowel disease such as ulcerative colitis or diverticulitis, and multiple sets of transrectal biopsies are risk factors for rectal injury. In those cases with risk factors for rectal injury, the dissection of the apex should be initiated laterally rather than in the midline.

Obturator nerve injury

The obturator nerve is most vulnerable during the pelvic lymphadenectomy. Injury to it is associated with the inability to adduct the thigh. Injury can be avoided if the nerve is always identified prior to ligating the nodal package inferiorly. The obturator nerve must be identified early in the course of the lymphadenectomy. The first step in the lymphadenectomy should be to bluntly sweep the lymph node package off the pelvic sidewall and immediately identify the obturator nerve.

The author has no personal experience of injury to the obturator nerve. If identified intraoperatively, the nerve can be reapproximated using nonabsorbable sutures. Obturator nerve injuries are often recognized postoperatively when the patient complains of the inability to adduct the lower extremity. In these cases, the injury often spontaneously resolves with limited functional deficit. Physical therapy may facilitate the return of lower extremity function.

Ureteral injury

Ureteral injury is a rare complication occurring in between 0.05% and 1.6% of cases (Table 19.2).[5] Injury to the ureter may occur during an extended staging pelvic lymphadenectomy, during mobilization of the seminal vesicles, while dividing the prostatovesical junction, while obtaining hemostasis for brisk pelvic bleeding, or when performing the bladder neck reconstruction. Failure to observe a blue efflux from both ureteral orifices following administration of methylene blue or indigo carmine during the surgical procedure provides the opportunity to identify most ureteral injuries intraoperatively. If a blue efflux is not observed bilaterally, it is mandatory to pass a 5-Fr feeding tube in order to confirm that the ureter is intact and not ligated. Depending on the site and degree of injury, ureteroneocystotomy or ureteroureterotomy should be performed. At times, deligation may be adequate. A ureteral ligation or transaction not detected intraoperatively typically present with flank pain, a slight and transient increase in the serum creatinine, or persistent urinary drainage from the pelvic drains. Any one of these events should trigger a renal ultrasound in order to identify hydronephrosis and/or a contrast imaging study to identify urinary extravasation. A very slight rise in creatinine may be attributed to a ureteral ligation whereas a marked rise suggests a ureteral transection with intraperitoneal extravasation owing to an associated peritonotomy.

The author has personally encountered three ureteral injuries. One injury was identified intraoperatively and occurred while mobilizing the seminal vesicle. An ureteroneocystotomy with a psoas hitch reimplantation was performed without sequelae. The second injury occurred in an individual from Kenya who failed to divulge a history of schistosomiasis. The prostate and bladder were encased in extensive fibrosis and the ureter was ligated just outside the bladder. This individual postoperatively experienced flank pain and a slight elevation of the serum creatinine. A renal ultrasound revealed hydronephrosis. A ureteroneocystotomy was also performed without sequelae. A third patient presented 3 years following an uncomplicated radical prostatectomy. An abdominal CT scan was performed following a motor vehicle accident which revealed an atrophic kidney. Subsequent imaging studies demonstrated the site of ureteral obstruction to be just outside the bladder wall. The patient never experienced flank pain postoperatively despite what appears to have been a complete ligation of the ureter. Since the hydronephrotic kidney was atrophic and asymptomatic, no treatment was recommended.

Vascular injury

Injury to the external iliac vesicles rarely occurs during radical prostatectomy. In cases where there is a laceration, the vessels should be repaired with appropriate vascular sutures. In rare cases when the external iliac artery or vein is inadvertently ligated, these structures must be repaired immediately to avoid ischemia to the lower extremity.

Hemorrhage

Historically, radical prostatectomy was associated with significant bleeding. The description of the dorsal venous complex by Reiner and Walsh and a technique for its early control has greatly diminished the likelihood of encountering life-threatening intraoperative bleeding.[16] Significant intraoperative bleeding is most likely to occur in men with very large prostates,[17] excessive perivesical and periprostatic venous tributaries, or an unrecognized coagulopathy. If the prostate exceeds 100 g, a row of hemostatic prostatic capsular sutures are placed on the anterior surface of the prostate in order to reduce back-bleeding prior to ligating the dorsal venous complex distally. In some cases, the prostate is so large it is not feasible to suture/ligate the dorsal venous complex prior to dividing this structure. In these cases, the dorsal venous complex is sharply divided and hemostasis is secondarily achieved. The urethra is then divided without preplacement of the anastomotic sutures, and the apex is mobilized with care not to inadvertently enter the plane between the capsule and adenoma. The prostate is quickly mobilized off the rectum. With the Foley catheter retracted in a cephalad direction, the dorsal venous complex is controlled.

In cases where there are massive venous tributaries enveloping the bladder and prostate, attempts at achieving hemostasis with suture ligation may promote bleeding. Efforts to achieve hemostasis may become futile and the surgeon must proceed expeditiously to complete the prostatectomy. Packing of the pelvis with lap pads during the prostatectomy will significantly reduce blood loss.

In rare cases, the surgeon may encounter diffuse small vessel bleeding that is refractory to attempts at hemostasis. If the bleeding cannot be controlled with suture ligatures, empiric transfusion of platelets and clotting factors should be considered. The author recently experienced this scenario. An intraoperative coagulation profile was sent before the administration of platelets and clotting factors which revealed disseminated intravascular coagulopathy.

Postoperative complications

Hemorrhage

Significant and potentially life-threatening hemorrhage may occur during the immediate postoperative period. In many of these cases, the patient left the operating room after achieving meticulous hemostasis. The signs of life-threatening postoperative hemorrhage include hypotension, tachycardia, and low urine output. In the majority of cases, these signs of life-threatening postoperative bleeding occur in the first 2 to 4 h while the patient is in the recovery room. Central venous and arterial lines should be placed in order to facilitate monitoring of blood pressure and provide access for rapid volume replacement. If the hypotension, tachycardia, and low urine output do not respond rapidly to boluses of intravenous fluids, the surgeon should begin to make plans to return the patient to the operating room even if multiple units of blood products have not yet been transfused. If there is a transient response to fluid expansion, the patient must remain in a monitored setting. Serial hematocrits should be obtained. In cases of significant bleeding, the response to intravascular fluid replacement is often transient. The volume of pelvic drainage is a very unreliable indicator of significant bleeding. As the bleeding progresses, the abdomen becomes distended. The expanding hematoma exerts tension and may disrupt the anastomosis, which leads to greater abdominal distention as both urine and blood fill the pelvis. If the decision is made not to return the patient immediately to the operating room, the patient should remain or be transferred to a monitored setting with repeat hematocrits obtained until stabilization is demonstrated and hypotension resolves. In our experience, only six (0.2%) men have returned to the operating room for control of life-threatening bleeding. This is similar to Walsh et al's reported reoperation rate of 1% for the control of bleeding.[18] In our experience, the decision to return the patient to the operating room was always made within the first 8 postoperative hours. While it is difficult to provide absolute criteria for reoperation, this decision should be made before the patient has received extensive transfusions. As the amount of transfused blood products increases, the patient's clotting capacity further deteriorates. While significant bleeding may eventually subside, the pelvic hematoma will likely cause a protracted clinical course due to anastomotic disruption, ileus, infection, and clot retention. Re-exploration with evacuation of the hematoma and repair of the anastomosis often expedites recovery.

Prior to re-exploration, large-bore intravenous access must be obtained with restoration of intravascular volume. It is also prudent to place an arterial line for blood pressure monitoring. Depending on the volume of blood transfused, fresh frozen plasma, platelets, and calcium should be administered. In several cases requiring reoperation, we have identified an unrecognized coagulopathy such as factor II deficiency and von Willebrand disease. In these cases, no active bleeding site was identified in the operative field. Replacement of clotting factors was the primary requirement for achieving hemostasis.

The incision is reopened and blood clots evacuated. In many cases, the anastomosis is already disrupted due to the expanding hematoma. It is not possible to adequately explore the pelvis for bleeding with the anastomosis intact. Therefore, it is always taken down and meticulous hemostasis secured. In the rare case where bleeding is persistent and a specific site is not identified, the pelvis should be tightly packed and the incision closed with retention sutures. The author has resorted to this measure on only one occasion. The packing may be removed 24 h later when the patient is hemodynamically stabilized. In our cases where the decision to re-explore was made relatively early, patients were discharged within 48 h after the reoperation; and the catheter removed on the seventh postoperative day.

Anastomotic leakage

In the majority of cases, pelvic drains are removed by the second postoperative day.[6] Persistent drainage from the pelvic drains may be attributed to a lymphatic or urine leak. If drainage is excessive and not decreasing after 48 h, the drainage fluid should be tested for creatinine and glucose in order to differentiate between urine and serum (lymph).

If the fluid creatinine and glucose content is consistent with urine, an intravenous contrast imaging study should be performed to identify a ureteral injury. A cystogram should also be performed to exclude a bladder injury and to demonstrate that the catheter is indwelling within the bladder. The anastomotic leak may be attributed to a technically poor anastomosis, disruption of the bladder neck repair or a pelvic hematoma. The overwhelming majority of urine leaks due to partial disruption of the anastomosis will heal spontaneously with prolonged catheter drainage. If the catheter is not in the bladder, attempts should be made to reposition it endoscopically. If these endoscopic efforts are not successful, the patient should be brought to the operating theater for an open cystotomy.

A significant disruption of the anastomosis may exist despite no evidence of urinary extravasation from the pelvic drain sites. This phenomenon has been recognized more commonly since the routine use of cystograms to facilitate early removal of the catheter. In our experience, moderate or massive urinary extravasation was seen in only 10% of cases, 3 or 4 days after radical prostatectomy.[19]

These men often have gross hematuria and blood emanating around the catheter while straining to have a bowel movement. The longest time to demonstrate a dry anastomosis in our experience is 6 weeks postoperatively. Men who develop significant postoperative bleeding not necessitating re-exploration are at greater risk for developing partial disruption of the anastomosis requiring prolonged catheter drainage. The catheter should not be removed in this setting until healing of the anastomosis is confirmed.

In the setting of persistent lymphatic drainage, the pelvic drain should be left indwelling until the drainage is less than 50 ml/day. It is advisable to release the suction on the closed drainage system. Premature removal of the pelvic drains may result in a lymphocele which will require percutaneous or open drainage.

A lymphocele may develop if a lymph leak is not recognized. This occurs following a staging pelvic lymphadenectomy. A lymphocele may present with lower extremity edema, flank pain due to hydronephrosis or scrotal edema. Percutaneous drainage with or without instillation of a sclerosing agent often is the initial management of a symptomatic lymphocele.[20,21] Historically, a recurrent or untreated lymphocele required open exploration with unroofing and drainage into the peritoneal cavity. In the modern era, a recurrent lymphocele is best managed laparoscopically.[21]

Long-term complications

Bladder neck contracture

Bladder neck contracture is a relatively common complication following radical prostatectomy (Figure 19.1). The incidence has been reported to be as high as 27%.[22] The incidence of postoperative

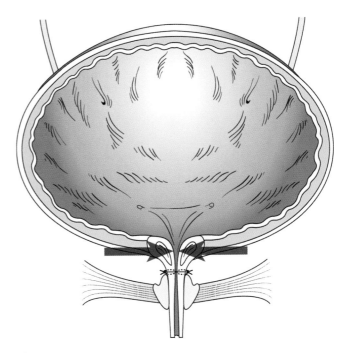

Figure 19.1
Bladder neck contractures may develop after radical prostatectomy. The point of narrowing is usually just above the anastomosis and usually responds well to treatment.

bladder neck contracture depends on surgical technique, the definition of a bladder neck contracture, and how aggressively the diagnosis is pursued. Lower rates exist among those experts who do not consider bladder outlet obstruction responding to a single dilation as a bladder neck contracture.

Bladder neck contractures almost always present within the first 3 months following radical prostatectomy.[23] A diminished urinary stream is the most common symptom of a bladder neck contracture. Deterioration of urinary continence also suggests a bladder neck contracture.

The etiology of a bladder neck contracture is likely multifactorial. Undoubtedly, technical issues must influence its development. Many experts recommend everting the bladder neck to facilitate a mucosa-to-mucosa apposition in order to decrease the incidence of a bladder neck contracture.[24] Catalona et al[9] reported that bladder neck contractures occurred more commonly when the bladder neck is reconstructed too tightly, which is consistent with the author's personal observations. We have reported that men who form keloids of the abdominal incision also have a greater risk of developing a bladder neck contracture, suggesting that in some cases the etiology is not technical but rather a generalized hypertrophic healing response.[23]

Some experts have speculated that the development of a bladder neck contracture is dependent on achieving a water-tight anastomosis.[25] Since February 2000, it has been our practice to perform cystograms between 3 to 8 days postoperatively in order to facilitate early removal of the urinary catheter. In one series, 77%, 17%, 7%, and 3% of men were noted to have none, slight, moderate or severe extravasation on a cystogram performed 7 days following radical prostatectomy, respectively.[26] In men with moderate-to-severe extravasation, the urinary catheters were left indwelling until a follow-up cystogram showed complete resolution of the extravasation. In our experience, the incidence of bladder neck contracture is independent of the degree of extravasation on the initial cystogram. These observations suggest that urinary extravasation may have an impact on stricture formation only if the catheter is removed prematurely. Performing a cystogram between 3 and 8 days postoperatively not only provides the opportunity to remove the catheter early, but identifies the small cohort of men who likely benefit from prolonged catheter drainage.

Our bladder neck contracture rate in the year 2001 was 16.6%. To decrease this rate, we reconstructed the bladder neck to a caliber of 30 Fr instead of 20 Fr, and removed the catheter only in the absence of extravasation. We consider these measures lowered the bladder neck contracture rate in 2003 to 7.7%.

A bladder neck contracture is suspected when the patient complains of a poor urinary flow rate. It is important to determine whether the perceived decreased flow rate is due simply to small voided volumes or bladder outlet obstruction. Uroflowmetry, in cases of bladder neck contracture, will demonstrate a prolonged urinary flow pattern and a decreased flow rate. The bladder neck contracture is confirmed with flexible cystoscopy. The overwhelming majority of bladder neck contractures will resolve following a simple dilation.[23] Under direct vision, a flexible guidewire is passed through the constricted urethral lumen and advanced into the bladder. The bladder neck contracture is dilated to an 18 Fr, using Nottingham dilating catheters. The anastomosis and bladder is inspected to ensure that a calculi has not formed on a retained anastomotic suture. The patient is instructed to self-catheterize using an 18-Fr red-rubber catheter once a day for a month, every other day the following month, and once a week for the next month. Refractory strictures will typically recur within 3 months of the initial dilation. In these cases, a second dilation is performed. Bladder neck contractures refractory to two dilations are treated with endoscopic incision or resection.

Incontinence

Between 2.5% and 87% of men fail to regain continence following radical prostatectomy.[27] The broad range of continence rates may be attributed to varying expertise of surgeons, different definitions of continence, different methodologies for assessing continence, and the timing of reporting continence outcomes. Lepor et al,[28] utilizing a validated self-administered questionnaire, reported that 96% of men achieved urinary continence two years following radical prostatectomy.

Incontinence following radical prostatectomy is almost always stress induced and is caused by damage to the rhabdosphincter.[29] Therefore, every effort should be made to maximally preserve the rhabdosphincter while dividing the prostatourethral junction. In an effort to maximize urethral length and its surrounding periurethral smooth and skeletal muscle, the prostatourethral junction should be divided as close to the prostate as possible. A frozen section is sent from the urethral (apical) soft-tissue margin in order to minimize the likelihood that the cancer is not completely removed.[30]

We have shown that men who develop bladder neck contractures are more prone to develop incontinence.[23] Therefore, every effort should be made to prevent bladder neck contractures.

All men are encouraged to perform pelvic floor (Kegel) exercises immediately after the urinary catheter is removed. The NYU Continence Index is a useful instrument for predicting the time interval to regain continence and final continence status.[31] If the continence score is less than 14, we recommend initiating a formal biofeedback program immediately following catheter removal. By 3 months postoperatively, 80% of men will have regained their urinary continence.[28] For those men who fail to do so, uroflowmetry and a urine culture should be obtained to rule out bladder neck contracture and urinary tract infection (UTI), respectively. If uroflowmetry is normal and there is no UTI, a formal biofeedback program is initiated.

Continence may continue to improve over a 2-year interval.[28] Men with moderate-to-severe incontinence (more than two pads/day, moderate-to-severe bother, frequent or total incontinence) 1 year following radical prostatectomy, are encouraged to undergo a male sling (generally recommended for men with moderate incontinence) or placement of an artificial urinary sphincter (men with severe incontinence).

Erectile dysfunction

Erectile dysfunction is the most common complication confronting men following radical prostatectomy. The likelihood of preserving sexual function following radical prostatectomy is dependent on age, baseline sexual function, number of neurovascular bundles preserved (Figure 19.2), expertise of the surgeon, and baseline sexual activity. Overall preservation of erection following radical prostatectomy ranges between 20% and 65%.[32] The potency rates presented in the literature are highly variable and dependent on the skill and experience of the surgeon, methodology utilized for ascertaining potency, patient selection, definition of potency, number of neurovascular bundles preserved, and use of oral and intracavernous agents. Post-prostatectomy potency rates in the modern era have improved, presumably due to the development of the nerve-sparing technique,[24] and the availability of phosphodiesterase (PDE) inhibitors.[32] Several experts have reported and illustrated their techniques for performing nerve-sparing prostatectomy.[24,34]

Walsh et al[18] have provided compelling evidence that excision of a single neurovascular bundle significantly lowers potency rates.

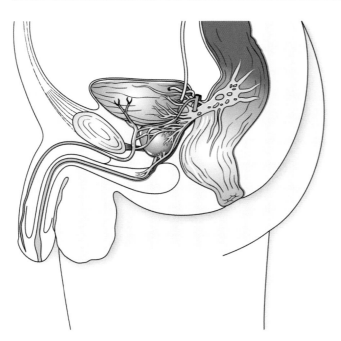

Figure 19.2
Anatomic representation of the neurovascular bundles which travel posterolateral to the prostate on either side and may be preserved at the time of surgery.

Obviously, the surgeon must balance preserving potency against curing the cancer. A significant proportion of men with extracapsular extension do not develop progressive disease, especially when a negative margin is achieved.[35] Lepor et al[36] have proposed an algorithm for guiding decisions regarding preservation or excision of the neurovascular bundle based on preoperative Gleason score, presence of perineural invasion, and tumor volume.

There is reason to believe that administration of PDE inhibitors immediately after RRP may increase potency rates. Padma-Nathan et al[37] reported the results of a randomized placebo controlled trial comparing return of sexual function in men randomized to receive 50 mg/day of oral sildenafil versus placebo for 9 months following radical prostatectomy. Those men randomized to sildenafil achieved better sexual function off all treatment 1 year following radical prostatectomy. The rationale for daily sildenafil is to prevent cavernosal muscle soft-tissue atrophy by stimulating penile smooth muscle activity during nocturnal erections. Based on this study, we offer an oral PDE inhibitor immediately after catheter removal.

Men must be counseled that the return of erections may take up to 2 years. If substantial erectile function has returned 3 months following radical prostatectomy, men are not encouraged to pursue intracavernosal therapy since the ability to obtain erections adequate for intercourse will likely return imminently. If erectile function is minimal at 3 months, men interested in resuming sexual activity are encouraged to pursue a penile injection program. There is evidence that penile injection therapy not only restores erectile function but also increases the likelihood erections will return.[38]

The most significant way to impact potency rates following radical prostatectomy is to optimally perform the nerve-sparing technique. This mandates a bloodless surgical field. Care must be taken while dividing the prostatourethral junction not to injure the neurovascular bundle which is attenuated and in close proximity to the prostatourethral junction. In most cases, the author incises the visceral layer of the pelvic fascia beginning at the apex of the prostate

and extending the incision toward the bladder neck. The incision in the visceral pelvic fascia is extended along the anterior surface of the prostate in cases with low volume disease in order to maximally preserve the autonomic innervation to the penis. In cases with significant fibrosis at the apex, the incision in the visceral pelvic fascia is started at the bladder neck and extended to the apex. The neurovascular bundle is sharply and/or bluntly mobilized off the prostate to the level of the vascular pedicle and only significant bleeders are controlled with surgical clips. The advantage of open versus laparoscopic radical prostatectomy is the ability to rely on palpation to ensure the prostate is not inadvertently incised. The Denonvilliers' fascia is then incised, exposing the vas deferens and seminal vesicles. The medial margin of the vascular pedicle to the prostate is identified immediately lateral to the prostate. The lateral pedicle is then divided as close to the prostate as possible without entering the gland.

Several surgeons have advocated nerve grafting in order to improve potency rates following uni- or bi-lateral excision of the neurovascular bundles.[39,40] Unfortunately, these studies have serious methodologic design flaws and, therefore, the benefit of nerve grafting remains unanswered.

References

1. Young HH. The early diagnosis and radical cure of carcinoma of the prostate: Being a study of 40 cases and presentation of a radical operation which was carried out in four cases. Bull Johns Hopkins Hosp 1905;16:315.
2. Millin T. Retropubic Urinary Surgery. London: Livingstone, 1947.
3. Walsh PC, Lepor H. The role of radical prostatectomy in the management of prostatic carcinoma. Cancer 1987;60(Suppl):526–537.
4. Catalona WJ, Scott WW. Carcinoma of the prostate. In Walsh PC, Gittes RF, Perlmutter AD, Stamey TA (eds): Campbell's Urology, vol 5. Philadelphia: WB Saunders, 1986, pp 1463–1534.
5. Shekarriz B, Upadhyay J, Wood PP. Intraoperative, perioperative and long-term complications of radical prostatectomy. Urol Clin North Am 2001;28:639–653.
6. Lepor H, Nieder AM, Ferrandino MN. The intraoperative and postoperative complications following radical retropubic prostatectomy in a consecutive series of 1,000 cases. J Urol 2001;166:1729–1733.
7. Lepor H, Kaci L. Contemporary evaluation of operative parameters and complications related to open radical retropubic prostatectomy. Urology 2003;62:702–706.
8. Lerner SE, Blute ML, Lieber MM, et al. Morbidity of contemporary radical retropubic prostatectomy for localized prostate cancer. Oncology (Williston Park) 1995;9:379–382, discussion 382, 385–386, 389.
9. Catalona WJ, Carvalhal GF, Mager DE, et al. Potency, continence and complication rates in 1870 consecutive radical retropubic prostatectomies. J Urol 1999;162:433–438.
10. Gheiler EL, Lovisolo JA, Tiguert R, et al. Results of a clinical care pathway for radical prostatectomy patients in an open hospital-multiphysician system. Eur Urol 1999;35:210–216.
11. Leandri P, Rossignol G, Gautier JR, et al. Radical retropubic prostatectomy: Morbidity and quality of life. Experience with 620 consecutive cases. J Urol 1992;147:883–887.
12. Hull RD, Pineo GF. Prophylaxis of deep venous thrombosis and pulmonary embolism. Med Clin North Am 1998;82:477–493.
13. Harpster LE, Rommel FM, Sieber PR, et al. The incidence and management of rectal injury associated with radical prostatectomy in a community based urology practice. J Urol 1995;154:1435–1438.
14. McLaren RH, Barrett DM, Zincke H. Rectal injury occurring at radical retropubic prostatectomy for prostate cancer: Etiology and treatment. Urology 1993;42:401–405.
15. Borland RN, Walsh PC. The management of rectal injury during radical retropubic prostatectomy. J Urol 1992;147:905–907.

16. Reiner WG, Walsh PC. An anatomical approach to the surgical management of the dorsal vein and Santorini's plexus during radical retropubic surgery. J Urol 1979;121:198–200.

17. Hsu EI, Hong EK, Lepor H. The influence of body weight and prostate volume on intraoperative, perioperative, and postoperative outcomes following radical retropubic prostatectomy. Urology 2003;61:601–606.

18. Walsh PC, Partin AW, Epstein JI. Cancer control and quality of life following anatomical radical retropubic prostatectomy: Results at 10 years. J Urol 1994;152:1831–1836.

19. Patel R, Lepor H. Removal of the urinary catheter on postoperative days 3 or 4 following radical retropubic prostatectomy. Urology 2003; 61:156–160.

20. Gilliland JD, Spies JB, Brown SB, et al: Lymphoceles: Percutaneous treatment with povidone-iodine sclerosis. Radiology 1989;171:227–229.

21. Waples MJ, Wegenke JD, Vega RJ. Laparoscopic management of lymphocele after pelvic lymphadenectomy and radical retropubic prostatectomy. Urology 1992;39:82–84.

22. Surya BV, Provet J, Johanson KE, et al. Anastomotic strictures following radical prostatectomy: Risk factors and management. J Urol 1990;143:755–758.

23. Park R, Martin S, Lepor H. Anastomotic strictures following radical prostatectomy: Insights into incidence, effectiveness of intervention, impact on continence and factors predisposing to occurrence. Urology 2001;57:742–746.

24. Walsh PC. Anatomic radical retropubic prostatectomy. In Walsh PC, Retik AB, Vaughan ED, et al (eds): Campbell's Urology, ed 7. Philadelphia: WB Saunders, 1998, p 2565.

25. Novicki DE, Larson TR, Andrews PE, et al. Comparison of the modified vest and the direct anastomosis for radical retropubic prostatectomy. Urology 1997;49:732–736.

26. Lepor H, Nieder AM, Fraiman MC. Early removal of urinary catheter after radical retropubic prostatectomy is both feasible and desirable. Urology 2001;58:425–429.

27. Foote J, Yun S, Leach GE. Post prostatectomy incontinence. Pathology, evaluation and management. Urol Clin North Am 1991;18:229–241.

28. Lepor H, Kaci L. The impact of open radical retropubic prostatectomy on continence and lower urinary tract symptoms (LUTS):

29. A prospective assessment using validated self-administered outcome instruments. J Urol 2004;171:1216–1219.

30. Ficazzola MA, Nitti VW. The etiology of post-radical prostatectomy incontinence and correlation of symptoms with urodynamic findings. J Urol 1998;160:1317–1320.

31. Lepor H, Kaci L. The role of intraoperative biopsies during radical retropubic prostatectomy. Urology 2004;63:499–502.

32. Twiss C, Martin S, Shore R, et al. A continence index predicts the early return of urinary continence following radical retropubic prostatectomy. J Urol 2000;164:1241–1247.

33. McCullough AR. Prevention and management of erectile dysfunction following radical prostatectomy. Urol Clin North Am 2001;28:613–627.

34. Marks LS, Duda C, Dorey FJ, et al. Treatment of erectile dysfunction with Sildenafil. Urology 1999;53:19–24.

35. Lepor H. Radical retropubic prostatectomy. Urol Clin North Am 2001;28:509–520.

36. Han, M, Partin AW, Pound CR, et al. Long-term biochemical disease-free and cancer-specific survival following anatomic radical retropubic prostatectomy. The 15-year Johns Hopkins Experience. Urol Clin North Am 2001;28:555–565.

37. Shah O, Robbins DA, Mani N, et al. The NYU nerve sparing algorithm decreases the rate of positive surgical margins following radical retropubic prostatectomy. J Urol 2003;169:2147–2159.

38. Padma-Nathan H, McCullough AR, Giuliano F, et al. Postoperative nightly administration of Sildenafil citrate significantly improves the return of normal spontaneous erectile function after bilateral nerve-sparing radical prostatectomy. J Urol 2003;169(Suppl):375–376.

39. Montorsi F, Guazzoni G, Strambi L, et al. Recovery of spontaneous erectile function after nerve-sparing radical retropubic prostatectomy with and without early intracavernous injections of alprostadil. J Urol 1997;158:1408–1410.

40. Kim ED, Scardino PT, Hampel O, et al. Interposition of sural nerves restores function of cavernous nerves resected during radical prostatectomy. J Urol 1999;161:188–192.

41. Sawin KM, Canto EI, Shariat SF, et al. Sural nerve interposition grafting during radical prostatectomy. Rev Urol 2002;4:12–23.

20

External beam radiotherapy for the treatment of prostate cancer

Vincent S Khoo, David P Dearnaley

Introduction

External beam radiotherapy is a commonly used modality in the radical treatment of both early and locally advanced prostate cancer. It also has a role in men with biochemical prostate-specific antigen (PSA) relapse following radical prostatectomy and in metastatic disease (see Chapters 11 and 42, respectively). This chapter will discuss the rationale, treatments, and outcomes for both early and locally advanced prostate cancer, briefly chronicle the technical developments in external beam irradiation, outline the methods underpinning modern radiotherapy, and address the treatment issues pertinent to external beam radiotherapy. New and future developments will be described including hypo-fractionation, image-guided radiotherapy, and treatment individualization.

Treatment selection for prostate cancer

Careful clinical assessment and staging is essential to select the appropriate treatment for men presenting with prostate cancer. Patients with localized disease and no clinical evidence of metastatic disease are suitable for radical radiotherapy. Many factors need to be considered in the selection of treatment for the individual patient, including:

- Patient factors such as age, clinical symptoms, sexual function, co-morbid conditions such as inflammatory bowel disease, potential life-expectancy and individual preference
- Tumor factors such as tumor grade (Gleason scoring), tumor stage, and initial PSA value at presentation
- Treatment factors such as method of treatment, probability of local control, and morbidity profile of the therapy.

Currently, the optimal management in men with localized prostate cancer remains uncertain. This is because there is substantial biologic heterogeneity within each prostate cancer subgroup dictating local behavior and metastatic potential. This is reflected by the widely variable treatment outcomes for each individual disease stage. However, there is reasonable evidence to recommend rational guidelines for radiotherapy treatment. For men anticipated to have a life-expectancy of 10 or more years, it would be appropriate to offer curative treatment. This judgment is based on the balance of

probability that the cancer is likely to progress during this timespan in these individuals. It is also reasonable to consider curative treatment for men with shorter life-expectancy ($\geq$5 years) if they have poorly differentiated cancer,[1] as data from Chodak et al[2] suggest their disease is more likely to progress during this period.

Clinical parameters

The clinicopathologic factors used to estimate clinical outcomes, such as tumor grade (Gleason score), tumor stage, and initial PSA values at presentation, are discussed in earlier chapters. Using these factors, a variety of clinical algorithms or nomograms have been formulated to predict the extent of disease and clinical outcomes (see Chapters 55 and 56). Based on large surgical series, Partin's tables is one example of a nomogram that correlates clinical T stage, biopsy Gleason score, and presenting PSA for the prediction of final pathologic stage.[3] Nomograms are also available for men with clinically localized prostate cancer to classify patients into early and locally advanced disease groups, depending on the likelihood of pelvic lymph node involvement.[4] Nomograms are also available to predict PSA-based outcomes following external beam radiotherapy.[5,6] These algorithms can be used to tailor radiotherapy regimens to each clinical prognostic subgroup.

Comparison of radiotherapy versus surgery

The relative merits of radical external beam radiotherapy or surgery for the individual will depend on the factors mentioned above. There are no adequate large randomized trials comparing radical radiotherapy with radical prostatectomy. The only randomized trial comparing radiotherapy and radical prostatectomy showed superior results for radical prostatectomy in "time to first evidence of treatment failure."[7] However, this trial has been criticized for violations in randomization, inadequate staging and follow-up, and possible selection bias,[8] and was disregarded in the National Institutes of Health consensus recommendations.[9] This issue has fueled nonrandomized comparisons of men with early localized prostate cancer treated by radical radiotherapy techniques and radical surgery. However, issues that can hamper interpretation of retrospective and nonrandomized comparisons include case selection, lack of central pathologic review, uncertain quality assurance of treatment methods with variable lengths of follow-up and definitions of biochemical failure.

Recent comparisons have not shown any consistent differences between radical radiotherapy and prostatectomy approaches.[10–12] The largest comparison collated pooled data from six large US centers of 6877 men treated over a 10-year period between 1989 and 1998.[12] Although there was variation in outcomes within individual institutions using the same treatment, the overall 5-year PSA results were similar for patients within the same prognostic risk group regardless of the form of therapy. These data suggest that there is little difference between radical radiotherapy and radical prostatectomy for early-stage localized disease. In general, nomogram predictions give very similar outcomes for surgery and radiotherapy.

The situation is different for men with locally advanced prostate cancer (clinical stage T3/4). The results of radical prostatectomy alone are unsatisfactory. Two large surgical series report pathologic evidence of extracapsular extension or seminal vesicle disease in 36% to 41% of cases, positive nodal involvement in 42%, and only 9% to 22% had pathologic T2 stage.[13,14] The high probability of positive resection margins and/or residual disease means that radical prostatectomy alone is inadequate to control disease in these patients. A multicenter analysis of 345 men with clinical T3 disease treated with radical prostatectomy alone reported actuarial 10-year metastatic-free survival rates of only 32%.[15] The results for clinical T3 patients treated with radiotherapy appear to be better than those for surgery. Zagars et al[16] treated 551 men with clinical stage T3 disease using external beam radiotherapy alone and reported 10-year actuarial disease-free survival and local control rates of 46% and 81%, respectively. It is important to note that a proportion of clinical T3 patients will not be cured by prostate radiotherapy even if pelvic volumes are treated because clinical outcome will be influenced by the presence of subclinical metastatic disease at the outset.

period of time, during which both prescribed radiation dose and radiotherapy techniques have evolved considerably, and relate principally to clinically detected cancers in the pre-PSA era.

Local tumor control is related to clinical stage and is best for T1 disease and decreases with higher T stage (see Table 20.1). At 10 years, local control is reported at 92% to 96% for T1, 71% to 83% for T2, and 69% to 81% for T3 disease. Local control at 15 years is in the region of 83% for T1, decreasing to 65% to 68% for T2 and 44% to 75% for T3 disease. Tumor size can also influence local control rates. Analysis of the earlier RTOG studies revealed that tumors smaller than 25 cm^3 have local control rates of up to 75% compared to tumors greater than 25 cm^3 with local control rates of less than 50%.[17] Tumor sizes greater than 25 cm^3 are also more likely to be advanced T stage disease.

PSA testing has revolutionized and standardized reporting of treatment outcome. Serum PSA estimations at disease presentation have been shown to be a useful prognosticator, and PSA levels following radical radiotherapy can also be a sensitive indicator of disease recurrence. In a study of 120 patients treated with radical radiotherapy and mean follow-up of 12.6 years, Hanks et al[18] reported biochemical PSA control of up to 72% in T1 disease, 54% in T2A disease, and 28% in T3 disease. Additionally, low Gleason scores were associated with a 75% rate of PSA control compared to 18% for Gleason summed score of 7 and 0% in those cases with Gleason summed scores of 8 or 9. In a multi-institutional series of 1765 men with T1 and T2 cancers treated to a median dose of 69.4 Gy between 1988 and 1995, 5-year PSA control rates were 81%, 68%, 51%, and 31% for men with initial presenting PSA levels of less than 10 ng/ml, 10 to less than 20 ng/ml, 20 to less than 30 ng/ml, and 30 ng/ml or more, respectively. For the group with T1C cancers, PSA control rates were 87% and 47% for presenting PSA levels of less than 20 ng/ml and 20 ng/ml or more, respectively.[19]

There is emerging evidence that biochemical or clinical failures are less likely after 5 years if PSA levels remain controlled at this time point,[19–21] and that PSA control is a surrogate for clinically defined disease progression.[21]

Results of external beam radiotherapy

The long-term survival of patients with T1 to T3 prostate cancer treated with external beam radiotherapy in the USA Patterns of Care (POC) study group, Radiation Therapy Oncology Group (RTOG) randomized studies, and other large single institute series are shown in Table 20.1. The POC and RTOG study group results represent national outcome averages for the US and provide reasonable estimation of treatment outcomes following conventional and more modern external beam radiotherapy techniques, respectively. It is also important to note that these results span a long

Radiation-related complications

The likelihood of radiation-related complications is dependent on the dose delivered, irradiation technique used, volume of normal tissues or organs-at-risk irradiated, and tolerance/radiosensitivity of the respective normal tissues. Radiotherapy-related complications can be divided into acute side effects (i.e. those occurring during and/or within 3 months of radiotherapy) and late side effects (i.e. those occurring >3 months following radiotherapy but usually developing months to years post-irradiation).

Table 20.1 External beam radiotherapy in prostate cancer: Long-term results from Patterns of Care studies, RTOG studies and large single institute series.[16,17,113,114]

	Number	Local recurrence (%)			Disease-free survival (%)			Overall survival (%)		
		5 year	10 year	15 year	5 year	10 year	15 year	5 year	10 year	15 year
T1Nx	583	3–6	4–8	17	84–85	52–68	39	83–95	52–76	41–46
T2Nx	1117	12–14	17–29	32–35	66–90	27–85	15–42	74–78	43–70	22–36
T3NX	2292	12–26	19–31	25–56	32–60	14–46	17–40	56–72	32–42	23–27

Table 20.2 RTOG/EORTC grading criteria for acute effects[22]

Grade	Gastrointestinal symptoms	Genitourinary symptoms
0	No change	No change
1	Increased frequency or change in quality of bowel habits not requiring medication, rectal discomfort not requiring analgesics	Frequency of urination or nocturia twice the pretreatment habit, dysuria, urgency not requiring medication
2	Diarrhea requiring antidiarrheal medication, mucus discharge not requiring pads, rectal or abdominal pain requiring analgesics	Frequency of urination or nocturia less frequent than every hour, dysuria, urgency, bladder spasm requiring local anesthetic
3	Diarrhea requiring parenteral support, mucus or blood discharge necessitating pads, abdominal distention	Frequency with urgency and nocturia hourly or more frequently, dysuria, pelvic plain or bladder spasm requiring regular narcotics, gross hematuria with or without clot passage
4	Acute or subacute obstruction, fistula or perforation, gastro-intestinal bleeding requiring transfusion, abdominal pain or tenesmus requiring tube decompression or bowel diversion	Hematuria requiring transfusion, acute bladder obstruction not secondary to clot passage, ulceration or necrosis

Table 20.3 RTOG/EORTC grading criteria for late effects[22]

Grade	Gastrointestinal symptoms	Genitourinary symptoms
0	No change	No change
1	Mild diarrhea, mild cramping, bowel movements 5 times daily, slight rectal discharge or bleeding	Slight epithelial atrophy, minor telangiectasia, microscopic hematuria
2	Moderate diarrhea and colic, bowel movements >5 times daily, excessive mucus discharge or intermittent bleeding	Moderate frequency, generalized telangiectasia, intermittent microscopic hematuria
3	Obstruction or bleeding requiring surgery	Severe frequency and dysuria, severe telangiectasia (often with petechiae), frequent hematuria, reduction in bladder capacity(<150 ml)
4	Necrosis, perforation, fistula	Necrosis, contracted bladder (<100 ml), severe hemorrhagic cystitis

The RTOG and European Organization Research and Treatment of Cancer (EORTC) have collaborated to update toxicity grading criteria in order to provide a suitable framework for consistent reporting and thorough evaluation of late radiation complications—the late effects normal tissues (LENT) scoring system.[22] The RTOG grading scales for the assessment of acute and late radiation-related toxicity are shown in Tables 20.2 and 20.3, respectively.

Acute side-effects resulting from pelvic or prostate radiotherapy can include abdominal discomfort, rectal symptoms such as proctitis, diarrhea, bleeding, bladder symptoms such as urinary frequency, nocturia, dysuria, bleeding, and rarely skin reactions. The reported incidence of acute side effects range from 70% to 90% for mild symptoms, 20% to 45% for moderate, and 1% to 4% for severe or prolonged reactions.[23–25] The majority of acute complications resolve completely within 2 to 6 weeks following completion of external beam radiotherapy.

For external beam radiotherapy in prostate cancer, late rectal side effects are the major dose-limiting complications and include persistent rectal discharge, tenesmus and rectal urgency, and rectal bleeding, ulcer or stricture. Important late genitourinary complications include chronic cystitis, urinary incontinence, bladder ulceration, hematuria, urethral stricture, and impotence.

Late complications from conventional external beam radiotherapy have been reported by the POC study group. The overall incidence of major late complications, defined as those requiring hospital admission for investigation or management, was 4.5% (1.8% urologic and 2.8% gastrointestinal). These complications resulted from substandard radiotherapy techniques that are no longer used, such as very large fields or anteroposterior fields treating only one field each day.[26] The 10-year update from the POC study group reported actuarial 5- and 10-year major complication-free rates of 93% and 86%, respectively.[27]

The predominant type of late gastrointestinal complication is proctitis with grade 2 side effects occurring in 3% to 15% of cases.[28,29] Less than 1% of late rectal complications require colostomy.[28,30] The most common late urinary side effect is cystitis in 2% to 11% of cases, followed by urethral stricture in 2% to 10%, while urinary incontinence occurs in less than 1% to 2%.[28–31] The main predisposing factor for the development of urinary strictures and urinary incontinence is previous transurethral resections.[28–31]

An important prostate radiotherapy side effects is erectile dysfunction. Etiology of this complication is multifactorial and is influenced by factors such as pretreatment function, age, small vessel disease, and previous urologic surgery. Its incidence is estimated as between 30% and 40% of treated men.[32] Recent studies may be more reliable because of routine pre- and post-therapy evaluations of sexual function. Using quality-of-life questionnaires, up to 62% of men reported return of sexual function following conformal radiotherapy.[33]

Similarly, a RTOG study revealed that 76% of sexually potent men reported return of function following radiotherapy.[34] However, the impact on different patient age groups can vary substantially, with 75% of men between 55 and 59 years and 53% between 60 and 74 years being bothered by sexual dysfunction following surgery compared to 40% and 47%, respectively, after radiotherapy.[35]

Factors influencing treatment outcome with radiotherapy

An important determinant of radiotherapy treatment outcome is local control. Lack of local control has been associated with higher biochemical PSA failure and metastatic rates.[36] At the Royal Marsden Hospital, London, analysis of radically irradiated patients with clinically locally controlled disease at 5 years revealed a 57% metastatic-free survival rate compared to 26% in patients who have developed local failure (P≤0.01). Multivariate analysis of metastatic-free and overall survival in this cohort of patients revealed that local control remains a highly significant parameter when included as a time-dependent variable (P≤0.01). This finding is consistent with reports from other series,[37,38] and is applicable to patients who present with bulky disease or higher stage (T3/4), higher initial PSA levels, and poorly differentiated grades.

Strategies to improve local control include an increase in the prescribed dose or the use of neoadjuvant and/or adjuvant androgen deprivation. The use of hormonal therapy is covered in Chapters 35 to 38 and will not be discussed further here. A dose–response relationship has been demonstrated for local control. Retrospective studies have reported lower local control rates of 62% to 63% when prescribed doses were less than 60 Gy, increasing to 74% to 80% for doses between 60 and 70 Gy, and 81% to 88% when doses were greater than 70 Gy.[39,40] There is potential for an increase in radiation-related complication rates when dose is increased. Using conventional external beam radiation techniques, the overall incidence of side-effects increased from 6% to 11% when patients received more than 65 Gy.[41] However, other investigators have not noted such a substantial increase in rectal complications with doses up to 70 Gy.[16,31] Studies suggest that the threshold for dose-limiting rectal complications is higher. The RTOG studies report a significant increase in late morbidity with doses greater than 70 Gy,[30] while other investigators note that when dose to the anterior rectal wall exceeds 75 Gy, the incidence of grade 2 or greater proctitis/bleeding rises from less than 20% to around 60%.[42] However, newer radiotherapy techniques (described below) may permit acceptable escalation of dose without an increase in late complications.

Developments in external beam radiotherapy

A major advance in pelvic external beam irradiation was the introduction of higher energy x-rays in the 1960s, which superseded the use of orthovoltage or deep x-ray beams of 200 kV to 300 kV. This heralded the modern era of prostate radiotherapy. Subsequently, megavoltage beams of greater 4 MeV (usually 10–18 MeV), produced by linear accelerators, delivered enhanced clinical depth–dose beam profiles that enable skin sparing and improved dose coverage of the prostate gland and seminal vesicles within the pelvis. Optimal visualization of the tumor volume and its surrounding anatomic structures is necessary for any cancer treatment delivered in a localized manner, such as radiotherapy. The use of computed tomography (CT) scanning has allowed clinicians to more accurately define treatment volumes. Initial studies assessing the value of CT scanning when it was first introduced recorded that geographic miss of the gross tumor can be avoided in up to 40% of cases.[43]

Radiotherapy planning nomenclature

Modern radiotherapy planning techniques, such as conformal radiotherapy (CFRT) and intensity-modulated radiotherapy (IMRT), require definition of treatment volumes distinct from the simple visualization of gross tumor. The International Commission for Radiation Units (ICRU) Report 50 and 62 provides a series of definitions that incorporates parameters such as the extent of disease and its variation, organ motion due to physiologic activity, and uncertainties in patient and treatment set-up.[44,45] This nomenclature (Table 20.4; Figure 20.1) permits unambiguous specification of

---

Table 20.4 ICRU-50 and -62 treatment planning volumes

Nomenclature	Definition
Gross target volume (GTV)	Radiologically visible or clinically palpable extent of tumor
Clinical target volume (CTV)	GTV with a margin that includes the presumed microscopic extent of disease or subclinical nodal involvement
Planning target volume (PTV)	CTV with a margin added to account for patient movement, internal organ and target motion, uncertainties in patient set-up, and treatment beam penumbra. This can be subdivided into the following: • Internal margin (IM) is that which is added for variations in position and/or shape and size of the CTV • Set-up margin (SM) is that which is added to account for all the variations and uncertainties in patient-beam positioning. Therefore CTV + IM + SM define the PTV.
Treated volume (TV)	Volume of tissue actually treated to the prescribed dose as specified by the clinician (e.g. 95% isodose volume)
Irradiated volume (IV)	Volume of tissue irradiated to a clinically significant dose in relation to normal tissue tolerance (e.g. 50% isodose volume)
Planning organ-at-risk volume (PRV)	Margin added to the organ-at-risk (OAR) to account for the positional/shape variation and uncertainties of the location of the OAR

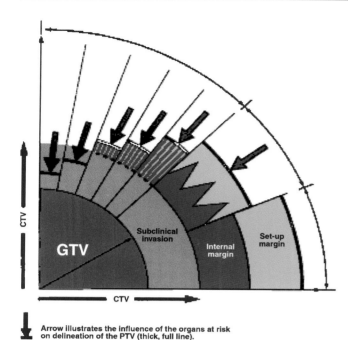

Figure 20.1
Schematic representation of the radiotherapy planning volume 50 and 62. CTV, clinical target volume; GTV, gross tumor volume; PTV, planning treatment volume.

From ICRU-62,45 with permission.

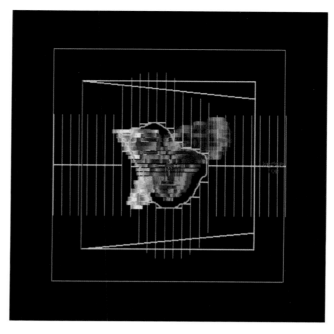

Figure 20.2
Beams-eye-view (BEV) for a lateral prostate radiotherapy field. Prostate (red), rectum (yellow), bladder (blue).

treatment volumes, uniformity in planning and treatment delivery, and consistency in reporting and comparison of results between different radiotherapy centers.

Cross-sectional imaging and conformal radiotherapy

Cross-sectional anatomic information has permitted the development of advanced radiotherapy techniques and is the basis of CFRT. CFRT uses CT to create three-dimensional (3D) models of the prostate gland and seminal vesicles in relation to their surrounding normal tissues or pelvic organs. This allows each radiotherapy beam to be shaped to the projected profile of the target within the axis of the beam (beams-eye-view, BEV) (Figure 20.2). By using multiple beams with each beam shaped in the BEV, the high dose region is made to conform to the shape of the planning target volume in 3D. This method can reduce unnecessary irradiation of the adjacent normal structures. Until recently, CT has been the main method of imaging for radiotherapy planning. Although CT provides geometrically stable images and electron density information needed for planning dose calculations, it is limited in defining soft tissues/organs in anatomic sites where there are many tissues/organs of similar electron densities, such as within the pelvis. As a result of the uncertainty in accurately determining organ boundaries, clinicians often provide larger treatment volumes to compensate for this uncertainty.

The use of magnetic resonance imaging (MRI) can overcome some of the limitation of CT scanning and improve the definition of prostate treatment volumes. Its applications in radiotherapy have

been reviewed.[46] The major advantage of MRI is its superior ability to distinguish between soft-tissue structures of similar tissue electron densities. This is particularly useful when imaging structures such as the prostate gland, rectum, and bladder in the pelvis. Comparative MRI versus CT planning studies using MRI-defined prostate volumes as the gold standard have reported that CT-defined prostate volumes tend to overestimate the planning volume by as much as 40%.[47] Thus, the use of MR-based prostate planning volumes can result in smaller treatment volumes, leading to more appropriate shaping of the treatment fields and thereby reducing the risk of treatment-related complications. Although there are potential problems of image distortion with MRI, these technical issues can be effectively and reliably corrected or minimized.[46] The value of MR spectroscopy in defining tumor volumes within the prostate gland for radiotherapy is being investigated.[48,49] This procedure offers the opportunity to selectively boost identified clonagenic tumor regions for potentially better local control and subsequently improved survival. Other imaging methods under investigation are discussed in Chapters 50 to 53.

Planning for prostate radiotherapy

CFRT is the minimum planning standard for prostate radiotherapy, providing reduced treatment-related toxicity compared to nonconformal techniques.[50] The radiotherapy treatment planning procedure involves a series of steps that start with obtaining 3D anatomic information of the patient in the treatment position, defining the target volumes, determining the optimal treatment plan, and implementing appropriate quality assurance, which includes treatment verification and monitoring of the patient during and following radiotherapy.

Patient positioning and immobilization

Patient positioning and immobilization are important to ensure that the patient can lie on the treatment table quietly and comfortably in a reliably immobile and reproducible manner for each treatment fraction. Usually, the patient lies supine and is supported with a foam head pad, and knee and ankle stocks help to maintain his position. Different treatment centers may use prone compared to supine positions, but a recent randomized trial demonstrated significantly less prostate motion and normal tissue irradiation with the supine position.[51]

Many immobilization devices are available to aid stabilization of the patient treatment position from body casts or cradles to ankle stocks. Although some investigators have shown that treatment set-up can be improved by immobilization of both the pelvis and legs,[52,53] a recent randomized trial revealed that the combination of knee supports and ankle stocks provided a high degree of accuracy, making pelvic immobilization unnecessary.[54]

Planning CT scanning

A CT scan in the treatment position is used to plan radiotherapy. Small skin tattoos are used to mark points on the patient's surface anteriorly and laterally. These skin points are used to align treatment room lasers for more reproducible patient set-up. The planning CT scan usually uses a slice interval of between 1 and 5 mm from below the ischial tuberosities to above the top of the bladder dome, or for the whole pelvis if pelvic treatment is intended.

The patient is usually instructed to keep his bladder comfortably "full" for the CT scan to reduce the proportion of the bladder and bowel within the planning target volume (PTV). At the Royal Marsden Hospital, patients are asked to empty their bladder 1 h prior to the start of the planning scan or treatment, and are asked to drink 300 to 400 ml of water during the waiting period. The bladder is thus partially filled but remains comfortable throughout scanning or treatment.

Rectal filling and emptying can influence prostate position during radiotherapy.[55] Strategies to achieve a more reliable rectal "state" include the use of daily laxatives or enemas prior to each radiotherapy fraction, endorectal balloons[56,57] or tensioned radioopaque marked urethral catheters.[58] These approaches have not been evaluated in controlled settings and some techniques may have issues with patient acceptability.

The position of the prostate may also be indirectly visualized using implanted intraprostatic markers. These radioopaque markers allow daily verification of the prostate location using electronic portal imaging devices, which can quantify the degree of positioning errors and permit online correction of these set-up errors.

Once the CT information has been obtained, these data are transferred to a radiotherapy planning workstation. It is important to ensure that all the relevant pelvic organs of interest for radiotherapy are adequately imaged so that they can be outlined for treatment planning and evaluation using dose–volume histograms. This is particularly crucial for IMRT to ensure that any organs to be treated or avoided can be optimized.

Definition of target volumes: prostate, seminal vesicles, and pelvis

Treatment planning nomenclature based on ICRU-62 recommendations[45] is not always relevant for prostate radiotherapy. For example, the gross target volume (GTV) cannot be defined either by clinical examination or standard prostate imaging used for treatment planning. By definition it is not defined in T1 tumors. The clinical target volume (CTV) should include the whole prostate gland with all or part of the seminal vesicles, depending on clinical risk and an appropriate margin to account for subclinical disease spread. Multimodality imaging, particularly using MRI, may be used to improve definition of the target volumes.[46,59]

There is considerable controversy as to what forms appropriate coverage of the seminal vesicles, from some clinicians not including them in the treatment volume to complete coverage of the whole extent of the seminal vesicles. One pathologic series suggested seminal vesicle involvement was sequential in 96% of cases with direct extension through the prostatic capsule or spread along the ejaculatory ducts.[60] This sequential pattern of spread was also advocated by others who suggested that seminal vesicle coverage can be limited to the proximal 20 to 25 mm because in 90% of cases pathologic involvement was limited to the proximal 20 mm.[61] Our local institution policy is to include the proximal 20 mm of the seminal vesicles if they are to be treated. Table 20.5 lists the planning protocols in recent and ongoing major clinical trials for treatment margins and inclusion of the seminal vesicles.

When coverage of the pelvic lymph nodes is intended, the internal and external iliac nodal groups, including the presciatic, presacral, and obturator groups, are usually included in the treatment volume. These nodal groups are selected based on their likely microscopic involvement from surgical series.[62,63] Some clinicians may also include part of the common iliac lymph nodes.

Definition of treatment margins

PTV margins depend on local institution policy and relate to local experience as well as known thresholds for systematic and random errors that may manifest during treatment planning and delivery. All treatment margins need to be added in 3D to ensure adequate coverage, particularly where there is considerable variation in the size of the outline between consecutive CT slices.[64] PTV margins may be nonuniform, varying from 7 to 10 mm isotropically, with tighter posterior margins (0–5 mm) to limit dose to the anterior wall of the rectum depending on the prescribed dose. Treatment margins usually change for different phases of the treatment, particularly if different treatment volumes and dose escalation is used (see Table 20.5).

Treatment planning

The use of Hounsfield units from the CT data allows for the assessment of tissue inhomogeneities and dose calculation. The number of treatment beams and their beam orientation largely depends on local facility expertise, experience, and protocols. Frequently three to four fields are used in Europe, while more than four fields are usually used in North America. The number of fields and their orientation may also change for different phases of the treatment. A recent comprehensive review for CFRT concluded that a three-field technique (an anterior and two wedged opposed lateral fields) gave equivalent or improved dose distributions.[65] For cases where there is asymmetry in the posterior extent of the PTV, individual optimization of the beam orientations, such as substituting a posterior oblique field for one lateral field, may provide better coverage and this may be automated using optimization algorithms.[66] The use of non-coplanar CFRT plans may not provide substantial

Table 20.5 Contemporary prostate cancer radiotherapy trials showing details of radiotherapy technique

Trial	Risk of SV involvement* (%)	Target + margin (mm)†			Dose‡ (Gy)			
		Phase I	Phase II	Phase III	Phase I	Phase II	Phase III	Total
Dutch	Low (<10)	P + 10	P + 5/0	-	68	0, 10	–	68, 78
	Mod (10-25)	P + SV + 10	P + 10	P + 5/0	50	18	0, 10	68, 78
	High (>25)	P + SV + 10	P + 5/0	–	68	0, 10	–	68, 78
	Involved	P + SV + 10	P + SV+ 5/0	–	68	0, 10	–	68, 78
PROTECT, UK	Low (<15)	P + bSV + 10/5	P + 0	–	56	18	–	74
	High (≥15)	P + SV	P + 0	–	56	18	–	74
RT-01, UK	Low (<15)	P + bSV + 10	P + 0	–	64	0, 10	–	64, 74
	High (≥15)	P + SV	P + 0	–	64	0, 10	–	64, 74
EORTC 22991	All ± nodes	P + SV + 10	P + bSV + 10	P + 5/0	46	24	0, 4, 8	70, 74, 78 (not randomized)
RTOG P-0126	All	P + SV + 10/5	P + 10/5	–	58	15, 24	–	73, 82
RTOG 9406	Low (<15)	P + 5–10	P + 5-10	–	68	0, 6, 11	–	68, 74, 79
	High (15)	P + SV + 5-10	P + 5-10	–	56	12, 8, 23	-	68, 74, 79
	Involved	P + SV + 5-10	-	–	68, 74, 79	-	–	68, 74, 79
MSKCC	All	P + SV + 10/6	P + SV + 10/6 Rectal block	–	65, 70, 76, 76	0, 0, 0, 5	–	65, 70, 76, 81
CHHIP, UK (high-dose arm)	Low (<15)	P + bSV + 10	P + 10/5	P + 5/0	56	16	4	74
	High (≥15)	P + SV + 10	P + 10/5	P + 5/0	56	16	4	74

bSV, base of seminal vesicle; P, prostate; SV, seminal vesicle.
*Risk of SV based on Roach formula and Partin tables.
†","/" Indicates margin: all around prostate/prostate-rectum interface.
‡Multiple figures in each risk group indicate different dose arms of trials.

additional dosimetric gains compared to coplanar CFRT plans to warrant the increased efforts required for non-coplanar planning.[67]

Comparative studies of CFRT versus IMRT reveal that IMRT techniques can permit better dose distributions for irregularly shaped or concave target volumes, such as those found in seminal vesicles wrapping around the rectum, and improved avoidance or sparing of adjacent dose-limiting normal structures, such as the rectum.[68–70] When treating pelvic lymph nodes, IMRT techniques have been shown to permit better avoidance of bowel compared to CFRT, and allow escalation of dose to nodal regions while respecting bowel tolerances.[71] The tolerance of such a strategy is being assessed in a trial setting at the Royal Marsden Hospital. If an IMRT technique is used to treat the prostate and/or pelvis, five equally spaced coplanar fields can provide equivalent plans as more complex field arrangements.[71]

In the prostate treatment planning process, particularly with IMRT techniques, it is necessary to define minimum dose coverage of the target and/or limitations of dose to susceptible organs at risk (OARs), such as the rectum, bladder, bowel or femoral heads. These clinical planning dose thresholds may also be used to determine the "goodness" of the treatment plan. In evaluating the acceptability of any plan, treatment parameters, such as dose statistics (mean, minimum or maximum doses), dose–volume histograms, and visual inspection of the dose distribution on each transaxial slice of the treatment volume, are used to ensure appropriate coverage of the target and maximal avoidance of the OARs. Reported dose thresholds for both acute and late toxicity are available for a variety of OARs, such as rectum,[72–80] bladder,[81] bowel[75,82] and femoral heads.[83] We have collated a set of suitable planning dose thresholds that guide our current assessment of plans for either prostate and/or pelvic radiotherapy at the Royal Marsden Hospital (Table 20.6). Future reporting of dose-related toxicity from randomized trials of dose escalation is likely to refine these dose thresholds.

Table 20.6 Suggested dose/volume thresholds for organs at risk used at the Royal Marsden Hospital

Dose (Gy) at 2 Gy/ fraction to 100%	Maximum volume (%)
Rectum*	
50	60
60	50
65	30
70	15
74	3
Bladder†	
50	50
60	25
74	5
Femoral heads‡	
50	50

*Rectum including outer wall and contents from rectosigmoid junction to ischial tuberosities.
†Defined as whole bladder including outer wall.
‡Defined as the round part of the femoral head.

Verification

Accurate and reliable delivery of radiation to the target is paramount for prostate radiotherapy. Treatment verification is needed to identify systematic and random errors in the treatment planning process in order to allow its correction. During treatment delivery, film-based portal x-rays or electronic portal images are used to compare patient positioning with reference simulator films or digitally reconstructed radiographs. Gross inaccuracies may be corrected by repositioning the patient in realtime.[84] However, these verification methods only permit identification of field boundaries relative to bony landmarks and not the spatial location of the prostate or other internal organs. The use of radioopaque markers implanted in the prostate will allow daily quantification of the prostate position. More recent methods for visualizing the spatial location of targets and OARs during radiotherapy and image-guided treatment strategies will be discussed later.

Results from conformal radiotherapy

The impact and value of CFRT was assessed in a randomized prostate radiotherapy trial at the Royal Marsden Hospital. This trial compared the use of conformal shaped fields versus conventional or unshaped rectangular fields at a dose of 64 Gy.[85] In men treated with CFRT, the incidence of clinically relevant late radiation sequelae, such as rectal proctitis requiring treatment (RTOG grade $\geq$2), was significantly reduced compared to conventional techniques (5% vs 15% respectively). More importantly, the close shaping of the conformal fields did not lead to any reduction in PSA-based local control between the randomized arms at a median follow-up of 3.6 years. These data set CFRT as the standard for prostate external beam irradiation. The use of CFRT to reduce the rate of treatment-related complications provides the potential for safe dose escalation. It has been postulated that if radiation dose can be safely escalated by 20%, this may result in demonstrable improvements in local tumor control rates by up to 10%.[86,87] This may subsequently increase the probability of cancer-specific survival for some cancer types such as prostate cancer.

The dose–response hypothesis fueled by data from the pre-PSA Patterns of Care analysis from the US suggested that higher doses provided improved disease-free intervals, especially for locally advanced disease.[26,88] However, depending on the level of dose escalation, radiotherapy using conventional techniques has been associated with an unreasonable and substantial increase in rectal bleeding, from 6% to 12% around 60 Gy to 11% to 20% with doses above 64 to 65 Gy.[26,31,41]

The result of dose escalation with CFRT was reviewed in a retrospective study from three USA institutions.[89] This study of 180 men reported a dose effect for men with high-grade T1/T2 disease with improved 5-year biochemical PSA control rates using doses of 70 Gy or greater. In a larger CFRT study of 743 patients with localized prostate cancer treated with escalating doses, PSA relapse-free survival rates in patients with intermediate or unfavorable prognosis (characterized by $\geq$1 or $\geq$2 higher prognostic indicators, respectively, i.e. $\geq$T3, PSA level >10 ng/ml, Gleason score >6) was significantly improved with doses of 75.6 Gy or greater (P = <0.05).[90]

Translation of improved local control into survival was reported for the first time by the RTOG.[91] The outcomes from four randomized RTOG trials comprising 1465 men treated between 1975 and 1992 with a median follow-up of 8 years showed an improvement in 10-year disease-specific survival and overall survival rates for high-grade prostate cancers treated to doses of 66 Gy or greater. This was associated with a 29% lower relative risk of death from prostate cancer and 27% reduced mortality rate (P = <0.05). No neoadjuvant or adjuvant androgen deprivation therapy was used. These data suggest that increases in radiation dose alone can confer a survival benefit in men with localized prostate cancer but this may be limited to those with higher grade disease.

However, improvements in outcome during the PSA era may in part be due to a shift in presentation to low-risk disease and earlier detection of high-grade disease.[92] Caution is needed in the interpretation

of results from sequentially treated cohorts of patient, such as those reported from phase I/II studies of dose-escalated prostate radiotherapy. Phase III randomized controlled trials are needed to properly define the use of higher dose radiotherapy, clinical prognostic parameters, reporting PSA control rates, and clinically important endpoints, including toxicity and quality-of-life data.

Two randomized controlled trials have reported results of dose escalation in prostate radiotherapy and the results of others are maturing. The first of these to report was from the MD Anderson Cancer Center; this randomized 305 men with T1 to T3 localized prostate cancer between 1993 and 1998 to either 70 or 78 Gy.[80] With a median follow-up of 60 months, the 6-year freedom-from-failure rates, including biochemical PSA failure rates, were 64% for 70 Gy and 70% for 78 Gy (P = 0.03). Subgroup multivariate analysis revealed that those patients with presenting a PSA level of greater than 10 ng/ml benefited from dose escalation with a freedom-from-failure rate of 62% compared to 43% in the 70-Gy arm (P = 0.01). However, late rectal side effects were also significantly increased in the 78-Gy arm with an actuarial risk of RTOG grade 2 or greater toxicity at 6 years of 26% compared to 12% in the 70-Gy arm (P = 0.001). This late complication was highly correlated to the volume of rectum treated beyond 70 Gy with a threshold at 25% of the irradiated rectal volume. This may be avoided by more stringent attention to limiting dose to the rectum by better radiation techniques.

The second trial to report results was from the Institute of Cancer Research/Royal Marsden Hospital, which in a randomized pilot study (which led into the UK Medical Research Council [MRC] RT-01 trial) included 125 men with T1 to T3 cancers treated for 3 to 6 months with neoadjuvant androgen suppression and then randomized to either 64 or 74 Gy.[93] This patient group had less favorable prognostic features than those patients included in the MD Anderson Cancer Center trial (e.g. initial presenting PSA level of 14 versus 8 ng/ml). After a median follow-up of 74 months, the 5-year PSA control rate was higher in the 74-Gy (71%) than in the 64-Gy (59%) group (hazard ratio, 0.64; P = 0.10). Bowel and bladder side effects were also increased in the higher dose group, particularly in the subgroup of patients who in a second randomization had the phase I radiotherapy volume treated with a 15-mm rather than a 10-mm margin.[93] The PSA control rates were very similar for these groups and as the 15-mm margin increased toxicity without any apparent clinical benefit, a 10-mm margin was used in the subsequent MRC RT-01 trial.

The MRC RT-01 trial has now completed recruitment of over 850 men with localized prostate cancer in 2003.[94,95] The Netherlands CKVO 96-10 trial completed recruitment of approximately 670 men in 2003 and randomized patients to either 68 or 78 Gy, also using CFRT methods.[96] The use of neoadjuvant androgen deprivation therapy was allowed in this trial. The French Collaborative trial recruited 306 patients with localized prostate cancer to a randomized trial of 70 versus 80 Gy. No androgen deprivation therapy was used in this trial.[97] Outcomes for biochemical PSA control rates and incidence of late complications from these trials are awaited with much interest and will provide further clarification for optimization of patient management.

Intensity-modulated radiotherapy

Whether dose escalation is being considered or not, it is crucial to ensure that any potential treatment-related complications are minimized. Advances in technology have enabled the development of more sophisticated radiotherapy treatment methods. Such technical developments include multileaf collimators (MLC) that allow automatic shaping of the radiotherapy field and routine use of electronic portal imaging devices (EPID) that permit daily online verification of the treatment fields. These devices together with modern computational power for sophisticated 3D radiotherapy dose-cube calculations and "inverse" planning algorithms have enabled the refinement of conformal techniques into a new treatment paradigm, IMRT.

IMRT expands the concept of CFRT by enabling the high-dose regions to be shaped around "concave" targets and not just to the profile of the target in the BEV. IMRT can produce deliberate inhomogeneous dose distributions, such as to tumor regions as defined by MR spectroscopy, for boosting or to conformally avoid important OARs, such as the rectum in prostate radiotherapy. Compared to CFRT where the beam fluence is constant across each treatment field, in the IMRT technique, the intensity of the beam fluence is varied across each treatment field. The effect of IMRT is to produce a series of many smaller beamlets for each treatment field, each of which can be controlled individually to provide different dose fluences; these beamlets are then combined to generate the overall desired dose distribution. The conceptual difference in beam fluences between conformal and intensity-modulated fields is schematically shown in Figure 20.3A and B, respectively. Inverse planning algorithms are needed to create and optimize the IMRT plan. These algorithms avoid previous manual trial-and-error methods of producing appropriate prostate radiotherapy plans by using an iterative computational process based on cost functions and/or physical dose parameters to obtain the optimum plan from the desired projected dose distribution for the ideal prostate with or without seminal vesicles radiotherapy plan.

Results

The delivery of appropriately designed nonuniform dose intensities with IMRT can produce better sculpturing of the high-dose region to complex irregular shapes, particularly concave-shaped target volumes such as the coverage of seminal vesicles or pelvic nodal volumes. One clinical example where IMRT is being used to cover a "U"-shaped target volume (Figure 20.4) to a relatively high dose (55–60 Gy) within the pelvis while dramatically sparing bowel dosage is our phase I/II trial of pelvic nodal irradiation in high-risk prostate cancer patients. Preliminary results from this study report acceptable early toxicity.[98]

IMRT plans can provide a very steep high-to-low-dose gradient at the edge of the target volume for improved avoidance of important adjacent normal structures in prostate radiotherapy, such as the rectum, bowel, and bladder. In this manner, external beam radiotherapy-related complications may be further reduced and higher dose escalation may be safely achieved compared to CFRT. Using this refined technique with appropriate and judicious shielding of the rectum, clinicians at the Memorial Sloan-Kettering Cancer Center treated 772 men to doses 81 Gy or greater and reported a relatively low incidence of late rectal complications.[99] With a median follow-up of 24 months, the 3-year actuarial likelihood of greater than late grade 2 rectal toxicity was 4%.

New strategies for external beam radiotherapy

Developments in radiotherapy fractionation

External beam prostate radiotherapy is usually given by conventional fractionation (i.e. 1.8–2.0 Gy/fraction) in many parts of the world. The dogma of conventional fractionation for prostate cancer has been challenged recently by several investigators.[100,101] In radiobiology, the components of lethal radiation damage to the cell are expressed by the interrelationship of two measures, α and β, which can be modeled. The most commonly used radiobiologic model utilizing α and β values is the linear-quadratic formula and this can be used to guide the rationale for different fractionation schemes. It has been suggested that the α:β ratio for prostate cancer is much lower than previously thought, being around 1.2 to 1.5 Gy. This is lower than for other tumor types where the a:b ratio can range from 4 to 30 Gy; an "average" α:β ratio value of 10 Gy is generically assumed for most tumors. This lower predicted a:b ratio is consistent with the slower growth rates or low labeling indices of around 1% noted in prostate cancer compared to other tumor types that have labeling indices of around 3% to 5%.[102,103]

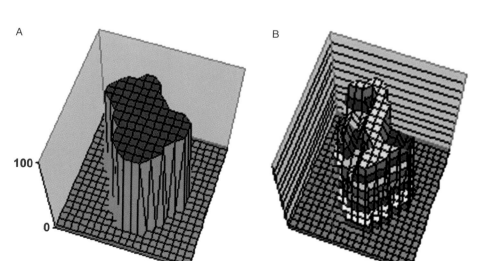

A

B

Figure 20.3

Comparison of beam fluences between a conformal radiotherapy (CFRT) and an intensity-modulated radiotherapy (IMRT) prostate field. *A*, CRFT field shaped in the beams-eye-view (BEV), showing uniform beam intensity across its treatment field. *B*, IMRT field showing variation in beam intensity across its treatment field with each color shading representing a different dose intensity.

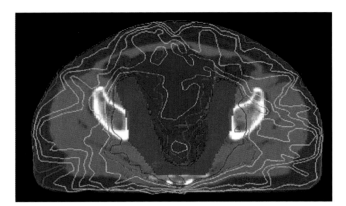

Figure 20.4
Example of an intensity-modulated radiotherapy (IMRT) plan used to treat pelvic lymph nodes at the Royal Marsden Hospital. In the transaxial plane, the 90% isodose (red line) is shaped around the planning target volume (solid red) and spares doses to the organs at risk (OARs) located adjacent and centrally (solid purple and blue, respectively).

The low α:β ratio of prostate cancer implies that these cancers possess higher fractionation sensitivity similar to that for late-responding normal tissues. This means that the use of hypofractionation (i.e. larger dose/fraction and fewer fractions) in prostate external beam radiotherapy may provide an improved therapeutic ratio by reducing the probability of late radiation morbidity for the same level of local control. Early indications for this are provided by a recent Australian trial that reported on a randomized comparison of 64 Gy in 32 fractions (2 Gy/fraction) with 55 Gy in 20 fractions (2.75 Gy/fraction) in men with early stage (T1–2N0M0) prostate cancer.[104] The interim analysis of the first 120 patients with a median follow-up of 43.5 months revealed similar PSA relapse-free survival rates and toxicities between the two radiation schedules. The follow-up is still too short to determine long-term control but is reasonable for defining the potential safety or toxicity of the program. A larger study from the National Cancer Institute of Canada PR-5 trial randomized 936 patients with T1/T2 prostate cancer to either 66 Gy in 33 fractions or 52.5 Gy in 20 fractions between 1994 and 1998.[105] With a median follow-up of 59 months, preliminary results in abstracted form showed comparable late toxicity between the arms (hypofractionated 2.6% vs conventional 3.6%), but the 5-year failure probability was higher in the hypofractionated arm than in the conventional fractionation arm (55.6% vs 48.6%, respectively; hazards ratio, 1.20). One potential explanation may be that the arms were not biologically equivalent in dose. This result is compatible with a α:β ratio of 1.5 assuming a γ 50 value of approximately 2.0.[106]

Local control rates will vary when different prognostic groups are considered, particularly with locally advanced cases. The hypofractionated schedule can also be dose escalated to improve the likelihood of local control, while maintaining the same level of radiation morbidity expected from the use of higher dose prescriptions (>74–78 Gy) using conventional fractionation schemes.

A large UK series has recently reported on 703 patients from 1995 to 1998 with clinical staged T1–4N0M0 prostate cancer treated to 50 Gy in 16 daily fractions (3.13 Gy/fraction) without hormonal manipulation.[107] Using this hypofractionated scheme to a relatively low total dose, the reported overall 5-year PSA relapse-free survival

and radiation morbidity rates are similar to those obtained with 65 to 70 Gy delivered using 1.8- to 2-Gy fractions. This study grouped the patients into three prognostic subsets based on PSA at presentation, clinical T stage, and Gleason score. The "good" group was defined as stage T1/2, PSA level of 10 ng/ml or less, and Gleason score less than 7; the "intermediate" group had one raised value; and the "poor" group had two or more raised values. With a median follow-up of 48 months, the 5-year PSA relapse-free survival rates were 82%, 56%, and 39% for the good, intermediate, and poor groups, respectively, with RTOG grade 2 or greater for bowel and bladder toxicity in 5% and 9%, respectively. These data on late complications confirms acceptable toxicity at this hypofractionated dose level and suggests that this is an acceptable regimen for good prognosis patients but may be less adequate for the other prognostic groups. The lower PSA relapse-free survival rates experienced by the intermediate and poor risk groups may be improved by dose escalation.

Several reservations have been directed towards the recent estimation for a much lower α:β ratio in prostate cancer:[108] the use of biochemical PSA-dependent results at 5 years which may not reflect long-term outcomes; data obtained at different centers and over time periods; estimations of the radiation damage repair half life and its effectiveness; as well as assumptions about the biologic and physical dose heterogeneity of the different patient groups. Nevertheless, the hypothesis is an attractive one not only for the potential improved therapeutic ratio but also for logistic and workflow issues. The advantages of hypofractionation are a shortened overall treatment time with reduced patient visits and departmental resources. This has prompted several groups around the world to reinvestigate the use of hypofractionation and dose escalation.

A variety of phase I/II studies are being undertaken to evaluate the use of hypofractionation regimens. One US collaborative study has reported on the use of 2.5 Gy/fraction prescribed to 70 Gy in 100 men with T1 to T3 prostate cancer.[109] With a median follow-up of 43 months, the overall biochemical PSA relapse-free survival at 4 years was reported to be 88%, with a 4-year actuarial late rectal RTOG grade 2 or 3 complication rate of 6%. Only 1 of the 100 patients suffered a grade 3 complication. The outcome from this study group demonstrated a favorable survival and toxicity profile.

At the Christie Hospital in Manchester, UK, Princess Margaret Hospital in Toronto and Notre-Dame Hospital in Montreal, Canada, 3 Gy/fraction to escalated doses of 60 to 66 Gy are being studied for different prognostic groups. A randomized phase III study comparing 74 Gy in 2 Gy/fraction with 57 Gy and 60 Gy using 3 Gy/fraction has begun at the Institute of Cancer Research/Royal Marsden Hospital, London, and with Department of Health support will aim to increase recruitment to a larger cohort of 450 men in a multicenter study. These centers have reported acceptable rates of toxicity in abstracted form and mature outcome for local control and late complication are awaited with much interest.

Verifying radiotherapy and four-dimensional treatment strategies

Currently, the technology for shaping treatment beam and radiation dose distributions far exceeds the ability to localize tumor extent and variability in internal target position using conventional means. Furthermore, there are inaccuracies in treatment and patient set-up during a fractionated course of radiotherapy that need to be addressed. Laser guidance systems and patient immobilization devices are often used to aid reproducibility of the treatment position. New approaches to these issues involve the development of systems that use patient surface or multiregion sensing with automated linkage to predefined topologic maps or treatment portals, and delivery simultaneously correlated to automated indexed treatment couches based on the realtime information gleaned from the patient on the therapy bed.

Traditional methods to verify static prostate radiation fields involved exposing radiographic film to a small test dose for each delivered field portal. Recently, this same task has been replaced by electronic portal imaging devices (EPIDs). This method conveniently avoids the need for film and provides digital advantages in terms of image processing, transfer, and storage. However, the disadvantage of these systems is that only the prostate radiation field shapes are verified. It is well known that the anatomic position of the prostate/seminal vesicles within the pelvis can vary from day to day and is influenced by the physiologic activity of the surrounding pelvic organs.[55] There is little information available from EPIDs to determine if the internal organs, such as the prostate and/or seminal vesicles, are within the treatment portal unless a radioopaque marker is implanted to provide a surrogate measure.

A variety of methods have been investigated to address the issue of prostate organ motion, each with their peculiar advantages and disadvantages. Some investigators have used rectal obturators or balloons,[57] while others have utilized special transurethral catheters with radioopaque markers[110] to help reproduce the treatment position. One disadvantage of these methods is the need for daily instrumentation, which may not be well tolerated by patients. Daily localization of the prostate gland can be performed using a portable ultrasound machine (BAT or B-mode acquisition targeting ultrasound system, Nomos Corporation), which provides spatial localization of the prostate correlated to the position of the patient on the therapy couch. This method relies heavily on operator expertise for reliability.

Another method is to use implanted markers within the prostate. The position of the radioopaque markers in relation to bony pelvic landmarks imaged using EPIDs can then be used to correct for errors in field placement. More recent approaches to this consider a four-dimensional (4D) strategy (with time as the fourth dimension) or the realtime element of the prostate position during radiation delivery. Again, implanted radioopaque markers in the prostate or body/pelvic surface contours with deformable organ modeling act as surrogates for prostate gland position to permit tracking and/or gating of radiation treatment in realtime. This approach is the subject of a research project, called ON-TARGET (ONline Tracking And Realtime Gated External beam Therapy), in several clinical subsites, including the prostate, at our institution. This ON-TARGET project uses the Elekta Synergy (Elekta Oncology Systems) in which an x-ray volumetric imager device capable of kilovoltage (kV) cone beam imaging forms part of the linear accelerator (LINAC). This digital kV flat panel device provides the opportunity for 3D cross-sectional and fluoroscopic imaging of the patient on a linear accelerator (Figure 20.5A). This system can also provide 3D information for treatment verification. Similar systems for 3D and kV imaging on the LINAC have been developed by Varian Oncology Systems with their On-Board Imager (Figure 20.5B) and by Siemens Artiste (Figure 20.5C). The latter system differs from both the Varian and Elekta systems by having its kV imager along the same axis as the gantry head instead of perpendicular to the irradiation axis.

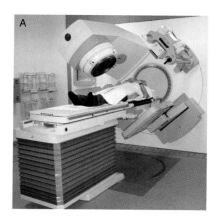

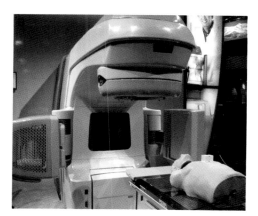

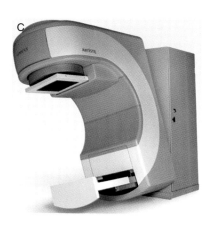

Figure 20.5

A kilovoltage x-ray imager (arrow) capable of obtaining cross-sectional volumetric and fluoroscopic images is mounted perpendicular to the gantry head of a linear accelerator. Examples are shown of *A*, Elekta Synergy XVI system; *B*, Varian On-Board Imager system; and *C*, Siemens Artiste system.

Courtesy of Elekta Oncology Systems (A), Varian Medical Systems (B), and Siemens Medical Solutions (C).

Another novel system that is in current usage incorporates a CT scanner within the LINAC, delivering treatment in a helical tomotherapy method (TomoTherapy Inc, Wisconsin).

Other available systems that can track the prostate include the system sponsored by Mitsubishi Electronics at the Hokkaido University School of Medicine and the CyberKnife (Accuray Inc, Sunnyvale, CA). The Hokkaido University system uses a linear accelerator synchronized with a fluoroscopic realtime tumor tracking system which has four sets of diagnostic x-ray television systems, each adjusted such that the central axis of the individual systems would cross at the isocenter of the linear accelerator (Figure 20.6). Together with a moving object recognition software system, this system has been reported to have an accuracy of ±1 mm in determining the position of the implanted marker every 0.033 s during radiotherapy.[111]

The CyberKnife is a 6-MV linear accelerator mounted on a computer-controlled robotic arm and is equipped with an orthogonal pair of diagnostic quality digital x-ray imaging devices that monitor the position of implanted markers (Figure 20.7). It has been reported that the CyberKnife allows delivery with a precision of less than 0.5 mm and a tracking error of less than 1 mm to the position of the radioopaque markers.[112]

The guiding principle of all these systems is that by accurate localization to the actual position of the target at the time of delivery, either gated or not, geographic miss and set-up errors will be avoided, treatment margins can be reduced, and dose escalation can be safely delivered. However, regardless of the system used and its possible complexity, it is imperative that protocols and adequate quality assurance are present to ensure safety of the system for patient use.

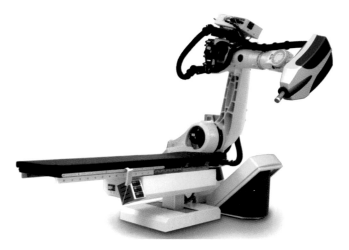

Figure 20.7
CyberKnife.
Courtesy of Accuray Inc.

Summary

External beam irradiation is a well established curative treatment modality for men with nonmetastatic prostate cancer and additionally has a role in palliation of patients with metastatic disease. Recent technologic developments have changed prostate radiotherapy practice. The widespread availability of cross-sectional CT imaging with the development of software to reconstruct anatomy and manipulate 3D images, together with hardware such as MLC, has enabled the routine use of conformal radiotherapy. The addition of multimodality morphologic imaging, such as pelvic MRI, has enhanced volume definition for treatment planning in prostate cancer.

Sophisticated computing has allowed the development of IMRT. These developments and techniques have permitted the safe escalation of radiation dose in prostate cancer. The published data suggest a dose–response relationship for different prognostic groups of patients with prcostate cancer. Early randomized data is encouraging but long-term results are needed to confirm this outcome.

Further refinements in radiotherapy strategy for prostate cancer will include consideration of the radiobiologic rationale for hypofractionation in prostate cancer and the assessment of volumes appropriate to the prognostic group for high-dose irradiation. The utilization of biologic images to include functional, biochemical, metabolic, and physiologic data may aid in defining more appropriate treatment volumes. Technologic advances have ushered the capability to consider 4D treatment strategies for online realtime and/or gated treatments to further enhance accuracy and reliability of high-dose radiation schemes. Further developments for 4D treatments are expected into the next decade. This will substantially alter the way the practice of radiotherapy is perceived and influence the manner in which patients are treated with radiotherapy.

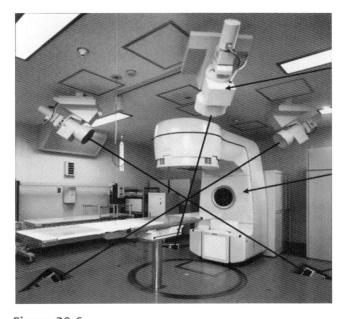

Figure 20.6
Hokkaido University motion-gated linear accelerator system and fluoroscopic realtime tumor tracking system.

Reprinted from Int J Radiation Oncology Biol Phys, 48, Shirato et al, Four-dimensional treatment planning and fluoroscopic real-time tumor tracking radiotherapy for moving tumor, 435–442, 2000, with permission from Elsevier.

References

1. Dearnaley DP, Melia J. Early prostate cancer—to treat or not to treat? Lancet 1997;349:892–893.
2. Chodak GW, Thisted RA, Gerber GS, et al. Results of conservative management of clinically localised prostate cancer. N Engl J Med 1994;330:242–248.

3. Partin AW, Kattan MW, Subong EN, et al. Combination of prostate-specific antigen, clinical stage, and Gleason score to predict pathological stage of localized prostate cancer. A multi-institutional update. JAMA 1997;277:1445–1451.

4. Roach M 3rd, Marquez C, Yuo HS, et al. Predicting the risk of lymph node involvement using the pre-treatment prostate specific antigen and Gleason score in men with clinically localized prostate cancer. Int J Radiat Oncol Biol Phys 1994;28:33–37.

5. Parker CC, Norman AR, Huddart RA, et al. Pre-treatment nomogram for biochemical control after neoadjuvant androgen deprivation and radical radiotherapy for clinically localised prostate cancer. Br J Cancer 2002;86:686–691.

6. Kattan MW, Zelefsky MJ, Kupelian PA, et al. Pretreatment nomogram for predicting the outcome of three-dimensional conformal radiotherapy in prostate cancer. J Clin Oncol 2000;18:3352–3359.

7. Paulson DF, Lin GH, Hinshaw W, et al. Radical surgery versus radiotherapy for adenocarcinoma of the prostate. J Urol 1982;128:502–504.

8. Hanks GE. More on the Uro-Oncology Research Group report of radical surgery vs. radiotherapy for adenocarcinoma of the prostate. Int J Radiat Oncol Biol Phys 1988;14:1053–1054.

9. NIH Consensus Development Conference. Management of clinically localized prostate cancer. Oncology (Huntingt) 1987;1:46–49, 54.

10. D'Amico AV, Whittington R, Malkowicz SB, et al. Biochemical outcome after radical prostatectomy or external beam radiation therapy for patients with clinically localized prostate carcinoma in the prostate specific antigen era. Cancer 2002;95:281–286.

11. Kupelian PA, Elshaikh M, Reddy CA, et al. Comparison of the efficacy of local therapies for localized prostate cancer in the prostate-specific antigen era: a large single-institution experience with radical prostatectomy and external-beam radiotherapy. J Clin Oncol 2002;20:3376–3385.

12. Vicini FA, Martinez A, Hanks G, et al. An interinstitutional and interspecialty comparison of treatment outcome data for patients with prostate carcinoma based on predefined prognostic categories and minimum follow-up. Cancer 2002;95:2126–2135.

13. Morgan WR, Bergstralh EJ, Zincke H. Long-term evaluation of radical prostatectomy as treatment for clinical stage C (T3) prostate cancer. Urology 1993;41:113–120.

14. van den Ouden D, Davidson PJT, Hop W, Schroder FH. Radical prostatectomy as a monotherapy for locally advanced (stage T3) prostate cancer. J Urol 1994;151:646–651.

15. Gerber GS, Thisted RA, Chodak GW, et al. Results of radical prostatectomy in men with locally advanced prostate cancer: multi-institutional pooled analysis. Eur Urol 1997;32:385–390.

16. Zagars GK, von-Eschenbach AC, Johnson DE, et al. Stage C adenocarcinoma of the prostate. An analysis of 551 patients treated with external beam radiation. Cancer 1987;60:1489–1499.

17. Pilepich MV, Krall JM, Sause WT, et al. Prognostic factors in carcinoma of the prostate—analysis of RTOG study 75-06. Int J Radiat Oncol Biol Phys 1987;13:339–349.

18. Hanks GE, Hanlon AL, Hudes G, et al. Patterns-of-failure analysis of patients with high pretreatment prostate-specific antigen levels treated by radiation therapy: the need for improved systemic and locoregional treatment. J Clin Oncol 1996;14:1093–1097.

19. Shipley WU, Thames HD, Sandler HM, et al. Radiation therapy for clinically localized prostate cancer: a multi-institutional pooled analysis. JAMA 1999;281:1598–1604.

20. Hanlon AL, Hanks GE. Failure pattern implications following external beam irradiation of prostate cancer: long-term follow-up and indications of cure. Cancer J 2000;6(Suppl 2):S193–197.

21. Vicini FA, Kestin LL, Martinez AA. The correlation of serial prostate specific antigen measurements with clinical outcome after external beam radiation therapy of patients for prostate carcinoma. Cancer 2000;88:2305–2318.

22. RTOG-EORTC. LENT SOMA Tables: Tables of contents. Radiother Oncol 1995;35:17–60.

23. Duncan W, Warde P, Catton CN, et al. Carcinoma of the prostate: results of radical radiotherapy (1970–1985). Int J Radiat Oncol Biol Phys 1993;26:203–210.

24. Amdur RJ, Parsons JT, Fitzgerald LT, et al. Adenocarcinoma of the prostate treated with external-beam radiation therapy: 5-year minimum follow-up. Radiother Oncol 1990;18:235–246.

25. Mithal NP, Hoskin PJ. External beam radiotherapy for carcinoma of the prostate: a retrospective study. Clin Oncol (R Coll Radiol) 1993;5:297–301.

26. Leibel SA, Hanks GE, Kramer S. Patterns of Care outcome studies: results of the national practice in adenocarcinoma of the prostate. Int J Radiat Oncol Biol Phys 1984;10:401–409.

27. Hanks GE, Diamond JJ, Krall JM, et al. A ten year follow-up of 682 patients treated for prostate cancer with radiation therapy in the United States. Int J Radiat Oncol Biol Phys 1987;13:499–505.

28. Hanks GE. External beam irradiation for clinically localised prostate cancer: Patterns of Care studies in the United States. NCI Monogr 1988;7:75–84.

29. Shipley WU, Zietman AL, Hanks GE, et al. Treatment related sequelae following external beam radiation for prostate cancer: a review with an update in patients with stages T1 and T2 tumor. J Urol 1994;152:1799–1805.

30. Lawton CA, Won M, Pilepich MV, et al. Long-term treatment sequelae following external beam irradiation for adenocarcinoma of the prostate: analysis of RTOG studies 7506 and 7706. Int J Radiat Oncol Biol Phys 1991;21:935–939.

31. Pilepich MV, Asbell SO, Krall JM, et al. Correlation of radiotherapeutic parameters and treatment related morbidity—analysis of RTOG Study 77-06. Int J Radiat Oncol Biol Phys 1987;13:1007–1012.

32. Dewit L, Ang KK, Van der Schueren E. Acute side effects and late complications after radiotherapy of localized carcinoma of the prostate. Cancer Treat Rev 1983;10:79–89.

33. Roach M, Chin DM, Holland J, et al. A pilot study of sexual function and quality of life following 3D conformal radiotherapy for clinically localised prostate cancer. Int J Radiat Oncol Biol Phys 1996;35:869–874.

34. Pilepich MV, Krall JM, al-Sarraf M et al. Androgen deprivation with radiation therapy compared with radiation therapy alone for locally advanced prostatic carcinoma: a randomized comparative trial of the Radiation Therapy Oncology Group. Urology 1995;45:616–623.

35. Potosky AL, Legler J, Albertsen PC, et al. Health outcomes after prostatectomy or radiotherapy for prostate cancer: results from the Prostate Cancer Outcomes Study. J Natl Cancer Inst 2000;92:1582–1592.

36. Horwitz EM, Vicini FA, Ziaja EL, et al. Assessing the variability of outcome for patients treated with localized prostate irradiation using different definitions of biochemical control. Int J Radiat Oncol Biol Phys 1996;36:565–571.

37. Leibel SA, Ling CC, Kutcher GJ, et al. The biological basis for conformal three-dimensional radiation therapy. Int J Radiat Oncol Biol Phys 1991;21:805–811.

38. Fuks Z, Leibel SA, Wallner JE, et al. The effect of local control on metastatic dissemination in carcinoma of the prostate: long term results in patients treated with I-125 implantation. Int J Radiat Oncol Biol Phys 1991;21:537–547.

39. Perez CA, Walz BJ, Zivnuska FR. Irradiation of carcinoma of the prostate localized to the pelvis: Analysis of tumor response and prognosis. Int J Radiat Oncol Biol Phys 1980;6:555–563.

40. Hanks GE, Martz KL, Diamond JJ. The effect of dose on local control of prostate cancer. Int J Radiat Oncol Biol Phys 1988;15:1299–1305.

41. Hanks GE, Krall JM, Martz KL, et al. The outcome of 313 patients with T1 (UICC) prostate cancer treated with external beam irradiation. Int J Radiat Oncol Biol Phys 1988;14:243–248.

42. Smit WGJM, Helle PA, van Putten LJ, Wijnmaalen AJ, et al. Late radiation damage in prostate cancer patients treated by high dose external beam radiotherapy in relation to rectal dose. Int J Radiat Oncol Biol Phys 1990;18:23–29.

43. Goitein M, Wittenberg J, Mendiondo M, et al. The value of CT scanning in radiation therapy treatment planning: A prospective study. Int J Radiat Oncol Biol Phys 1979;5:1787–1798.

44. ICRU-50. International Commission on Radiation Units and Measurements. ICRU Report 50: Prescribing, recording, and reporting

photon beam therapy. Bethesda, MD: International Commission on Radiation Units and Measurement 1993, pp 3–16.

45. ICRU-62. International Commission on Radiation Units and Measurements. ICRU Report 62: Prescribing, recording, and reporting photon beam therapy. Bethesda, MD: International Commission on Radiation Units and Measurement 1999, pp 3–20.

46. Khoo VS, Dearnaley DP, Finnigan DJ, et al. Magnetic resonance imaging (MRI): considerations and applications in radiotherapy planning. Radiother Oncol 1997;42:1–15.

47. Sannazzari GL, Ragona R, Ruo Redda MG, et al. CT-MRI image fusion for delineation of volumes in three-dimensional conformal radiation therapy in the treatment of localized prostate cancer. Br J Radiol 2002;75:603–607.

48. Pickett B, Vigneault E, Kurhanewicz J, Verhey L, Roach M. Static field intensity modulation to treat a dominant intra-prostatic lesion to 90 Gy compared to seven field 3-dimensional radiotherapy. Int J Radiat Oncol Biol Phys 1999;44:921–929.

49. Pouliot J, Kim Y, Lessard E, et al. Inverse planning for HDR prostate brachytherapy used to boost dominant intraprostatic lesions defined by magnetic resonance spectroscopy imaging. Int J Radiat Oncol Biol Phys 2004;59:1196–1207.

50. Dearnaley DP, Khoo VS, Norman A, et al. Comparison of radiation side-effects of conformal and conventional radiotherapy in prostate cancer: a randomised trial. Lancet 1999;353:267–272.

51. Bayley AJ, Catton CN, Haycocks T, et al. A randomized trial of supine vs. prone positioning in patients undergoing escalated dose conformal radiotherapy for prostate cancer. Radiother Oncol 2004;70:37–44.

52. Soffen EM, Hanks GE, Hwang CC, et al. Conformal static field therapy for low volume low grade prostate cancer with rigid immobilization. Int J Radiat Oncol Biol Phys 1991;20:141–146.

53. Fiorino C, Reni M, Bolognesi A, et al. Set-up error in supine-positioned patients immobilized with two different modalities during conformal radiotherapy of prostate cancer. Radiother Oncol 1998;49:133–141.

54. Nutting CM, Khoo VS, Walker V, et al. A randomized study of the use of a customized immobilization system in the treatment of prostate cancer with conformal radiotherapy. Radiother Oncol 2000;54:1–9.

55. Padhani AR, Khoo VS, Suckling J, et al. Evaluating the effect of rectal distension and movement on prostate gland position using cine MRI. Int J Radiat Oncol Biol Phys 1999;44:525–533.

56. D'Amico AV, Manola J, Loffredo M, et al. A practical method to achieve prostate gland immobilization and target verification for daily treatment. Int J Radiat Oncol Biol Phys 2001;51:1431–1436.

57. Wachter S, Gerstner N, Dorner D, et al. The influence of a rectal balloon tube as internal immobilization device on variations of volumes and dose–volume histograms during treatment course of conformal radiotherapy for prostate cancer. Int J Radiat Oncol Biol Phys 2002;52:91–100.

58. Fransson P, Bergstrom P, Lofroth PO, et al. Daily-diary evaluated side effects of dose-escalation radiotherapy of prostate cancer using the stereotactic BeamCath technique. Acta Oncol 2003;42:326–333.

59. Khoo VS, Padhani AR, Tanner SF, et al. Comparison of MRI sequences with CT for the radiotherapy planning of prostate cancer: a feasibility study. Br J Radiol 1999;72:590–597.

60. Ohori M, Scardino PT, Lapin SL, et al. The mechanisms and prognostic significance of seminal vesicle involvement by prostate cancer. Am J Surg Pathol 1993;17:1252–1261.

61. Kestin L, Goldstein N, Vicini F, et al. Treatment of prostate cancer with radiotherapy: should the entire seminal vesicles be included in the clinical target volume? Int J Radiat Oncol Biol Phys 2002;54:686–697.

62. Golimbu M, Morales P, Al-Askari S, et al. Extended pelvic lymphadenectomy for prostatic cancer. J Urol 1979;121:617–620.

63. Heidenreich A, Varga Z, Von Knobloch R. Extended pelvic lymphadenectomy in patients undergoing radical prostatectomy: high incidence of lymph node metastasis. J Urol 2002;167:1681–1686.

64. Khoo VS, Bedford JL, Webb S, et al. Comparison of 2D and 3D algorithms for adding a margin to the gross tumor volume in the conformal radiotherapy planning of prostate cancer. Int J Radiat Oncol Biol Phys 1998;42:673–679.

65. Khoo VS, Bedford JL, Webb S, et al. Class solutions for conformal external beam prostate radiotherapy. Int J Radiat Oncol Biol Phys 2003;55:1109–1120.

66. Rowbottom CG, Khoo VS, Webb S. Simultaneous optimization of beam orientations and beam weights in conformal radiotherapy. Med Phys 2001;28:1696–1702.

67. Bedford J, Henrys A, Dearnaley D, et al. Treatment planning evaluation of non-coplanar techniques for conformal radiotherapy of the prostate. Radiother Oncol 2005; 75:287–292.

68. De Meerleer GO, Vakaet LA, De Gersem WR, et al. Radiotherapy of prostate cancer with or without intensity modulated beams: a planning comparison. Int J Radiat Oncol Biol Phys 2000;47:639–648.

69. Fiorino C, Broggi S, Corletto D, et al. Conformal irradiation of concave-shaped PTVs in the treatment of prostate cancer by simple 1D intensity-modulated beams. Radiother Oncol 2000;55:49–58.

70. Bos LJ, Damen EM, de Boer RW, et al. Reduction of rectal dose by integration of the boost in the large-field treatment plan for prostate irradiation. Int J Radiat Oncol Biol Phys 2002;52:254–265.

71. Nutting CM, Convery DJ, Cosgrove VP, et al. Reduction of small and large bowel irradiation using an optimized intensity-modulated pelvic radiotherapy technique in patients with prostate cancer. Int J Radiat Oncol Biol Phys 2000;48:649–656.

72. Benk VA, Adams JA, Shipley WU, et al. Late rectal bleeding following combined x-ray and proton high dose irradiation for patients with stages T3–T4 prostate carcinoma. Int J Radiat Oncol Biol Phys 1993;26:551–7.

73. Lu Y, Song PY, Li SD, et al. A method of analyzing rectal surface area irradiated and rectal complications in prostate conformal radiotherapy. Int J Radiat Oncol Biol Phys 1995;33:1121–1125.

74. Boersma LJ, van den Brink M, Bruce AM, et al. Estimation of the incidence of late bladder and rectum complications after high-dose (70–78 Gy) conformal radiotherapy for prostate cancer, using dose–volume histograms. Int J Radiat Oncol Biol Phys 1998;41:83–92.

75. Storey MR, Pollack A, Zagars G, et al. Complications from radiotherapy dose escalation in prostate cancer: preliminary results of a randomized trial. Int J Radiat Oncol Biol Phys 2000;48:635–642.

76. Jackson A, Skwarchuk MW, Zelefsky MJ, et al. Late rectal bleeding after conformal radiotherapy of prostate cancer. II. Volume effects and dose–volume histograms. Int J Radiat Oncol Biol Phys 2001;49:685–698.

77. Wachter S, Gerstner N, Goldner G, et al. Rectal sequelae after conformal radiotherapy of prostate cancer: dose–volume histograms as predictive factors. Radiother Oncol 2001;59:65–70.

78. Fiorino C, Cozzarini C, Vavassori V, et al. Relationships between DVHs and late rectal bleeding after radiotherapy for prostate cancer: analysis of a large group of patients pooled from three institutions. Radiother Oncol 2002;64:1–12.

79. Fiorino C, Sanguineti G, Cozzarini C, et al. Rectal dose–volume constraints in high-dose radiotherapy of localized prostate cancer. Int J Radiat Oncol Biol Phys 2003;57:953–962.

80. Pollack A, Zagars GK, Starkschall G, et al. Prostate cancer radiation dose response: results of the M. D. Anderson phase III randomized trial. Int J Radiat Oncol Biol Phys 2002;53:1097–1105.

81. Gallagher MJ, Brereton HD, Rostock RA, et al. A prospective study of treatment techniques to minimize the volume of pelvic small bowel with reduction of acute and late effects associated with pelvic irradiation. Int J Radiat Oncol Biol Phys 1986;12:1565–1573.

82. Marks LB, Carroll PR, Dugan TC, et al. The response of the urinary bladder, urethra, and ureter to radiation and chemotherapy. Int J Radiat Oncol Biol Phys 1995;31:1257–1280.

83. Emami B, Lyman J, Brown A, et al. Tolerance of normal tissue to therapeutic radiation. Int J Radiat Oncol Biol Phys 1991;21:109–122.

84. Gildersleve J, Dearnaley DP, Evans PM, et al. Reproducibility of patient positioning during routine radiotherapy, as assessed by an integrated megavoltage imaging system. Radiother Oncol 1995;35:151–160.

85. Dearnaley DP, Khoo VS, Norman AR, et al. Comparison of radiation side-effects of conformal and conventional radiotherapy in prostate cancer: a randomised trial. Lancet 1999;353:267–272.

86. Williams MV, Denekamp J, Fowler JF. Dose response relationships for human tumours: implications for clinical trials of dose modifying agents. Int J Radiat Oncol Biol Phys 1984;10:1703–1707.

87. Thames HD, Schultheiss TE, Hendry JH, et al. Can modest escalations of dose be detected as increased tumor control? Int J Radiat Oncol Biol Phys 1992;22:241–246.

88. Hanks GE, Krall JM, Hanlon AL, et al. Patterns of Care and RTOG studies in prostate cancer: long-term survival, hazard rate observations, and possibilities of cure. Int J Radiat Oncol Biol Phys 1994;28:39–45.

89. Fiveash JB, Hanks G, Roach M, et al. 3D conformal radiation therapy (3DCRT) for high grade prostate cancer: a multi-institutional review. Int J Radiat Oncol Biol Phys 2000;47:335–342.

90. Zelefsky MJ, Leibel SA, Gaudin PB, et al. Dose escalation with three-dimensional conformal radiation therapy affects the outcome in prostate cancer. Int J Radiat Oncol Biol Phys 1998;41:491–500.

91. Valicenti R, Lu J, Pilepich M, et al. Survival advantage from higher-dose radiation therapy for clinically localized prostate cancer treated on the Radiation Therapy Oncology Group trials. J Clin Oncol 2000;18:2740–2746.

92. D'Amico AV, Chen MH, Oh-Ung J, et al. Changing prostate-specific antigen outcome after surgery or radiotherapy for localized prostate cancer during the prostate-specific antigen era. Int J Radiat Oncol Biol Phys 2002;54:436–441.

93. Dearnaley DP, Hall E, Lawrence D, et al. Phase III pilot study of dose escalation using conformal radiotherapy in prostate cancer: PSA control and side effects. Br J Cancer 2005;92:488–498.

94. Seddon B, Bidmead M, Wilson J, et al. Target volume definition in conformal radiotherapy for prostate cancer: Quality assurance in the MRC RT–01 trial. Radiother Oncol 2000;56:73–83.

95. Sydes MR, Stephens RJ, Moore AR, et al. Implementing the UK Medical Research Council (MRC) RT01 trial (ISRCTN 47772397): methods and practicalities of a randomised controlled trial of conformal radiotherapy in men with localised prostate cancer. Radiother Oncol 2004;72:199–211.

96. Lebesque J, Koper P, Slot A, Tabak H, et al. Acute and late GI and GU toxicity after prostate irradiation to doses of 68 Gy and 78 Gy: results of a randomized trial. Int J Radiat Oncol Biol Phys 2003;57:S152.

97. Beckendorf V, Bachaud JM, Bey P, et al. [Target–volume and critical-organ delineation for conformal radiotherapy of prostate cancer: experience of French dose-escalation trials]. Cancer Radiother 2002;6(Suppl 1):78s–92s.

98. Staffurth J, Dearnaley D, McNair H, et al. Early results of a phase 2 trial of pelvic nodal irradiation in prostate cancer IMRT. Clin Oncol 2003;15:S17.

99. Zelefsky MJ, Fuks Z, Hunt M, et al. High-dose intensity modulated radiation therapy for prostate cancer: early toxicity and biochemical outcome in 772 patients. Int J Radiat Oncol Biol Phys 2002;53:1111–1116.

100. Brenner DJ, Hall EJ. Fractionation and protraction for radiotherapy of prostate carcinoma. Int J Radiat Oncol Biol Phys 1999;43:1095–1101.

101. Fowler J, Chappell R, Ritter M. Is alpha/beta for prostate tumors really low? Int J Radiat Oncol Biol Phys 2001;50:1021–1031.

102. Haustermans KM, Hofland I, Van Poppel H, et al. Cell kinetic measurements in prostate cancer. Int J Radiat Oncol Biol Phys 1997;37:1067–1070.

103. Rew DA, Wilson GD. Cell production rates in human tissues and tumours and their significance. Part II: clinical data. Eur J Surg Oncol 2000;26:405–417.

104. Yeoh EE, Fraser RJ, McGowan RE, et al. Evidence for efficacy without increased toxicity of hypofractionated radiotherapy for prostate carcinoma: early results of a Phase III randomized trial. Int J Radiat Oncol Biol Phys 2003;55:943–955.

105. Lukka H, Hayter C, Warde P, et al. A randomized trial comparing two fractionation schedules for patients with localized prostate cancer. Int J Radiat Oncol Biol Phys 2003;57:S126.

106. Cheung R, Tucker SL, Dong L, et al. Dose–response for biochemical control among high-risk prostate cancer patients after external beam radiotherapy. Int J Radiat Oncol Biol Phys 2003;56:1234–1240.

107. Livsey JE, Cowan RA, Wylie JP, et al. Hypofractionated conformal radiotherapy in carcinoma of the prostate: five-year outcome analysis. Int J Radiat Oncol Biol Phys 2003;57:1254–1259.

108. Nahum AE, Movsas B, Horwitz EM, et al. Incorporating clinical measurements of hypoxia into tumor local control modeling of prostate cancer: implications for the alpha/beta ratio. Int J Radiat Oncol Biol Phys 2003;57:391–401.

109. Djemil T, Reddy CA, Willoughby TR, et al. Hypofractionated Intensity-Modulated Radiotherapy (70 Gy at 2.5 Gy per fraction) for localized prostate cancer. Int J Radiat Oncol Biol Phys 2003;57:S275–276.

110. Bergstrom P, Lofroth PO, Widmark A. High-precision conformal radiotherapy (HPCRT) of prostate cancer—a new technique for exact positioning of the prostate at the time of treatment. Int J Radiat Oncol Biol Phys 1998;42:305–311.

111. Shimizu S, Shirato H, Kitamura K, et al. Use of an implanted marker and real-time tracking of the marker for the positioning of prostate and bladder cancers. Int J Radiat Oncol Biol Phys 2000;48:1591–1597.

112. King CR, Lehmann J, Adler JR, Hai J. CyberKnife radiotherapy for localized prostate cancer: rationale and technical feasibility. Technol Cancer Res Treat 2003;2:25–30.

113. Perez CA, Pilepich MV, Garcia D, et al. Definitive radiation therapy in carcinoma of the prostate localized to the pelvis: experience at the Mallinckrodt Institute of Radiology. NCI Monogr 1988;7:85–94.

114. Goffinet DR, Bagshaw MA. Radiation therapy of prostate carcinoma: thirty year experience at Stanford University. In Schroder FH (ed): EORTC Genitourinary Group Monograph 8: Treatment of Prostate Cancer—Facts and Controversies. New York: Wiley–Liss, 1990, pp 209–222.

115. Shirato H, Shimizu S, Kitamura K, et al. Four-dimensional treatment planning and fluoroscopic real-time tumor tracking radiotherapy for moving tumor. Int J Radiation Oncol Biol Phys 2000;48:435–442.

21

Brachytherapy for the treatment of prostate cancer

Jamie A Cesaretti, Nelson N Stone, Johnny Kao,
Richard G Stock

Introduction

In its modern form, transperineal brachytherapy using computer-based dosimetry is capable of both curing prostate cancer and decreasing the morbidity long associated with all definitive prostate cancer treatments.[1] The application of trans-rectal ultrasound guided transperineal technique using a two-dimensional (2D) probe, first reported by Holm in 1983, heralded the era of modern image-guided prostate brachytherapy.[2] Since that time, the implant technique has evolved to its present form, allowing the brachytherapist to visualize the dose distribution in real time while radioactive sources are placed, resulting in tumoricidal doses within the prostate and minimizing radiation dose to uninvolved normal anatomy. In addition to precise source placement, brachytherapy fully utilizes the innate advantage of radiation therapy in cancer treatment by allowing for preservation of normal anatomy and functional relationships in order to preserve physiologically complex functions such as orgasm, urination and ejaculation.[3]

The application of intraoperative radiation dosimetry allows the physician to directly visualize the dosing consequences of each seed placement. These innovations allow the prostate implant to become an interactive process reliant on the combined input of the multidisciplinary care team as the procedure progresses in the surgical suite.[4]

Historical contributions

Shortly after the discovery of radium by Marie Curie in 1898, Alexander Graham Bell suggested that inserting radioactive sources directly into a tumor might be a highly effective approach to cancer therapy.[5] The use of radioactive sources to treat patients with prostate cancer was pioneered early in the 20th century by such luminaries as Hugh Hampton Young at Johns Hopkins School of Medicine and Benjamin Stockwell Barringer at the Memorial Hospital in New York City.[6] These practitioners beginning with Young's acquisition of the then extremely valuable 102 mCi of refined radium, and the development of gold-encapsulated harvested radon seeds by the Memorial Hospital physicist Giocchino Failla, carried out numerous innovative brachytherapy applications over the following decades. Several of the concepts of therapeutic radiation usage have been consistently applied since its inception. In a paper in JAMA from 1917, Young revealed a prescient appreciation of normal tissue toxicity by noting the location, date, and dose of each treatment he delivered to the patient. He was careful to not repeat transrectal radiation treatments to the same position on the rectal mucosa, and used a technique that allowed the entire prostate to be treated over a period of several days. The combinations of several different treatments were intended to add to adequate treatment of the whole prostate[7] (Figure 21.1).

In the 1970s Whitmore et al developed retropubic iodine-125 (^{125}I) radioactive seed implantation at the time of laparotomy.[8] The placement of seeds was performed freehand and was not image guided resulting in significant underdosed areas. Long-term disease control was disappointing, particularly for patients with poor dosimetry.[9] Advances in imaging—notably 2D transrectal ultrasound, computed tomography (CT)-based post-implant dosimetry and, more recently, magnetic resonance imaging (MRI) using an endorectal coil—have contributed significantly to higher quality since the mid-1980s.

Physics of brachytherapy

Radioactive sources obey physical laws, several of which are useful for the practicing urologist to fully understand. The isotopes commonly used in therapy are manmade radioactive elements, which decay at a constant rate. The isotopes chosen to treat prostate cancer emit gamma ray energy. A gamma ray has no mass, travels at the speed of light, and can display both the properties of a wave or a particle. The energy spectra of the gamma rays emitted by the isotopes used in brachytherapy are well characterized. Of particular relevance to the brachytherapist is that the dose falloff from a radioactive source obeys the inverse square law, that is it is proportional to $1/r^2$, where r is the distance from the source. In general, high-energy gamma ray sources are used for temporary implants or high dose rate (HDR) applications and low-energy sources are used for low dose rate (LDR) permanent implants. The modern treatment planning systems used by radiation oncologists are programmed to obey these physical rules as they assist in determining optimal source placement.

Iodine-125

Iodine-125 has a physical half-life of 59.4 days and relatively low photon energy of 0.028 MeV. The implications of this are that the sources require less lead shielding to protect the operating room staff and that the actual physical geometry of the seed and its

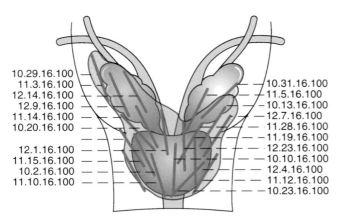

Figure 21.1
An example of an early understanding of dose-volume and time relationships in the application of brachytherapy by Hugh Hampton Young, MD. Young used a single radium source to apply multiple treatments over several months. The dwell time of the application and the date of the treatment are noted relative to this patient's locally advanced prostate cancer (in the public domain).
From Young HH. The use of radium in cancer of the prostate and bladder: A presentation of new instruments and new methods of use. JAMA 1917;68:1174–1177.

encasement significantly influence the dosimetry characteristics of the source. As the field continues to progress, new isotopes may prove to be useful, in addition to novel seed architecture.[10] The model 6711 seed (Oncura, Amersham, Buckinghamshire, England) is in common usage throughout the United States; the encapsulation consists of a 0.05-mm thick titanium tube welded at both ends forming a cylinder-like seed; the seed is 4.5 mm in length and 0.8 mm in diameter. A silver wire is at the center of the seed, making it readily identifiable during post-implant fluoroscopy. The initial dose rate of ^{125}I is lower than palladium-103 ([103]P), but due to its longer half-life, the dose is given over a longer period of time. Clinical differences between [103]P and ^{125}I in terms of outcome and symptom spectrum are minimal.[11]

Palladium-103

Palladium-103 has a physical half-life that is 17 days and photon energy of 0.021 MeV. In terms of shielding, 0.008 mm of lead thickness is required to reduce the amount of radiation emitted by 50% compared with 0.025 mm of lead for [125]I. [103]Pd has a much shorter half-life than ^{125}I, therefore, the initial dose rate of [103]Pd (20 cGy/h) must be higher than that for [125]I (7 cGy/h) in order for them to give approximately similar doses. In addition, the amount of radioactivity per seed must be more with [103]Pd than ^{125}I at the time of implant in order for the radiotherapist to be able to proscribe roughly similar levels of absorbed dose. It is important to also understand that there are significant variations in brachytherapy practice; some centers prefer to use fewer sources with a higher activity per seed, while others prefer to use a greater number of low energy sources to achieve the optimal absorbed dose. However, in most cases the total amount of activity prescribed, in mCi, is quite consistent for most centers.[12]

Iridium-192

Iridium-192 (^{192}Ir) has a physical half-life of 73.8 days, which is much longer than [103]Pd and on par with [125]I. The important physical feature of ^{192}Ir is its relatively high gamma energy, which is much higher than the LDR isotopes at 0.38 MeV. The ^{192}Ir source is used for fractionated HDR brachytherapy by using temporary indwelling catheters. The ^{192}Ir source requires much more shielding in order to protect the operative staff—it requires over a centimeter of lead to decrease the transmitted dose by 96.9% of the source intensity. [192]Ir has become the preferred source for HDR temporary implants.[13] A potential advantage for HDR is improved dose distributions due to the ability to vary dwell times of radioactive sources.[14] A major disadvantage of the HDR technique is the need for inpatient hospitalization for the duration of the implant.

Radiobiology

The characterization of the radiation sensitivity of cancer and human normal tissues has a long history from which many of the fundamental concepts of modern cancer biology have evolved. Fundamentally, the target of radiation in the cancer cell is DNA, resulting in potentially lethal double strand breaks. A complex cellular pathway is mobilized in order to maintain genomic integrity by repairing DNA lesions.[15] These DNA repair processes are able to successfully repair most types of DNA damage within a few hours. Unrepaired DNA double strand breaks will result in cell death.[16] The four major differences between the way cancer cells and normal cells respond to radiation are repair, reassortment, reoxygenation, and repopulation. Cancer cells are usually more sensitive than normal cells because they are less proficient at repairing DNA damage, are more likely to become synchronized in radiosensitive phases of the cell cycle, and become reoxygenated during the course of radiation therapy. Since the proliferative rate of prostate cancers are relatively slow, repopulation, the regrowth of tumor cells during a course of radiation, is considered a minor issue for prostate cancer. However, some clinicians choose to employ [103]Pd, with its higher initial dose rate, rather than ^{125}I to treat high grade tumors.[16,84]

Based on significant scientific and empirical evidence, the optimal approach to external beam radiation therapy (EBRT) has been to treat most cancers with standard fractions of radiation, 1.8 to 2 Gy, 5 days per week over several weeks. The alpha/beta model attempts to predict the effect of various dose-fractionation schemes on tumor and late toxicity. Most tumor cells and early reacting normal tissues (lymphocytes, gastrointestinal epithelium) have a high alpha/beta ratio (>10) whereas many types of late reacting normal tissues (skin, bone, bladder) have low alpha/beta ratios.[2–3] This model predicts that repeated small doses of radiation delivers a biologically more effective dose to tumor cells while allowing normal tissues to recover. There is some evidence that indicates that the alpha/beta ratio for prostate cancer cells may be very low, on the order of 1.5 to 2.[19] The implication of this finding is that long courses of fractionated radiotherapy or permanent seed implantation may not be the best treatment strategy for men with prostate cancer. Several radiobiologists have made a persuasive case to treat prostate cancer with very large doses of radiation per fraction over a short time period.[20,21] This concept provides the radiobiologic rationale for the recent interest in HDR brachytherapy.[22]

It is important to note that not all radiation oncologists and radiation biologists agree about the alpha/beta ratio for prostate cancer, and its implications.[23] The most important counterargument to the widespread adaptation of HDR is the considerable clinical success obtained using both LDR brachytherapy and dose escalation with EBRT using standard radiation fraction sizes realized over the past decade.[24–26] Additionally, it is not known whether HDR will result in greater late toxicity than permanent seed implant, as predicted by the alpha/beta model. To date, follow up is too short to assess the rate of late toxicity in patients treated by HDR.[22,27]

Treatment planning

Brachytherapy treatment planning is an anatomy-based concept that is entirely dependent upon properly measuring distance and volume relationships within and beyond the prostate gland. The placement of needles through a template into the prostate gland under ultrasound guidance, allows for markedly increased accuracy of seed placement compared with the obsolete retropubic freehand technique and has become the standard of care for brachytherapy.[14] Because the prostate gland has a characteristic barrel type shape, it is amenable to several different dosimetric solutions in terms of how to place radioactive sources to cover the volume.

Historically, brachytherapy planning was significantly influenced by two schools of thought, which evolved prior to the era of the modern computational power and 3D imaging. The Patterson–Parker method refers to a set of rules and tables developed in the 1940s in Manchester, UK.[28] The goal of the brachytherapy implant rules was to limit dose inhomogeneity within the implanted volume while treating the volume with a tumoricidal dose. In brief, the method places radioactive sources non-uniformly in order to achieve a uniform dose distribution. In terms of spherical shapes, such as an idealized prostate, this meant that most of the total activity of an implant was placed on the outer edges of the implanted volume. A competing system of interstitial implantation developed in the US was called the Quimby system. This system was characterized by placing all of the radioactive sources uniformly throughout the implanted structure. In general, this implant technique resulted in a non-uniform dose distribution with very high central region doses.

However, with this geometry the risk of encountering an underdosed region or "cold spot" due to seed migration is low.

Modern brachytherapy treatment planning systems allow for preoperative images from either ultrasound or CT to be captured and manipulated as 3D objects. The current planning system known as the computer system calculates 3D doses to the implanted volume. However, our current philosophy of implanting 75% to 80% of the activity in the peripheral needles and 20% to 25% of the activity in the interior needles is reminiscent of the Patterson–Parker philosophy. When pursuing a preplanned strategy, details such as hip and leg position become very important in order to assure that, at the time of implant, the plan generated by the physicist can be successfully produced at the time of implant. This method has been well described and is widely used in the US.[29] Using the preplanned approach, seeds may be implanted by either preloaded needles or the Mick applicator.[14]

Another solution is to use intraoperative images captured at the time of implant to plan the procedure in real time.[4] This method also allows the operator to account for variations in patient set-up, intra- and interoperative prostate gland movement, and prostate swelling secondary to the trauma caused by needle placement. The seeds can be placed in the gland using the Mick applicator (Mick TP-200, Mick Radionuclear Instruments. Mount Vernon, NY), under the guidance of the biplanar transrectal ultrasound probe.[30] As the procedure progresses, the treating team can determine optimal placement of seeds in order to cover the prostate gland, and avoid the urethra and rectum[4] (Figure 21.2).

Dosing and constraints

In radiation oncology the concept of radiation dosing and dose constraints are of fundamental importance to successful and optimal treatment. From a modern perspective when using 3D planning the dose of radiation can be defined for the entire 3D structure. Modern treatment planning systems require the user to delineate, by outlining, structures of interest on a computer screen. In prostate cancer treatment, these structures include the prostate, urethra,

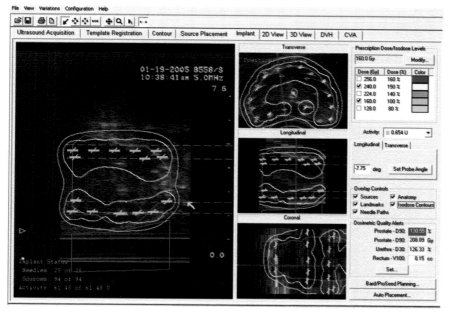

Figure 21.2
Sagittal image of prostate and rectum encompassed by prescription dose. Seed placement (hashed rectangles) is continually modified throughout the case in order to conform prescription dose and limit high-dose regions (interior isodose clouds).

bladder wall, and rectal wall. The dose to these structures can be quantified and analyzed in a number of different ways that emphasize important concepts in radiation oncology: low-dose regions or "cold spots" may lead to tumor relapse, while high-dose regions or "hot spots" in normal tissues may result in late complications.

Dose using the Standard International (SI) unit Gray (Gy, equivalent to 100 rads) can be expressed in terms of a percentage of the volume of interest. For example, D90 for the prostate is the minimum dose received by at least 90% of the prostate gland. When a typical D90 is 144 Gy, the D100 (or dose to 100% of the prostate gland) for the implant could be markedly less—on the order of 80 to 100 Gy. The reason that the D90 is often chosen as a reference value is that it is representative of the quality of the implant; also clinical correlation has been made in terms of a dose-response relationship by several investigators.[31] If one were to prescribe a dose of 144 Gy to the D95 or D100; the D90 in such an implant would be significantly hotter than 144 Gy. Such an approach has the potential of allowing concern over dose to a relatively small portion of the gland drive up the dose to the entire gland. If one were to automate such an approach using a dose constraint prescribing 144 Gy to the D100, the D90 could be as high as 240 to 280 Gy. It is also important to pay special attention to the 10% not accounted for in the D90 dosing parameter. This is done by looking at each 2D slice of a prostate implant while it is being completed. If the 90% dosing line dips into the prostate where there is a known cancerous nodule then that part of the cancer will be underdosed even though the D90 might be within an acceptable range. Therefore, successful brachytherapy requires not only thoughtful consideration by the therapeutic physics staff; but also active participation by the brachytherapist with special attention given to such details.

Determination of the volume of normal tissue receiving the prescription dose is a useful way to quantify the effects of radiation toxicity. If we know that a patient is at a much higher risk of radiation proctitis when more than 2 cm^3 is exposed to the prescription dose, then this information can be incorporated into a treatment planning system and used as a dose constraint. For normal tissues, quantifying dose constraints in terms of tissue volume is advantageous relative to quantification in terms of percentage of a volume because a significant portion of any given volume can be at no or very little risk of being exposed to radiation from brachytherapy. The bladder and the rectum are good examples of tissues that are better analyzed in terms of radiation late effects based upon the amount of tissue in each cubic centimeter receiving the prescription dose; the posterior rectum and the superior bladder should not be included in dosing considerations because they receive minimal radiation doses after implant (unless of course the patient is also receiving EBRT). In contrast, the external radiation beam must traverse normal tissues to reach the prostate.

The V100 refers to the volume of a structure in percent receiving the prescription dose. For example, if the prescription dose for an ^{125}I implant is 144 Gy, and the post-implant dosimetry study shows that the entire prostate received 144 Gy, the V100 would be 100%. A common use for V is to help the brachytherapist determine the extent of the intraprostatic hot spots of an implant. If the V150 (the volume of the prostate receiving 150% of the prescription dose) is equal to 80% and the prescription dose was 144 Gy, then the majority of the gland would be covered by 216 Gy, putting the patient at considerable risk for urinary morbidity.[30,32] If the V150 of an implant was 40% and the D90 160 Gy, this would be an optimal use of brachytherapy sources, the brachytherapist, or the planning module, would have had significant success in decreasing the intraprostatic doses and still covering the entire gland with the target dose.

Patient selection

There are several strategies one can use to decide which patients are best suited for prostate brachytherapy. Most clinicians recognize that the long-term cure rate is favorable with early stage prostate cancer regardless of the treatment strategy employed, and the selection of therapy often must be made based on expected toxicity profile and patient preferences.[33] Advice given to patients is often variable and usually represents components from the extremes of therapeutic philosophies.[34] The patients often welcome a frank discussion of tailored risks associated with the brachytherapy procedure. Certain clinical situations might require additional discussions, for example in patients with prior transurethral resection of the prostate (TURP) where there may be an increased risk of urinary toxicity and concerns of poor implant quality.[35,36] Other risks, including proctitis, incontinence, and erectile dysfunction are discussed, with a focus on our own institutional results.

Patients who present with localized prostate cancer may have a spectrum of diseases. Low-, moderate-, and high-risk prostate cancer should be recognized as different diseases that require different approaches. A patient with low-risk prostate cancer—defined as a prostate-specific antigen (PSA) of 10 ng/mL or less, a Gleason score of 6 or less, and clinical stage T2a or less—will do well with radical prostatectomy or brachytherapy. These patients have a high likelihood that disease is confined to the prostate.[37] Radical prostatectomy is not a cancer operation in which wide surgical margins are easily achieved, therefore, patients at risk for extracapsular disease are often not cured by a prostatectomy. A similar situation exists for brachytherapy. Due to the inverse square2 law, the radioactivity travels only a short distance from the sources. While brachytherapy adequately treats minimal (<3 mm) extracapsular extension typically seen in modern prostatectomy series, a seed implant in a high-risk patient is not likely to achieve an adequate peripheral radiation dose in a patient with significant extracapsular extension.[38] Thus, the ideal patient for brachytherapy monotherapy is the same as for radical prostatectomy.

Patients who present with more advanced features will require additional therapy if implantation is elected. Further work-up is required before the selection of therapy is made. Patients who present with a Gleason score of 7 or higher, or PSA above 10 ng/mL, or clinical stage greater than T2b should have a seminal vesicle biopsy to exclude extraprostatic extension to this area. Several investigators have shown that this biopsy can identify patients with disease in the seminal vesicles. Linzer et al compared a cohort of radical prostatectomy patients with those undergoing seminal vesicle biopsy.[39] In six biopsies performed of the seminal vesicle, no difference was found between these patients and the radical prostatectomy group in likelihood of positive biopsies. The chance of finding extension to the seminal vesicles was at least 20% in men with these high-risk features.

Physicians and patients who are considering brachytherapy as a treatment option do not often think about the indications for a pelvic lymph node dissection, because brachytherapy is considered a minor outpatient procedure, whereas the node dissection can have much more morbidity. High-risk patients, however, can be considered candidates for brachytherapy combined with either hormonal therapy or EBRT or both. Such patients may benefit from having the pelvic lymph nodes analyzed. Lymph node dissection can be limited to those patients with a positive seminal vesicle biopsy (33% positive) or with perineural invasion found in the biopsy specimen (27%). If the seminal vesicle biopsy is negative and the prostate biopsy specimen is free of perineural invasion, fewer than 2% will have nodal metastases.[40] An advantage of this approach is to obviate the need for nodal irradiation in patients with high-risk disease.[37,40]

In addition to disease-related selection criteria, other factors can influence the decision to offer brachytherapy. Many so-called inclusion or exclusion criteria were developed when the limitations of preplanning did not afford the flexibility of real-time planning to overcome certain technical problems, most often those related to patient anatomy. Prostate size was often limited to 50 cm³ or less because of the fear of pubic arch interference. Stone, however, has shown that patients with prostate volumes greater than 50 cm³ can have excellent results from implants when the real-time method is used.[41] Patients with prior TURP were also considered inappropriate candidates for brachytherapy because of the high risk of incontinence.[42] This complication is rare even in a patient with a prior TURP if a peripheral seed distribution is used and accurate urethral imaging guides seed deposition no closer than 5 mm to the urethra.[41] Some mistakenly call this method urethral-sparing and speculate that it is risky to place lower doses around the urethra where prostate cancer may exist. Others have likened this technique to cryoablation, where a warming catheter protects the urethra from freezing. In actuality, the urethra typically will still receive a higher dose than the prostate and is only spared the very high doses (>2× prescription dose) typically seen with a uniform seed placement.

Hormonal therapy and brachytherapy

Androgen deprivation (AD) in conjunction with EBRT has gained widespread acceptance, especially in patients with locally advanced prostate cancer.[43–46] Androgen deprivation with brachytherapy has been less well studied, although it has become accepted clinical practice for some indications. Large prostate size is probably the most agreed-upon indication for the use of hormonal therapy. The absolute prostate size for which AD should be advocated, the type of AD to use (luteinizing hormone-releasing hormone [LHRH] agonists alone or in combination with an antiandrogen), or the length of time a patient should remain on AD are not known. Data from several studies seem to indicate that a minimum of 3 months of AD will result in a 30% to 45% volume reduction. Most trials used a combination of LHRH agonists plus an antiandrogen; two trials showed an advantage with the addition of an antiandrogen to the LHRH agonist. Several also showed that patients with larger glands had a greater degree of shrinkage than those with smaller glands. If a recommendation is to be made, patients with a prostate volume greater than 50 cm³ can be considered for a short course of AD to facilitate the implantation and reduce the likelihood of postimplantation voiding difficulties.[47]

More controversy exists concerning the use of AD in patients with locally advanced disease.[48–52] Several well-performed randomized studies with AD and EBRT have demonstrated the advantages of short- and long-term AD in improving both local and systemic disease control.[43–46] In patients receiving either ¹²⁵I or ¹⁰³Pd brachytherapy, Stone has shown a clear advantage in local control when high-risk patients are treated with 6 months of AD. Of 268 men who had biopsy 2 years after implantation, 2% of those receiving AD (n = 96) had a positive biopsy, compared with 16.3% of those treated with implants alone.[53] Lee, et al has demonstrated that only high-risk patients benefit from the addition of AD and that the local control rates for low-risk patients treated by implants alone are no different from for those treated with implants plus AD.[48]

Technology

There are many similarities between EBRT and brachytherapy. Both deliver radiation therapy from X-rays (photons), and both may result in acute and chronic late radiation injuries. While ¹²⁵I and ¹⁰³Pd emit low energy X-rays, modern linear accelerators deliver high energy, penetrating radiation beams (6–18 MV). The most conformal dose distributions are obtained by an inadequate implant because of the physical advantage of the inverse square law. While high-energy radiation beams must traverse normal tissues to treat the target volume, relative rectal and bladder sparing may be achieved by 3-D conformal radiation therapy (3D-CRT) and intensity modulated radiation therapy (IMRT). Doses from EBRT have increased over the last 10 years as treatment-planning systems have become more sophisticated (3D-CRT and IMRT), and dose response studies have shown the need for increased doses with longer follow-up, or in patients with more advanced local disease.[54,55] Treatment planning with EBRT usually includes a generous margin, although margins have been scaled back as doses have increased and setup accuracy has improved with widespread adoption of B-mode abdominal ultrasound, fiducial markers, or rectal balloons. The recommended doses for ¹²⁵I and ¹⁰³Pd are 145 Gy and 124 Gy, respectively. These recommendations came from the American Association of Physicists in Medicine guidelines and are based on physics work relating to the radiobiologic characteristics of these isotopes and constructing a biologic equivalent dose (BED) to that of EBRT.[56]

The best dosing recommendations are those that have been substantiated by clinical investigation. Although ample dosing data are available for EBRT, only a few studies have addressed proper doses for prostate brachytherapy. Stock et al published the first dose response study for ¹²⁵I implants.[31] One hundred thirty-four men treated with ¹²⁵I monotherapy and followed for biochemical failure (defined as PSA > 1.0 ng/mL) were analyzed. Computed tomographic scans of the prostate were taken within 1 month of implantation, and dose volume histograms of the prostate were analyzed. Patients who had received a D90 of 140 Gy had a 92% biochemical relapse-free survival rate, compared with 48% who received a dose less than 140 Gy. Potters found similar results in an evaluation of dose and biochemical outcomes using the definition of PSA failure promulgated by the American Society for Therapeutic Radiology and Oncology (ASTRO).[57]

Stone et al also demonstrated the importance of the delivered radiation dose and biopsy results.[53] With ¹²⁵I brachytherapy, a D90 of at least 160 Gy resulted in less than 5% with a positive biopsy. No patients treated with ¹⁰³Pd to a dose of at least 120 Gy had a positive biopsy. Long-term follow up of these patients show that most achieve complete eradication of local disease by 5 years. If the D90 was at least 140 Gy (¹²⁵I), 97.2% had a negative biopsy, compared with 88.8% if the delivered dose was less.[53]

Computed tomography-based postimplantation dosimetry at approximately 1 month after implantation (to allow for postimplantation edema to subside) is a mandatory component of a high quality implant program.[58,59] Detailed analysis of prostate, urethra, and rectal doses will yield prognostic information for both disease and quality-of-life outcomes. For example, early urinary morbidity (irritative voiding symptoms) is more likely to occur when prostate and urethral doses are high.[60] The risk of radiation proctitis have also been correlated with rectal doses. Snyder et al has shown that if the volume of the rectum irradiated by 160 Gy (¹²⁵I) is kept below 1.3 cm³, grade 2 radiation proctitis will occur in less than 5% of patients.[61] This information should be used prospectively when planning the implantation to reduce this complication.

Treatment results

Assessment of treatment success following prostate brachytherapy has usually been reported based on a non-rising PSA rather than a nadir value. Most investigators have adopted the ASTRO consensus definition of three consecutive PSA rises to classify a patient as having biochemical failure.[62] Critz et al suggested that a nadir value of 0.1 or 0.2 ng/mL is more appropriate, while other definitions of biochemical failure are currently undergoing evaluation.[63,65] A PSA decline can take as long as 5 years following ^{125}I implantation.[66] During this time, 35% of patients will experience a temporary rise of PSA of at least 0.2 ng/mL followed by sustained biochemical remission.[67] The average time to PSA bounce is 24 months. Grimm has shown that if patients are followed at least 7 years, the PSA nadir and ASTRO definitions yield the same results.[68]

Low-risk patients (PSA ≤ 10 ng/mL, Gleason score <7, and clinical stage ≤ T2a) are the best candidates for brachytherapy monotherapy. Most reports demonstrate prostate-specific antigen failure-free rates between 80 and 95% at 5 years[69,70] (Table 21.1). It should be emphasized that implant quality is strongly correlated to outcome. Several studies have established that biochemical relapse-free survival is highly correlated with implant dose.[31,57] Patients implanted with ^{125}I who received a D90 of at least 140 Gy had a significantly improved rate of disease-free survival over those implanted with a lower dose. Grimm stratified patients based on date of implantation.[26] Patients treated before 1988 had an inferior outcome compared with the more contemporary patients (65% versus 87% free of failure). Although no dosimetry data were available for those earlier patients, implant quality was no doubt inferior.

Emerging MR spectroscopy data from University of California, San Francisco demonstrate that 100% of patients treated by brachytherapy had metabolic resolution of disease compared with an 86% metabolic complete response for high dose (72 Gy) EBRT. These radiographic findings translated to lower nadir PSA levels in the brachytherapy group.[71] While these data suggest that a 144 Gy implant is biologically more potent than 72 Gy of EBRT, whether this will translate to a disease control or survival advantage is unknown. Due to limited numbers of events seen in the low-risk patient population, a sizeable randomized trial would be needed to definitively address this question. A randomized trial comparing prostate brachytherapy versus radical prostatectomy, known as the SPIRIT trial, sponsored by the American College of Surgical Oncologists has been closed due to lack of accrual.

Patients presenting with intermediate- or high-risk prostate cancer may also be candidates for permanent prostate brachytherapy, usually in combination with EBRT and/or hormonal therapy. This issue is still controversial, suggesting the need for randomized studies to determine the optimal regimen. In a widely quoted retrospective comparison of three selected databases, D'Amico et al reported inferior PSA control for patients treated with brachytherapy ± hormonal therapy compared with surgery or EBRT for intermediate- and high-risk patients.[72] Lack of dosimetric data, use of orthogonal films rather than CT for postimplant dosimetry, and a limited experience in implant technique contributed to the unusually poor results in the brachytherapy arm. In stark contrast, experienced brachytherapy teams from Mount Sinai, Seattle Prostate Cancer Center, and Memorial Sloan Kettering Cancer Center have reported results comparable or superior to surgery or definitive EBRT for intermediate- and high-risk patients.[48,69,73] Nonetheless, there has been significant interest in adding EBRT and/or hormonal therapy to interstitial brachytherapy with the goal of further improving outcomes in patients with intermediate- and high-risk disease by addressing

Table 21.1 Freedom from prostate-specific antigen (PSA) failure among low-risk patients

Author	Patient (#)	Prognostic group (PSA, ng/mL)	Rate (%)	Time (years)	PSA definition of failure (ng/mL)
Stone[107]	146	PSA ≤ 10, Stage ≤ 2b, Gleason ≤ 6	91	10	ASTRO
Blasko[42]	NA	PSA 0–10	78	8	PSA > 1.0
Ragde[97]	98	Stage T1–2		10	PSA > 0.5
D'Amico[49]	123	PSA ≤ 10, Stage ≤ 2a, Gleason ≤ 6	88 (estimate from survival curve)	5	ASTRO
Grado[98]	114	Gleason 2–4	95	5	2 rises > nadir
Dattoli[99]	60	PSA 4.1–10	80	5	PSA > 1.0
Potters[100]	52	PSA ≤ 10, Stage T1–2, Gleason ≤ 6	91	5	ASTRO
Stokes[101]	72	PSA ≤ 10, Gleason ≤ 6, Stage ≤ 2a	76	5	ASTRO or PSA nadir > 1
Zelefsky[73]	146	PSA ≤ 10, Stage ≤ 2b, Gleason ≤ 6	82	5	ASTRO
Critz[102]*	451	PSA 4.1–10	93	5	PSA > 0.2
Beyer[104]	128	PSA 0–4	85	7	ASTRO or PSA > 10 or + biopsy
Lederman[105]*	164	PSA ≤ 20, Stage ≤ 2b, Gleason ≤ 6	88	6	PSA > 1.0
Sharkey[106]	528	PSA ≤ 10 and Gleason < 7	87	6	PSA > 1.5
Kwok[107]	41	PSA ≤ 10, Stage ≤ 2a, Gleason ≤ 6	85	5	ASTRO
Kollmeier[24]	75	PSA ≤ 6, Stage ≤ 2a, Gleason ≤ 6	88 94 (D90 >144)	8 8	ASTRO ASTRO
Wallner[108]	57 58	PSA 4–10, Stage ≤ 2a, Gleason ≤ 6	89(^{125}I) 91([103]Pd)	3 3	PSA > 0.5

*Indicates treatment with adjuvant EBRT.
ASTRO, definition of PSA failure promulgated by the American Society for Therapeutic Radiology and Oncology.

regional and/or micrometastatic disease. Lee et al has demonstrated 94% biochemical control in men with intermediate-risk prostate cancer treated with either ^{125}I or ^{103}Pd with 6 months of hormonal therapy and also receiving a high-dose implant (>140 Gy for ^{125}I and >100 Gy for ^{103}Pd).[48] For patients with high-risk disease, Stock reported 86% biochemical control at 5 years for patients treated by androgen ablation (9 months), brachytherapy, and external beam radiotherapy.[74]

Currently our approach is to treat patients with intermediate-risk disease with brachytherapy combined with either short-term hormonal therapy or EBRT. For high-risk disease, brachytherapy is combined with hormonal therapy and EBRT to maximize the likelihood of disease control. We prefer to deliver brachytherapy prior to EBRT, although there are no published data, to the authors' knowledge, addressing whether the sequence of treatment affects outcome. In addition to interstitial brachytherapy, temporary HDR-brachytherapy, 3D-CRT, IMRT, or proton therapies are methods of dose escalation in intermediate and high-risk patients.

Other centers using the combination therapy in high-risk patients also report promising results.[75,76]

In summary, brachytherapy alone is at least as effective as either surgery or high-dose EBRT for low-risk patients. For intermediate- and high-risk patients, brachytherapy in combination with EBRT and/or hormonal therapy is at least or more effective as surgery or external beam radiotherapy[70,75,77] (Tables 21.2 and 21.3).

Treatment morbidity

The ideal treatment for prostate cancer would eradicate the tumor and would not severely alter the patient's quality of life. Brachytherapy, an organ-preserving approach, can accomplish these goals because the radiation is placed inside the prostate and travels only a short distance from the gland. However, both early and late complications can occur following the seed implantation and are related to both technical and patient factors.

Needle and seed placement during the procedure can result in edema and bleeding within the prostate, leading to obstructive symptoms and, in some cases, to urinary retention, especially in patients with some degree of obstructive prostatism. The incidence of urinary retention ranges is usually between 4% and 7%.[4,42,76,78] The need for catheterization is generally days to weeks. In a study of 451 patients, Terk et al found that a high urinary symptom score, rather than prostate size, is the most significant predictor of postimplant retention.[79] Patients who had an International Prostate Symptom Score (IPSS) greater than 15 had a 25% likelihood of developing urinary retention. Pre- and post-treatment prostate volume and American Urological Association symptom score predicted for retention.[80]

Irritative voiding symptoms are quite common following permanent seed implantation. Patients treated with ^{125}I tend to develop urinary symptoms 1 to 2 months after implantation, whereas patients treated with ^{103}Pd may experience symptoms within 1 to 2 weeks of the implantation. Kleinberg reported urinary symptoms in 80% of patients, with complaints starting within 2 months of the implantation and lasting for 1 year in 45%.[81] Desai found that postimplantation urinary symptoms peak 1 month following implantation and gradually return to normal by 24 months.[60] Urinary symptoms were also highly correlated to the dose received by the prostate and urethra. Stone et al determined the late urinary morbidity of 250 men treated with ^{125}I who prospectively completed an IPSS assessment.[3] There were no significant changes between the pretreatment individual, total, and quality-of-life scores and post-treatment scores an average of 3 years following implantation.

Late urinary complications include stricture and incontinence. Patients who have had prior prostate surgery, such as a TURP, may be at greater risk for urinary incontinence. The Seattle group report an almost 20% rate of incontinence among patients that had a prior TURP.[36] The preplanned technique combined with a uniform

Table 21.2 Freedom from prostate-specific antigen (PSA) failure among moderate risk patients

Author	Patient (#)	Prognostic group (PSA, ng/mL)	Rate (%)	Time (years)	PSA definition of failure (ng/mL)
Blasko[42]	NA	PSA 10–20	67	8	PSA > 1.0
Ragde[97]*	152	Stage T1–T3	66	10	PSA > 0.5
D'Amico[49]	53	(1 feature: PSA 10.1–20, Stage 2b, Gleason 7)	34	5	ASTRO
Grado[98]*†	262	Gleason 5–6	82	5	2 rises > nadir
Dattoli[99]*	29	PSA 10–20	75	5	PSA > 1.0
Potters[100]*	NA	PSA > 10, Stage > T2, Gleason > 6	85	5	ASTRO
Stokes[101]	75	PSA 10–20, Stage 2b, Gleason ≤ 6	64	5	ASTRO or PSA nadir > 1
Critz[102]*	144	PSA 10.1–20	75	5	PSA > 0.2
Singh[103]*	47	(1 feature: PSA > 10, Gleason ≥ 7)	85	3	ASTRO
Beyer[104]	345	PSA 4.1–10	66	7	ASTRO or PSA > 10 or + biopsy
Lederman[105]*	124	PSA ≥ 20, Stage ≥ 2c, Gleason ≥ 7	75	6	PSA > 1.0
Sharkey[106]	287	PSA > 10 or Gleason ≥ 7	77	6	PSA > 1.5
Kwok[107]	33	(1 feature: PSA >10, Stage ≥ 2b, Gleason ≥ 7)	63	5	ASTRO
Kollmeier[24]	70	(1 feature: PSA 10.1–20, Stage 2b, Gleason 7)	81	8	ASTRO

*Indicates treatment with adjuvant EBRT; †87% of reported patients were treated with adjuvant external beam radiation therapy.
ASTRO, definition of PSA failure promulgated by the American Society for Therapeutic Radiology and Oncology.

Table 21.3 Freedom from prostate-specific antigen (PSA) failure among high risk patients

Author	Patient (#)	Prognostic group (PSA, ng/mL)	Rate (%)	Time (years)	PSA definition of failure (ng/mL)
Blasko[42]	NA	PSA > 20	36	8	PSA >1.0
D'Amico[49]	42	(1 feature: PSA > 20, Stage 2c, Gleason > 7)	15(est)	2	ASTRO
Grado[98]*	114	Gleason ≥ 7	58	5	2 rises > nadir
Dattoli[99]*	35	PSA > 20	70	5	PSA >1.0
Potters[100]*	NA	(>1 feature: PSA >10, Stage > T2, Gleason > 6)	85	5	ASTRO
Stokes[101]	39	Stage 2c or 3, Gleason ≥ 7	36	5	ASTRO or PSA nadir > 1
Critz[102]*	44	PSA > 20	75	5	PSA > 0.2
Singh[103]*	18	(2 features: PSA > 10, Gleason > 6)	85	3	ASTRO
Beyer[104]	144	PSA 10.1–20 PSA > 20	53	7	ASTRO or PSA > 10
	73		33	7	or + biopsy
Lederman[105]*	59	(>1 feature: PSA ≥ 20, Stage ≥ 2c, Gleason ≥ 7)	51	5	PSA >1.0
Sharkey[106]	59	PSA > 10 and Gleason ≥ 7	40	6	PSA > 1.5
Kwok[107]	28	(>1 feature: PSA > 10, Stage ≥ 2b, Gleason > 6)	24	5	ASTRO
Stock[74]*	38	PSA > 20 Gleason 8–10	79	5	ASTRO
	37		76	5	

*Indicates treatment with adjuvant EBRT.
ASTRO, definition of PSA failure promulgated by the American Society for Therapeutic Radiology and Oncology.

seed-loading pattern resulted in urethral doses higher than 400 Gy that led to significant urethral damage.[82] The incidence of urethral stricture is approximately 10% with the uniform seed-loading pattern. The peripheral loading technique with real-time seed placement avoids placing the sources too close to the urethra and has been shown to reduce the risk of incontinence greatly, to less than 1%, even after TURP.[83] Among patients without TURP, the incidence of incontinence after brachytherapy is less than 1% irrespective of the seed loading pattern.[14]

Radiation proctitis has been reported to occur in 2% to 12% of patient following seed implantation and results from the proximity of the anterior rectal wall to the posterior aspect of the prostate, where a large number of seeds are placed.[78,80,84,99] Although proctitis is usually mild, with most patients complaining of intermittent painless rectal bleeding, 1% to 2% of patients will develop more serious complications of ulceration and fistula.[87] Patients who are treated with the combined EBRT and implantation can be expected to have a higher rate of radiation proctitis. Snyder found a relationship between the volume of the rectum irradiated and the incidence of grade 2 proctitis.[61] If the rectal volume irradiated by 160 Gy was less than 1.3 cm^3, fewer than 5% of the patients developed grade 2 proctitis by 5 years after implantation. Han measured rectal surface area encompassed by the dose and determined that rectal bleeding is more common when larger surface areas are covered by the prescribed dose.[88]

More severe rectal complications such as ulcer (grade 3) or fistula formation (grade 4) have been more commonly reported in patients who have had rectal bleeding treated by some form of caustic therapy. Theodorescu reported 7 fistulas out of 724 men treated with implantation alone or in combination with EBRT.[89] Six of the seven patients had rectal bleeding managed by biopsy and electrocautery. Gelbum noted that 50% of the grade 3 rectal complications had an antecedent rectal biopsy and that the biopsied patients took twice as long to heal.[80] Most experienced brachytherapists caution patients against biopsy and fulguration of bleeding areas in the anterior rectal wall. It is prudent to caution the patients not to have any rectal

procedures performed without getting clearance from the physicians who performed the implantation.

All forms of treatment for localized prostate cancer can cause erectile dysfunction. Brachytherapy has historically been associated with lower impotence rates than seen with radical prostatectomy or EBRT. Because the radiation dose from the seeds falls off so rapidly, the total dose of radiation delivered to the penile vessels and neurovascular bundles is less than that delivered with EBRT, and probably causes far less trauma than that caused by prostatectomy. The data for the newer ultrasound-guided implants tend to bear out this finding, with potency rates of 34% to 86%.[42,76,85,90,91] Stock demonstrated at 59% of patients with potency prior to implant retained erectile function.[91] Patients with good erectile function before implantation have much greater likelihood of maintaining an adequate erection following the implantation. Stock showed that age and hormonal therapy are less important than pretreatment erectile function in determining long-term potency.[91] Merrick found that the addition of EBRT also had a negative effect on erectile function.[92]

The introduction of sildenafil citrate has had a significant effect on treatment-related impotence. Incrocci performed a placebo-controlled study in patients receiving conformal EBRT.[93] Successful intercourse was reported by 55% of the patients after sildenafil citrate versus 18% after placebo (P < 0.001). When sildenafil citrate was included in Merrick's 6-year potency analysis, potency rates increased from 39% to 92%.[92] Potters found that 62% of the men who were impotent following brachytherapy had a favorable response to sildenafil citrate.[94]

Health-related quality-of-life (HRQOL) assessment for brachytherapy patients may provide additional quality-of-life information to help patients select the appropriate treatment for prostate cancer. Wei assessed 1400 men treated by brachytherapy, EBRT, or radical prostatectomy.[95] The RAND 36, functional assessment of cancer therapy—general (FACT-G), functional assessment of cancer therapy—prostate (FACT-P), and the Expanded Prostate Cancer Index (EPIC) were mailed to patients after initial therapy. These investigators found that long-term HRQOL domains for brachytherapy were no better than for radical prostatectomy or EBRT. Unfortunately, no baseline studies were available, and dosimetry data on the implants were not reported, making interpretation of this data problematic. Davis performed a similar study in more than 500 patients using five HRQOL instruments.[96] Little difference was found between the three treatments in general health assessment, although treatment-specific differences were noted for bowel, urinary, and sexual function.

Summary

Prostate brachytherapy has become an accepted treatment modality for localized prostate cancer. Long-term biochemical and biopsy data confirm the early positive impressions that brachytherapy is as valid a treatment option as radical prostatectomy or EBRT. Quality-of-life data also look promising, but more follow-up data are needed. Is brachytherapy as good as or perhaps better than radical prostatectomy? This question cannot be answered yet. Well-controlled, randomized studies are needed. In the meantime, the clinician will have to rely on the available published data.

References

1. Stone NN. Brachytherapy or radical prostatectomy: is there a preferred method for treating localized prostate cancer? BJU Int 2004;93:5.
2. Holm HH, Juul N, Pedersen JF, et al. Transperineal [125]iodine seed implantation in prostatic cancer guided by transrectal ultrasonography. J Urol 1983;130:283–286.
3. Stone NN, Stock RG. Prospective assessment of patient-reported long-term urinary morbidity and associated quality of life changes after ^{125}I prostate brachytherapy. Brachytherapy 2003;2:32–39.
4. Stock RG, Stone NN, Wesson MF, et al. A modified technique allowing interactive ultrasound-guided three-dimensional transperineal prostate implantation. Int J Radiat Oncol Biol Phys 1995;32:219–225.
5. Bell AG. The uses of radium. Am Med 1903;6:261.
6. Aronowitz JN. Dawn of prostate brachytherapy: 1915–1930. Int J Radiat Oncol Biol Phys 2002;54:712–718.
7. Young HH. The use of radium in cancer of the prostate and bladder: A presentation of new instruments and new methods of use. JAMA 1917;68:1174–1177.
8. Whitmore WF Jr, Hilaris B, Grabstald H, et al. Implantation of ^{125}I in prostatic cancer. Surg Clin North Am 1974;54:887–895.
9. Zelefsky MJ, Whitmore WF Jr. Long-term results of retropubic permanent [125]iodine implantation of the prostate for clinically localized prostatic cancer. J Urol 1997;158:23–29; discussion 29–30.
10. Nath R, Yue N. Dosimetric characterization of a newly designed encapsulated interstitial brachytherapy source of iodine-125-model LS-1 BrachySeed. Appl Radiat Isot 2001;55:813–821.
11. Wallner K, Merrick G, True L, et al. [125]I versus [103]Pd for low-risk prostate cancer: preliminary PSA outcomes from a prospective randomized multicenter trial. Int J Radiat Oncol Biol Phys 2003;57:1297–1303.
12. Bice WS Jr, Prestidge BR, Grimm PD, et al. Centralized multiinstitutional postimplant analysis for interstitial prostate brachytherapy. Int J Radiat Oncol Biol Phys 1998;41:921–927.
13. Mate TP, Gottesman JE, Hatton J, et al. High dose-rate afterloading [192]Iridium prostate brachytherapy: feasibility report. Int J Radiat Oncol Biol Phys 1998;41:525–533.
14. Blasko JC, Mate T, Sylvester JE, et al. Brachytherapy for carcinoma of the prostate: techniques, patient selection, and clinical outcomes. Semin Radiat Oncol 2002;12:81–94.
15. Shiloh Y. ATM and related protein kinases: safeguarding genome integrity. Nat Rev Cancer 2003;3:155–168.
16. Shiloh Y, Lehmann AR. Maintaining integrity. Nat Cell Biol 2004;6:923-8.
17. Ling CC, Li WX, Anderson LL. The relative biological effectiveness of I-125 and Pd-103. Int J Radiat Oncol Biol Phys, 1995. 32:373–378.
18. Ling CC. Permanent implants using Au-198, Pd-103 and I-125: radiobiological considerations based on the linear quadratic model. Int J Radiat Oncol Biol Phys 1992;23:81–87.
19. Brenner DJ, Martinez AA, Edmundson GK, et al. Direct evidence that prostate tumors show high sensitivity to fractionation (low alpha/beta ratio), similar to late-responding normal tissue. Int J Radiat Oncol Biol Phys 2002;52:6–13.
20. Fowler JF, Ritter JF, Chappell RJ, et al. What hypofractionated protocols should be tested for prostate cancer? Int J Radiat Oncol Biol Phys 2003;56:1093–1104.
21. Brenner DJ, Hall EJ. Fractionation and protraction for radiotherapy of prostate carcinoma. Int J Radiat Oncol Biol Phys 1999;43:1095–1101.
22. Martinez A, Gonzalez J, Spencer W, et al. Conformal high dose rate brachytherapy improves biochemical control and cause specific survival in patients with prostate cancer and poor prognostic factors. J Urol 2003;169:974–979; discussion 979–980.
23. Wang JZ, Guerrero M, Li XA. How low is the alpha/beta ratio for prostate cancer? Int J Radiat Oncol Biol Phys 2003;55:194–203.
24. Kollmeier MA, Stock RG, Stone N. Biochemical outcomes after prostate brachytherapy with 5-year minimal follow-up: importance of patient selection and implant quality. Int J Radiat Oncol Biol Phys 2003;57:645–653.
25. Zelefsky MJ, Fuks Z, Hunt M, et al. High dose radiation delivered by intensity modulated conformal radiotherapy improves the outcome of localized prostate cancer. J Urol 2001;166:876–881.
26. Grimm PD, Blasko JC, Sylvester JE, et al. 10-year biochemical (prostate-specific antigen) control of prostate cancer with ^{125}I brachytherapy. Int J Radiat Oncol Biol Phys 2001;51:31–40.
27. Gardner BG, Zietman AL, Shipley WU, et al. Late normal tissue sequelae in the second decade after high dose radiation therapy with combined photons and conformal protons for locally advanced prostate cancer. J Urol 2002;167:123–6.
28. Meredith J. Radium dosage. The Manchester System. London: Livingston, 1967.
29. Blasko JC, Grimm PD, Ragde H. Brachytherapy and organ preservation in the management of carcinoma of the prostate. Semin Radiat Oncol 1993;3:240–249.
30. Stock RG, Stone NN, Lo YC, et al. Postimplant dosimetry for ^{125}I prostate implants: definitions and factors affecting outcome. Int J Radiat Oncol Biol Phys 2000;48:899–906.
31. Stock RG, Stone NN, Tabert A, et al. A dose-response study for I-125 prostate implants. Int J Radiat Oncol Biol Phys 1998;41:101–108.
32. Stone NN, Stock RG. Prospective assessment of patient-reported long-term urinary morbidity and associated quality of life changes after ^{125}I prostate brachytherapy. Brachytherapy 2003;2:32–39.
33. Jani AB, Hellman S. Early prostate cancer: clinical decision-making. Lancet 2003;361:1045–1053.
34. Fowler FJ Jr, McNaughton Collins M, Albertsen PC, et al. Comparison of recommendations by urologists and radiation oncologists for treatment of clinically localized prostate cancer. JAMA 2000;283:3217–3222.
35. Cesaretti JA, Stone NN, Stock RG. Does prior transurethral resection of prostate compromise brachytherapy quality: a dosimetric analysis. Int J Radiat Oncol Biol Phys 2004;60:648–653.
36. Blasko JC, Ragde H, Grimm PD. Transperineal ultrasound-guided implantation of the prostate: morbidity and complications. Scand J Urol Nephrol Suppl 1991;137:113–118.
37. Partin AW, Kattan MW, Subong EN, et al. Combination of prostate-specific antigen, clinical stage, and Gleason score to predict pathological stage of localized prostate cancer. A multi-institutional update. JAMA 1997;277:1445–1451.
38. Davis BJ, Pisansky TM, Wilson TM, et al. The radial distance of extraprostatic extension of prostate carcinoma: implications for prostate brachytherapy. Cancer 1999;85:2630–2637.
39. Linzer DG, Stock RG, Stone NN, et al. Seminal vesicle biopsy: accuracy and implications for staging of prostate cancer. Urology 1996;48:757–761.

40. Stone NN, Stock RG, Unger P. Laparoscopic pelvic lymph node dissection for prostate cancer: comparison of the extended and modified techniques. J Urol 1997;158:1891–1894.
41. Stone NN, Stock RG. Prostate brachytherapy in patients with prostate volumes >/= 50 cm³: dosimetric analysis of implant quality. Int J Radiat Oncol Biol Phys 2000;46:1199–1204.
42. Blasko JC, Ragde H, Luse RW, et al. Should brachytherapy be considered a therapeutic option in localized prostate cancer? Urol Clin North Am 1996;23:633–650.
43. Bolla M, Collette L, Blank L, et al. Long-term results with immediate androgen suppression and external irradiation in patients with locally advanced prostate cancer (an EORTC study): a phase III randomised trial. Lancet 2002;360:103–106.
44. D'Amico AV, Manola J, Loffredo M, et al. 6-month androgen suppression plus radiation therapy vs radiation therapy alone for patients with clinically localized prostate cancer: a randomized controlled trial. JAMA 2004;292:821–827.
45. Pilepich MV, Winter K, John MJ, et al. Phase III radiation therapy oncology group (RTOG) trial 86-10 of androgen deprivation adjuvant to definitive radiotherapy in locally advanced carcinoma of the prostate. Int J Radiat Oncol Biol Phys 2001;50:1243–1252.
46. Lawton CA, Winter K, Murray K, et al. Updated results of the phase III Radiation Therapy Oncology Group (RTOG) trial 85-31 evaluating the potential benefit of androgen suppression following standard radiation therapy for unfavorable prognosis carcinoma of the prostate. Int J Radiat Oncol Biol Phys 2001;49:937–946.
47. Marshall DT, et al. Hormonal therapy reduces the risk of post-implant urinary retention in symptomatic prostate cancer patients with glands larger than 50 cc. 2004;60(Suppl. 1):S451.
48. Lee LN, Stock RG, Stone NN. Role of hormonal therapy in the management of intermediate- to high-risk prostate cancer treated with permanent radioactive seed implantation. Int J Radiat Oncol Biol Phys 2002;52:444–452.
49. D'Amico AV, Whittington R, Malkowicz SB, et al. Biochemical outcome after radical prostatectomy, external beam radiation therapy, or interstitial radiation therapy for clinically localized prostate cancer. JAMA 1998;280:969–974.
50. Martinez A, Galalae R, Gonzalez J, et al. No apparent benefit at 5 years from a course of neoadjuvant/concurrent androgen deprivation for patients with prostate cancer treated with a high total radiation dose. J Urol 2003;170:2296–2301.
51. Potters L, Torre T, Ashley R, et al. Examining the role of neoadjuvant androgen deprivation in patients undergoing prostate brachytherapy. J Clin Oncol 2000;18:1187–1192.
52. Merrick GS, Butler WM, Galbreath RW, et al. Does hormonal manipulation in conjunction with permanent interstitial brachytherapy, with or without supplemental external beam irradiation, improve the biochemical outcome for men with intermediate or high-risk prostate cancer? BJU Int 2003;91:23–29.
53. Stone NN, Stock RG, Unger P, et al. Biopsy results after real-time ultrasound-guided transperineal implants for stage T1–T2 prostate cancer. J Endourol 2000;14:375–380.
54. Pollack A, Zagars GK, Starkschall G, et al. Prostate cancer radiation dose response: results of the M. D. Anderson phase III randomized trial. Int J Radiat Oncol Biol Phys 2002;53:1097–1105.
55. Zelefsky MJ, Fuks Z, Hunt M, et al. High dose radiation delivered by intensity modulated conformal radiotherapy improves the outcome of localized prostate cancer. J Urol 2001;166:876–881.
56. Nath R, Anderson LL, Luxton G, et al. Dosimetry of interstitial brachytherapy sources: recommendations of the AAPM Radiation Therapy Committee Task Group No. 43. American Association of Physicists in Medicine. Med Phys 1995;22:209–234.
57. Potters L, Huang D, Calugaru E, et al. Importance of implant dosimetry for patients undergoing prostate brachytherapy. Urology 2003;62:1073–1077.
58. Nag S, Bice W, DeWyngaert K, et al. The American Brachytherapy Society recommendations for permanent prostate brachytherapy postimplant dosimetric analysis. Int J Radiat Oncol Biol Phys 2000;46:221–230.
59. Stock RG, Stone NN. Importance of post-implant dosimetry in permanent prostate brachytherapy. Eur Urol 2002;41:434–439.
60. Desai J, Stock RG, Stone NN, et al. Acute urinary morbidity following I-125 interstitial implantation of the prostate gland. Radiat Oncol Investig 1998;6:135–141.
61. Snyder KM, Stock RG, Hong SM, et al. Defining the risk of developing grade 2 proctitis following ¹²⁵I prostate brachytherapy using a rectal dose-volume histogram analysis. Int J Radiat Oncol Biol Phys 2001;50:335–341.
62. Consensus statement: guidelines for PSA following radiation therapy. American Society for Therapeutic Radiology and Oncology Consensus Panel. Int J Radiat Oncol Biol Phys 1997;37:1035–1041.
63. Critz FA, Levinson AK, Williams WH, et al. Prostate specific antigen nadir achieved by men apparently cured of prostate cancer by radiotherapy. J Urol 1999;161:1199–1203; discussion 1203–1205.
64. Critz FA, Levinson AK, Williams WH, et al. Prostate-specific antigen nadir: the optimum level after irradiation for prostate cancer. J Clin Oncol 1996;14:2893–2900.
65. Thames H, Kuban D, Levy L, et al. Comparison of alternative biochemical failure definitions based on clinical outcome in 4839 prostate cancer patients treated by external beam radiotherapy between 1986 and 1995. Int J Radiat Oncol Biol Phys 2003;57:929–943.
66. Critz FA. Time to achieve a prostate specific antigen nadir of 0.2 ng/ml after simultaneous irradiation for prostate cancer. J Urol 2002;168:2434–2438.
67. Stock RG, Stone NN, Cesaretti JA. Prostate-specific antigen bounce after prostate seed implantation for localized prostate cancer: descriptions and implications. Int J Radiat Oncol Biol Phys 2003;56:448–453.
68. Grimm PD, Blasko JC, Sylvester JE, et al. 10-year biochemical (prostate-specific antigen) control of prostate cancer with ¹²⁵I brachytherapy. Int J Radiat Oncol Biol Phys 2001;51:31–40.
69. Blasko JC, Grimm PD, Sylvester JE, et al. Palladium-103 brachytherapy for prostate carcinoma. Int J Radiat Oncol Biol Phys 2000;46:839–850.
70. Sylvester J, Blasko JC, Grimm PD, et al. Neoadjuvant androgen ablation combined with external-beam radiation therapy and permanent interstitial brachytherapy boost in localized prostate cancer. Mol Urol 1999;3:231–236.
71. Pickett B, et al. Efficacy of external beam radiotherapy compared to permanent prostate implant in treating low risk prostate cancer based on endorectal magnetic resonance spectroscopy imaging and PSA. 2004;60(Suppl. 1):S185.
72. D'Amico AV, Whittington R, Malkowicz SB, et al. Biochemical outcome after radical prostatectomy, external beam radiation therapy, or interstitial radiation therapy for clinically localized prostate cancer. JAMA 1998;280:969–974.
73. Zelefsky MJ, Hollister T, Raben A, et al. Five-year biochemical outcome and toxicity with transperineal CT-planned permanent I-125 prostate implantation for patients with localized prostate cancer. Int J Radiat Oncol Biol Phys 2000;47:1261–1266.
74. Stock RG, Cahlon O, Cesaretti JA, et al. Combined modality treatment in the management of high-risk prostate cancer. Int J Radiat Oncol Biol Phys 2004;59:1352–1359.
75. Blasko JC, Grimm PD, Sylvester JE, et al. The role of external beam radiotherapy with I-125/Pd-103 brachytherapy for prostate carcinoma. Radiother Oncol 2000;57:273–278.
76. Dattoli M, Wallner K, Sorace R, et al. ¹⁰³Pd brachytherapy and external beam irradiation for clinically localized, high-risk prostatic carcinoma. Int J Radiat Oncol Biol Phys 1996;35:875–879.
77. Zelefsky MJ, Fuks Z, Hunt M, et al. High dose radiation delivered by intensity modulated conformal radiotherapy improves the outcome of localized prostate cancer. J Urol 2001;166:876–881.
78. Arterbery VE, Wallner K, Roy J, et al. Short-term morbidity from CT-planned transperineal I-125 prostate implants. Int J Radiat Oncol Biol Phys 1993;25:661–667.
79. Terk MD, Stock RG, Stone NN. Identification of patients at increased risk for prolonged urinary retention following radioactive seed implantation of the prostate. J Urol 1998;160:1379–1382.

80. Gelblum DY, Potters L, Ashley R, et al. Urinary morbidity following ultrasound-guided transperineal prostate seed implantation. Int J Radiat Oncol Biol Phys 1999;45:59–67.

81. Kleinberg L, Wallner K, Roy J, et al. Treatment-related symptoms during the first year following transperineal ^{125}I prostate implantation. Int J Radiat Oncol Biol Phys 1994;28:985–990.

82. Wallner K, Roy J, Harrison L. Dosimetry guidelines to minimize urethral and rectal morbidity following transperineal I-125 prostate brachytherapy. Int J Radiat Oncol Biol Phys 1995;32:465–471.

83. Stone NN, Ratnow ER, Stock RG. Prior transurethral resection does not increase morbidity following real-time ultrasound-guided prostate seed implantation. Tech Urol 2000;6:123–127.

84. Wallner K, Roy J, Zelefsky M, et al. Short-term freedom from disease progression after I-125 prostate implantation. Int J Radiat Oncol Biol Phys 1994;30:405–409.

85. Wallner K, Roy J, Harrison L. Tumor control and morbidity following transperineal iodine 125 implantation for stage T1/T2 prostatic carcinoma. J Clin Oncol 1996;14:449–453.

86. Merrick GS, Butler WM, Dorsey AT, et al. Rectal function following prostate brachytherapy. Int J Radiat Oncol Biol Phys 2000;48:667–674.

87. Stone NN, Stock RG. Complications following permanent prostate brachytherapy. Eur Urol 2002;41:427–433.

88. Han BH, Wallner KE. Dosimetric and radiographic correlates to prostate brachytherapy-related rectal complications. Int J Cancer 2001;96:372–378.

89. Theodorescu D, Gillenwater JY, Koutrouvelis PG. Prostatourethral-rectal fistula after prostate brachytherapy. Cancer 2000;89:2085–2091.

90. Kao J, Jani A, Vijayakumar S. Sexual functioning after treatment for early stage prostate cancer. Sexuality and Disability 2002;20:239–260.

91. Stock RG, Kao J, Stone NN. Penile erectile function after permanent radioactive seed implantation for treatment of prostate cancer. J Urol 2001;165:436–439.

92. Merrick GS, Bulter WM, Galbreath RW, et al. Erectile function after permanent prostate brachytherapy. Int J Radiat Oncol Biol Phys 2002;52:893–902.

93. Incrocci L, Koper PC, Hop WC, et al. Sildenafil citrate (Viagra) and erectile dysfunction following external beam radiotherapy for prostate cancer: a randomized, double-blind, placebo-controlled, cross-over study. Int J Radiat Oncol Biol Phys 2001;51:1190–1195.

94. Potters L, Torre T, Feam PA, et al. Potency after permanent prostate brachytherapy for localized prostate cancer. Int J Radiat Oncol Biol Phys 2001;50:1235–1242.

95. Wei JT, Dunn RL, Sandler HM, et al. Comprehensive comparison of health-related quality of life after contemporary therapies for localized prostate cancer. J Clin Oncol 2002;20:557–566.

96. Davis JW, Kuban DA, Lynch DF, et al. Quality of life after treatment for localized prostate cancer: differences based on treatment modality. J Urol 2001;166:947–952.

97. Ragde H, Elgamal AA, Snow PB, et al. Ten-year disease free survival after transperineal sonography-guided iodine-125 brachytherapy with or without 45-gray external beam irradiation in the treatment of patients with clinically localized, low to high Gleason grade prostate carcinoma. Cancer 1998;83:989–1001.

98. Grado GL, Larson TR, Balch CS, et al. Actuarial disease-free survival after prostate cancer brachytherapy using interactive techniques with biplane ultrasound and fluoroscopic guidance. Int J Radiat Oncol Biol Phys 1998;42:289–298.

99. Dattoli M, Wallner K, True L, et al. Prognostic role of serum prostatic acid phosphatase for ^{103}Pd-based radiation for prostatic carcinoma. Int J Radiat Oncol Biol Phys 1999;45:853–856.

100. Potters L, Cha C, Ashley R, et al. The role of external beam irradiation in patients undergoing prostate brachytherapy. Urol Oncol 2000;5:112–117.

101. Stokes SH. Comparison of biochemical disease-free survival of patients with localized carcinoma of the prostate undergoing radical prostatectomy, transperineal ultrasound-guided radioactive seed implantation, or definitive external beam irradiation. Int J Radiat Oncol Biol Phys 2000;47:129–136.

102. Critz FA, Williams WH, Levinson AK, et al. Simultaneous irradiation for prostate cancer: intermediate results with modern techniques. J Urol 2000;164:738–741.

103. Singh A, Zelefsky MJ, Raben A, et al. Combined 3-dimensional conformal radiotherapy and transperineal Pd-103 permanent implantation for patients with intermediate and unfavorable risk prostate cancer. Int J Cancer. 2000;90:275–280.

104. Beyer DC and Brachman DG. Failure free survival following brachytherapy alone for prostate cancer: comparison with external beam radiotherapy. Radiother Oncol. 2000;57:263–267.

105. Lederman GS, Cavanagh W, Albert PS, et al. Retrospective stratification of a consecutive cohort of prostate cancer patients treated with a combined regimen of external-beam radiotherapy and brachytherapy. Int Jnl Radiat Oncol Biol Phys 2001;49:1297–1303.

106. Sharkey J, Cantor A, Solc Z, et al. Brachytherapy versus radical prostatectomy in patients with clinically localized prostate cancer. Curr Urol Rep 2002;3:250–257.

107. Kwok Y, DiBiase SJ, Amin PP, et al. Risk group stratification in patients undergoing permanent ^{125}I prostate brachytherapy as monotherapy. Int J Radiat Oncol Biol Phys 2002;53:588–594.

108. Wallner K, et al. ^{125}I versus ^{103}Pd for low-risk prostate cancer: preliminary PSA outcomes from a prospective randomized multicenter trial. Int J Radiat Oncol Biol Phys 2003;57:1297–1303.

22

High dose rate ^{192}Ir as monotherapy or as a boost: the new prostate brachytherapy

Alvaro Martinez, Jeffrey Demanes, Razvan Galalae, Jose Gonzalez, Nils Nuernberg, Carlos Vargas, Rodney Rodriguez, Mitchell Hollander, Gary Gustafson

Introduction

Since the mid-1980s, surgery and radiotherapy have been the treatment modalities most frequently used to treat patients with prostate cancer. However, it is important to recognize the prominence brachytherapy treatments have achieved. To this respect, The American Urologic Society,[1] and the American College of Radiology[2] patterns of care of utilization have reported the significant increase of utilization of brachytherapy during the last decade. We will limit the extent of our data analysis and comments to a type of brachytherapy called high dose rate (HDR) brachytherapy, whether used as a monotherapy or as a boost therapy combined with pelvic external beam with or without androgen deprivation therapy (ADT).

Prostate brachytherapy has been performed using one of two treatment techniques, low dose rate (LDR) or high dose rate (HDR). Low dose rate brachytherapy involves the permanent implantation of multiple radioactive seeds into the prostate. This signifies that the patient remains radioactive and must comply with the state rules and regulations for patients harboring radioactive material. High dose rate brachytherapy, on the other hand, uses a single high-intensity radioactive source stored in a "robot-like machine" called a remote afterloader. The afterloader sends and retracts this single source of radiation in a very short period of time, typically 10 to 15 minutes. Hence, the patients are no longer radioactive after the completion of treatment.

Advantages of high dose rate brachytherapy

High dose rate brachytherapy has a number of advantages over LDR, which are both patient- and target-specific. They are summarized below:

1. The overall treatment time is reduced from many weeks with LDR to several minutes with HDR. This eliminates the uncertainties related to volume changes occurring over weeks (typical with LDR) due to trauma and swelling or subsequent shrinkage due to postradiation fibrosis.

2. HDR significantly improves the radiation dose distribution secondary to the ability to modulate and accurately control the spatial source position and vary the source dwell time during treatment.

3. The intraoperative (or real-time) optimization used with HDR allows ideal selection of needle placement in real-time and better source position targeting, hence modulating the intensity with the potential for limiting treatment toxicity.

4. HDR can significantly reduce the cost of treatment because the radioactive sources are not purchased per case treated, as is done with LDR.

5. There are advantages in radiation safety and protection with HDR, since the patient is not radioactive when he returns home. The HDR single radiation source is retracted into the robot at the completion of treatment.

6. There are multiple radiobiologic considerations favoring HDR since the treatment is given in several minutes for which repopulation, cell cycle, and recovery of sublethal damage cannot occur.

For patients with early-stage prostate cancer, radical prostatectomy, external beam radiotherapy (EBRT), and brachytherapy are commonly used treatment modalities. Although the most appropriate definition of biochemical failure may be controversial, the Cleveland Clinic Foundation,[3] and William Beaumont Hospital, Michigan,[4] have reported similar outcomes for patients with favorable prognostic features undergoing either radical prostatectomy or EBRT at a single institution. In addition, several other investigators have reported excellent results with interstitial prostate brachytherapy,[6–11] with biochemical control rates comparable to those of patients treated with either radical prostatectomy or external beam irradiation. While most monotherapy series have utilized LDR technique with iodine-125 (^{125}I) seeds or palladium-103 (^{103}Pd) seeds, HDR brachytherapy with iridium-192 (^{192}Ir) is gaining popularity.[10–13]

A wide variety of treatment approaches has been used for patients with unfavorable prostate cancer. However, treatment remains a challenge. Survival rates from series in which radical prostatectomy is performed for stage C or T3 disease,[14–16] and/or low-dose EBRT are given remain suboptimal.[17] To improve on these results three radiotherapeutic strategies have been tested: 1) the addition of hormonal ablation before standard radiotherapy[18–20]; 2) the addition of particle beam as a boost to EBRT[21,22]; and 3) dose-escalating conformal radiotherapy. Dose escalation has been accomplished by using three-dimensional (3D) conformal EBRT,[23,24] or brachytherapy using a conformal HDR boost.[25,26]

Assessing high dose rate brachytherapy

In 1991, the William Beaumont Hospital (WBH) Human Investigation Committee (HIC) approved a prospective clinical trial that was designed to test the hypothesis that for patients with intermediate and/or poor prognostic factors local failure is related to the large volume of cell mass and radioresistant cell clones, both of which require biologically higher radiation dosages, than those conventionally used. Thus, we selected a hypofractionated 3D conformal HDR brachytherapy boost as the method of dose escalation. We have published our results previously.[25,26] We reported an update combining the data from Kiel University and WBH, using a similar treatment program.[27] In this report, we are adding the data from the California Endocuritherapy Cancer Center (CET). In total, 1660 patients were treated with HDR brachytherapy as a boost or as monotherapy: CET treated 889 patients, WBH 527 patients, and Kiel 244 patients.

Materials and methods

Hypofractionated treatment program

The radiotherapeutic approach at the three institutions involved a hypofractionated regimen delivering a very high biologic equivalent dose to EBRT. Our treatment schedule (Figure 22.1) was designed for 5 weeks instead of the conventional 8-week course of EBRT

High dose rate brachytherapy as a boost

Our treatment technique has been previously described.[25,26,28,29] The pelvis was treated with an isocentric dose of 46 Gy in 23 fractions using a 4-field technique. All patients underwent pretreatment pelvic computed tomography (CT) with contrast to assist in

defining the prostate and normal tissue volumes. Pelvic EBRT was interdigitated with transrectal ultrasound (TRUS)-guided transperineal conformal interstitial ^{192}Ir implants. The overall treatment time was compressed to only 5 weeks (see Figure 22.1). Patients with a prostate gland volume of more than 65 cm³ or length of 5.5 cm were initially ineligible for the protocol. These patients underwent downsizing with a short course of hormonal therapy (<6 months) and were the subject of a separate analysis.[30] The dosimetry was done in real-time intraoperatively. The optimal needle positions within the reference plane were determined intraoperatively using our real-time, interactive optimization program.[28,29] After placement of all needles, cystoscopy was performed to reconfirm the prostate treatment length with adequate depth by virtue of bladder mucosa tenting. To reconfirm the gland apex during cystoscopy, the TRUS probe was placed in the sagittal plane. The veru montanum (1 cm behind) was used to correlate with the TRUS probe position in the longitudinal plane. On each transverse TRUS image, the 100% isodose line encompassed the contoured prostate volume (Figure 22.2). The urethra was limited to less than 125% of the prostate dose and a dose–volume histogram (DVH) was used to assess dosimetry quality as seen in Figure 22.3. The rectal dose was limited to 75% of the prostate dose.

When the trial began in 1991, the linear-quadratic formula was used to calculate the biologic effective dose (BED).[31] The α/β value ratio for tumor control probability was 10, and for normal tissue complications, 4. There is evidence now that the α/β ratio for prostate cancer is much lower. In 1998, we published the validation of this low α/β value. The value 1.2 was derived from this EBRT and HDR clinical trial.[32] The WBH dose-escalation trial with the corresponding α/β ratios and length of follow up are depicted on Table 22.1.

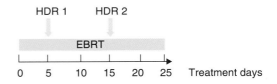

Figure 22.1
Treatment schedule for prostate cancer patients treated with pelvic external beam radiotherapy (EBRT) and a high dose rate (HDR) brachytherapy boost. External beam radiotherapy: total dose 46 Gy in 23 fractions of 2 Gy/fraction; technique—pelvis 4-field 3D conformal radiotherapy, including pelvic nodes. High dose rate boost: 11.5 Gy on day 5 and day 15 of EBRT without interruption.

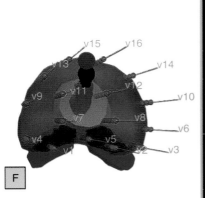
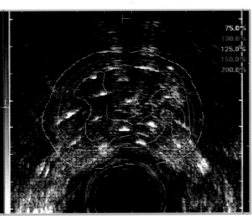

Figure 22.2
Swift PTV rendering of the prostate, urethra and seminal vesicles with needle trajectory on the left. Real time transrectal ultrasound (TRUS) image with final implant dosimetry on the right. 100% isodose line in red, 125% in green.

High dose rate brachytherapy as monotherapy

The twice per day accelerated hypofractionated regimen was selected based on HDR favorable radiobiologic considerations described above and physical dose-delivery advantages of TRUS guidance,[10] with conformal intensity modulated real-time dosimetry of prostate HDR brachytherapy.[11,26,8,29] Figures 22.2 and 22.3 depict an HDR intraoperative implant using the Nucletron Swift guidance system. Patients with clinical stage II (T1c–T2a) disease, Gleason score less than 7, and pretreatment PSA of less than 12 ng/mL were treated with monotherapy. The majority of patients presented with what would be considered low-risk or favorable prostate cancer. Once it was determined that the patient met all clinical and anatomic criteria for monotherapy, the HDR and LDR brachytherapy treatment options were discussed and then the patient selected the brachytherapy modality. A short course of neoadjuvant androgen deprivation (<6 months) was utilized for downsizing the gland volume, in 31% of WBH patients in equal proportions between permanent seeds and HDR, and in 30% of the CET patients.[13] All procedures were done under spinal anesthesia.

Table 22.1 Biologic equivalent dose between an external beam radiotherapy (EBRT) alone versus a combined treatment with EBRT and high dose rate (HDR) prostate brachytherapy

Dose level, Gy (# sessions)	# of patients	Mean follow-up years	BED* (Gy) $\alpha/\beta = 10$	BED* (Gy) $\alpha/\beta = 12$
Low				
5.50 (3)	19	8.8	67.1	80.2
6.00 (3)	15	8.7	70.0	86.1
6.5 (3)	25	6.7	72.6	92.5
8.25 (2)	26	4.7	72.0	94.2
High				
8.75 (2)	25	4.6	74.2	99.9
9.5 (2)	38	4.5	78.0	108.9
10.50 (2)	46	3.3	82.9	122.0
11.5 (2)	32	1.9	87	136.3

*Biological equivalent dose to external beam.

William Beaumont Hospital experience

Between January 1996 and December 2002, 253 patients with clinically localized prostate cancer, were treated with accelerated hypofractionated brachytherapy as the sole treatment modality. Of the patients, 92 were treated with HDR brachytherapy alone using ^{192}Ir, and 161 patients were treated with LDR brachytherapy alone using [103]Pd.

For the implant procedure, as well as for pain control during the entire treatment time, spinal anesthesia was administered following placement of an epidural catheter. In the same manner as in the boost technique, using both transverse and sagittal views, TRUS was used to visualize and identify the base and apex of the prostate, as well as normal structures, such as urethra, rectum, and bladder. Images were captured, and the urethra was mapped at each 5 mm transverse slice from base to apex. The transverse image with the largest cross-sectional area was considered the "reference plane."

Dosimetry was continuously updated in real-time, based on the actual location of needles, to compensate for organ distortion and motion and to assure conformal coverage of the gland.[28] Gold seed markers were then placed under TRUS guidance at the base and at the apex of the prostate to assess and measure possible interfraction needle displacement. Before delivery of the radiation, the entire prostate was imaged again, with final needle and urethral positions captured by TRUS, and a final treatment plan was created.

The prescription dose was 950 cGy delivered four times for a total dose of 3800 cGy. Two fractions were delivered daily over 2 days, with at least 6 hours separating each fraction.

California Endocuritherapy Cancer Center experience

Between January 1996 and December 2002, 77 patients with clinically localized prostate cancer were treated with interstitial brachytherapy as the sole treatment modality.[13] After recovery, the patient underwent a dual method of simulation radiography consisting of plain film localization for applicator adjustment and quality control and a CT scan was performed. The images were downloaded to the "treatment-planning" computer and a 3D reconstruction was

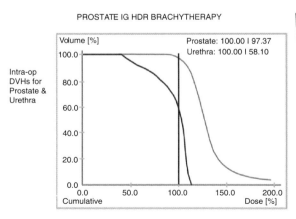
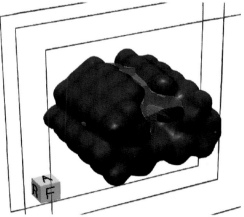

Figure 22.3
Swift dose–volume histogram (DVH) for prostate and urethra on the left. Prostate 100% isodose cloud (red) rendering on the right with sparing of urethra (green).

carried out. The dose was prescribed to a point 5 to 6 mm beyond the prostate capsule laterally and 3 mm posteriorly. A dose-volume histogram and virtual images of the anatomy, clinical target volume (CTV), and planning target volume (PTV) were obtained. A series of six HDR fractions was administered twice per day in two separate procedures 1 week apart. Each fraction delivered 7 Gy for a total dose of 42 Gy. Postoperative management was similar to that described for the WBH experience.

Results

High dose rate brachytherapy as a boost

For the WBH dose-escalation trial and stratifying the patients by dose level (low-dose level <95 Gy; high-dose level >95 Gy), the ASTRO 5-year biochemical control (BC) was 87% for high dose and 52% for low dose (Figure 22.4). Mean follow-up was 8.1 years (range 2–12 years) for the low dose level and 4.2 years (range 0.5–8.2 years) for the high dose level. The mean dose for the biochemically-controlled patients was 108.2 Gy versus 92.5 Gy for biochemical failures (t-test, $P = 0.001$).

The collaborative long-term outcome results with HDR brachytherapy as a boost with or without adjuvant/concurrent hormonal therapy are presented. A total of 1491 patients were treated at WBH, CET, and Keil University. The mean follow up was 4.9 years with a range of 0.5 to 15.7 years. At 5 years, 589 have been followed; at 8 years, 216 patients; and at more than 10 years, 97 patients were followed.

For all 1491 patients, the 5 and 10-year actuarial analysis of biochemical control, freedom from clinical failure, disease-free survival, cause-specific survival, and overall survival, are shown in Table 22.2. Of significance is that the percentage drop in outcome from 5 years to 10 years is very small for all the above tested categories. Also, the freedom from clinical failure of 85% at 10 years is very remarkable for these patients with intermediate- and high-risk prostate cancer.

For the three institutions collaborative group (n = 1491), the 10 year cause-specific survival (CSS) and overall survival are depicted

in Figure 22.5. Despite the unfavorable group of patients treated, at 10 years only 16% have died of prostate cancer.

Since this is a long-term analysis, we want to emphasize clinical failures, CSS, and distant metastatic rates. In Figure 22.6, the clinical failure rate by poor risk factors is depicted. The risk factors were patients with a stage higher than T2b, PSA greater than 10 ng/mL and Gleason score of more than 7. A clear spread of failures ($P < 0.001$) can be seen as risk factors increased. However, a remarkably low 10-year clinical failure rate of 27% was seen for those 204 patients with all three poor prognostic factors. The CSS by risk factors is illustrated in Figure 22.7. The number of risk factors has a significant influence in cancer death ($P < 0.001$). At 10 years, for those patients with all three poor risk factors, the cancer mortality rate was only 16%.

Figure 22.8 depicts the 5-year and 10-year distant metastatic rate for 934 patients, of whom 528 patients did not receive, and 406 patients did receive, a short course (<6 months) of total ADT. Only patients with a minimum follow up of 18 months, or three times the exposure to ADT were analyzed. A detrimental effect can be seen with the use of a short course of ADT ($P = 0.035$). We explain this finding as a negative impact of delaying the initiation of the curative treatment by high-dose radiation. Figure 22.9 and Table 22.3 are subset analysis of these patients. In Figure 22.9 we are demonstrating a very negative influence of less than 6 months of ADT for those 204

Table 22.2 Clinical outcome for patients with intermediate and high-risk prostate cancer treated with a combination of external beam radiotherapy (EBRT) with a high dose rate (HDR) brachytherapy boost (n = 1491)

	5 years (%)	10 years (%)
Biochemical no evidence of disease	85	82
Freedom from clinical failure	93	85
Disease free survival	85	69
Cause-specific survival	97	93
Overall survival	90	76

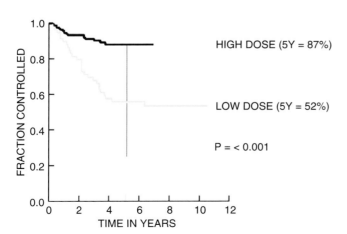

Figure 22.4
Actuarial analysis of biochemical failure (ASTRO definition) stratified by high dose rate (HDR) brachytherapy dose level.

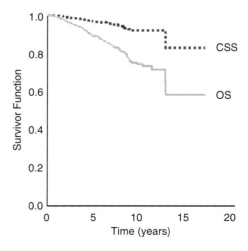

Figure 22.5
Overall survival (OS) and cause-specific survival (CSS, cancer mortality) for all 1491 prostate cancer patients treated with a high dose rate (HDR) prostate brachytherapy boost.

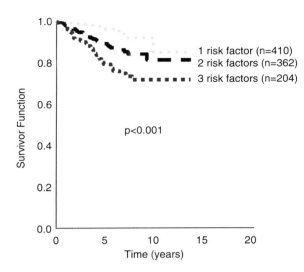

Figure 22.6
Assessment of clinical failures stratified by patients harboring one, two or all three poor prognostic factors for patients treated with a high dose rate (HDR) prostate brachytherapy boost.

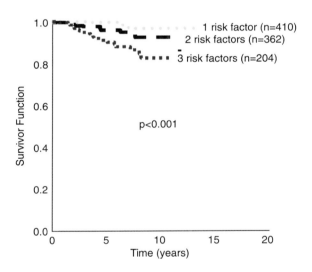

Figure 22.7
Assessment of cause-specific survival (cancer mortality) stratified by patients harboring one, two, or all three poor prognostic factors for patients treated with a high dose rate (HDR) prostate brachytherapy boost.

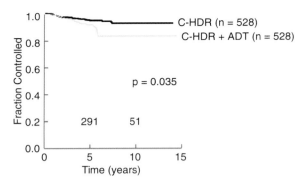

Figure 22.8
Actuarial analysis of distant metastasis for patients with intermediate- and high-risk prostate cancer treated with a high dose rate (HDR) prostate brachytherapy boost with or without androgen deprivation therapy (ADT).

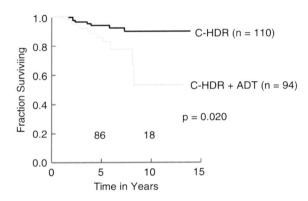

Figure 22.9
Actuarial analysis of cause-specific survival (cancer deaths) for patients with all three poor prognostic factors treated with a high dose rate (HDR) prostate brachytherapy boost with or without androgen deprivation therapy (ADT).

patients with all three poor prognostic factors ($P = 0.02$). Table 22.3 depicts a subset analysis of patients under 70 years of age to 1) be comparable in age with radical prostatectomy series; and 2) diminish the influence of elderly patients with significant co-morbidities affecting survival. If one looks at the worst group (Gleason score 8–10, PSA > 15 ng/mL, and palpable disease >T2a), there is a clear detrimental effect in terms of increased metastatic rate ($P = 0.007$), increased cancer mortality ($P = 0.01$), and decrease survival ($P = 0.01$). These findings are rather distressing and emphasize the importance of not delaying curative treatment in these patients with a high probability of developing metastasis if not treated in a timely fashion.

To place our collaborative HDR boost results in perspective, we selected a recently published radical prostatectomy study by Hull et al.[33] They reported the results on 1000 consecutive patients treated with a radical retropubic prostatectomy. Gleason grade utilized for analysis was the one on the biopsy/transurethral resection of the prostate, and not the one at prostatectomy, and was assigned by one pathologist. This improves the validity of the comparison with our clinical data base.[34] The median follow-up for prostatectomy patients was 3.9 years, while our HDR series was 4.9 years. Table 22.4 depicts the 10-year freedom from distant metastasis stratified by Gleason score. While the 10-year results for Gleason scores up to 6 are equivalent in both studies, there is a clear superiority for Gleason 7 (58% versus 92%) and for Gleason 8 to 10 (58% versus 84%), favoring the EBRT with an HDR boost.

High dose rate brachytherapy as monotherapy

A total of 330 prostate cancer patients were treated with either HDR ^{192}Ir or LDR [103]Pd brachytherapy alone. The median follow-up for all patients was 4.1 years (range 0.8–12.3 years).

Table 22.3 Outcome analysis in terms of distant metastasis, cause-specific survival and overall survival for the high-risk group in patients ≤ 70 years stratified by androgen deprivation therapy

		Cases	Mets, 5 year	Cause-specific survival, 5 year	Overall survival, 5 year
All cases	No AD	308	5%	98%	91%
P-value	AD	252	10%	93%	89%
			0.04	0.02	0.4
Gleason score 8–10 or PSA ≥ 15 ng/mL or ≥T2a	No AD	250	6%	98%	91%
P-value	AD	198	12%	92%	90%
			0.03	0.02	0.9
Gleason score 8–10 and ≥T2a	No AD	49	13%	93%	89%
P-value	AD	48	27%	78%	78%
			0.04	0.2	0.1
Gleason score 8–10 and PSA ≥ 15 ng/mL and ≥T2a	No AD	16	13%	93%	92%
P-value	AD	18	40%	65%	60%
			0.007	0.01	0.01

Table 22.4 Comparative outcome for prostate cancer treated patients, 10-year freedom from distant metastasis stratified by Gleason score, between radical prostatectomy versus external beam radiotherapy (EBRT) with a high dose rate (HDR) brachytherapy boost

	10-year freedom from distant metastasis	
	Surgery* (n = 987)	Brachytherapy† (n = 528)
Gleason score:		
2–6	95% (n = 723)	99% (n = 194)
7	58% (n = 226)	92% (n = 236)
8–10	58% (n = 38)	84% (n = 98)
Median follow-up	3.9 years	4.9 years

*Hull et al. J Urol 2002;167:528–534.
†Martinez et al.[34]

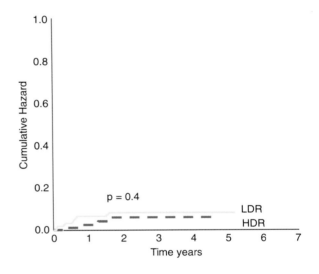

Figure 22.10
Actuarial chronic genitourinary and gastrointestinal grade 3 toxicity comparison between high dose rate (HDR) and low dose rate (LDR, permanent seeds) monotherapy treated patients.

Acute toxicity

High dose rate brachytherapy alone was associated with statistically significant reductions in the acute rates of dysuria, from 65% with [103]Pd seeds to 38% with HDR monotherapy (P < 0.001), as well as urinary frequency and/or urgency, from 94% for [103]Pd to 53% for HDR (P < 0.001) and urinary retention from 43% for [103]Pd to 29% for HDR (P = 0.012). In addition to reduced acute genitourinary symptoms, HDR was also associated with lower rates of rectal pain, 18% for LDR versus 7% for HDR (P = 0.025). The majority of acute toxicities in both groups were grade 1. Hormonal androgen ablation for gland downsizing was given to 31% of patients in both groups.

Chronic toxicity

Again, HDR brachytherapy alone was associated with reduced urinary frequency and urgency, 54% for [103]Pd versus 32% for HDR (P < 0.001). The majority of toxicities were grade 1. There were no differences in the remaining chronic toxicity rates of urinary inconti-

nence or retention, hematuria, diarrhea, rectal pain, or rectal bleeding between the two treatment groups. The rate of urethral stricture requiring dilatation was 3% with HDR compared with 1% with [103]Pd (P = 0.3). The median time to development of urethral stricture was 17 months, with a range of 4 to 37 months. Figure 22.10 shows, the cumulative proportion of chronic grade 3 toxicity by treatment modality. No difference was noted between the two treatment types.

Potency

Regardless of the use of adjuvant hormonal therapy all cases were included. This included 51 patients treated with HDR brachytherapy alone and 71 patients treated with permanent [103]Pd. The 4-year probability of impotency was 38% for all patients with available

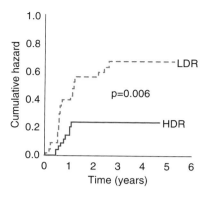

Figure 22.11

Probability of erectile dysfunction stratified by treatment modality high dose rate (HDR) versus low dose rate (LDR, permanent seeds) for monotherapy treated patients with favorable prostate cancer.

Table 22.5 Actuarial 5-year outcome for the favorable group prostate cancer patients treated with monotherapy divided by high dose rate (HDR) versus low dose rate (LDR, permanent seeds) prostate brachytherapy

5-year actuarial	HDR brachytherapy, %WBH+CET (n = 169)	LDR brachytherapy, %WBH (n = 161)	p-value*
Overall survival	99	93	0.35
Cause-specific survival	100	100	–
Biochemical control	99	98	0.602

*Kaplan–Meier log rank.

Box 22.1 Summary of high dose rate (HDR) brachytherapy

HDR prostate brachytherapy
- Allows the delivery of very high doses of radiation (>95 Gy BED) to the prostate with significant sparing of radiation dose to
  rectum and urethra, therefore, decreasing toxicity.
- Similar results were obtained at three different institutions when used as a boost and at two institutions when utilized as monotherapy to replace permanent seeds.
- Does not leave the patient radioactive after the procedure, nor irradiate intraoperatively the urologists, radiation oncologists, anesthesiologists, and operating room personnel.

HDR as a boost
- Excellent long-term outcomes for patients with intermediate- and high-risk factors, particularly with Gleason scores >8.
- The use of a short course of neoadjuvant androgen deprivation therapy has a detrimental effect increasing distant metastasis and cancer related metastasis and decreasing survival. Most likely related to the delay in curative therapy by high dose radiation.
- When HDR boost was compared with retropubic prostatectomy, HDR improved the 10-year freedom from distant metastasis for patients harboring Gleason scores 7 and 8–10.
- There is an improved outcome with doses (BED) above 95 Gy.

Box 22.1 Continued

HDR as monotherapy
- At 5 years, equal biochemical control, cause-specific survival, and overall survival when compared with permanent seeds.
- HDR produced less grade 1 chronic genitourinary toxicity compared with permanent seeds.
- Very large improvement in erectile dysfunction rates, from 41% with permanent seeds to 61% with HDR.
- Cost effective since the seeds do not have to be purchased for each patient.

data. As shown in Figure 22.11, the probability was 61% for LDR patients, and 21% for HDR patients ($P = 0.006$). The mean times to impotency for the HDR and LDR treatments were 3.9 years and 3.2 years, respectively.

Monotherapy outcomes

The 5-year actuarial outcomes for monotherapy can be seen in Table 22.5. No difference was noted in terms of ASTRO definition for biochemical control, cancer mortality, or overall survival.

Acknowledgment

This work is supported in part by the Department of Defense award PC031163.

References

1. Mettlin CJ, Murphy GP, McDonald CJ, et al. The national Cancer Data Base Report on increased use of brachytherapy for the treatment of patients with prostate carcinoma in the USA. Cancer 1999;86:1877–1882.
2. Lee WR, Moughan J, Owen JB, et al. The 1999 patterns of care study of radiotherapy in localized prostate carcinoma. A comprehensive survey of prostate carcinoma. A comprehensive survey of prostate brachytherapy in the United States. Cancer 2003;98:1987–1994.
3. Kupelian P, Katcher J, Levin H, et al. External beam radiotherapy versus radical prostatecomy for clinical Stage T1-T2 prostate cancer: Therapeutic implications of stratification by pretreatment PSA levels and biopsy Gleason scores. Cancer J Sci Am 1997;3:78–87.
4. Martinez AA, Gonzalez JA, Chung AK, et al. A comparison of external beam radiation therapy versus radical prostatectomy for patients with low risk prostate carcinoma diagnosed, staged and treated at a single institution. Cancer 2000;88:425–432.
5. D'Amico AV, Whittington R, Malkowski SB, et al. Biochemical outcome after radical prostatectomy, external beam radiation therapy or interstitial radiation therapy for clinically localized prostate cancer. JAMA 1998;280:969–974.
6. Blaska JC, Grimm PD, Sylvester JE, et al. Palladium-103 brachytherapy for prostate carcinoma. Int J Radiat Oncol Biol Phys 2000;46:839–850.
7. Stock RG, Stone NN, Tabert A, et al. A dose-response study for I-125 prostate implants. Int J Radiat Oncol Biol Phys 1998;41:101–108.
8. Wallner K, Merrick G, True L, et al. I-125 versus Pd-103 for low risk prostate cancer. Morbidity outcomes from a perspective randomized multicenter trial. Cancer J Sci Am 2002;8:67–73.

9. Beyer DC, Priestley JB. Biochemical disease-free survival following I-125 prostate implantation. Int J Radiat Oncol Biol Phys 1997; 37:559–563.

10. Martinez AA, Pataki I, Edmundson G, et al. Phase II prospective study of the use of conformal high-dose rate brachytherapy as monotherapy for the treatment of favorable stage prostate cancer: A feasibility report. Int J Radiat Oncol Biol Phys 2001;49:61–69.

11. Grills IS, Martinez A, Hollander M, et al. High does rate brachytherapy as prostate cancer monotherapy reduces toxicity compared to low dose rate Palladium seeds. J Urol 2004;171:1098–1104.

12. Yoshioka Y, Nose T, Yoshida K, et al. High-dose rate interstitial brachytherapy as monotherapy as monotherapy for localized prostate cancer: Treatment description and preliminary results of phase I/II clinical trial. Int J Radiat Oncol Biol Phys 2000;48:675–681.

13. Demanes JD, Rodriguez RR, Altieri GA. Hose dose rate prostate brachytherapy the California Endocurietherapy (CET) Method. Radiother Oncol 2000;57:289–296.

14. Morgan WR, Bergstralh EJ, Zincke H. Long-term evaluation of radical prostatectomy as treatment for clinical state C (T3) prostate cancer. Urology 1993;41:113–120.

15. Gerber GS, Thisted RA, Chodak GW, et al. Results of radical prostatectomy in men with locally advanced prostate cancer: Multi-institutional pooled analysis. Eur Urol 1997;32:385–390.

16. Oefelein MG, Smith ND, Grayhack JT, et al. Long-term results of radical retropubic prostatectomy in men with high grade carcinoma of the prostate. J Urol 1997;158:1460–1465.

17. Hanks GE, Diamond JJ, Krall JM, et al. A ten-year follow-up of 682 patients treated for prostate cancer with radiation therapy in the United States. Int J Radiat Oncol Biol Phys 1987;13:499–505.

18. Pilepich MV, Caplan R, Byhardt CA, et al. Phase III trial of androgen suppression using goserelin in unfavorable-prognosis carcinoma of the prostate treated with definitive radiotherapy: Report of Radiation Therapy Oncology Group Protocol 85-35. J Clin Oncol 1997;15:1013–1021.

19. Bolla M, Gonzalez D, Warde P, et al. Improved survival in patients with locally advanced prostate cancer treated with radiotherapy and goserelin. N Engl J Med 1997;337:295–300.

20. Roach M, Lu J, Pilepich M, et al. Predicting survival and the role of androgen suppressive therapy (AST): Radiation Therapy Oncology Group (RTOG) phase III randomized prostate cancer trials. Int J Radiat Oncol Biol Phys 1998;42–177.

21. Shipley WU, Verhey JJ, Munzenrider JE, et al. Advanced prostate cancer: The results of a randomized comparative trial of high dose irradiation boosting with conformal protons compared with conventional dose irradiation using photons alone. Int J Radiat Oncol Biol Phys 1995;32:3–12.

22. Forman JD, Duclos M, Sharma R, et al. Conformal mixed neutron and photon irradiation in localized and locally advanced prostate cancer: Preliminary estimates of the therapeutic ratio. Int J Radiat Oncol Biol Phys 1996;35:259–266.

23. Zelefsky MJ, Leibel, SA, Gaudin, PB, et al. Dose escalation with three-dimensional conformal radiation therapy affects the outcome in prostate cancer. Radiology 1998;209:169–174.

24. Hanks GE, Lee WR, Hanlon Al, et al. Conformal technique dose escalation for prostate cancer: Biochemical evidence of improved cancer control with higher doses in patients with pretreatment prostate-specific antigen 10 ng/ml. Int J Radiat Oncol Biol Phys 1996;35:861–868.

25. Martinez AA, Kestin LL, Stromberg J, et al. Interim report of image-guided conformal high dose rate brachytherapy for patients with unfavorable prostate cancer. The William Beaumont phase II dose-escalating trial. Int J Radiat Oncol Biol Phys 2000;47:343–352.

26. Martinez AA, Gonzales J, Spencer W, et al. Conformal high dose rate brachytherapy improves biochemical control and cause specific survival in patients with prostate cancer and poor prognostic factors. J Urol 2003;169:974–980.

27. Galalae R, Martinez A, Mate T, et el. Long term outcome by risk factors using conformal HDR brachytherapy boost with or without neoadjuvant androgen deprivation for localized prostate cancer. Int J Radiat Oncol Biol Phys 2004;58:1048–1055.

28. Edmundson G, Rizzo N, Teahan M, et al. Concurrent treatment planning for outpatient high dose rate prostate template implants. Int J Radiat Oncol Biol Phys 1993;27:1215–1223.

29. Edmundson GK, Yan D, Martinez A. Intraoperative optimization of needle placement and dwell times for conformal prostate brachytherapy. Int J Radiat Oncol Biol Phys 1995;33:1257–1263.

30. Martinez AA, Galalae R, Gonzalez J, et al. No apparent benefit at 5 years from a course of neoadjuvant/concurrent androgen deprivation for prostate cancer patients treated to a high total radiation dose. J Urol 2003;170:2296–2301.

31. Brenner DJ, Hall EJ. Fractionation and protraction for radiotherapy of prostate carcinoma. Int J Radiat Biol Phys 1999;43:1095–1101.

32. Brenner DJ, Martinez AA, Edmundson GK, et al. Direct evidence that prostate tumors show high sensitivity to fraction (low α/β ratio) comparable to late-responding normal tissues. Int J Radiat Oncol Biol Phys 2002;52:6–13.

33. Hull GW, Rabbani F, Abbas F, et al. Cancer control with radical prostatectomy alone in 1000 consecutive patients. J Urol 2202;167: 528–534.

34. Martinez AA, Demanas J, Galalae R, et al. Lack of benefit from a short course of androgen deprivation for unfavorable prostate cancer patients treated with an accelerated Hypofractionated regime. Int J Radiat Oncol Biol Phys 2005;62:1322–1331.

23

MRI-guided partial prostatic irradiation in select patients with clinically localized adenocarcinoma of the prostate

Michele Albert, Mark Hurwitz, Clair Beard, Clare M Tempany, Robert A Cormack, Anthony V D'Amico

Introduction

The introduction of the serum prostate-specific antigen (PSA) has changed the presentation of prostate cancer worldwide. Patients now present at a younger age, with lower grade disease, and are more likely to have organ-confined cancers found upon pathologic evaluation of the radical prostatectomy specimen.[1] This migration toward smaller volume disease raises the possibility of more tailored therapy.

Brachytherapy is the therapeutic delivery of radiation to a diseased site by the insertion, either temporarily or permanently, of sources containing radioactive material. The current method of prostate brachytherapy in the United States commonly uses transrectal ultrasound (TRUS) imaging to guide radioactive seed placement.[2] Using this approach, the goal is to deliver 100% of the prescription dose to the entire prostate gland.

Since the late 1990s, a real-time intraoperative magnetic resonance image (IMRI) guided prostate brachytherapy technique[3] has been designed and implemented. This utilized both MRI[4,5] and dose and volume histogram (DVH) analysis performed in real time, intraoperatively. Using this technique, regions of the prostate gland (i.e., peripheral zone [PZ], transition zone [TZ], periurethral, anterior base) can be delineated using MRI providing the opportunity to focus the radiation dose delivery to specific zone(s) of the prostate gland, based on the likelihood of cancer presence using the individual patient's pretreatment clinical characteristics. In particular, several investigators have identified a subset of patients—based on the pretreatment PSA level, biopsy Gleason score, and clinical T-category—in which the presence of cancer in the anterior base is rare.[6,7]

A direct correlation with the development of acute urinary morbidity and brachytherapy dose to the entire prostate gland has been documented.[8] Given that the IMRI technique limits dose to the anterior base and the transition zone anterior to the urethra to under 100%, while delivering 100% or more of the prescription dose to the peripheral zone of the prostate gland, this approach has permitted the treatment of patients with large prostate glands (>60 cm³) with a resultant low risk of self-limited acute urinary retention,[9] and no need for neoadjuvant hormonal therapy to achieve prostate gland shrinkage. However, such an approach for patients with moderate prostate gland enlargement intentionally did not treat a portion of the prostate gland to high dose. Therefore, whether not treating part of the prostate gland in these patients to high dose led to a decrement in PSA outcome when compared at 5 years with patients treated with maximal therapy (i.e., radical prostatectomy [RP]) was the subject of this study.

Patient population, staging, and treatment

Between 1997 and 2002, of 406 and 227 patients who underwent RP or an IMRI-guided prostate brachy monotherapy procedure, respectively, at the Brigham and Women's Hospital (BWH) for the 2002 American Joint Commission on Cancer (AJCC),[10] and who had clinical category T1c, PSA less than 10 ng/mL and biopsy Gleason 3 + 4 or less, and who had perineural invasion biopsy negative adenocarcinoma of the prostate, 322 and 196 had a 2-year minimum follow up respectively.[11] No patient received neoadjuvant or adjuvant androgen suppression or radiation therapy. Patients who had a history of a transurethral resection of the prostate (TURP), urinary daytime frequency less than every 2 hours, and/or nocturia exceeding 4 that was not medically correctable with an α_{1A}-blocker were not eligible for brachytherapy. However, patients who had a previous abdominal perineal resection were not excluded because the IMRI-guided technique did not require a rectum to guide source placement because the imaging apparatus was extrinsic to the patient.[12] In addition, long-term quality-of-life data were available on 152 of the 196 patients who underwent brachytherapy and 50 patients who underwent external-beam radiation therapy to 45 Gy plus a brachytherapy boost to 77 Gy. Internal Review Board (IRB)-approved informed consent was obtained on all patients. All biopsy slides were reviewed by a single genitourinary pathology group at the BWH, and all patients had at least a sextant biopsy. The prostate gland volume (PG Vol) was determined in each case using a 1.5 tesla staging endorectal MRI study and an ellipsoid approximation where PG Vol = $\pi/6 \times$ length $\times$ width $\times$ height. The median age (range) of the surgical and IMRI brachytherapy patients at the time of initial therapy was 60 (44–75) and 62 (49–79) years respectively. Table 23.1 lists the pretreatment clinical characteristics of the RP and IMRI brachytherapy cohorts. The pretreatment medical management,[3]

Table 23.1 Percent distribution of the pre-treatment clinical characteristics of the 406 surgery and 227 brachytherapy managed patients comprising the study cohort*

Clinical characteristic	Surgery (%)	Brachytherapy (%)	$P_{Chi-square}$
PSA (ng/mL)			0.0005
<4	9	91	
4–9.99	19	81	
Biopsy Gleason score			<0.0001
≤5	20	8	
6	65	81	
3 + 4	15	11	
Age (years)†			<0.0001
<60	48	32	
60–64	24	33	
65–69	21	17	
≥70	7	18	
% Positive biopsies			0.25
<34	73	78	
34–50	17	12	
>50	11	10	
Prostate volume (cm³)			<0.0001
<20	1	6	
20 –44.9	26	58	
45–59.9	38	20	
60–99.9	30	15	
≥100	5	1	

PSA, prostate-specific antigen.
*Percentages may not sum to 100 due to rounding. †Age at the time of initial therapy.

intraoperative magnetic resonance unit,[13] and IMRI technique[14] have been previously described and mandated that the end of operating-room dosimetry provided a V100 of at least 100%.

Follow-up

For the 322 RP- and 196 brachytherapy-managed patients whose minimum follow-up was 2 years the median follow up was 4.2 and 3.95 years, respectively. Patients generally had a serum PSA measurement and digital rectal examination performed every 3 months for 2 years, then every 6 months for an additional 3 years, then annually thereafter. The median (range) number of PSA values per patient whose minimum follow up was 2 years was 14 (8–26). Prostate-specific antigen failure was defined using the American Society for Therapeutic Radiology and Oncology (ASTRO) consensus criteria.[15] Determinations of PSA were made no more frequently then every 3 months, and three consecutive increments were necessary to constitute a rise in order to avoid overcalling PSA failure in brachytherapy-managed patients due to the PSA bounce phenomenon.[16] A PSA level postoperatively was not considered detectable until it exceeded 0.2 ng/mL. No patient died of prostate cancer during the study period, and no patient was lost to follow-up.

Assessment of late toxicity

Rectal function

Patients were asked whether they had experienced any rectal bleeding at each follow-up by a specialty oncology nurse. All rectal bleeding was analyzed with colonoscopy, and evidence of proctitis needed to be confirmed endoscopically before grading the rectal bleeding as an event related to radiation. In all cases, the date that the patient reported the first evidence of rectal bleeding was noted as the event date. The following scales were used to quantify the rectal bleeding: grade 1 (G1) no clinical evidence of rectal bleeding but with evidence of mild proctitis seen on screening colonoscopy; grade 2 (G2) cortisone enemas necessary for eradication of rectal bleeding; and grade 3 (G3) argon plasma coagulation (APC)[17,18] necessary for the eradication of bleeding. Other late gastrointestinal (GI) toxicity such as diarrhea and rectal urgency was not collected in this study.

Erectile function

At baseline and then at each follow-up, patients were asked about their ability to have an erection sufficient for vaginal intercourse and, specifically, how this ability compared with their erectile function prior to treatment. Erectile function was noted as being the same as the baseline, worse than the baseline, or better than the baseline. Information on the use of erectile function aids and their efficacy was collected. A standardized questionnaire was not used.[19] The date that the patient reported the first evidence of any decrease in erectile function compared with baseline was noted as the event date.

Urinary function

Prior to treatment and at the time of each follow-up, patients were asked whether they had noted any blood in the urine. All patients who presented with hematuria were evaluated with a urine analysis and culture to rule out a urinary tract infection (UTI).

Once a UTI had been excluded then a cystoscopy was performed to determine the etiology of the hematuria. In addition, patients were asked about the strength of their urinary stream and the frequency of voiding, nocturia, hesitancy, and urgency, as well as the presence of any urinary incontinence. In cases where a significant change had occurred in their voiding pattern, a cystoscopy and a urodynamic study was performed to assess for a urethral stricture or the need for a TURP.

Statistical methods

A Cox regression multivariable analysis[20] was performed to evaluate the ability of the treatment received (RP versus brachytherapy), pre-treatment PSA level (continuous), percent positive biopsies (continuous), prostate gland volume (continuous), and biopsy Gleason score (continuous but could only take on integer values from 2 to 7 inclusive) to predict time to post-treatment PSA failure. In addition, a Cox regression analysis was performed to evaluate the ability of the categorical variables of initial treatment received (RP versus brachytherapy), PSA level (≤4 ng/mL versus >4 and <10 ng/mL), biopsy Gleason score (3 + 4 versus ≤6), percent positive biopsies (≥34% versus <34%), and prostate gland volume (≥45 cm³ versus <45 cm³) to predict time to post-treatment PSA failure. The cut-points for the categorical variables were selected based on data suggesting their predictive value from previously reported studies for PSA, biopsy Gleason score, and the percent positive biopsies.[21] The cut-point for prostate gland volume was selected based on the currently accepted maximum prostate gland volume recommended by the American Brachytherapy Society for a TRUS-guided brachytherapy procedure.[22]

A chi-square metric was used to evaluate whether the distribution in age, PSA level, biopsy Gleason score, and percent positive prostate biopsies at the time of treatment were significantly different between surgically and brachytherapy-managed patients. Estimates of PSA failure following RP or IMRI-guided brachytherapy were calculated using the method of Kaplan and Meier[23] and are graphically displayed for patients with a minimum follow-up of 2 years. Comparisons of PSA failure-free survival were made using a log rank test, and time zero was defined as the date of diagnosis for all patients.

Quality-of-life data are available on 152 and 50 patients who underwent IMRI-guided prostate brachytherapy as monotherapy or as a boost in conjunction with 45 Gy neoadjuvant external-beam radiation therapy, respectively. Freedom from rectal bleeding, freedom from radiation cystitis, freedom from urethral stricture, freedom from the need for a post-implant TURP, and freedom from any decrease in erectile function compared with the baseline were computed using the actuarial method of Kaplan and Meier.[23] Comparisons were made using a log rank test. One and four patients were not evaluable for rectal toxicity and erectile dysfunction respectively due to lack of information in the patient's chart.

Prostate-specific antigen control

As shown in Table 23.1, there were statistically significant differences in the distribution of the PSA level ($P = 0.0005$), biopsy Gleason score ($P < 0.0001$), and the prostate gland volume ($P < 0.0001$) between surgically and brachytherapy-managed patients. However, only the percent positive prostate biopsies ($P_{Cox} = 0.02$) was a significant predictor of time to post-treatment PSA failure in the Cox regression multivariable analyses in which the pretreatment predictors were analyzed first as continuous and then categorical variables as noted in Table 23.2. Importantly, the distribution of the percent positive biopsies amongst RP- and brachytherapy-managed patients was not significantly different ($P_{chi\,square} = 0.25$) as shown in Table 23.1.

The median (range) PSA nadir for the brachytherapy managed patients was 0.5 (<0.2–1.2) ng/mL. Initial therapy received did not predict for time to post-therapy PSA failure ($P_{Cox} = 0.18$). Specifically, for patients with a minimum 2-year follow up and a median follow-up ranging from 3.95 to 4.2 years, Figure 23.1 illustrates that the 5-year estimates of PSA control were 93% versus 95% ($P_{log\,rank} = 0.16$) following RP or brachy monotherapy respectively.

A few points are worth noting. First, while a Cox proportional-hazards model was used to adjust for significant predictors of the time to PSA failure following initial therapy when comparing the two treatment groups, factors not yet discovered that predict for time to PSA failure following RP or IMRI-guided brachytherapy may be imbalanced between the two treatment arms and can confound the results of this study. Therefore, the findings should be viewed as hypothesis generating and not conclusive.

Table 23.2 P-values from the Cox regression multivariable analyses evaluating the ability of the initial therapy received and pretreatment clinical characteristics to predict time to prostate-specific antigen (PSA) failure following treatment

Pretreatment predictor	P value	
	Continuous	*Categorical**
Surgery vs brachytherapy	0.18[†]	0.18
Percent positive biopsies	0.02	0.02
PSA level	0.26	0.18
Biopsy Gleason score	0.42	0.57
Prostate gland volume	0.49	0.62

***Categories:** percent positive biopsies (≥34% vs <34%); PSA (4–9.99 ng/mL vs <4 ng/mL); Gleason score (3 + 4 vs ≤6); prostate volume (≥45 cm³ vs <45 cm³). [†]evaluated as a categorical variable with surgery as the baseline.

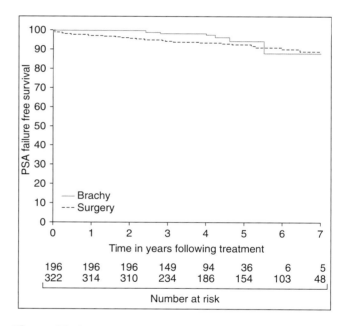

196	196	196	149	94	36	6	5
322	314	310	234	186	154	103	48

Number at risk

Figure 23.1
Prostate-specific antigen (PSA) failure-free survival for patients with a minimum follow up of 2 years stratified by initial therapy received. Surgery versus brachytherapy: $P_{log\,rank} = 0.16$.

Second, no matter what definition of PSA failure is used, there remains a bias in favor of radiation because of the time it takes to nadir before a rise can be scored compared with surgery where any value more than 0.2 ng/mL would be considered detectable. This bias has been previously described and noted,[21] and is also noted in this study. Specifically, careful examination of Figure 23.1 will reveal that the brachytherapy-managed patient's PSA control curve is slightly above the surgical control curve during the early years of follow-up reflecting this potential bias.

Third, following brachytherapy, PSA bouncing has been described and in this study population nearly two thirds of patients were reported to experience this effect.[16] As a result, PSA failure could potentially be overestimated in the brachytherapy group. To minimize this problem, PSA determinations were made no more frequently then every 3 months and three consecutive increments in the PSA of at least 0.2 ng/mL needed to be observed in order to define a PSA failure.

Interestingly however, the prostate gland volume was not a significant predictor of time to post-therapy PSA failure when considered as a continuous ($P_{Cox} = 0.49$) or categorical ($P_{Cox} = 0.62$) variable above and below a gland volume of 45 cm^3 using a Cox regression multivariable analysis as shown in Table 23.2. Therefore, in the patients selected for implant monotherapy in this study who also had moderate benign prostatic hyperplasia (BPH; n = 81/227, 36% of all study patients had prostate gland volumes of at least 45 cm^3), delivering radiation doses to regions of the TZ anterior to the urethra that were less than prescription dose did not appear to negatively impact on PSA outcome.

This lack of impact of prostate gland volume on PSA outcome may be explained by suggesting that patients with moderate BPH would also be expected to have smaller volume cancers compared with patients without BPH and the same PSA level, because some of the serum PSA in patients with BPH was contributed from the benign component of the prostate gland. Another potential explanation may be that for the select group of patients with low-risk disease treated in this study, prostate cancer residing in the TZ may be an infrequent finding. However, given the slow rate of progression expected for the low-risk patients selected for treatment in this study, further follow-up will be needed to evaluate whether these results are maintained.

Radiation proctopathy

Estimates of grade 3 rectal bleeding stratified by implant mono or combined modality therapy are shown in Figure 23.2. Four years following initial therapy, estimates of the rates of grade 1, 2, and 3 rectal bleeding were 80% versus 85% ($P_{\log rank} = 0.88$), 18% versus 22% ($P_{\log rank} = 0.16$), and 8% versus 30% ($P_{\log rank} = 0.0001$) for patients who received implant versus combined modality, respectively. All patients who sustained grade 2 or 3 rectal bleeding were controlled using cortisone enemas or APC.

Erectile dysfunction

Figure 23.3 illustrates the estimated rate of patients experiencing any decrease in their ability to have an erection sufficient for vaginal intercourse compared with baseline stratified by initial therapy. While there was a significant difference ($P_{\log rank} = 0.03$) in patients receiving mono as opposed to combined therapy in the estimate of erectile dysfunction, essentially all patients (82–93%) were estimated to experience some degree of erectile dysfunction compared with baseline within 4 years following therapy. However, as shown in Figure 23.4, when erectile function aids were utilized, which was sildenafil citrate (Viagra®) in 95% of the cases, at least two thirds of patients reported rates of erectile function comparable to or superior to baseline by 4 years following either implant or combined modality therapy ($P_{\log rank} = 0.46$).

Radiation cystitis

In two prior reports,[24,25] a decrease in acute urinary retention and urinary obstructive and irritative symptoms have been reported for IMRI-guided compared with TRUS-guided prostate brachytherapy. In this study, there were no events with regard to bladder or urethral dysfunction after implant monotherapy. Specifically, no patient required a post-implant TURP. In addition urethral strictures and radiation cystitis was not documented. However, two patients who received combined modality therapy presented with radiation cysti-

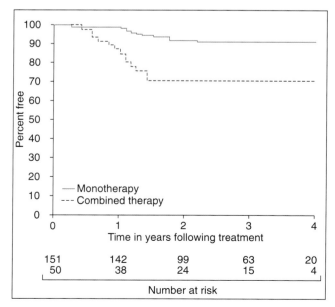

Figure 23.2
Estimates of grade 3 rectal bleeding following magnetic resonance imaging (MRI)-guided implant monotherapy or combined modality therapy. $P_{\log rank} = 0.0001$.

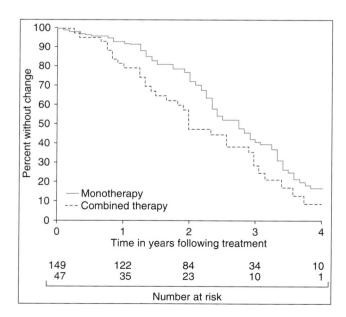

Figure 23.3
Estimates of erectile function compared with baseline following magnetic resonance imaging (MRI)-guided implant monotherapy or combined modality therapy. $P_{\log rank} = 0.03$.

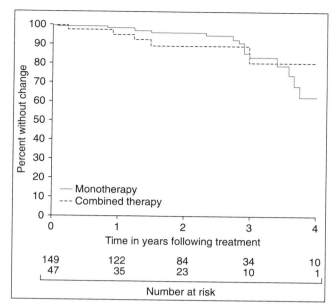

Figure 23.4

Estimates of erectile function with sildenafil citrate (Viagra) compared with baseline following magnetic resonance imaging (MRI)-guided implant monotherapy or combined modality therapy. $P_{\log rank} = 0.46$.

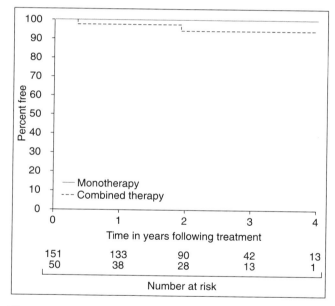

Figure 23.5

Estimates of freedom from any late urinary dysfunction following magnetic resonance imaging (MRI)-guided implant monotherapy or combined therapy. $P_{\log rank} = 0.01$.

tis. Specifically, cystoscopy performed after a single episode of gross hematuria confirmed this finding. The first patient presented in the setting of a UTI and the hematuria resolved and did not recur following administration of an antibiotic. The other patient's hematuria resolved after bladder irrigation. Neither patient has had recurrent symptoms 3 years following the initial presentation of gross hematuria. Figure 23.5 illustrates the 100% versus 95% ($P_{\log rank} = 0.01$) estimates of freedom from radiation cystitis at 4 years

following treatment for patients who received mono or combined modality therapy respectively.

The quality-of-life results suggest that the ability of the IMRI-guided approach to keep the dose to any point on the urethra at less than 200 Gy was urethral sparing. In particular, urethral and/or bladder toxicity were rare. Specifically, there were no reports of gross hematuria or need for a post-implant TURP, or documentation of urethral stricture for patients treated with monotherapy, and only two patients (5%) were estimated to have radiation cystitis by 4 years following combined modality therapy, both of which were resolved with minimal intervention (antibiotics by mouth and bladder irrigation). These very low rates of late urinary toxicity coupled with the low rates of acute urinary retention[25] and need for post-implant Flomax support the urethral sparing effect of IMRI-guided brachytherapy.

Conclusion

Five-year estimates of PSA control following either RP or partial prostatic irradiation using an IMRI-guidance technique[3] in select patients are not significantly different. Longer follow-up will determine if these results are maintained. While estimates of grade 3 rectal bleeding were low following implant monotherapy, they were significantly higher following combined modality therapy. Nearly all patients experienced a decrease in erectile function compared with the baseline, however, the vast majority of patients returned to at least baseline function with the use of sildenafil citrate (Viagra). Urethral and bladder toxicity were rare which may be attributed to the urethral sparing technique of the IMRI-guided approach.

References

1. Catalona WJ, Smith DS, Ratliff TL, et al. Detection of organ-confined prostate cancer is increased through prostate-specific antigen-based screening. JAMA 1993;270:948–954.
2. Ragde H, Korb LJ, Elgamal AA, et al. Modern prostate brachytherapy. Prostate specific antigen results in 219 patients with up to 12 years of observed follow up. Cancer 2000;89:135–141.
3. D'Amico AV, Cormack R, Tempany CM, et al. Real time magnetic resonance image guided interstitial brachytherapy in the treatment of select patients with clinically localized prostate cancer. Int J Rad Oncol Biol Phys 1998;42:507–516.
4. Jolesz FA, Kikinis R. Intraoperative imaging revolutionizes therapy. Diagn Imaging 1995;17:62–68.
5. Silverman SG, Jolesz FA, Newman RW, et al. Design and implementation of an interventional MR imaging suite. AM J Roentgenol 1997;168:1465–1471.
6. D'Amico AV, Davis A, Vargas SO, et al. Defining the implant treatment volume for patients with low risk prostate cancer: does the anterior base need to be treated? Int J Radiat Oncol Phys 1999;43:587–590.
7. Takashima R, Egawa S, Kuwao S, et al. Anterior distribution of Stage T1c nonpalpable tumors in radical prostatectomy specimens. Urology 2002;59:692–697.
8. Desai J, Stock RG, Stone NN, et al. Acute urinary morbidity following I-125 interstitial implantation of the prostate gland. radiation oncology investigations. 1998;6:135–141.
9. Thomas MD, Cormack R, Tempany CM, et al. Identifying the predictors of acute urinary retention following magnetic-resonance image guided prostate brachytherapy. Int J Radiat Oncol Biol Phys 2000;47:905–908.

10. Greene FL, Page DL, Fleming ID, et al. American Joint Committee on Cancer, Manual for staging cancer, 6th ed. New York: Springer-Verlag, 2002, pp 337–346.

11. Gleason DF, and the Veterans Administration Cooperative Urological Research Group. Histologic grading and staging of prostatic carcinoma. In: Tannenbaum M (ed.): Urologic pathology. Philadelphia, PA: Lea & Febiger, 1977, pp 171–187.

12. D'Amico AV, Cormack RA, Tempany CM. MRI-guided diagnosis and treatment of prostate cancer. N Engl J Med 2001;344:776–777.

13. Hirose M, Bharatha A, Hata N, et al. Quantitative MR imaging assessment of prostate gland deformation before and during MR imaging-guided brachytherapy. Acad Radiol 2002;9:906–912.

14. Cormack RA, Tempany CM, D'Amico AV. Optimizing target coverage by dosimetric feedback during prostate brachytherapy. Int J Radiat Oncol Biol Phys 2000;48:1245–1249.

15. Cox JD, for the American Society for Therapeutic Radiology and Oncology Consensus Panel. Consensus Statement: Guidelines for PSA Following Radiation Therapy. Int J Radiat Oncol Biol Phys 1997;37:1035–1041.

16. Das P, Chen M, Valentine K, et al. Utilizing the magnitude of PSA bounce following magnetic resonance image guided prostate brachytherapy to distinguish recurrence, benign precipitating factors and idiopathic bounce. Int J Radiat Oncol Biol Phys 2002;54:698–703.

17. Smith S, Wallner K, Domonitz JA, et al. Argon plasma coagulation for rectal bleeding after prostate brachytherapy. Int J Rad Oncol Biol Phys 2001;51:636–642.

18. Venkatesh KS, Ramanujam P. Endoscopic therapy for radiation proctitis-induced hemorrhage in patients with prostatic carcinoma using argon plasma coagulator application. Surg Endosc 2002;16:707–710.

19. Rosen RC, Riley A, Wagner G, et al. The international index of erectile function (IIEF): a multidimension scale for assessment of erectile dysfunction. Urology 1997;49:822–830.

20. Neter J, Wasserman W, Kutner M. Simultaneous inferences and other topic in regression analysis-1. In Neter J, Wasserman W, Kutner M (eds): Applied Linear Regression Models. Homewood, Ill: Richard D Irwin Inc, 1983, pp 150–153.

21. D'Amico AV, Whittington R, Malkowicz SB, et al. Biochemical outcome following radical prostatectomy or external beam radiation therapy for clinically localized prostate cancer in the PSA era. Cancer 2002;95:281–286.

22. Nag S. Brachytherapy for prostate cancer: summary of American Brachytherapy Society recommendations. Semin Urol Oncol 2000;18:133–136.

23. Kaplan EL, Meier P. Non-parametric estimation from incomplete observations. J Am Stat Assoc 1958;53:457–500.

24. Thomas MD, Cormack R, Tempany CM, et al. Identifying the predictor of acute urinary retention following magnetic-resonance-guided prostate brachytherapy. Int J Rad Oncol Biol Phys 2000;47:905–908.

25. Seo PH, Clark JA, Mitchell SP, et al. Early symptoms and symptom distress after standard ultrasound guided brachytherapy or MRI-guided brachytherapy in early stage prostate cancer. Proc Am Soc Clin Oncol 2001;20:157b [abstract #2377].

24

Hyperthermia for treatment of localized prostate cancer

Serdar Deger

Introduction

Standard therapy for localized prostate cancer is radical prostatectomy. Experience since the mid-1990s has shown that radical surgery could not achieve local tumor control in patients with extracapsular extension of prostate cancer.[1] Looking at long-term results of radical prostatectomy, clinicopathologic parameters influence cancer-specific and overall survival.[2] Unfavorable risk factors like extraprostatic extension and seminal vesical involvement affect long-term biochemical recurrence-free survival.[3]

In the early 1990s radiation therapy was technically improved so that a dose increase within the prostate gland could be achieved.[4–6] Many institutions had suggested that better progression-free survival could be achieved with escalated treatment doses achieved by improvements in treatment planning and delivery technology.[7–11] Intensity modulated radiotherapy (IMRT) is a new form of external beam radiotherapy to achieve higher doses in the prostate without increasing side effects.[12]

Another possibility to raise the radiation dose in the prostate gland is high dose rate brachytherapy. Different institutions were able to demonstrate local tumor control in patients with unfavorable prognostic parameters.[13–15] These data suggested that increasing the intraprostatic dose while reducing side effects could be a treatment strategy for local advanced prostate cancer. To achieve higher doses in the prostate while reducing the nominal radiation brought hyperthermia into this concept. Adding hyperthermia to radiation therapy seems to be an additional strategy to effectively achieve a higher dose in the treatment of prostate cancer.

Cytotoxic effects of hyperthermia were first demonstrated in 1979 by Raaphorst. The extent of the hyperthermic cytotoxicity depends on the thermal dose, which is a function of the administered amount of heat and the duration of the exposure to the heat.[16,17]

Hyperthermia has been the subject of several recent reviews on results of both phase I/II and randomized studies, demonstrating the benefit of adding hyperthermia.[18,19] Randomized studies have shown that the addition of hyperthermia to radiotherapy does improve the clinical outcome. Additional hyperthermia improved local tumor control rates, palliative effects, and/or overall survival rates for breast cancer,[20] cervical cancer,[21] head and neck tumors,[22] glioblastoma multiforme,[23] and melanoma.[24]

Hyperthermia in prostate cancer

Regarding prostate cancer, Ryu reported on radiosensitization using hyperthermia in 1996.[25] Li et al studied apoptosis in irradiated and heated PC-3 prostate cancer cells. They found that apoptosis was an important mode of death in heated cells, but not in irradiated cells. No significant apoptosis was observed when cells were heated to 42°C for 240 minutes; therefore, a heating temperature of 43°C and above may be required to induce significant apoptosis in a clinically feasible duration of time. They concluded that apoptosis-inducing modalities such as hyperthermia may supplement radiation therapy in the future management of prostate cancer.[26]

Peschke et al studied three different sublines (anaplastic, moderately differentiated, and well differentiated) of a Dunning rat prostate carcinoma R3327 model, in which local tumor hyperthermia alone induced growth delay in both differentiated tumors, while the anaplastic tumor subline did not respond. Combining hyperthermia with radiation intensified cell damage in anaplastic tumors.[28,29] This study group also worked on radiation dose rate, sequence, and frequency of heating. They found a clear thermal enhancement of low dose rate irradiation, with maximal sensitization when hyperthermia was given just before irradiation.[29] Mittelberg also reported synergistic effects between hyperthermia and radiation. He concluded that injury of heated and irradiated Dunning cells is likely to be induced by separate mechanisms, which may explain the observed synergy.[30]

It is difficult to achieve adequate hyperthermia temperatures within the prostate under clinical circumstances. Different forms of heat application have been published. The combination of hyperthermia with radiation therapy to treat prostate cancer has been investigated since the 1970s. Several single institution and collaborative group results were disappointing.[31–33] Anscher et al[31] reported 3-year disease-free survival rates of 25%. The main problem of this study was the inability to achieve adequate therapeutic temperatures within the prostate.

The option to overcome the limitations of external heating systems is interstitial hyperthermia. The interstitial application modality of hyperthermia seems to be interesting for urologist. In the early 1990s, a transrectal ultrasound device was developed specially for prostate hyperthermia.[34,35] A phase I trial combining transrectal hyperthermia using a transrectal ultrasound device with external beam radiation therapy was performed at the University of Arizona by Fosmire et al.[36] The ultrasound power is delivered from a water cooled 16-element partial-cylindrical intracavitary array. Fosmire et al measured an average temperature, using thermocouples, of only 41.9 ± 0.9°C over 30 min. Using this device, a phase II trial of hyperthermia and external beam radiation therapy with or without hormonal therapy for locally advanced prostate cancer was performed by Hurwitz on nine patients with clinical T2b to T3b prostate cancer.[37] The total dose was 6660 cGy ± 5% of the prescribed target volume using a 3D conformal technique. Acute toxicity was limited to National Cancer Institute Common Toxicity Criteria grade 1. No excess toxicity was noted with full course of radiation therapy with or without hormonal therapy. This study group reported on approximately 30 patients having rectal toxicity using the described method in 2002.[38] A cooling water bolus was maintained between 33°C and 37°C to keep the maximum rectal wall temperature within treatment guidelines. Rectal toxicity was correlated with maximum allowable rectal wall temperature of >40°C (7 of 11 patients had an acute grade 2 proctitis). Both papers, however, do not include oncologic data.

Using the same ultrasound device, long-term toxicities with the combination of hyperthermia and radiation for treatment of prostate cancer in 26 patients with stage T3 or N+ prostate cancer with a median follow-up of 71 months were reported by Algan et al.[39] They had no additional toxicity. Disease free survival rate was 39% in a patient population with a median pretreatment prostate-specific antigen (PSA) level of 29 ng/mL.

Using regional radiofrequency systems resulted in relatively low temperatures in the tumor.[40] A phase I study was reported in 1994, which included 36 patients with prostate cancer (5 with locally recurrent, 15 with T2, and 16 T3 prostate cancer), treated with radiofrequency-induced hyperthermia and high dose rate brachytherapy from 1987 until 1992.[41] In this study 2D-steered 0.5-MHz radiofrequency-induced interstitial hyperthermia was administered in combination with 50 Gy external radiation for 5 weeks, followed by 30 Gy high dose rate brachytherapy using iridium-192 (^{192}Ir). Two hyperthermia sessions of 45 min were planned, immediately before and after brachytherapy. Between 7 and 32 1.5-mm steel trocar hyperthermia electrodes were positioned transperineally in the prostate. The treatment was well tolerated.

To overcome the problem of too low local temperatures in the prostate using a radiofrequency system, a multielectrode current source (MECS) interstitial hyperthermia system was developed. This system uses segmented radiofrequency electrodes. Each individual electrode controls the locally measured tissue temperature.[42,43]

In 2003, van Pulpen et al[44] published data from 26 patients, treated between 1997 and 2001 with T3 to T4, Nx prostate cancer. Of 14 patients, 5 received weekly regional hyperthermia treatments within a phase II study, using the coaxial transverse electrical magnetic system with a mean follow up of 3 years. Twelve patients received one interstitial hyperthermia treatment within a phase I trial, using the multielectrode current source system. Radiation therapy was administered to a total dose of 70 Gy in 2-Gy fractions over 7 weeks using a conformal three-field technique. There was no severe toxicity. All patients survived; 27% of patients had a biochemical relapse. Three of these patients were in the regional and four patients were in the interstitial group. The actuarial probability of freedom from biochemical relapse was 79% for the regional and 57% for the interstitial group. Actuarial probability of freedom from biochemical relapse was 70% at 36 months for all patients.

Kalapurakal et al reported a phase I/II study in 13 patients with locally advanced, hormone-refractory prostate cancer using thermoradiotherapy[45] between 1997 and 2002. Eight patients had a recurrence of the disease after radiotherapy and five had recurrence without having prior radiotherapy. All patients had clinical symptomatic disease. The patients with prior radiation received 39.6 Gy and those without prior external beam radiation received 66.6 Gy. Hyperthermia was applied in 8 to 10 sessions, using MECS. Despite the size of these large tumors, radiotherapy and hyperthermia resulted in significant tumor shrinkage, rapid serum prostate-specific antigen decline, durable treatment responses, and durable palliation of symptoms in a median follow-up of 13 to 14 months for both groups.

An innovative technique for interstitial hyperthermia is the use of implantable ferromagnetic thermoseeds. They are heated by induction in a magnetic field based on the so-called Curie temperature, at which the material loses its magnetic dipole momentum. Paramagnetism occurs when the temperature of an alloy rises above this level. Ferromagnetism is based on the quantum-mechanic nature of the inner electrons of a material and leads to the generation of a dipole. When the magnetic field oscillates and the ferromagnetic material is exposed to a surrounding field, atomic dipoles straighten out and heat is generated. The material heats up until the Curie temperature is reached and the ferromagnetic characteristics are lost. The selection of alloys allows for a self-regulating system according to the respective Curie temperatures.[46–48] As the thermoseeds remain in the prostate, hyperthermia induction can, therefore, be repeated as often as necessary, even in case of local tumor recurrence.

Different studies worked with animal models using ferromagnetic thermoseeds for prostate treatment.[49–51] Deger et al[52] described a combination of interstitial hyperthermia with external radiation therapy for prostate cancer patients. They used ferromagnetic cobalt–palladium alloy thermoseeds. This study group examined several alloys (e.g., nickel–copper) to come to the optimal biocompatibility, and cobalt–palladium was the most promising alloy.[47,53,54] Other investigators also reported palladium–nickel and ferrite core/metallic sheath thermoseeds.[55,56]

Using thermoseeds overcomes the problem of routine clinical application of hyperthermia. Advantages of thermoseeds are exactly defined energy application in the tumor with protection of benign tissue, more effective local therapy, homogeneous energy distribution and compact measure matrix, as well as better representation of invasively measured temperatures.

Deger et al used thermoseeds with a Curie temperature of 55°C in a phase II trial.[57,58] They added a 3D-conformal radiotherapy of 68.4 Gy given simultaneously to the hyperthermia in daily fractions of 1.8 Gy. A patented coil system of 50 kHz was utilized to establish the magnetic field. Patients received 1-hour hyperthermia at intervals of 1 week for 6 sessions. Temperatures were measured using thermocouples. The intraprostatic, urethral, and rectal temperatures were between 42°C and 48°C, between 38°C and 43°C, and between 37°C and 39.5°C, respectively.[59] A median follow-up of 36 months was published for this patient population in 2004. There was no seed migration observed on follow-up X-rays and no major side effects during hyperthermia. The initial median PSA value was 11.6 ng/mL, which regressed after 12, 24, and 36 months to 1.1 ng/mL, 0.9 ng/mL, and 0.6 ng/mL, respectively. Forty-two percent of the patients reached a PSA nadir of 0.5 ng/mL in a median time of 12 months. Nine patients progressed at a median time of 20 months. Three patients had local and six patients had systemic progression.[60] Prostate-specific antigen follow-up data of this patient group were equal to the data of the patients who were treated with a high dose rate brachytherapy, and better than the data of those patients who received conformal radiation therapy in the same institution.[61]

Another exciting new tool for applying interstitial hyperthermia is nanoparticle technology. Jordan et al reported that magnetic fluid hyperthermia (MFH) selectively heats up tissue by coupling alternating current magnetic fields to targeted magnetic fluids, so that boundaries of different conductive tissues do not interfere with power absorption.[62]

This is a completely new approach to deep tissue hyperthermia application. It couples the energy magnetically to nanoparticles in the target region. A new aminosilan-type nanoparticle preparation (manu-factured at the Institute of New Materials [INM] Saarbruecken, Germany) is taken up by prostate carcinoma cells but not by normal prostate cells. Preliminary data indicate that the malignant cells take up nine times more particles than normal cells do.[62] Johannsen et al[63] published the first experimental data using this technology on a rat model of prostate cancer. They used an orthotopic Dunning R3327 prostate cancer model on male Copenhagen rats. The animals either received MFH treatment following intratumoral administration of magnetic fluids or were used as either tumor growth controls to determine iron distribution in selected organs or as histologic controls without MFH treatment. The MFH treatments were carried out at 45°C or 50°C using an alternating current (AC) magnetic field applicator system. Sequential treatments with MFH were possible following a single intratumoral injection of magnetic fluid. Intratumoral temperatures of 50°C and more were obtained and were monitored online using fluoro-optic thermometry. Four days after MFH treatments, 79% of the injected dose of ferrites was still present in the prostate.

Interstitial hyperthermia in combination with conformal radiotherapy may be a powerful new method to improve the results of external radiation therapy for localized prostate cancer. Most studies describe feasibility and toxicity. Quality-of-life studies are urgently needed in this area. Van Pulpen et al[64] published a prospective quality-of-life study in patients with locally advanced prostate cancer, treated with radiotherapy with or without regional or interstitial hyperthermia. They concluded that after radiotherapy with or without hyperthermia only a temporary deterioration of quality of life occurs, concerning social, psychological, and disease-related symptoms. Additional hyperthermia does not seem to decrease quality of life.

Nevertheless, the addition of hyperthermia to different treatment strategies like chemotherapeutics[65,66] or thermo- or radiosensitizing modalities[67–69] has further research potential for the new treatment strategies of localized prostate cancer.

References

1. Zietman AL, Shipley WU, Willet CG. Residual disease after radical surgery or radiation therapy for prostate cancer—clinical significance and therapeutic implications. Cancer 1993;71:959–969.
2. Roehl KA, Han M, Ramos CG, et al. Cancer Progression and survival rates following anatomical radical retropubic prostatectomy in 3478 consecutive patients: long term results. J Urol 2004;172:910–914.
3. Khan MA, Partin AW, Mangold LA, et al. Probability of biochemical recurrence by analysis of pathologic stage, Gleason score, and margin status for localized prostate cancer. Urology 2003;62:866–871.
4. Hanks GE, Schultheiss TE, Hunt MA, et al. Factors influencing incidence of acute grade 2 morbidity in conformal and standard radiation treatment of prostate cancer. Int J Radiat Oncol Biol Phys 1995;31:25–29.
5. Schultheiss TE, Hanks GE, Hunt MA, et al. Incidence of and factors related to late complications in conformal and conventional radiation treatment of cancer of the prostate. Int J Radiat Oncol Biol Phys 1995;32:643–650.
6. Hanks GE, Hanlon AL, Schultheiss TE, et al. Conformal beam treatment of prostate cancer. Urology 1997;50:87–92.
7. Pollack A, Zagars GK. External beam radiotherapy dose response of prostate cancer. Int J Radiat Oncol Biol Phys 1997;39:1011–1018.
8. Pollack A, Smith LG, von Eschenbach AC. External beam radiotherapy dose response characteristics of 1127 men with prostate cancer treated in the PSA era. Int J Radiat Oncol Biol Phys 2000;48:507–512.
9. Hanks GE, Hanlon AL, Schultheiss TE, et al. Dose escalation with 3D conformal treatment: five year outcomes, treatment optimization, and future directions. Int J Radiat Oncol Biol Phys 1998;41:501–510.
10. Zelefsky MJ, Leibel SA, Gaudin PB, et al. Dose escalation with three-dimensional conformal radiation therapy affects the outcome in prostate cancer. Int J Radiat Oncol Biol Phys 1998;41:491–500.
11. Lyons JA, Kupelian PA, Mohan DS, et al. Importance of high radiation doses (72 Gy or greater) in the treatment of stage T1-T3 adenocarcinoma of the prostate. Urology 2000;55:85–90.
12. Roach M 3rd. Reducing the toxicity associated with the use of radiotherapy in men with localized prostate cancer. Urol Clin North Am 2004;31:353–366.
13. Deger S, Boehmer D, Tuerk I, et al. High dose rate brachytherapy of localized prostate cancer. Eur Urol 2002;41:420–426.
14. Martinez A, Gonzalez J, Spencer W, et al. Conformal high dose rate brachytherapy improves biochemical control and causes specific survival in patients with prostate cancer and poor prognostic factors. J Urol 2003;169:974–980.
15. Galalae RM, Kovacs G, Schultze J, et al. Long term outcome after elective irradiation of the pelvic lymphatics and local dose escalation using high dose rate brachytherapy for locally advanced prostate cancer. Int J Radiat Oncol Biol Phys 2002;52:81–90.
16. Raaphorst GP, Romano SL, Mitchell JB, et al. Intrinsic differences in heat and/or x-ray sensitivity of seven mammalian cell lines cultured and treated under identical conditions. Cancer Res 1979;39:396–401.
17. Sapareto SA, Dewey WC. Thermal dose determination in cancer therapy. Int J Radiat Oncol Biol Phys 1984;10:787–800.
18. Hildebrandt B, Wust P, Ahlers O, et al. The cellular and molecular basis of hyperthermia. Crit Rev Oncol Hematol 2002;43:33–56.
19. Van der Zee J. Heating the patient: A promising approach? Ann Oncol 2002;13:1173–1184.
20. Vernon CC, Hand JW, Field SB, et al. Radiotherapy with or without hyperthermia in the treatment of superficial breast cancer: Results from five randomized controlled trials. International Collaborative Hyperthermia Group. Int J Radiat Oncol Biol Phys 1996;35:731–744.
21. Van der Zee J, Gonzalez Gonzalez D, Van Rhoon GC, et al. Comparison of radiotherapy alone with radiotherapy plus hyperthermia in locally advanced pelvic tumours: A prospective, randomised, multicentre trial. Lancet 2000;355:1119–1125.
22. Valdagni R, Amichetti M. Report of long-term follow-up in a randomized trial comparing radiation therapy and radiation therapy plus hyperthermia to metastatic lymph nodes in stage IV head and neck patients. Int J Radiat Oncol Biol Phys 1994;28:163–169.
23. Sneed PK, Stauffer PR, McDermott MW, et al. Survival benefit of hyperthermia in a prospective randomized trial of brachytherapy boost +/- hyperthermia for glioblastoma multiforme. Int J Radiat Oncol Biol Phys 1998;40:287–295.
24. Overgaard J, Gonzalez Gonzalez D, Hulshof MCCM, et al. Randomised trial of hyperthermia as adjuvant to radiotherapy for recurrent or metastatic malignant melanoma. Lancet 1995;345:163–169.
25. Ryu S, Brown SL, Khil MS, et al. Preferential radiosensitization of human prostatic carcinoma cells by mild hyperthermia. Int J Radiat Oncol Biol Phys 1996;34:133–138.
26. Li WX, Franklin WA. Radiation- and heat-induced apoptosis in PC-3 prostate cancer cells. Radiat Res 1998 Aug;150:190–194.
27. Peschke P, Hahn EW, Wenz F, et al. Differential sensitivity of three sublines of the rat Dunning prostate tumor system R3327 to radiation and/or local tumor hyperthermia. Radiat Res 1998;150:190–194.
28. Peschke P, Klein V, Wolber G, et al. Morphometric analysis of bromodeoxyuridine distribution and cell density in the rat Dunning prostate tumor R3327-AT1 following treatment with radiation and/or hyperthermia. Histol Histopathol 1999;14:461–469.
29. Peschke P, Hahn EW, Wolber G, et al. Interstitial radiation and hyperthermia in the Dunning R3327 prostate tumour model: therapeutic efficacy depends on radiation dose-rate, sequence and frequency of heating. Int J Radiat Biol 1996;70:609–616.
30. Mittelberg KN, Tucker RD, Loening SA, et al. Effect of radiation and hyperthermia on prostate tumor cells with induced thermal tolerance and the correlation with HSP70 accumulation. Urol Oncol 1996;2:146–151.
31. Anscher MS, Samulski TV, Dodge R, et al. Combined external beam irradiation and external regional hyperthermia for locally advanced adenocarcinoma of the prostate. Int J Radiat Oncol Biol Phys 1997;37:1059–1065.

32. Emami B, Scott C, Perez CA, et al. Phase III study of interstitial thermoradiotherapy compared with interstitial radiotherapy alone in the treatment of recurrent or persistent human tumors. A prospectively controlled randomized study by the Radiation Therapy Group. Int J Radiat Oncol Biol Phys 1996;34:1097–1104.

33. Myerson RJ, Scott CB, Emami B, et al. A phase I/II study to evaluate radiation therapy and hyperthermia for deep-seated tumours: a report of RTOG 89-08. Int J Hyperthermia 1996;12:449–459.

34. Hynynen K. Ultrasound heating technology. In Seegenschmiedt MH, Fessenden P, Vernon CC (eds): Thermo-Radiotherapy and Thermo-Chemotherapy, vol. 1. Berlin: Springer-Verlag, 1995, p 253.

35. Diederich CJ, Hynynen K. The development of intracavitary ultrasonic applicators for hyperthermia:a design and experimental study. Med Phys 1990;17:626–634.

36. Fosmire H, Hynynen K, Drach GW, et al. Feasibility and toxicity of transrectal ultrasound hyperthermia in the treatment of locally advanced adenocarcinoma of the prostate. Int J Radiat Oncol Biol Phys 1993;26:253–259.

37. Hurwitz MD, Kaplan ID, Svensson GK, et al. Feasibility and patient tolerance of a novel transrectal ultrasound hyperthermia system for treatment of prostate cancer. Int J Hyperthermia 2001;17:31–37.

38. Hurwitz MD, Kaplan ID, Hansen JL, et al. Association of rectal toxicity with thermal dose parameters in treatment of locally advanced prostate cancer with radiation and hyperthermia. Int J Radiat Oncol Biol Phys 2002;53:913–918.

39. Algan O, Fosmire H, Hynynen K, et al. External beam radiotherapy and hyperthermia in the treatment of patients with locally advanced prostate carcinoma. Cancer 2000;89:399–403.

40. Raaymakers BW, Van Vulpen M, Lagendijk JJ, et al. Determination and validation of the actual 3D temperature distribution during interstitial hyperthermia of prostate carcinoma. Phys Med Biol 2001;46:3115–3131.

41. Prionas SD, Kapp DS, Goffinet DR, et al. Thermometry of interstitial hyperthermia given as an adjuvant to brachytherapy for the treatment of carcinoma of the prostate. Int J Radiat Oncol Biol Phys 1994;28:151–162.

42. van der Koijk JF, Lagendijk JJ, Crezee J, et al. The influence of vasculature on temperature distributions in MECS interstitial hyperthermia: Importance of longitudinal control. Int J Hypertherm 1997;13:365–385.

43. Kaatee RS, Crezee J, Kanis AP, et al. Design of applicators for a 27 MHz multielectrode current source interstitial hyperthermia system; impedance matching and effective power. Phys Med Biol. 1997;6:1087–1108.

44. Van Vulpen M, De Leeuw AA, Raaymakers BW, et al. Radiotherapy and hyperthermia in the treatment of patients with locally advanced prostate cancer: preliminary results. BJU Int. 2004;93:36–41.

45. Kalapurakal JA, Pierce M, Chen A, et al. Efficacy of irradiation and external hyperthermia in locally advanced, hormone-refractory or radiation recurrent prostate cancer: a preliminary report. Int J Radiat Oncol Biol Phys. 2003;57:654–664.

46. Case JA, Tucker RD, Park JB. Defining the heating characteristics of ferromagnetic implants using calorimetry. J Biomed Mater Res 2000;53:791–798.

47. Le UT, Tucker RD, Park JB. The effects of localized cold work on the heating characteristics of thermal therapy implants. J Biomed Mater Res 2002;63:24–30.

48. Tucker RD, Ehrenstein T, Loening SA. Thermal ablation using interstitial temperature self regulating cobalt - palladium seeds. A new treatment alternative for localized prostate cancer ? In Schnorr D, Loening SA, Dinges S, Budach V (eds): Lokal fortgeschrittenes Prostatakarzinom. Berlin: Blackwell, 1995, 221–240.

49. Paulus JA, Tucker RD, Loening SA, et al. Thermal ablation of canine prostate using interstitial temperature self-regulating seeds:new treatment for prostate cancer. J Endourol 1997;11:295–300.

50. Tompkins DT, Vanderby R, Klein SA, et al. The use of generalized cell-survival data in a physiologically based objective function for hyperthermia treatment planning: a sensitivity study with a simple tissue model implanted with an array of ferromagnetic thermoseeds. Int J Radiat Oncol Biol Phys 1994;30:929–943.

51. Tompkins DT, Vanderby R, Klein SA, et al. Temperature-dependent versus constant-rate blood perfusion modelling in ferromagnetic thermoseed hyperthermia: results with a model of the human prostate. Int J Hyperthermia 1994;10:517–536.

52. Deger S, Boehmer D, Roigas J, et al. Interstitial hyperthermia using thermoseeds in combination with conformal radiotherapy for localized prostate cancer. Front Radiat Ther Oncol 2002;36:171–176.

53. Ferguson SD, Paulus JA, Tucker RD, et al. Effect of thermal treatment on heating characteristics of Ni-Cu alloy for hyperthermia: preliminary studies. J Appl Biomater 1993;4:55–60.

54. Paulus JA, Parida GR, Tucker RD, et al. Corrosion analysis of NiCu and PdCo thermal seed alloys used as interstitial hyperthermia implants. Biomaterials. 1997;18:1609–1614.

55. Cetas TC, Gross EJ, Contractor Y. A ferrite core/metallic sheath thermoseed for interstitial thermal therapies. IEEE Trans Biomed Eng 1998;45:68–77.

56. Meijer JG, van Wieringen N, Koedooder C, et al. The development of PdNi thermoseeds for interstitial hyperthermia. Med Phys 1995;22:101–104.

57. Deger S, Boehmer D, Tuerk I, et al. Thermoradiotherapy with interstitial thermoseeds in treatment of local prostatic carcinoma. Initial results of a phase II study. Urologe A 2001;403:195–198.

58. Deger S, Boehmer D, Tuerk I, et al. Interstitial hyperthermia using self-regulating thermoseeds combined with conformal radiation therapy. Eur Urol 2002;2:147–153.

59. Tucker RD, Loening SA, Huidobro C, et al. The use of permanent interstitial temperature self regulating rods for the treatment of prostate cancer. [Abstract] Rad Oncol 2000;55:132.

60. Deger S, Taymoorian K, Boehmer D, et al. Thermoradiotherapy using interstitial self-regulating thermoseeds: an intermediate analysis of a phase II trial. Eur Urol 2004;45:574–579.

61. Deger S, Boehmer D, Tuerk I, et al. High dose rate brachytherapy of localized prostate cancer. Eur Urol 2002;41:420–426.

62. Jordan A, Scholz R, Maier-Hauff K, et al. Presentation of a new magnetic field therapy system for the treatment of human solid tumors with magnetic fluid hyperthermia. J Magn Magn Mater 2001;225:118–126.

63. Johannsen M, Jordan A, Scholz R, et al. Evaluation of magnetic fluid hyperthermia in a standard rat model of prostate cancer. J Endourol 2004;18:495–500.

64. Van Vulpen M, De Leeuw JR, Van Gellekom MP, et al. Prospective quality of life study in patients with locally advanced prostate cancer, treated with radiotherapy with or without regional or interstitial hyperthermia. Int J Hyperthermia 2003;19:402–413.

65. Roigas J, Wallen ES, Loening SA, et al. Estramustine phosphate enhances the effects of hyperthermia and induces the small heat shock protein HSP27 in the human prostate carcinoma cell line PC-3. Urol Res 2002;30:130–155.

66. Roigas J, Wallen ES, Loening SA, et al. Effects of combined treatment of chemotherapeutics and hyperthermia on survival and the regulation of heat shock proteins in Dunning R3327 prostate carcinoma cells. Prostate 1998;34:195–202.

67. Asea A, Mallick R, Lechpammer S, et al. Cyclooxygenase inhibitors are potent sensitizers of prostate tumours to hyperthermia and radiation. Int J Hyperthermia 2000;17:401–414.

68. Asea A, Ara G, Teicher BA, et al. Effects of the flavonoid drug quercetin on the response of human prostate tumours to hyperthermia in vitro and in vivo. Int J Hyperthermia 2001;17:347–356.

69. Lee YJ, Lee H, Borrelli MJ. Gene transfer into human prostate adenocarcinoma cells with an adenoviral vector: Hyperthermia enhances a double suicide gene expression, cytotoxicity and radiotoxicity. Cancer Gene Ther 2002;9:267–274.

25

Initial management of high risk early stage prostate cancer: radiation

Eric M Horwitz, Steven J Feigenberg, Alan Pollack

Introduction

Because there are many treatment options for nonmetastatic prostate cancer, it is vitally important to define risk and determine a patient's prognosis to aid in the treatment design. Risk is defined many ways, although the single most important prognostic variable is a person's pretreatment PSA level.[1] Other important variables include Gleason score, T stage, and radiation dose.[2] At Fox Chase Cancer Center (FCCC) and elsewhere, these variables are used to categorize men into multiple risk groups.[3–5] Patients with low-risk disease include those with PSA (10 ng/mL, Gleason score 2 to 6 and T1c/T2a disease. The high-risk group consists of patients having one of the following high-risk features: Gleason score 8 to 10, PSA greater than 20 ng/mL, or T3/T4 disease. Intermediate-risk patients do not fit into either of the above risk groups. Treatment options for low- and high-risk disease are discussed elsewhere. The focus of this chapter is on radiation treatment options for men with intermediate risk prostate cancer.

Over the last few decades, the goal for radiation oncologists has been to improve the therapeutic index by increasing radiation dose to the cancer or target (prostate in this case) while restricting or decreasing dose to the surrounding normal tissue (bladder and rectum). This will allow the delivery of a lethal dose of radiation to the cancer while protecting the normal tissue and minimizing side effects. This can be accomplished using a variety of radiation techniques.

Radiation treatment techniques

Planning for patients treated with conventional radiation therapy (RT) is the least complex of these techniques. These patients undergo simulation (planning) and treatment in the supine position. Custom immobilization devices are usually not utilized. Rectal and bladder contrast and retrograde urethrograms to aid in the localization of the prostate are not mandatory during the simulation. Treatment fields are based upon bony landmarks from orthogonal radiographs. Radiation dose distributions for conventional treatment plans are typically generated in a single plane, and the dose is prescribed at the isocenter and normalized at the 100% isodose line.

For patients treated with three-dimensional conformal radiation therapy (3DCRT), the planning begins first by defining treatment volumes including both the target (prostate) and the surrounding normal structures (bladder and rectum most importantly) based on a 3D data set. Target volumes are defined according to the International Commission on Radiation Units and Measurements (ICRU) report 50.[6] Three-dimensional conformal radiation therapy is the process where the radiation dose is planned and delivered so that the high-dose volume conforms to an accurately defined target volume. This process minimizes the volume of normal tissue receiving a clinically significant radiation dose, thereby reducing the probability of normal tissue complications.

As with 3DCRT, planning for treatment with intensity modulated radiation therapy (IMRT) begins by defining the target and normal tissues. This technique can achieve tighter dose distributions through the use of non-uniform intensity radiation beams. Each beam is divided into multiple segments or beamlets. The target volume and critical normal organs are defined and the upper and lower dose limits for the target and normal structures selected. The quality of the plan is assessed using dose–volume histograms (DVHs), which graphically represent the specific dose of radiation the volume an organ receives (Figure 25.1).

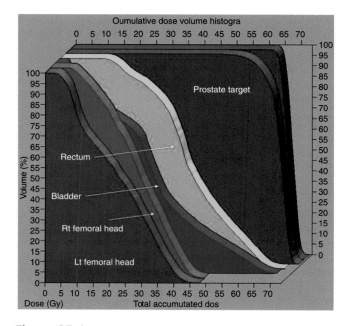

Figure 25.1

Dose–volume histogram (DVH) for an intensity modulated radiotherapy (IMRT) treatment plan.

Radiation dose escalation

Beginning in the 1980s, prospective dose-escalation studies were conducted at Fox Chase Cancer Center (FCCC) and the University of Michigan and Memorial Sloan-Kettering Cancer Center (MSKCC).[7–9] At Fox Chase, the first patients to benefit from increased dose were those with intermediate features. Pinover et al reported the Fox Chase experience treating patients with pre-treatment prostate-specific antigen (PSA) levels greater than 10 ng/mL. Patients were placed in good (T1–T2a, Gleason score 2–6, absence of perineural invasion) or poor risk strata based on palpation T stage, Gleason score and the presence of perineural invasion and biochemical non-evidence of disease (bNED) control was calculated based upon radiation dose received. Patients were stratified into three groups according to dose: less than 72.50 Gy; 72.50 to 75.99 Gy; and greater than or equal to 76 Gy. Median dose in these three groups was 70.67 Gy, 72.78 Gy, and 77.34 Gy, respectively. bNED control was 91% versus 76% at 5 years for good risk patients treated with greater than or equal to 71.5 Gy and less than 71.5 Gy, respectively. The same trend was observed for the poor risk patients (98%, 79%, and 72% for ≥74.5, 71.5–74.5, and <71.5 Gy, respectively).[10]

The long-term results from the original group of prostate cancer patients treated in the first prospective FCCC radiation dose-escalation study with an 8 to 12 year follow-up was reported by Hanks et al.[7] Between 1989 and 1992, 232 patients with clinically localized prostate cancer were treated with 3DCRT alone at FCCC on a prospective dose-escalation study and 229 patients were evaluable. The median total dose for all patients was 74 Gy (range: 67–81 Gy). The median follow-up for patients alive was 110 months (range: 89–147 months). bNED control was defined using the American Society of Therapeutic Radiology and Oncology (ASTRO) definition and for all patients included in this series was 55% at 5 years, 48% at 10 years, and 48% at 12 years.[11] Only for patients with pretreatment PSA levels of 10 to 20 ng/mL were statistically significant differences in bNED control seen for all patients stratified by dose from less than 71.5, 71.5 to 75.6, and more than 75.6 Gy (19%, 31%, 84%, respectively; p = 0.0003) (Table 25.1). For the 229 patients with follow-up, 124 (54%) were clinically and biochemically free of disease. Sixty-nine patients were alive at the time of last follow-up and 55 patients were dead of intercurrent disease. On multivariate analysis, radiation dose was a statistically significant predictor of

bNED control for all of the patients. Freedom from distant metastases (DM) for all patients was 89%, 83%, and 83% at 5, 10, and 12 years, respectively. For patients with pretreatment PSA levels less than 10 ng/mL, all four covariates (radiation dose, Gleason score, pretreatment PSA, and T stage) were significant predictors of DM. Based on the RTOG morbidity scale, there was no difference in the frequency of grade 2 and 3 genito-urinary (GU) and grade 3 gastrointestinal (GI) morbidity when patients in this dataset were stratified by radiation dose. There was, however, a significant increase in grade 2 GI complications as radiation dose increased.

Long-term data from institutions including FCCC, MSKCC, the Cleveland Clinic and M.D. Anderson Cancer Center (MDACC) show increased rates of bNED control, especially for patients with pretreatment PSA levels less than 10 ng/mL (Figures 25.2 and 25.3).[4,7,12,13] The 10-year update of the MSKCC dose comparison trial was reported by Zelefsky et al; MSKCC risk groups are similar to those at FCCC

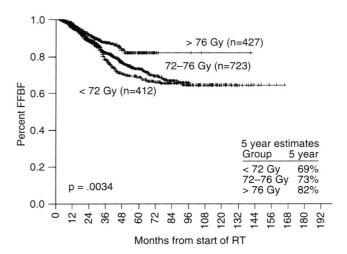

Figure 25.2

Biochemical non-evidence of disease (bNED) control for all Fox Chase Cancer Center patients treated in the prostate-specific antigen (PSA) era with 3D conformal radiotherapy (3DCRT). They are subdivided into three dose groups: <72 Gy, 72–76 Gy, and >76 Gy. (FFBF, freedom from biochemical failure; RT, radiotherapy.)

Table 25.1 Eight-year biochemical non-evidence of disease (bNED) control rates at Fox Chase Cancer Center stratified by pretreatment prostate-specific antigen (PSA) level, radiation dose, and prognostic group

Pretreatment PSA (ng/mL)	Dose group (Gy)	Median dose (Gy)	All patients	Favorable (events)	Unfavorable (events)
<10	<70	69	68%	5/23 (73%)	3/7 (44%)
	70–71.9	71	74%	3/22 (85%)	5/11 (51%)
	>72	76	69%	4/16 (75%)	5/15 (64%)
Significance			p = 0.9518	p = 0.7219	p = 0.7388
10–20	<71.5	70	19%	7/13 (30%)	6/8 (0%)
	71.5–75.75	72	31%	5/11 (37%)	6/10 (36%)
	>75.75	76	84%	1/17 (92%)	3/11 (73%)
Significance			p = 0.0003	p = 0.0065	p = 0.0265
>20	<71.5	70	8%	8/10 (13%)	8/9 (44%)
	71.5–75.75	73	23%	5/6 (17%)	10/15 (51%)
	>75.75	76	11%	4/7 (38%)	16/18 (64%)
Significance			p = 0.34	p = 0.3180	p = 0.3745

and are based on the presence or absence of the following parameters: PSA less than 10 ng/mL, stage T1 to T2, and Gleason score less than 7 disease. The favorable risk group has all three parameters present, the intermediate risk group has two parameters present, and the unfavorable risk group has none or only one parameter present. Eight hundred twenty eight patients were treated as part of this prospective study, and 10-year bNED control rates for good-, intermediate-, and poor-risk patients were 70%, 49%, and 35%, respectively. Differences in bNED control were associated with dose within each group. For low-risk patients, bNED control was 83% versus 57% for patients treated with 75.6 Gy versus less than 70.2 Gy. These rates were 50% versus 42% for intermediate-risk patients and 42% versus 24% for poor-risk patients (Table 25.2).[14]

In 1999, the results using external beam radiation therapy (EBRT) alone in 1765 men with T1 and T2 prostate cancer from six

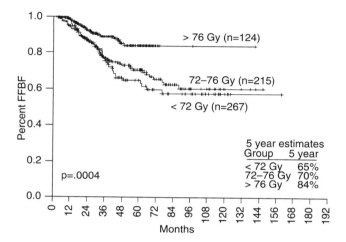

Figure 25.3

Biochemical non-evidence of disease (bNED) control for the intermediate-risk patients treated at Fox Chase Cancer Center in the prostate-specific antigen (PSA) era with 3D conformal radiotherapy (3DCRT). They are subdivided into three dose groups: <72 Gy, 72 Gy–76 Gy, and >76 Gy. (FFBF, freedom from biochemical failure.)

institutions (FCCC, Massachusetts General Hospital, Mallinckrodt Institute of Radiology, the University of Michigan, Eastern Virginia Medical School, and Stanford University) was summarized and reported. The biochemical durability of radiation therapy as well as the effect of prognostic factors on outcome was described.[15] As a follow-up to this experience, nine institutions (the original six along with MDACC, William Beaumont Hospital, and the Mayo Clinic College of Medicine) pooled data on nearly 5000 patients treated with EBRT alone between 1986 and 1995, with a median follow-up of more than 6 years. The results of this collaborative effort were first reported in 2003.[2,16] Kuban et al reported long-term biochemical and clinical outcomes for patients with stage T1 to T2 prostate cancer using the ASTRO definition. bNED control for the entire group was 59% at 5 years and 53% at 8 years. For patients who had received at least 70 Gy, bNED control was 61% and 55%. The greatest risk of failure was at 1.5 to 3.5 years post-treatment. In multivariate analysis for bNED failure, pretreatment PSA, Gleason score, radiation dose, T stage, and treatment year were all significant prognostic factors. The effect of radiation dose was most significant in the intermediate risk group.[2]

A more detailed analysis of the effect of dose on bNED control was reported by Kupelian using this same large dataset. Because differences in bNED control have been observed in some series attributed solely to differences in length of follow-up, the dose response was analyzed in patients treated during a 2-year period, 1994 and 1995; for this study, 1061 were treated with less than 72 Gy and 264 patients with greater than or equal to 72 Gy. The median follow-up for the first group was 5.8 years and for the second group was 5.7 years. The median radiation doses for the 2 groups were 68.4 Gy and 75.6 Gy, respectively. For all 1325 patients, the 5- and 8-year bNED control rates were 64% and 62%, respectively. The 5-year bNED control rates for the low- and high-dose groups were 63% and 69%, respectively (p = 0.046). Pretreatment PSA (p < 0.001), Gleason score (p < 0.001), radiation dose (p < 0.001), and T stage (p = 0.007) were independent predictors of outcome on multivariate analysis. The authors concluded that while controlling for follow-up duration, higher than conventional radiation doses were associated with improved bNED control rates when controlling for pretreatment PSA, Gleason score, and clinical T stage.[17]

The first national prospective phase I/II study investigating dose escalation was completed in 2000. RTOG 94-06 enrolled

Table 25.2 Sequential radiotherapy dose escalation studies

Institution	Dose (Gy)	Group	bNED control (length of follow-up)	p-value
CC[35]	<72	All	54% (5 year)	<0.001
	≥72	All	85% (5 year)	
FCCC[7]	<71.5	PSA 10–20	19% (8 year)	0.0003
	71.5–75.75	PSA 10–20	31% (8 year)	
	>75.75	PSA 10–20	84% (8 year)	
MDACC[36]	≤67	All	54% (4 year)	<0.0001
	>67–77	All	71% (4 year)	
	>77	All	77% (4 year)	
MSKCC[37]	64.8–70.2	Int risk*	55% (4 year)	0.04
	75.6–81.0	Int risk*	79% (4 year)	

*Intermediate risk—patients with prostate-specific antigen (PSA) >10 ng/mL, or Gleason score 7, or T2b/T2c disease.
bNED, biochemical non-evidence of disease; CC, the Cleveland Clinic; FCCC- Fox Chase Cancer Center; MDACC, M.D. Anderson Cancer Center; MSKCC, Memorial Sloan-Kettering Cancer Center.

1055 analyzable patients from 34 institutions into five sequential dose levels—68.4 Gy, 73.8 Gy, 79.2 Gy, 74 Gy, and 78 Gy. Prostate-specific antigen failure was defined prior to the adoption of the ASTRO definition and included a failure to fall below 4 ng/mL by 1 year after the start of treatment or two consecutive rises at least 1 month apart during the first year after the start of treatment. The first long-term clinical results became available in 2004. The 5-year rates for the first three groups and 3-year rates for the last two groups for clinical and biochemical failure were 44%, 53%, 49%, 29%, and 26%, respectively. Local failure without PSA endpoints for the five groups was 5% for groups 1 to 3, 4% for group 4, and 2% for group 5. The 5-year clinical disease-free survival (DFS) for groups 1 to 3 was 86%, 82%, and 81%, respectively and 90% for groups 4 and 5 at 3 years. The results from this study support those seen in single institution studies.[18]

The strongest evidence to support a particular treatment is class I evidence from a randomized prospective trial. The first and most mature study in the PSA era was from M.D. Anderson Cancer Center.[19] In this study, 301 men were randomized between 70 Gy and 78 Gy. All were initially treated with a four-field box to 46 Gy, prescribed to the isocenter. The 150 patients randomized to 70 Gy received the remaining dose through a smaller volume using a four-field arrangement, while the 151 patients who received 78 Gy were treated with a six-field 3D conformal boost. The clinical target volume (CTV) consisted of the prostate and seminal vesicles. With 60 months median follow-up, patients with an initial pretreatment PSA greater than 10 ng/mL experienced the greatest benefit, whereas the additional 8 Gy had no effect on the more favorable patients (pretreatment PSA ≤ 10 ng/mL). Freedom from biochemical failure (FFBF) and clinical failures for patients with pretreatment PSA levels greater than 10 ng/mL are shown in Figure 25.4. The freedom from failure results (based on biochemical criteria) supported the

conclusions of the sequential dose escalation trials. The FFBF rates were significantly higher for those randomized to 78 Gy (70% versus 64% at 6 years; p = 0.03). The greatest benefit was observed in men with a pretreatment PSA greater than 10 ng/mL who had a 19% absolute gain in FFBF at 6 years when treated to 78 Gy. This translated into a borderline reduction in distant metastasis (2% versus 12% at 6 years; p = 0.056); although there were only eight patients with distant metastasis at the time of the analysis. For patients with a pretreatment PSA less than or equal to 10 ng/mL, no dose-related difference in FFBF or any other endpoint were observed.

Results from the second phase III randomized prospective trial were reported by Zietman et al; in this study, 393 patients were randomized to receive a boost to the prostate of either 19.8 Gray equivalent (GyE) (70.2 GyE total) or 28.8 GyE (79.2 GyE total) using protons. All patients first received 50.4 Gy using 3DCRT techniques with photons. Patients eligible for treatment on this study included those with T1b to T2b tumors and a pretreatment PSA level less than 15 ng/mL. Fifteen percent of patients had Gleason score 7 tumors and 8% had Gleason score 8 to 10. The 5-year bNED failure rate was 37.3% for the low-dose arm and 19.1% for the high-dose group. This difference was statistically significant (p = 0.00001). When patients were stratified by risk group, this difference remained statistically significant for both low (34.9% versus 17.2%; p = 0.002) and intermediate groups (39.5% versus 21.3%; p = 0.01). Although this study used protons to deliver the radiation boost in the experimental arm, this study clearly demonstrated an improvement in clinical and biochemical outcome with higher radiation doses. This was the second randomized prospective trial to confirm that patients with both low- and intermediate-risk prostate cancer achieve higher rates of bNED control with high doses of radiation.[20]

Although no national prospective trial involving IMRT has been reported, several series utilizing this technique have been published. As with the 3DCRT data, patients with intermediate risk features benefit the most from an escalation of radiation dose. The largest published experience with the longest follow-up of biochemical outcome and toxicity using IMRT to treat prostate cancer comes from MSKCC. The 3-year bNED control rates for 772 patients treated with IMRT at MSKCC were 92%, 86%, and 81% for patients with low risk, intermediate risk and high risk, respectively (Figure 25.5).[21] The risk group stratification used for the MSKCC IMRT experience was the same as the system used with the 3DCRT experience. A subset of these patients treated between 1996 and 1998 with long follow-up was reported and confirmed the durability of results as well as low rate of complications. For this group of 171 patients, the median follow-up was 6.3 years and all these patients received 81 Gy. The 5-year bNED control rates for the low-, intermediate-, and high-risk disease were 91%, 73%, and 64%, respectively (p = 0.008).

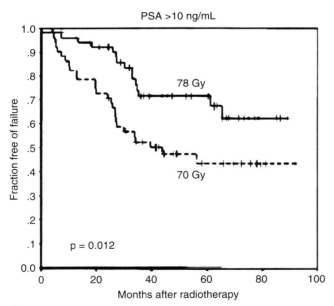

Figure 25.4
The biochemical and clinical failures curves for patients in the M.D. Anderson Cancer Center randomized trial who had a pretreatment prostate-specific antigen (PSA) > 10 ng/mL and were treated to 70 or 78 Gy.

With permission from Pollack A, Zagars GK, Starkschall G, et al. Prostate cancer radiation dose response: Results of the M.D. Anderson phase III randomized trial. Int J Radiat Oncol Biol Phys 2002;53:1097–1105.

Toxicity

Conventional and 3D conformal radiation therapy toxicity

Normal tissue complication risk has been well-established and is related to radiation dose, volume,[19,22–24] and other dosimetric and clinical parameters. Bladder complications can manifest much later than rectal complications.[25] Several authors have reported on techniques to reduce rectal toxicity.[23,26]

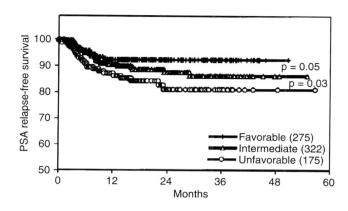

Figure 25.5

Biochemical non-evidence of disease (bNED) control for favorable, intermediate- and high-risk patients treated with intensity modulated radiotherapy (IMRT) at Memorial Sloan-Kettering Cancer Center.

With permission from Zelefsky MJ, Fuks Z, Hunt M, et al. High-dose intensity modulated radiation therapy for prostate cancer: early toxicity and biochemical outcome in 772 patients. Int J Radiat Oncol Biol Phys 2002;53:1111–1116.

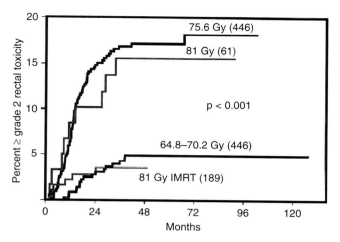

Figure 25.6

Freedom from grade 2 or higher rectal complications for patients treated with 3D conformal radiotherapy (3DCRT) and intensity modulated radiotherapy (IMRT) at Memorial Sloan-Kettering Cancer Center.

Used with permission from Zelefsky MJ, Fuks Z, Hunt M, et al. High-dose intensity modulated radiation therapy for prostate cancer: early toxicity and biochemical outcome in 772 patients. Int J Radiat Oncol Biol Phys 2002;53:1111–1116.

The late GI and GU complications following treatment with conventional or 3DCRT at FCCC were reported by Schultheiss et al. Seven hundred twelve patients treated between 1986 and 1994 with conventional (150 patients) or conformal (562 patients) techniques were analyzed for factors using a modified RTOG/SWOG scoring system to predict late GI (rectal bleeding requiring ≥ 3 procedures to correct or proctitis) and GU (cystitis or stricture) morbidity. One hundred fifteen patients experienced grade 2 or higher GI toxicity a mean of 13.7 months after treatment. Fifteen of these patients experienced grade 3 or 4 toxicity. Forty three cases of grade 2 or higher late GU toxicity were observed a mean of 22.7 months after treatment. On multivariate analysis only radiation dose (>74 Gy) significantly predicted late grade 3 GI toxicity. Radiation dose, use of increased rectal shielding, hormone therapy before RT, history of obstructive symptoms, and acute GU symptoms significantly predicted for late grade 2 GU toxicity on multivariate analysis. After the presence of minor rectal bleeding was noted in 1993, techniques were developed to reduce the radiation dose to the anterior rectal wall.[23] The need for endoscopic coagulation for bleeding was reduced from 5% to 2% at 75 to 76 Gy.[27] In the MSKCC 3DCRT series, the risk of grade 2 and grade 3 or higher rectal toxicity at 10 years was 17% and 1.5%, respectively. For GU side effects, the 10 year rates were 17% and 1.5%, respectively (Figure 25.6).[14]

Michalski et al reported toxicity data from 3DOG/RTOG 94-06, the prospective phase I dose escalation trial determining the maximally tolerated radiation dose in men treated with 3DCRT in a multi-institutional setting. Two hundred ninety two patients treated between 1994 and 1997 at the first two dose levels of 68.4 and 73.8 Gy were analyzed for rates of acute and chronic GI and GU toxicity. Acute and chronic grade 1 toxicity for both dose groups ranged from 30% to 46%. Rates of acute grade 2 toxicity ranged from 34% to 45%. Chronic grade 2 toxicity rates were 8% to 16%. Acute grade 3 rates were between 1% and 3%, while there were no acute grade 4 or 5, or chronic grade 3, 4, or 5 complications.[28] The first data from the final dose group (78 Gy, Level V), demonstrate that grade 3 acute effects were 2% for Group 1 and 4% for Group 2. No grade 4 or 5 complications were reported.[29]

Similar results were observed from two European randomized prospective trials that compared toxicity data with different radiation dose levels using 3D conformal techniques. In the first study, Lebesque et al described the acute and late GI and GU toxicity rates from a two arm phase III study, which randomized men between 68 and 78 Gy. Between 1997 and 2003, 669 men in the Netherlands were randomized to these two doses using 3DCRT. Data was available for 606 men and RTOG scoring was used to measure acute effects while RTOG/EORTC and SOMA/LENT scoring was used for late effects. No statistically significant differences in rates were observed for grade 2 and grade 3 GI and GU of complications between the two arms.[30] In the second study, 306 men with intermediate-risk prostate cancer were randomized in a French phase II prospective trial between 70 and 80 Gy from 1999 through 2002. There was also no statistically significant difference in acute toxicity between the two arms. Overall GU and GI grade 3 toxicity rates were 6% and 2%, respectively, for both groups. The target volume (prostate) size was the only independent predictor of acute grade 2 and 3 toxicity.[31]

In the MDACC randomized prospective trial, the 5-year actuarial freedom from a grade 2 or higher rectal complication was 26% for those in the 78 Gy arm and 12% for those in the 70 Gy arm. Dose–volume histogram analysis identified that exposure of more than 25% of the rectal volume to greater than or equal to 70 Gy resulted in a 5 year risk of grade 2 or higher rectal complications of 54%, as opposed to 84% when 25% or less was exposed. In a more detailed follow-up analysis of patients treated with 3DCRT at MDACC, Huang et al confirmed that the proportion of the rectum receiving over certain marker doses (e.g., 70 Gy) was found to be more significant than absolute rectal volume (Figure 25.7).[32] Kupelian et al, on the other hand, reported that the absolute rectal volume radiated was an independent predictor of grade 2 or higher complications. When more than 15 cm³ of the rectal volume received the prescription dose, the 2-year rate of rectal bleeding was 22%, versus 5% for 15 cm³ or less.[33]

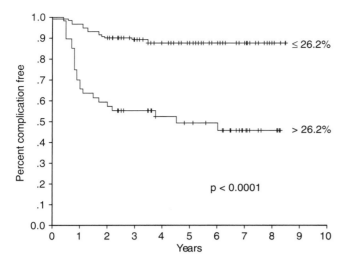

Figure 25.7
Freedom from grade 2 or higher rectal complications for patients treated with 3D conformal radiotherapy (3DCRT) in the M.D. Anderson Cancer Center randomized trial. The patients are divided by <26.2% versus >26.2% of the rectal volume received ≥70 Gy in dose–volume histogram analysis.

With permission from Pollack A, Zagars GK, Starkschall G, et al. Prostate cancer radiation dose response: Results of the M.D. Anderson phase III randomized trial. Int J Radiat Oncol Biol Phys 2002;53:1097–1105.

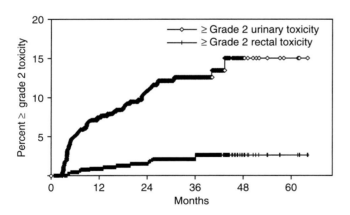

Figure 25.8
Freedom from grade 2 or higher late rectal and urinary complications after intensity modulated radiotherapy (IMRT) to 81 and 86.4 Gy at Memorial Sloan-Kettering Cancer Center.

With permission from Zelefsky MJ, Fuks Z, Hunt M, et al. High-dose intensity modulated radiation therapy for prostate cancer: early toxicity and biochemical outcome in 772 patients. Int J Radiat Oncol Biol Phys 2002;53:1111–1116.

Intensity modulated radiotherapy toxicity

The MSKCC group has had the most experience in the treatment of prostate cancer with IMRT. Zelefsky et al found that grade 2 or higher rectal complication rate at 3 years was 14% for 81 Gy (n = 189) using 3DCRT, compared with 2% using IMRT (n = 61)

(see Figure 25.6). Seven patients developed grade 2 rectal bleeding. At 6 years there was a 4% risk of developing rectal bleeding, and two patients developed grade 3 rectal bleeding. Eighteen patients developed grade 2 urinary toxicity. At 6 years, the risk was 10%, and there were no cases of grade 4 toxicity. The results look promising, although the follow-up in the IMRT patients was shorter. The reduction in morbidity using IMRT seems to be related to a reduction in rectal complications and longer follow up is needed to confirm these results (Figure 25.8).[21,34]

References

1. Horwitz EM, Hanlon AL, Pinover WH, et al. Defining the optimal radiation dose with three-dimensional conformal radiation therapy for patients with nonmetastatic prostate carcinoma by using recursive partitioning techniques. Cancer 2001;92:1281–1287.
2. Kuban DA, Thames HD, Levy LB, et al. Long-term multi-institutional analysis of stage T1-T2 prostate cancer treated with radiotherapy in the PSA era. Int J Radiat Oncol Biol Phys 2003;57:915–928.
3. Chism DB, Hanlon AL, Horwitz EM, et al. A comparison of the single and double factor high-risk models for risk assignment of prostate cancer treated with 3D conformal radiotherapy. Int J Radiat Oncol Biol Phys 2004;59:380–385.
4. Khuntia D, Reddy CA, Mahadevan A, et al. Recurrence-free survival rates after external-beam radiotherapy for patients with clinical T1-T3 prostate carcinoma in the prostate-specific antigen era: what should we expect? Cancer 2004;100:1283–1292.
5. Kattan MW, Zelefsky MJ, Kupelian PA, et al. Pretreatment nomogram that predicts 5-year probability of metastasis following three-dimensional conformal radiation therapy for localized prostate cancer. J Clin Oncol 2003;21:4568–4571.
6. International Commission on Radiation Units and Measurements. ICRU Report 50: Prescribing, recording, and reporting photon beam therapy. Bethesda, MD: International Commission on Radiation Units and Measurements, 1993.
7. Hanks GE, Hanlon AL, Epstein B, et al. Dose response in prostate cancer with 8-12 years' follow-up. Int J Radiat Oncol Biol Phys 2002;54:427–435.
8. Symon Z, Griffith KA, McLaughlin PW, et al. Dose escalation for localized prostate cancer: substantial benefit observed with 3D conformal therapy. Int J Radiat Oncol Biol Phys 2003;57:384–390.
9. Zelefsky MJ, Ben-Porat L, Scher HI, et al. Outcome predictors for the increasing PSA state after definitive external-beam radiotherapy for prostate cancer. J Clin Oncol 2005;23:826–831.
10. Pinover WH, Hanlon AL, Horwitz EM, et al. Defining the appropriate radiation dose for pretreatment PSA < or = 10 ng/mL prostate cancer. Int J Radiat Oncol Biol Phys 2000;47:649–654.
11. American Society for Therapeutic Radiology and Oncology Consensus Panel. Consensus statement: Guidelines for PSA following radiation therapy. Int J Radiat Oncol Biol Phys 1997;37:1035–1041.
12. Zelefsky MJ, Marion C, Fuks Z, et al. Improved biochemical disease-free survival of men younger than 60 years with prostate cancer treated with high dose conformal external beam radiotherapy. J Urol 2003;170:1828–1832.
13. Cheung R, Tucker SL, Lee AL, et al. Assessing the impact of an alternative biochemical failure definition on radiation dose response for high-risk prostate cancer treated with external beam radiotherapy. Int J Radiat Oncol Biol Phys 2005;61:14–19.
14. Zelefsky M, Fuks Z, Chan H, et al. Ten-year results of dose escalation with 3-dimensional conformal radiotherapy for patients with clinically localized prostate cancer. Int J Radiat Oncol Biol Phys 2003;57:S149–150.
15. Shipley WU, Thames HD, et al. Radiation therapy for clinically localized prostate cancer: a multi-institutional pooled analysis. JAMA 1999;281:1598–1604.

16. Thames H, Kuban D, Levy L, et al. Comparison of alternative bio-chemical failure definitions based on clinical outcome in 4839 prostate cancer patients treated by external beam radiotherapy between 1986 and 1995. Int J Radiat Oncol Biol Phys 2003;57:929–943.

17. Kupelian P, Kuban D, Thames H, et al. Improved biochemical relapse-free survival with increased external radiation doses in patients with localized prostate cancer: The combined experience of nine institutions in patients treated in 1994 and 1995. Int J Radiat Oncol Biol Phys 2005;61:415–49.

18. Michalski JM, Winter K, Roach M, et al. Clinical outcome of patients treated with 3D conformal radiation therapy 3DCRT for prostate cancer on RTOG 94-06. Int J Radiat Oncol Biol Phys 2004;60:169.

19. Pollack A, Zagars GK, Starkschall G, et al. Prostate cancer radiation dose response: Results of the M.D. Anderson phase III randomized trial. Int J Radiat Oncol Biol Phys 2002;53:1097–1105.

20. Zietman AL, DeSilvio M, Slater JD, et al. A randomized trial comparing conventional dose (70.2 GyE) and high-dose (79.2 GyE) conformal radiation in early stage adenocarcinoma of the prostate: Results of an interim analysis of PROG 95-09. International Journal of Radiation Oncology Biology and Physics 2004;60:131–132.

21. Zelefsky MJ, Fuks Z, Hunt M, et al. High-dose intensity modulated radiation therapy for prostate cancer: early toxicity and biochemical outcome in 772 patients. Int J Radiat Oncol Biol Phys 2002;53:1111–1116.

22. Shipley WU, Verhey LJ, Munzenrider JE, et al. Advanced prostate cancer: The results of a randomized comparative trial of high dose irradiation boosting with conformal protons compared with conventional dose irradiation using photons alone. Int J Radiat Oncol Biol Phys 1995;32:3–12.

23. Lee WR, Hanks GE, Hanlon AL, et al. Lateral rectal shielding reduces late rectal morbidity following high dose three-dimensional conformal radiation therapy for clinically localized prostate cancer: further evidence for a significant dose effect. Int J Radiat Oncol Biol Phys 1996;35:251–257.

24. Boersma LJ, van den Brink M, Bruce AM, et al. Estimation of the incidence of late bladder and rectum complications after high-dose (70–78 GY) conformal radiotherapy for prostate cancer, using dose-volume histograms. Int J Radiat Oncol Biol Phys 1998;41:83–92.

25. Gardner BG, Zietman AL, Shipley WU, et al. Late normal tissue sequelae in the second decade after high dose radiation therapy with combined photons and conformal protons for locally advanced prostate cancer. J Urol 2002;167:123–126.

26. Dearnaley DP, Khoo VS, Norman AR, et al. Comparison of radiation side-effects of conformal and conventional radiotherapy in prostate cancer: a randomised trial. Lancet 1999;353:267–272.

27. Schultheiss TE, Lee WR, Hunt MA, et al. Late GI and GU complications in the treatment of prostate cancer. Int J Radiat Oncol Biol Phys 1997;37:3–11.

28. Michalski JM, Winter K, Purdy JA, et al. Preliminary evaluation of low-grade toxicity with conformal radiation therapy for prostate cancer on RTOG 9406 dose levels I and II. Int J Radiat Oncol Biol Phys 2003;56:192–198.

29. Michalski J, Winter K, Purdy JA, et al. Toxicity following 3D radiation therapy for prostate cancer on RTOG 9406 dose level V. Int J Radiat Oncol Biol Phys 2003;57:S151.

30. Lebesque J, Koper P, Slot A, et al. Acute and late GI and GU toxicity after prostate irradiation to doses of 68 Gy and 78 Gy; results of a randomized trial. Int J Radiat Oncol Biol Phys 2003;57:S152.

31. Beckendorf V, Guerif S, Le Prise E, et al. The GETUG 70 Gy vs. 80 Gy randomized trial for localized prostate cancer: feasibility and acute toxicity. Int J Radiat Oncol Biol Phys 2004;60:1056–1065.

32. Huang EH, Pollack A, Levy L, et al. Late rectal toxicity: dose-volume effects of conformal radiotherapy for prostate cancer. Int J Radiat Oncol Biol Phys 2002;54:1314–1321.

33. Kupelian PA, Reddy CA, Carlson TP, et al. Dose/volume relationship of late rectal bleeding after external beam radiotherapy for localized prostate cancer: absolute or relative rectal volume? Cancer J 2002;8: 62–66.

34. Zelefsky MJ, Fuks Z, Hunt M, et al. High dose radiation delivered by intensity modulated conformal radiotherapy improves the outcome of localized prostate cancer. J Urol 2001;166:876–881.

35. Lyons JA, Kupelian PA, Mohan DS, et al. Importance of high radiation doses (72 Gy or greater) in the treatment of stage T1-T3 adenocarcinoma of the prostate. Urology 2000;55:85–90.

36. Pollack A, Smith LG, von Eschenbach AC. External beam radiotherapy dose response characteristics of 1127 men with prostate cancer treated in the PSA era. Int J Radiat Oncol Biol Phys 2000;48:507–512.

37. Zelefsky MJ, Leibel SA, Gaudin PB, et al. Dose escalation with three-dimensional conformal radiation therapy affects the outcome in prostate cancer. Int J Radiat Oncol Biol Phys 1998;41:491–500.

26

Management of biochemical recurrence following radiation therapy

Timothy S Collins, Daniel J George

Introduction

The introduction and use of the prostate-specific antigen (PSA) test has had a profound impact on the diagnosis and management of patients with prostate cancer. Prostate-specific antigen has gained wide acceptance as a screening tool for early detection of prostate cancer, yet it was originally developed as a tumor marker.[1] As a tumor marker, PSA has demonstrated exceptional sensitivity and specificity for disease progression. One of the most important applications of PSA is its use in patients following definitive local therapy.

Following radical prostatectomy (RP), radiation therapy is the second most common treatment modality chosen for clinically localized prostate cancer. According to the SEER database, approximately 30% of patients in the United States are treated with external-beam radiation, initially.[2] In addition, various forms of brachytherapy, either as monotherapy or in combination with external-beam radiation, have gained widespread acceptance and use as an alternative standard therapy. Unfortunately, despite early detection and risk stratification, a significant percentage of patients will relapse following primary therapy, with estimates ranging from 10% to 50% depending on pretreatment prognostic factors.[3] Often the first evidence of disease recurrence is detected by the PSA test. To better manage patients with rising PSA following local therapy, clinicians must have a thorough understanding of several important issues. This chapter will cover biochemical recurrence after primary radiation therapy including its definition, natural history, diagnostic considerations, and treatment options.

Definition of biochemical recurrence

Unlike post-prostatectomy, the definition of biochemical failure post-radiation is less straightforward. Since the goal of a prostatectomy is to remove all prostate tissue, the PSA in most patients declines to undetectable levels soon after surgery. In contrast, the decline of PSA following radiation therapy is more gradual, and, frequently, it does not drop to undetectable levels. Following external-beam radiation therapy or brachytherapy, PSA levels decline over the first 12 months with more subtle decreases occurring over 12 to 24 months.[4,5] Confounding this parameter further is the incidence of false elevations of PSA following radiation therapy. In as many as 30% of cases, a transient rise in PSA level, or bounce, has been described following brachytherapy and external-beam radiation.[6,7]

In addition, the use of adjuvant androgen-deprivation therapy (ADT) frequently suppresses PSA levels and may alter the kinetics of PSA progression as testosterone levels recover.[8,9] Overall, the interpretation of biochemical relapse following radiation therapy can be complex and ambiguous.

In order to standardize the definition of biochemical failure after radiation therapy, an expert committee was formed. From this effort, the American Society for Therapeutic Radiology and Oncology (ASTRO) issued a consensus statement detailing guidelines for PSA following radiation therapy[10] (Box 26.1). In addition to these guidelines, the authors presented recommendations for study publications. For publications, they recommended: 1) a minimum observation period of 24 months; 2) PSA levels should be measured every 3 to 4 months during the first 2 years and every 6 months thereafter; and 3) the results of patients who have had less than three consecutive rises should be reported separately from those with three or more. While such definitions still do not justify broad comparisons of nonrandomized studies, they do help in the extrapolation of data into clinical settings.

Natural history

A substantial proportion of patients will develop a biochemical recurrence following external-beam radiation. For example, Shipley et al demonstrated a 5-year estimate of freedom from biochemical failure rate of 65.8% in a multi-institutional pooled analysis.[11] Similarly, Kuban et al reported PSA disease-free survival (DFS) rates of 59% at 5 years and 53% at 8 years.[12] In addition, there is emerging evidence that longer term follow-up periods may be needed to fully appreciate the true rate of biochemical recurrence. In a recent long-term study with a minimum follow-up period of 22.9 years, it was found that recurrences developed throughout the length of the study.[13] In fact, over half of the recurrences occurred after 10 years and some even occurred after 20 years.

Predictors of biochemical recurrence and patient outcomes

Several clinical factors have been used to predict who is at risk for a biochemical recurrence following primary radiation therapy. It is

---

Box 26.1 ASTRO guidelines for PSA following radiation therapy

- Biochemical failure is not justification per se to initiate additional treatment. It is not equivalent to clinical failure. It is, however, an appropriate early end point for clinical trials.
- Three consecutive increases in PSA is a reasonable definition of biochemical failure after radiation therapy. For clinical trials, the date of failure should be the midpoint between the post-irradiation nadir PSA and the first of the three consecutive rises.
- No definition of PSA failure has, as yet, been shown to be a surrogate for clinical progression or survival.
- Nadir PSA is a strong prognostic factor, but no absolute level is a valid cut point for separating successful and unsuccessful treatments. Nadir PSA is similar in prognostic value to pretreatment prognostic variables.

ASTRO, American Society for Therapeutic Radiology and Oncology
From Cox JD for the American Society for Therapeutic Radiology and Oncology Concensus Panel. Concensus Statement Guidelines for PSA following radiation therapy. Int J Radiat Oncol Biol Phys 1997;37:1035–41.

---

important to recognize that biochemical recurrence will include patients with localized only relapse, microscopic metastatic disease progression, and combinations of both. In almost all cases, PSA recurrence will precede symptoms by several years. Differentiating local recurrence only from distant relapse, and potentially more aggressive disease progression, is critical to determining the most appropriate treatment course.

Primary tumor features

Several large reports have studied predictors of long-term outcomes following primary radiation therapy. Zagars et al analyzed the outcomes of 938 men treated with definitive external-beam radiation from 1987 to 1995.[14] In a multivariate regression model, pretreatment PSA, treatment stage, and Gleason scores were independent predictors of rising PSA, local recurrence, and incidence of metastases. Similarly, Kuban et al reported the long-term outcomes for patients treated for T1/T2 prostate cancer from 1986 to 1995 at nine institutions.[15] In multivariate analysis, several factors were found to be prognostic for biochemical failure including pretreatment PSA, Gleason score, radiation dose, tumor stage, and treatment year. Finally, Kupelian et al reviewed the biochemical relapse-free survival in 2991 patients receiving local therapy at two institutions.[16] In this group of patients, which included surgery, radiation, and brachytherapy, baseline PSA, Gleason score, and year of therapy were all found to be independent predictors of relapse.

Prediction models

Numerous prostate cancer nomograms have been developed to help predict patient outcomes. For an excellent review on the topic, one should turn to a recent publication cataloging 42 published nomograms.[17] For the nomograms designed to predict PSA recurrence following external-beam radiation and brachytherapy, the three most common predictors used in the nomograms include the biopsy Gleason score, clinical stage, and pretreatment PSA.

Prostate-specific antigen doubling time

The prostate-specific antigen doubling time (PSADT) has emerged as an important prognostic tool in patients with a biochemical recurrence following local therapy. Following RP, Partin et al studied several clinical parameters to help predict PSA recurrence.[18] In an updated report from the same group, PSADT was shown to predict distant failure and prostate cancer specific survival.[19] At 10 years following RP, prostate cancer-specific survival was 85% in the group with PSADT of more than 10 months and 47% in the group with PSADT of less than 10 months.

Prostate-specific antigen doubling time has also been studied in patients following radiation therapy. For example, Lee et al reported an outcome study of 151 patients with a biochemical recurrence following radiation therapy.[20] In this study, multivariate analysis showed that the time to PSA elevation and post-treatment PSADT were important predictors of the development of distant metastases. Furthermore, in a second retrospective report, D'Amico et al demonstrated that patients with a short PSADT (defined as 3 months or less) following radiation therapy was an important predictor of prostate cancer specific death[21–23] (Figure 26.1).

In addition to its use as a prognostic tool, PSADT may also be used to help guide management decisions. For example, Pinover et al reported on their institutions' experience using PSADT to manage patients following radiation therapy.[24] In their report, the use of ADT in men with a PSADT of less than 12 months was associated with a statistically significant improvement in 5-year freedom from distant metastasis (FDM) rate (57% versus 78%; $P = 0.0026$). Furthermore, the FDM rates in patients with PSADT of more than 12 months were similar in both the ADT group (88%) and observation group (92%) lending support for the strategy of reserving early ADT for patients with high-risk features such as a short PSADT.

100-day prostate-specific antigen

Developing surrogate markers with shorter periods of follow-up allows researchers to study newer treatment strategies in shorter periods of time. Johnstone et al recently published the results of a study which looked at the PSA value of patients 100 days after definitive radiotherapy for localized prostate cancer.[25] Patients with a PSA at 100 days of less than 4 ng/mL had significantly greater 8-year biochemical no evidence of disease (bNED) rates compared with patients with 100-day PSA value greater than 4 ng/mL (62% versus 20%, respectively; $P < 0.001$). As the authors point out, these results will need to be followed up in order to validate the 100-day PSA as a surrogate marker for long-term disease outcomes.

Diagnostic considerations

Once biochemical recurrence has been established, further clinical and radiographic staging may be indicated. Diagnostic options include digital rectal exam for localized recurrence, radionuclide bone scan, computed tomography (CT), magnetic resonance imaging (MRI), indium-111-labeled CYT-356 (ProstaScint) scan, and prostate re-biopsy. Decisions on which tests are needed are made based on an individual patient's PSA, symptoms, and further treatment goals. Clearly, one important goal of this work-up is to

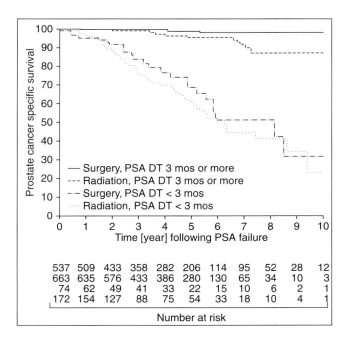

Figure 26.1
Prostate cancer-specific survival after prostate-specific antigen (PSA) -defined recurrence stratified by treatment received and the value of the post-treatment PSA doubling time (PSADT). A pairwise two-sided log-rank test was used. *P* values are as follows: for a PSADT <3 months (surgery versus radiation), *P* = 0.38; for PSA-DT ≥ 3 months (surgery versus radiation), *P* < 0.001; for PSADT <3 months versus PSADT of ≥ 3 months (surgery), *P* < 0.001; for PSADT <3 months versus PSADT of ≥ 3 months (radiation), *P* < 0.001.
Adapted from D'Amico AV, Moul JW, Carroll PR, Sun L, Lubeck D, Chen MH. Surrogate end point for prostate cancer-specific mortality after radical prostatectomy or radiation therapy. J Natl Cancer Inst 2003;95:1376–1383 (by permission of Oxford University Press).

determine whether the cancer has recurred locally, in distant metastatic sites, or both.

Bone scan

Although the radionuclide bone scan is the most sensitive test to detect bone metastases, clinicians must remember that the yield of this study is often very low in patients with a biochemical recurrence following radiation therapy. The yield of a bone scan in patients with biochemical recurrence has been better studied in the post-RP population. In one series of 132 patients, only 9.4% (12 of 127 patients who had bone scans) had a positive bone scan within 3 years of biochemical recurrence following RP.[26] In a second series, the probability of a positive bone scan was determined to be 5% or lower in patients until serum PSA levels reach the range of 30 to 40 ng/mL.[27]

Unfortunately, less data has been published in patients after radiation therapy. In one series of patients after either RP or radiation therapy, a PSA value of less than 8 ng/mL excluded bone metastases with a predictive value of a negative test of 98.5%.[28] A second retrospective study, studied the utility of bone scan in patients at time of biochemical failure after RP (n = 24) and radiotherapy (n = 20).[29]

Bone scans were more commonly positive post-radiotherapy (6 of 20; 30%) than post-RP (1 of 20; 5%). In the post-radiation group, the PSA ranged from 1.31 to 23.6 ng/mL (median 13.9 ng/mL) in patients with a positive bone scan and from 1.02 to 9.53 ng/mL (median 5.5 ng/mL) in patients with a negative bone scan. Taken together, a rational approach would be to consider bone scan in patients who: 1) have bone pain symptoms; 2) are candidates for local salvage procedures; or 3) have a PSA over 5 ng/mL.[30,31]

Computed tomography and magnetic resonance imaging

Abdominal and pelvic CT or MRI scan are other important imaging studies used to help determine the extent of spread of a patient's cancer at time of biochemical recurrence. Similar to the bone scan, the yield of CT or MRI can be expected to be quite low at the time of biochemical recurrence. In the Johnstone series, only 10 patients underwent CT imaging at time of biochemical recurrence following external-beam radiotherapy.[29] Of these 10 patients, three had positive findings including one with an abdominal wall metastasis, one with a positive pelvic lymph node, and one with bone metastases that were also seen with bone scan. Similar to the bone scan, CT or MRI imaging should be considered in patients with symptoms, those with higher PSA levels, and those who are candidates for potentially morbid local salvage procedures.

ProstaScint scan

The ProstaScint scan (Cytogen, Princeton, NJ) is a murine monoclonal antibody-based imaging modality that has been FDA approved for use in the staging of newly diagnosed prostate cancer patients who are at high risk for metastases, and for patients with a biochemical recurrence following prostatectomy. Although the ProstaScint scan has been used in patients following primary radiation therapy, the test has not been FDA approved for this indication.[32,33] Preliminary studies evaluating ProstaScint scan following definitive radiation therapy demonstrated positive prostatic uptake in 21 of 24 patients imaged and confirmed with positive biopsies in 10 of 15 patients.[34] Further studies are needed to evaluate the positive predictive value in this setting.

Prostate re-biopsy

A consensus panel convened by ASTRO recommended that systematic prostate re-biopsy is not routinely necessary after radiation therapy.[35] One caveat is in patients being considered for local salvage therapy, such as salvage prostatectomy. Under these circumstances, confirmation of localized disease recurrence may be necessary prior to committing patients to a potentially morbid procedure.

Management strategies

The management of a biochemical recurrence requires a careful understanding of the nature of recurrence (local versus distant), prognostic features, and patient preferences. In patients suspected of local recurrence only, management options include observation, salvage prostatectomy, cryotherapy, brachytherapy, and hormonal therapy. For patients suspected of having microscopic metastatic disease, hormonal therapy is the most commonly employed initial treatment modality; however, alternative approaches using chemotherapy or investigational agents are being studied.

Surgery

Salvage RP remains an option in a subset of patients with a local recurrence following radiation therapy. Traditionally, the use of salvage prostatectomy has been limited due to high reported rates of perioperative complications including incontinence rates of 40% to 50% and rectal injury rates of 10% to 15%.[36] Despite these limitations, salvage prostatectomy can result in long-term DFS in 30% to 47% of patients.[37–40]

Patients should be carefully selected prior to salvage prostatectomy. For example, Rogers et al studied PSA as a predictor of treatment outcome in patients who underwent prostatectomy following radiation.[41] In their report, 2 of the 13 patients (15%) with a PSA level below 10 ng/mL had an advanced pathologic stage (seminal vesicle invasion or lymph node metastasis) at time of surgery compared with 12 of 14 (86%) of patients with a PSA of 10 ng/mL or higher. Using prognostic factors including PSA below 10 ng/mL and Gleason score less than 7, salvage prostatectomy results approach those of RP in untreated patients with similar pathologic findings.[42]

Currently, a multicenter phase II study is ongoing (CALGB 9687) to gain an up-to-date understanding of the utility and side-effect profile of salvage prostatectomy for patients with a local recurrence following radiation therapy.

Brachytherapy

Brachytherapy has also been used for patients with a biochemical recurrence following primary radiation therapy (Figure 26.2). Grado et al reported the results of a retrospective study on the effectiveness and side effect profile of 49 patients who had undergone salvage brachytherapy.[43] The actuarial biochemical DFS at 3 and 5 years was 48% and 34%, respectively. In patients with a post-brachytherapy PSA nadir under 0.5 ng/mL, the actuarial biochemical DFS rates at 3 and 5 years were 77% and 56%, respectively. The reported serious complication rate was low. For example, although acute urinary symptoms (frequency, nocturia, urgency) were common, these symptoms were generally transient and often managed medically. More serious complications included persistent gross hematuria in two patients (4%), significant post-treatment pain in three patients (6%), and the development of rectal ulcers in two patients (4%). Nonetheless, salvage brachytherapy remains highly investigational. One caveat to these results is that this data represents a single institutional effort and should be replicated in a larger, multicenter setting before more standard application is considered.

Cryotherapy

A further option for patients with a local recurrence of their prostate cancer is salvage cryoablation of the prostate. Pisters et al reported

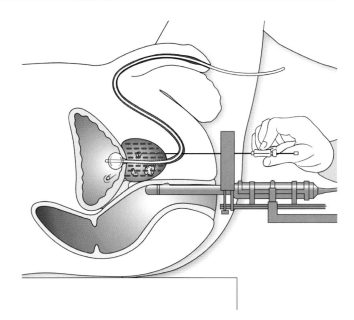

Figure 26.2
Brachytherapy needles are placed under ultrasound control. Although the technique is an established treatment for primary disease, it is only occasionally used as therapy for recurrence after external beam radiotherapy.

on 150 patients who underwent salvage cryotherapy for a biochemical recurrence following primary radiation.[44] In their first report, a double freeze-thaw cycle was found to be more effective than a single freeze-thaw cycle in achieving a negative post-cryotherapy biopsy and lower biochemical failure rates. Unfortunately, complication rates were high, including urinary incontinence (73% of patients), obstructive symptoms (67%), impotence (72%), and severe perineal pain (8%). A second analysis was later reported to better define predictive factors, such as pretreatment PSA and Gleason scores, which were associated with better outcomes.[45] The 2-year actuarial DFS rates were significantly higher in patients with pre-cryotherapy PSA values of under 10 ng/mL compared with those above 10 ng/mL (74% versus 28%, respectively; $P < 0.00001$). Similarly, 2-year DFS rates were significantly higher in patients with a Gleason score of less than 8 compared with over 9 (58% versus 29%, respectively; $P < 0.004$). Chin et al reported on an additional 118 patients treated with salvage cryotherapy.[46] Similar to the above series, worse outcomes were seen in patients with either a PSA above 10 ng/mL or a Gleason score of 8 or more. While new-generation techniques may decrease the morbidity rates associated with salvage cryotherapy, these results would suggest that candidates for cryotherapy should have a Gleason score of their recurrent tumor below 8 and PSA value below 10 ng/mL.

Hormonal therapy

Timing

The decision of when to start ADT remains controversial, and currently there is wide variation in clinical practice patterns. However, several studies since the mid-1990s support the hypothesis that ADT started before overt bone metastases have formed is associated with improved disease-specific survival. In 1997, Bolla et al published results of an 8-year study of 415 patients with locally advanced prostate cancer treated with 50 Gy of pelvic irradiation with a 20 Gy boost to the prostate versus a combination of the same radiation therapy plus 3 years of continuous ADT.[47,48] Their results demonstrated a significant improvement in the 5-year local control rate (97% versus 77%; $P < 0.001$) and overall survival (79% versus 62%; $P = 0.001$), both in favor of the combination group. All but two patients received ADT at the time of disease progression in the radiotherapy alone arm, suggesting that the timing of ADT (immediate versus disease progression) contributed in part to the improved survival. Further support for early versus delayed androgen deprivation therapy comes from Messing et al, who demonstrated a survival advantage for men with N1 disease following prostatectomy who were treated with androgen deprivation therapy immediately versus at the time of disease progression.[49] However, both of these studies defined disease progression as radiographic evidence of either local regional or metastatic disease recurrence. Whether PSA recurrence alone would identify relapse early enough to negate any survival advantage seen in the groups receiving immediate ADT is unclear.

Recent studies have begun to evaluate the possible benefit of early versus delayed androgen deprivation therapy in the post-PSA era. In particular, investigators have used PSA parameters (velocity, doubling time, and various thresholds) to evaluate in which patients early treatment impacts outcome. For example, Moul et al published results from the Department of Defense Center for Prostate Disease Research Database demonstrating that in 1352 men with PSA recurrence following RP early ADT resulted in a delay in clinical metastases in patients with a Gleason score greater than 7 and a PSA doubling time of less than 12 months (HR = 2.12; $P = 0.01$).[50] Conversely, no improvement in time to clinical metastases was detected for patients with Gleason score 7 or less tumors and PSA doubling times of more than 12 months. Unfortunately, further studies are needed to clarify the stratification of patients for intervention versus observation in this setting and currently this issue remains unresolved. In fact, a recent ASCO recommendation guideline report was unable to come up with specific recommendations on the issue of early versus deferred therapy.[51]

Clinicians must balance the side effects of ADT with the possibility for improved long-term outcomes. Potential side effects for ADT include hot flashes, muscle weakness, loss of libido, and erectile dysfunction. In addition, long-term complications include osteoporosis, depression, and anemia. Furthermore, the early use of ADT has financial considerations as these treatments are expensive and patients may remain on them for many years.

Intermittent androgen deprivation

As an alternative to continuous androgen ablation, the strategy of intermittent androgen deprivation (IAD) has received considerable interest. Preclinical studies have demonstrated that IAD may delay the onset of androgen-independence in prostate cancer models.[52–54] Several nonrandomized studies have demonstrated the feasibility of different strategies of IAD.[55–60] Each of these studies demonstrated the ability of IAD to give patients time off of therapy and presumably freedom from some of the negative side effects of ADT. Specific improvements in quality of life have been reported in a few reports.[61,62] Preliminary results from two randomized studies comparing IAD with continuous ADT have been reported.[63,64] To further define the utility of IAD, two large, cooperative group phase III studies are currently open in two different populations.[65] In the first,

JPR7, men with a PSA relapse without evidence of clinical metastases are being randomized to either intermittent or continuous androgen deprivation. In the second, SWOG-9346, men with distant metastatic disease will receive either intermittent or continuous combined androgen deprivation comprising bicalutamide and goserelin. Results of both of these trials will help clinicians gain a better understanding of the use of IAD as a hormonal strategy.

Other strategies

As a further way to avoid some of the side effects of total androgen ablation, other hormonal strategies are currently under investigation. One of these strategies is the combination of a 5α-reductase inhibitor with an antiandrogen. For example, finasteride has been combined with flutamide in at least three studies in men with advanced prostate cancer.[66–68] In all three reports, more than half of men with sexual potency at baseline maintained their erectile function on therapy. In a larger study, Barqawi et al studied the use of low-dose flutamide and finasteride in 71 men with a PSA-only recurrence following primary local therapy.[69] In this report, 45 patients (58%) achieved a nadir PSA of 0.1 ng/mL or less. Importantly, the therapy was well tolerated with the most common side effects being breast tenderness (90%), gynecomastia (72%), gastrointestinal disturbances (22%), and fatigue (10%). To date, these strategies have not been compared in a randomized study with standard ADT but, nonetheless, remain an option for some patients.

In a related approach, Scandinavian investigators performed a large, randomized, placebo-controlled trial randomizing patients to receive either high-dose bicalutamide (150 mg/day p.o.) versus placebo. Patients in this study also received standard care (RP, radiotherapy, or watchful waiting). With a 5.3 year median follow-up, bicalutamide improved overall survival (HR = 0.68; 95% CI 0.50–0.92) in patients with locally advanced disease (T3/4, M0, any N; or any T, M0, N+).[70] This type of approach may have utility in the setting of PSA relapse following local therapy in patients who wish to avoid the side effects of ADT.

Chemotherapy is actively being investigated in patients with biochemical relapse for prostate cancer. Recent studies have demonstrated a clear survival benefit to docetaxel-based chemotherapy regimens in men with metastatic hormone-refractory prostate cancer.[71,72] High-risk prognostic criteria, including PSADT of less than 3 months, may aid in patient selection for these studies, and combinations before, after, or concomitantly with ADT will need further evaluation. For the time being, chemotherapy is not considered a standard approach for management of hormone-naive prostate cancer patients with disease recurrence.

Summary

The management of patients with a biochemical recurrence following primary radiation therapy requires a thoughtful and balanced approach from a multidisciplinary team of prostate cancer specialists. In discussing options of therapy, clinicians need to consider each individual clinical situation. Clinicians continue to be faced with questions such as:

- What is the preferred salvage therapy in patients with suspected local-only recurrence?
- When is the appropriate time to start hormonal therapy?

- What is the relative efficacy of intermittent versus continuous androgen deprivation therapy?
- Are there better tolerated alternatives to complete androgen deprivation?
- Is there benefit to combining chemotherapy to ADT in patients at risk for developing androgen-independent prostate cancer and prostate cancer-specific mortality?

Hopefully, the results of ongoing and future trials will investigate these areas and lead to a more evidenced-based clinical approach.

References

1. Wang MC, Papsidero LD, Kuriyama M, et al. Prostate antigen: a new potential marker for prostatic cancer. Prostate 1981;2:89–96.
2. Stephenson RA. Prostate cancer trends in the era of prostate-specific antigen. An update of incidence, mortality, and clinical factors from the SEER database. Urol Clin North Am 2002;29:173–181.
3. D'Amico AV, Whittington R, Malkowicz SB, et al. Biochemical outcome after radical prostatectomy, external beam radiation therapy, or interstitial radiation therapy for clinically localized prostate cancer. JAMA 1998;280:969–974.
4. Iannuzzi CM, Stock RG, Stone NN. PSA kinetics following I-125 radioactive seed implantation in the treatment of T1-T2 prostate cancer. Radiat Oncol Investig 1999;7:30–35.
5. Critz FA. Time to achieve a prostate specific antigen nadir of 0.2 ng/ml after simultaneous irradiation for prostate cancer. J Urol 2002;168:2434–2438.
6. Stock RG, Stone NN, Cesaretti JA. Prostate-specific antigen bounce after prostate seed implantation for localized prostate cancer: descriptions and implications. Int J Radiat Oncol Biol Phys 2003;56:448–453.
7. Sengoz M, Abacioglu U, Cetin I, et al. PSA bouncing after external beam radiation for prostate cancer with or without hormonal treatment. Eur Urol 2003;43:473–477.
8. Tyldesley S, Coldman A, Pickles T. PSA doubling time post radiation: the effect of neoadjuvant androgen ablation. Can J Urol 2004;11:2316–2321.
9. Merrick GS, Butler WM, Wallner KE, et al. Temporal effect of neoadjuvant androgen deprivation therapy on PSA kinetics following permanent prostate brachytherapy with or without supplemental external beam radiation. Brachytherapy 2004;3:141–146.
10. Consensus statement: guidelines for PSA following radiation therapy. American Society for Therapeutic Radiology and Oncology Consensus Panel. Int J Radiat Oncol Biol Phys 1997;37:1035–1041.
11. Shipley WU, Thames HD, Sandler HM, et al. Radiation therapy for clinically localized prostate cancer: a multi-institutional pooled analysis. JAMA 1999;281:1598–1604.
12. Kuban DA, Thames HD, Levy LB, et al. Long-term multi-institutional analysis of stage T1-T2 prostate cancer treated with radiotherapy in the PSA era. Int J Radiat Oncol Biol Phys 2003;57:915–928.
13. Swanson GP, Riggs MW, Earle JD. Long-term follow-up of radiotherapy for prostate cancer. Int J Radiat Oncol Biol Phys 2004;59:406–411.
14. Zagars GK, Pollack A, von Eschenbach AC. Prognostic factors for clinically localized prostate carcinoma: analysis of 938 patients irradiated in the prostate specific antigen era. Cancer 1997;79:1370–1380.
15. Kuban DA, Thames HD, Levy LB, et al. Long-term multi-institutional analysis of stage T1-T2 prostate cancer treated with radiotherapy in the PSA era. Int J Radiat Oncol Biol Phys 2003;57:915–928.
16. Kupelian PA, Potters L, Khuntia D, et al. Radical prostatectomy, external beam radiotherapy <72 Gy, external beam radiotherapy > or =72 Gy, permanent seed implantation, or combined seeds/external beam radiotherapy for stage T1-T2 prostate cancer. Int J Radiat Oncol Biol Phys 2004;58:25–33.
17. Ross PL, Scardino PT, Kattan MW. A catalog of prostate cancer nomograms. J Urol 2001;165:1562–1568.
18. Pound CR, Partin AW, Eisenberger MA, et al. Natural history of progression after PSA elevation following radical prostatectomy. JAMA 1999;281:1591–1597.
19. Partin AW, Eisenberger MA, Sinibaldi VJ, et al. Prostate specific antigen doubling time (PSADT) predicts for distant failure and prostate cancer specific survival (PCSS) in men with biochemical relapse after radical prostatectomy (RP). J Clin Oncol 2004;22:14S [abstract].
20. Lee WR, Hanks GE, Hanlon A. Increasing prostate-specific antigen profile following definitive radiation therapy for localized prostate cancer: clinical observations. J Clin Oncol 1997;15:230–238.
21. D'Amico AV, Cote K, Loffredo M, et al. Determinants of prostate cancer specific survival following radiation therapy during the prostate specific antigen era. J Urol 2003;170:S42–S46.
22. D'Amico AV, Moul JW, Carroll PR, et al. Surrogate end point for prostate cancer-specific mortality after radical prostatectomy or radiation therapy. J Natl Cancer Inst 2003;95:1376–1383.
23. D'Amico AV, Moul J, Carroll PR, et al. Prostate specific antigen doubling time as a surrogate end point for prostate cancer specific mortality following radical prostatectomy or radiation therapy. J Urol 2004;172:S42–S46.
24. Pinover WH, Horwitz EM, Hanlon AL, et al. Validation of a treatment policy for patients with prostate specific antigen failure after three-dimensional conformal prostate radiation therapy. Cancer 2003;97:1127–1133.
25. Johnstone PA, Williams SR, Riffenburgh RH. The 100-day PSA: usefulness as surrogate end point for biochemical disease-free survival after definitive radiotherapy of prostate cancer. Prostate Cancer Prostatic Dis 2004;7:263–267.
26. Kane CJ, Amling CL, Johnstone PA, et al. Limited value of bone scintigraphy and computed tomography in assessing biochemical failure after radical prostatectomy. Urology 2003;61:607–611.
27. Cher ML, Bianco FJ, Jr., Lam JS, et al. Limited role of radionuclide bone scintigraphy in patients with prostate specific antigen elevations after radical prostatectomy. J Urol 1998;160:1387–1391.
28. Freitas JE, Gilvydas R, Ferry JD, et al. The clinical utility of prostate-specific antigen and bone scintigraphy in prostate cancer follow-up. J Nucl Med 1991;32:1387–1390.
29. Johnstone PA, Tarman GJ, Riffenburgh R, et al. Yield of imaging and scintigraphy assessing biochemical failure in prostate cancer patients. Urol Oncol 1998;3:108–112.
30. Lee WR, Hanks GE, Hanlon A. Increasing prostate-specific antigen profile following definitive radiation therapy for localized prostate cancer: clinical observations. J Clin Oncol 1997;15:230–238.
31. Moul JW. Biochemical recurrence of prostate cancer. Curr Probl Cancer 2003;27:243–272.
32. Sodee DB, Malguria N, Faulhaber P, et al. Multicenter ProstaScint imaging findings in 2154 patients with prostate cancer. The ProstaScint Imaging Centers. Urology 2000;56:988–993.
33. Elgamal AA, Troychak MJ, Murphy GP. ProstaScint scan may enhance identification of prostate cancer recurrences after prostatectomy, radiation, or hormone therapy: analysis of 136 scans of 100 patients. Prostate 1998;37:261–269.
34. Fang DX, Stock RG, Stone NN, et al. Use of radioimmunoscintigraphy with indium-111-labeled CYT-356 (ProstaScint) scan for evaluation of patients for salvage brachytherapy. Tech Urol 2000;6:146–150.
35. Cox JD, Gallagher MJ, Hammond EH, et al. Consensus statements on radiation therapy of prostate cancer: guidelines for prostate re-biopsy after radiation and for radiation therapy with rising prostate-specific antigen levels after radical prostatectomy. American Society for Therapeutic Radiology and Oncology Consensus Panel. J Clin Oncol 1999;17:1155.
36. Russo P. Salvage radical prostatectomy after radiation therapy and brachytherapy. J Endourol 2000;14:385–390.
37. Brenner PC, Russo P, Wood DP, et al. Salvage radical prostatectomy in the management of locally recurrent prostate cancer after 125I implantation. Br J Urol 1995;75:44–47.
38. Rogers E, Ohori M, Kassabian VS, et al. Salvage radical prostatectomy: outcome measured by serum prostate specific antigen levels. J Urol 1995;153:104–110.

39. Gheiler EL, Tefilli MV, Tiguert R, et al. Predictors for maximal outcome in patients undergoing salvage surgery for radio-recurrent prostate cancer. Urology 1998;51:789–795.

40. Amling CL, Lerner SE, Martin SK, et al. Deoxyribonucleic acid ploidy and serum prostate specific antigen predict outcome following salvage prostatectomy for radiation refractory prostate cancer. J Urol 1999;161:857–862.

41. Rogers E, Ohori M, Kassabian VS, et al. Salvage radical prostatectomy: outcome measured by serum prostate specific antigen levels. J Urol 1995;153:104–110.

42. Stephenson AJ, Scardino PT, Bianco FJ, et al. Salvage therapy for locally recurrent prostate cancer after external beam radiotherapy. Curr Treat Options Oncol 2004;5:357–365.

43. Grado GL, Collins JM, Kriegshauser JS, et al. Salvage brachytherapy for localized prostate cancer after radiotherapy failure. Urology 1999;53:2–10.

44. Pisters LL, von Eschenbach AC, Scott SM, et al. The efficacy and complications of salvage cryotherapy of the prostate. J Urol 1997;157:921–925.

45. Pisters LL, Perrotte P, Scott SM, et al. Patient selection for salvage cryotherapy for locally recurrent prostate cancer after radiation therapy. J Clin Oncol 1999;17:2514–2520.

46. Chin JL, Pautler SE, Mouraviev V, et al. Results of salvage cryoablation of the prostate after radiation: identifying predictors of treatment failure and complications. J Urol 2001;165:1937–1941.

47. Bolla M, Gonzalez D, Warde P, et al. Improved survival in patients with locally advanced prostate cancer treated with radiotherapy and goserelin. N Engl J Med 1997;337:295–300.

48. Bolla M, Collette L, Blank L, et al. Long-term results with immediate androgen suppression and external irradiation in patients with locally advanced prostate cancer (an EORTC study): a phase III randomised trial. Lancet 2002;360:103–106.

49. Messing EM, Manola J, Sarosdy M, et al. Immediate hormonal therapy compared with observation after radical prostatectomy and pelvic lymphadenectomy in men with node-positive prostate cancer. N Engl J Med 1999;341:1781–1788.

50. Moul JW, Wu H, Sun L, et al. Early versus delayed hormonal therapy for prostate specific antigen only recurrence of prostate cancer after radical prostatectomy. J Urol 2004;171:1141–1147.

51. Loblaw DA, Mendelson DS, Talcott JA, et al. American Society of Clinical Oncology recommendations for the initial hormonal management of androgen-sensitive metastatic, recurrent, or progressive prostate cancer. J Clin Oncol 2004;22:2927–2941.

52. Akakura K, Bruchovsky N, Goldenberg SL, et al. Effects of intermittent androgen suppression on androgen-dependent tumors. Apoptosis and serum prostate-specific antigen. Cancer 1993;71:2782–2790.

53. Sato N, Gleave ME, Bruchovsky N, et al. Intermittent androgen suppression delays progression to androgen-independent regulation of prostate-specific antigen gene in the LNCaP prostate tumour model. J Steroid Biochem Mol Biol 1996;58:139–146.

54. Hsieh JT, Wu HC, Gleave ME, et al. Autocrine regulation of prostate-specific antigen gene expression in a human prostatic cancer (LNCaP) subline. Cancer Res 1993;53:2852–2857.

55. Higano CS, Ellis W, Russell K, et al. Intermittent androgen suppression with leuprolide and flutamide for prostate cancer: a pilot study. Urology 1996;48:800–804.

56. Crook JM, Szumacher E, Malone S, et al. Intermittent androgen suppression in the management of prostate cancer. Urology 1999;53:530–534.

57. Strum SB, Scholz MC, McDermed JE. Intermittent androgen deprivation in prostate cancer patients: factors predictive of prolonged time off therapy. Oncologist 2000;5:45–52.

58. Grossfeld GD, Chaudhary UB, Reese DM, et al. Intermittent androgen deprivation: update of cycling characteristics in patients without clinically apparent metastatic prostate cancer. Urology 2001;58:240–245.

59. De La Taille, Zerbib M, Conquy S, et al. Intermittent androgen suppression in patients with prostate cancer. BJU Int 2003;91:18-22.

60. Youssef E, Tekyi-Mensah S, Hart K, et al. Intermittent androgen deprivation for patients with recurrent/metastatic prostate cancer. Am J Clin Oncol 2003;26:e119–e123.

61. Klotz LH, Herr HW, Morse MJ, et al. Intermittent endocrine therapy for advanced prostate cancer. Cancer 1986;58:2546–2550.

62. Rashid MH, Chaudhary UB. Intermittent androgen deprivation therapy for prostate cancer. Oncologist 2004;9:295–301.

63. Tunn U, Eckart O, Kienle E. Can intermittent androgen deprivation be an alternative to continuous androgen withdrawal in patients with a PSA relapse? First results of the randomized prospective phase III clinical trial EC 507. J Urol 2003;169:1481.

64. Schasfoort E, Heathcote P, Lock T. Intermittent androgen suppression for the treatment of advanced prostate cancer. J Urol 2003;169:1483 [abstract].

65. http://www.cancer.gov/search/ResultsClinicalTrials.aspx?protocolsearch=1850073.

66. Fleshner NE, Fair WR. Anti-androgenic effects of combination finasteride plus flutamide in patients with prostatic carcinoma. Br J Urol 1996;78:907–910.

67. Brufsky A, Fontaine-Rothe P, Berlane K, et al. Finasteride and flutamide as potency-sparing androgen-ablative therapy for advanced adenocarcinoma of the prostate. Urology 1997;49:913–920.

68. Ornstein DK, Rao GS, Johnson B, et al. Combined finasteride and flutamide therapy in men with advanced prostate cancer. Urology 1996;48:901–905.

69. Barqawi AB, Moul JW, Ziada A, et al. Combination of low-dose flutamide and finasteride for PSA-only recurrent prostate cancer after primary therapy. Urology 2003;62:872–876.

70. Iversen P, Johansson JE, Lodding P, et al. Bicalutamide (150 mg) versus placebo as immediate therapy alone or as adjuvant to therapy with curative intent for early nonmetastatic prostate cancer: 5.3-year median followup from the Scandinavian Prostate Cancer Group Study Number 6. J Urol 2004;172:1871–1876.

71. Petrylak DP, Tangen CM, Hussain MH, et al. Docetaxel and estramustine compared with mitoxantrone and prednisone for advanced refractory prostate cancer. N Engl J Med 2004;351:1513–1520.

72. Tannock IF, de Wit R, Berry WR, et al. Docetaxel plus prednisone or mitoxantrone plus prednisone for advanced prostate cancer. N Engl J Med 2004;351:1502–1512.

27

Cryotherapy as primary therapy for prostate cancer

Ulrich K Fr Witzsch

Introduction

Cryoablation of the prostate has been used clinically for more than half a century. Early results were unsatisfactory due to poor oncologic outcome and high morbidity. Technical evolution and clinical experience has led to improved results with less morbidity.

Cryobiology

Generally there are five effects discussed that might be of importance in destroying the prostate cancer cells[1,2]:

1. As the temperature falls, extracellular ice is created. The unfrozen intracellular water flows into the extracellular space causing dehydration, which is reversed during thawing. Water inflow into the hyperosmolaric intracellular space leads to rupture of the cell.
2. At lower temperatures intracellular ice forms. The ice crystals are needle shaped if the speed of freezing is fast. The sharper the ice, the more likely it is to destroy the cell membranes and organelles. During thawing, shear forces also destroy cell membranes.
3. Ice clots obstruct the blood vessels. These emboli or thrombi interrupt blood and oxygen supply to the tissue.
4. Apoptosis is induced by freezing.
5. Immunologic processes are initiated. The exact role of immunology in cryotherapy is still under investigation.

Experimental data[3] proves that the velocity of freezing correlates with the temperatures which must be achieved to be 100% lethal. The higher the velocity of freezing, the higher the temperature that destroys all cells. It has also been shown experimentally that repeated freeze thaw cycles are more effective than a single cycle (Table 27.1).

Cryoablation

Clinical experience and experimental data[4] show that maximum ablation occurs with: 1) fast freezing; 2) slow thawing; and 3) repetitive freeze thaw cycles.

The speed of freezing is dependent on the density and efficacy of the probes. Size wise the relation between effective (kill) zone and affected (side effect) zone is always the same. Creating big iceballs leads to a larger zone of morbidity than do small iceballs.

Due to this fact, it is obvious that multiple small iceballs covering the prostate homogeneously leads to a smaller zone of possible morbidity than a few big iceballs. Also, it is obvious that due to the circular form of the iceballs in larger ones warm areas are more probable between the killing zones than with more and smaller ones. Coverage of the prostate with numerous small iceballs is, therefore, known as "high-resolution cryotherapy."

Cryotechnology

The aim of cryotherapy is to ablate the prostate cancer tissue precisely, predictably, and in a controlled fashion.[5] This is most likely achieved with multiple small iceballs created by cryoneedles rather than thicker probes.

Influenced by technical inventions, cryotechnology developed considerably over the last few decades. The technology can be divided into three generations according to cryogen and type of probes:

1. First generation technology used liquid nitrogen for freezing. The probes had to be surgically placed.
2. Second generation uses high-pressure argon. Probes are still thick and have to be placed surgically with an insertion kit.
3. The most recent advance has been third generation devices.[6] Cryoneedles, miniaturized 17G double lumen needles, replace cryoprobes. The needles can be easily inserted into the prostate. High-pressure argon gas is expanded in the tip of the needle leading to cooling. High-pressure helium gas can be alternated in the same needle to produce a warming effect. The expanded gas returns back via the second lumen of the needle.

The change of temperature of gases while expanding is known as the Joule–Thompson effect. Using cooling and warming at the same location leads to higher controllability of the procedure. The iceballs created are approximately 2 cm × 3 cm, and they extend 0.5 cm from the tip of the needle. The needle tips are echogenic and, therefore, visible with ultrasound.

Procedure

Initially a cystoscopy is done to measure the distance between the ureteral orifices and the bladder neck. Then a suprapubic catheter (SPC) is placed, and an extrastiff (Amplat2-) guide wire is inserted

Table 27.1 Temperature that has to be reached to kill 100% of prostate cancer cells depending on velocity of freezing (Tatsutani)

	Velocity of freezing		
	1°C/min	5°C/min	25°C/min
One cycle	<−40°C	<−40°C	−40°C
Two cycles	−40°C	−35°C	−18°C

via the cystoscope for placement of the transurethral warming catheter later on in the procedure.

The transrectal ultrasound probe (TRUS) is placed in the rectum, and the preoperative measurements and landmarks of the prostate are re-identified. The TRUS probe will remain in place until the end of procedure for continuous real-time monitoring.

Needle placement

On average, *14 cryoneedles* are placed homo-geneously in the prostate (Figure 27.1). The density of needles is higher in the dorsal aspect of the prostate for more effective treatment and better control of the peripheral zone. Needle placement is constantly monitored with TRUS. The placement is guided by a grid-like template. Cryotherapy grids differ from brachytherapy grids because they offer the possibility of placing needles in Denonvilliers' space or outer rectal wall. This is achieved by a distance of less than 5 mm between the lower aspect of the grid and the TRUS probe. An inflatable stand off should be used over the TRUS probe to improve the image and position the prostate gland to facilitate needle placement.

Two needles are placed in Denonvilliers' space just above the rectal wall. These needles are used only in the warming mode to avoid freezing into the rectal wall while a sufficient temperature is reached in the dorsal aspect of the prostate.[7]

Temperature probes are placed in the prostate at positions where the cancer location is suspected. A temperature probe is placed between the *warming needles* just above the rectal wall.

A transurethral *warming catheter* is placed via the guide wire. This prevents urethral sloughing and also protects the external urethral sphincter area.

Freezing and thawing

Reviewing the literature several modes of freezing and thawing are used.

We decided to freeze down to target temperature (−40°C) and keep this for 10 minutes. The prostate disappears in TRUS (blacked out). Then passive thawing (by switching the argon flow off) is started. When a plateau in temperature change is reached, active thawing (by turning helium flow on) is started. One minute of active thawing is interrupted by one of passive thawing—the so-called "barcode thawing". After reaching positive temperatures and regaining echoes in TRUS, the next cycle of freezing is started. Two freeze thaw cycles are performed at each location. It may be necessary to reduce the time of freezing or to keep the temperature above certain levels to protect sensitive areas. It may also be useful to keep the temperature below a certain level but not cool further. This

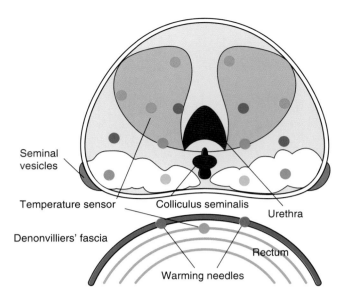

Figure 27.1
Placement of the cryoneedles within the prostate.

ensures both cancer eradication and the minimization of side effects. All this is possible with the software of third generation technology.

Pull back

For prostates longer than 3 cm a pull-back maneuver is required. This means the needles have to be pulled back for the distance by which the prostate extends over 3 cm. After each repositioning of the needles, two more freeze thaw cycles are applied.

Protection

Protection of sensitive areas is performed by special modes of operating. Warm water is applied to the perineal skin if the moisture in the operating room is frosting the needles. If the temperature in the rectal wall is falling too low, the inflatable stand off can be irrigated with warm water.

Perioperative care

Preoperatively, a complete staging should be done. We prefer a full bowel preparation the day before the procedure and an enema on the morning of the procedure. Prophylactic antibiotics are prescribed as for transurethral resection of the prostate (TURP) with i.v. broad spectrum penicillin.

Postoperatively, we check the patient every second week for 6 weeks for urinary tract infections. If this occurs the patient receives antibiotic therapy according to the urine culture. Prostate-specific antigen (PSA) is checked every 3 months. The PSA nadir will be reached after 3 to 6 months after an significant rise on the first postoperative day. At postoperative visits, the patient is regularly checked for local side effects and residual urine after voiding. The SPC is removed once the residual urine is below 50 mL but not before the end of the first week.

Side effects

Antibiotic prophylaxis and therapy have made post-cryoablation infection a rare occurrence. Urethral sloughing also appears in a reduced percentage of cases. Perineal fistulas or fistulas between the urinary tract and the rectum are unknown in primary cryoablation of the prostate with third generation technology.

After early removal of the SPC, urinary retention may occur due to delayed swelling of the organ. If the residual urine remains high a TURP for removal of devitalized tissue is indicated. This should not be done before the third postoperative month because, until then, spontaneous improvement is still possible.

Results

Long-term results—first and second generation

Bahn et al[8] reported their 7-year experience. Five hundred and ninety patients were treated for localized or locally advanced prostate cancer. Thirty-two patients were retreated for recurrence. Patients were classified in three risk groups:

- Low risk: PSA <10 ng/mL, stage <T2b, and Gleason score <7.
- Medium risk if one risk factor was present.
- High risk if two or three risk factors were present.

Seven-year biochemical-free survival was 61%, 68%, and 61% in the low, medium, and high risk groups, respectively at a PSA threshold of 0.5 ng/mL; at a threshold of 1.0 ng/mL biochemical-free survival of 87%, 79%, and 71% was achieved, and using the ASTRO criteria 92%, 89%, and 89% maintained free of biochemical relapse.

After an average of 16 months 5.1% of patients regained potency. Incontinence (any leakage) was reported in 15.9% although only 4.3% used pads. Transurethral resection of the prostate was performed on 5.5 % of the patients and two fistulas occurred.

Long-term results—second generation

Donnelly et al[9] report on results of a prospective nonrandomized clinical trial between December 1994 and February 1998. Eighty seven cryoprocedures were performed on 76 consecutive patients. All patients had histologically confirmed cancer of the prostate and PSA levels below 30 ng/mL. All patients had a negative bone scan. Patients with high risk for lymph node metastasis underwent laparoscopic lymph node dissection. Exclusion criteria were gland size greater than 60 mL, prior radiotherapy, and evidence of metastatic disease. After treating the first 30 patients, glands greater than 45 mL were downsized with 3 months of maximal androgen blockade.

Five probes were used. The first 10 patients only received a second freeze cycle if the prostate was longer than 4.5 cm. Starting with the eleventh patient, two freeze cycles were standard in all treatments. Eighty eight percent of the patients had T1 to T2 stage, Gleason score was less than 7 in 45% and 7 in 38%, and PSA was below

10 ng/mL in 62%. Transurethral resection of necrotic tissue due to sloughing was required in 3.9%. Incontinence was reported in 1.3% and testicular abscesses in 1.3%. The erectile dysfunction rate was 100%, initially, but five patients regained potency spontaneously and 13 with sexual aids.

Sixty five patients received one, ten patients received two, and one patient received three treatments. After all those treatments, 72 patients were negative for follow-up biopsies of the prostate area. One patient died of prostate cancer. At five years, PSA level was less than 0.3 ng/mL at 60% in the low-risk, 77% in the moderate-risk, and 48% in the high-risk group.

Short-term results—third generation

Cytron et al[7] first described results on 31 patients treated in a cryoablation technique with active rectal wall protection. The 12-month median PSA was 0.4 ng/mL, and no fistulas occurred. Potency was preserved in 20% of the patients who were potent preoperatively. Prolonged catheterization was required in 10% of the patients, two cases of urinary tract infection had to be treated with antibacterial agents, and one patient suffered bulbar urethral trauma due to improper placement of the transurethral warming catheter.

Personal results

Between September 2001 and October 2004 we treated 80 patients with cryotherapy for prostate cancer, 38 of whom were primary patients. Treatment was only considered primary in the absence of any other treatment for prostate cancer such as hormonal, radiation, or radical prostatectomy. A neoadjuvant treatment of less than 3 months was not considered as prior treatment.

All patients underwent a transrectal TRUS-guided biopsy, a bone scan, and, if the risk for lymph node metastases was high, either computed tomography (CT), magnetic resonance imaging (MRI), or a laparoscopic pelvic lymph node dissection. All patients treated were considered to have localized prostate cancer. The majority received cryotherapy because they had high comorbidity or were elderly, leading to a statistical life expectancy of less than 10 years. Two patients who were suitable for radical prostatectomy chose to have cryotherapy after receiving repetitively complete information on the outcome of all treatments for localized prostate cancer. Patients were categorized as favorable (n = 12) and unfavorable (n = 26) (Figure 27.2). Favorable patients had PSA <10 ng/mL, clinical stage less than T3, and combined Gleason score below 7.

Figure 27.3 shows the tumor stages based on clinical staging. Eight patients underwent a TURP unrelated to cryotherapy prior to the treatment. A prior TURP is not a contraindication for cryoablation of the prostate in experienced hands. Median preoperative PSA was 7.8 ng/mL, and median preoperative volume of the gland was 30 mL (12–80 mL).

Median treatment time was 135 minutes. A pull back was necessary in 85% due to length of the prostate being greater than 35 mm. The transurethral warming catheter remained in place for 20 minutes after finishing the last freeze cycle. Perioperative antibiotic prophylaxis was given for the time the SPC remained in place.

There were no serious adverse events. Especially, there were no perineal or rectal fistulas as described for earlier generation technology.

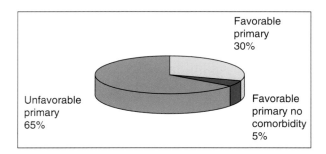

Figure 27.2
Categorization of patients as favorable or unfavorable based on prostate-specific antigen level, tumor stage, and Gleason score.

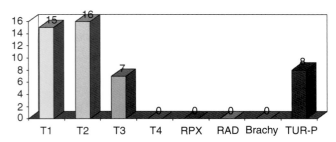

Figure 27.3
Tumor stages based on clinical staging (T1–T4), and previous treatments undergone by the patients in Figure 27.2. (RAD, radiotherapy; RPX, radical prostatectomy; Brachy, brachytherapy; TUR-P, transurethral resection of the prostate.)

Table 27.2 Prostate-specific antigen (PSA) levels at intervals after cryotherapy

Time after cryotherapy (months)	3	6	12	18	24
PSA (ng/mL)	<0.1	0.4	0.2	0.1	0.2

Forty two percent of the patients had gross hematuria, which spontaneously subsided the next day without special therapy except increased fluid intake. The first two patients had a scrotal hematoma. This can be avoided by applying pressure to the perineum for at least 5 minutes after removal of the needles. Since then, only superficial hematomas of the perineal skin, if any, were observed.

The suprapubic catheter remained open until the gross hematuria has subsided (if present) and was clamped the next day so that the patient could perform a residual voiding chart. The SPC remained in place at least for 1 week or until the patients could void properly (residual volume <50 mL). In case of residual volume of more then 50 mL, a transurethral removal of necrotic tissue was performed in 13% of the patients not earlier than 6 weeks after the cryoablation. These patients all had a preoperative IPSS score of 16 or more. It is unlikely that patients with low preoperative IPSS score will not be able to void properly.

Urethral sloughing was not reported, to our knowledge. One patient reported a stress incontinence, which improved under medication and pelvic floor training. Two patients reported a prolonged time of incontinence after TURP.

At 3 months, 64% of the patients had achieved a PSA level below 0.1 ng/mL. Table 27.2 shows the postoperative median PSA level over time.

Indications

Clinical experience gained during the last decades leads to several possible indications for primary cryoablation of the prostate:

- Primary patients with high comorbidity and increased anesthetic risk.
- Primary patients with suspected locally extended disease, which makes positive margins in radical prostatectomy probable. In these patients, an extended freezing may lead to good oncologic outcomes and minimizes the side effects, such as incontinence.
- Patients who are on hormone ablation for a while and their PSA is rising again. If the staging is negative, cryoablation may be an option for local tumor control even though there is not sufficient data on this subgroup available in the literature.
- Patients who definitely do not want radical surgery or other therapies.

Discussion

The minimally invasive nature of cryoablation earns it a place in the range of therapeutic options for localized prostate cancer. Adhering to the concept of "nihil nocere" it is a good option if other therapeutic modalities have absolute or relative contraindications. Also, it opens a therapeutic option with curative possibilities if other modalities have a low probability of curative results such that the side effects of those other therapies would be more probable than cure. Clinical studies tend to suggest that even if there is a difference in the outcome regarding the risk of preoperative occult metastasis or postoperative progression this is lower for cryoablation in relation to other therapeutic options.[10,11]

The time of stay in the hospital is not comparable between centers. It depends very much on the structure of the health system, availability of facilities, and mentality of the patients. In Germany, for example, patients tend to stay longer in the hospital due to historical developments and patients demands. Also, numbers for presence of side effects are hard to compare due to inter-institutional and intercultural differences. It seems to be disappointing for European patients if the "bad tissue" is not passed out, whereas sloughing seems to bother patients in North America very much.

Clinical results improve with the development of the technology. The learning curve can be reduced with technical improvement and structured training programs including workshops, nurses training, proctoring sessions, and support by clinical application specialists.

Conclusion

Cryotherapy for primary prostate cancer is a minimally invasive alternative to other therapeutic options. Technical and clinical evolution has reduced the side effects and improved the results. It will not replace radical prostatectomy or other therapeutic modalities, but it closes a gap in the concept of local tumor control in well-selected patients.

References

1. Hoffmann NE, Bischof JC. The cryobiology of cryosurgical injury. Urology 2002;60 (Suppl 2A):40–49.
2. Gage AA, Baust J. Mechanisms of tissue injury in cryosurgery. Cryobiology 1998;37:171–186.
3. Tatsutani K, Rubinsky B, Onik G, et al. Effect of thermal variables on frozen human primary prostatic adenocarcinoma cells. Urology 1996;48:441–447.
4. Larson T, Robertson D, Corica A, et al. In vivo interstitial temperature mapping of the human prostate during cryosurgery with correlation to histopathological outcomes. Urology 2000;55:547–552.
5. Patel B, Parsons C, Bidair M, et al. Cryoablation for carcinoma of the prostate. J Surg Oncol 1996;63:256–264.
6. Moore Y, Sofer P. Successful treatment of locally confined prostate cancer with the seed net™ system—preliminary multicenter results. Clin Appl Notes 2001;June:1–7.
7. Cytron S, Paz A, Kravchick S, et al. Active rectal wall protection using direct transperitoneal cryo-needles for histologically proven prostate adenocarcinomas, Eur Urol 2003;44:315–321.
8. Bahn D, Lee F, Badalament R, et al. Targeted cryoablation of the prostate: 7-year outcomes in the primary treatment of prostate cancer. Urology 2002;60 (Suppl 2A):3–11.
9. Donnelly B, Saliken J, Ernst D, et al. Prospective trial of cryosurgical ablation of the prostate: five-year results. Urology 2002;60:645–649.
10. Zisman A, Pantuck A, Cohen J, et al. Prostate cryoablation using direct transperineal placement of ultrathin probes through a 17- gauge brachytherapy template—technique and preliminary results. Urology 2001;58:988–993.
11. Long J, Bahn D, Lee F, et al. Five-year retrospective, multi-institutional pooled analysis of cancer-related outcomes after cryosurgical ablation of the prostate. Urology 2001;57:518–523.

28

Cryotherapy as salvage therapy for prostate cancer

Dan Leibovici, Louis L Pisters

Overview

The routine use of prostate-specific antigen (PSA) analysis in men over 50 years of age since the early 1990s has revolutionized the diagnosis of prostate cancer. With the advent of PSA, early detection of prostate cancer is often possible before any symptoms or palpable abnormalities occur in the prostate. As a result, patients typically present for treatment with organ-confined disease, and are subjected to a primary therapy modality with curative intent.[1,2] Despite this, cancer recurrence following initial therapy is not uncommon. It has been estimated that each year in the USA alone, 50,000 men have PSA recurrence after either radical prostatectomy or radiation therapy.[3] This typically precedes any clinical finding by 3 to 5 years.[4] Although PSA elevation following primary therapy is a very sensitive predictor of subsequent clinical disease progression, it does not reliably distinguish between local recurrence and systemic (metastatic) disease. The distinction between these two entities is crucial in determining the next line of therapy and the patient's prognosis. Generally, systemic disease is not amenable to curative therapy, and the goals of treatment in that setting are to preserve quality of life and minimize morbidity. Conversely, an isolated local recurrence following primary treatment has the potential of being cured by salvage therapy.

Finding the source of PSA elevation following primary therapy for prostate cancer has been challenging. Digital rectal examination or transrectal ultrasound are neither sensitive nor specific in the detection of local recurrence.[5,6] Conversely, prostate biopsy may be the single most reliable test to confirm local recurrence of prostate cancer. Nevertheless, it provides no information about the presence or absence of systemic disease in conjunction with a local recurrence. Cross-sectional imaging with computerized tomography also lacks sensitivity in detecting local recurrence following initial therapy.[7] Conversely, magnetic resonance imaging (MRI) with an external and an endorectal coil provides high-resolution anatomic images and has been found to be more accurate in the diagnosis of local cancer recurrence than any other imaging modality.[8] However, the experience with MRI in this setting has been limited, and larger studies are needed to confirm its role in detection of local recurrence. Although any of the above modalities could diagnose local cancer recurrence, none of them can distinguish between isolated local recurrence, which might be amenable to salvage therapy, and a combination of local recurrence and microscopic metastasis. Radionuclide bone scan is rarely positive in the presence of serum PSA below 20 ng/mL and, potentially, would miss microscopic metastatic disease in its early phase.[9] Monoclonal antibody based radioisotope scans were developed with the purpose of locating the site of recurrent tumor. Despite its initial promise, this modality did

not show the expected accuracy in ruling out metastatic disease, although the predictive value of a positive extrapelvic scan was high.[10,11] The velocity with which serum PSA increases after an initial failed primary treatment, specifically the PSA doubling time, may more reliably distinguish between an isolated localized tumor recurrence and metastatic disease.[12]

Recurrence of prostate cancer following initial therapy may reflect the aggressive biologic nature of the original tumor or, conversely, may be caused by a technical malfunction occurring at the time of the initial treatment procedure, leading to failure to eradicate an otherwise curable cancer. In the latter case, the residual cancer may still be curable if subjected to a salvage procedure. This curative prospect, albeit small, justifies the use of aggressive means that would not normally be applied to patients with metastasis. The decision to use a salvage procedure versus hormonal treatment largely depends on patient factors such as performance status, comorbidities, and personal preferences; but also depends on the type of initial therapy that has been given. Data from a national disease registry of patients with prostate cancer, (Cancer of the Prostate Strategic Urologic Research Endeavor [CaPSURE]) shows that the type of salvage therapy following initial radical prostatectomy is equally divided between androgen deprivation therapy (ADT) and radiation therapy, whereas ADT is applied as salvage therapy following radiation therapy in more than 90% of cases.[13] The available interventional procedures done in the other 10% of the patients who have failed radiation therapy include: salvage radical prostatectomy, salvage cystoprostatectomy or total pelvic exenteration, hyperthermia, and cryosurgery. The chapter will discuss cryosurgery as a post-radiation salvage procedure for prostate cancer.

General principles of salvage cryotherapy

Assuming that the prostate is the single site of tumor recurrence, any procedure resulting in complete ablation of the recurrent tumor has curative potential. Typically, this can be achieved either by surgical excision (i.e., salvage radical prostatectomy), or by in-situ ablation of the entire prostate, including the organ-confined tumor. Cryotherapy consists of in-situ tissue ablation by application of extremely cold temperature. This is accomplished by direct transperineal insertion of cryogenic probes into the prostate that are precisely positioned under transrectal ultrasound guidance. Cryogenic temperature is created inside and around the probe tip by flow of pressurized argon gas through a narrow nozzle over an abrupt pressure gradient. According to the Joule–Thompson principle, the flow of argon gas under such conditions is associated with a thermal sink. Following activation, an iceball is created around the tip of each probe, and sequentially additional cryogenic probes are activated until the freezing has encompassed the entire prostate. The number of probes used varies depending on the shape and size of the prostate. Typically, between 6 and 8 probes are used to conform the ice ball to the shape of the gland.[14] The freezing process is monitored in real time by transrectal ultrasound, and the temperature is measured at specific sites, such as the external urinary sphincter. Caution is used to prevent cryogenic injury to the rectal wall and urinary sphincter, and the urethra is kept warm by a designated warming catheter, which prevents urethral sloughing and stricture. The cryogenic temperature within the coalescent iceball is not homogenous but follows a thermal gradient, and isotherms corresponding to different temperatures can be calculated.[15] The biologic ablative effect of freezing corresponds to the volume of tissue included within lethal isotherms. Cryogenic tissue injury is caused by several putative mechanisms, including osmotic changes as the result of extracellular water transforming into ice, shearing forces exerted upon the cell membrane by extracellular ice crystals, intracellular freezing, tissue ischemia, and immune responses targeting the ablated tumor cells.[16] To achieve cure in the patient with recurrent prostate cancer, the entire tumor must be included within the lethal isotherm. This implies that the tumor needs to be confined to the prostate on the one hand and cryosurgery needs to be adequately performed on the other. Previous exposure of the urethra, rectum, or bladder to radiation renders these organs more susceptible to cryogenic-induced injury; consequently, the side effects of cryosurgery in the salvage setting are more pronounced than in primarily treated patients.

Cancer control achieved by cryosurgery in the salvage setting

Salvage cryosurgery following previous radiation therapy

The risk for recurrence of prostate cancer following initial radiation therapy depends on tumor factors such as Gleason grade, pretreatment PSA level, and T stage. In addition, the previously administered radiation dose appears to affect outcome, especially in patients in the intermediate- and high-risk groups.[17,18] Among patients who present for radiation therapy with T1 to T2 tumors 47% will experience biochemical progression at 8 years following treatment, and 14% to 34% will die of disease.[19,20] Furthermore, higher failure rates have been observed in high-risk patients (T3 or Gleason 8–10), who are most commonly treated with radiation therapy.[21] Following radiation therapy, tissue fibrosis occurs within the treated fields causing obliteration of anatomic planes, and making surgical dissection a major technical challenge and more prone to complications. As a result, many patients are left with the choices of watchful waiting or hormonal treatment, neither of which are curative approaches. Cryosurgery, on the other hand, offers the advantage of complete prostate ablation without the need to dissect through previously irradiated tissues. In comparison with salvage radical prostatectomy, salvage cryosurgery is much easier to perform, easier to learn, and more tolerable for the patient, making it a particularly appealing treatment approach in the patients who need a salvage procedure following radiation therapy.

The most important clinical endpoint in assessing the efficacy of cancer therapy is disease-specific survival. Because prostate cancer is a relatively slow growing malignancy, long follow-up is necessary to evaluate this endpoint. Surrogate endpoints such as serum PSA following therapy and post-cryosurgery prostate biopsy may not be as accurate as disease-specific survival in assessing the effect of therapy, because some of these patients may have been treated with hormone ablation leading to low PSA levels, and biopsies are often not specific. Most reported series on cryosurgery as salvage therapy for recurrent prostate cancer have a short follow-up, and consequently caution is needed in inferring the results to all patients.

As shown in Table 28.1, salvage cryosurgery following radiation therapy achieves a nadir PSA of less than 0.5 ng/mL and negative biopsies for most patients. With longer follow-up however, disease recurrence as evidenced by biochemical relapse occurs in some of the patients. The biochemical progression-free survival rate at 2 years after salvage cryosurgery ranges between 55% and 74%.[24,28,29] The risk of biochemical failure increases with higher pretreatment PSA levels and Gleason grades, and in patients with a PSA nadir greater than 0.1 ng/mL. Salvage cryosurgery may fail either due to incomplete ablation of the prostate reflecting technical limitations, or due to extraprostatic or seminal vesicle involvement beyond the reach of the freezing process. Ideally, a better staging method would improve patient selection leading to the restriction of this modality for the patients who are most likely to benefit from it.

There are limited long-term reports of the results of salvage cryosurgery. In 2002, Izawa et al reported on 131 patients who underwent salvage cryosurgery following initial radiation therapy.[30] In patients with Gleason grade 8 or less tumors, the 5-year disease-specific

Table 28.1 Efficacy of cryosurgery in controlling recurrent prostate cancer after failure of radiation therapy

# of patients	Median FU (months)	Undetectable PSA [<0.05 ng/mL], n (%)	PSA <0.5 ng/mL, n (%)	Negative FU biopsies, n (%)	Patients receiving ADT, n (%)	Reference
33	16.8	NA	39	26 (79)	16 (48)	Miller[22]
150	17	47 (31)	63 (42)	116 (77)	40 (27)	Pisters[23]
106	43	NA	114 (97)	91 (86)	71 (67)	Chin[24,25]
43	21.9	NA	26 (60)*	NA	43 (100)†	De la Taille[26]
18	20	NA	13 (72)	NA	0	Han[27]

FU, follow-up duration; PSA, prostate specific antigen.
*These patients had a nadir PSA level <0.1 ng/mL. †All received 3 months of neoadjuvant hormonal therapy that was discontinued at the time of cryosurgery.

survival rate was 87% compared with 63% in patients with Gleason grade 9 or 10. Similarly, the disease-free survival rate was 57% versus 23% in patients with presalvage PSA level below or above 10 ng/mL, respectively. Although the results of salvage radical prostatectomy in terms of biochemical progression-free survival have been reported to exceed those of salvage cryosurgery, because there have been no randomized controlled trials directly comparing the two modalities, the comparison of efficacy between the two procedures remains inconclusive.[31,32]

Androgen deprivation therapy has been used in conjunction with cryosurgery in the salvage setting. Its main effect appears to be that of downsizing the prostate, which decreases the distance between cryogenic probes and may facilitate a more efficient tissue ablation. There is no evidence, however, that ADT improves disease-specific survival in patients who undergo salvage cryosurgery.

A specific technical difficulty may be encountered when performing salvage cryosurgery following initial brachytherapy. Because the prostate is loaded with seeds, their echogenic appearance on ultrasound may interfere with that of the cryogenic probes and may render the accurate positioning of the cryogenic probes difficult. This problem is manageable, however, and cryosurgery can be done safely in this setting. Many of the patients treated with external beam radiation therapy have poor risk and thereby may not be cured by a procedure targeting the primary tumor alone. In contrast, most of the patients undergoing brachytherapy have low-risk disease, and consequently, cancer recurrence in this subset is more likely to result from technical failure than from the adverse biology of the disease. Due to this inherent difference in patient selection, salvage cryosurgery after previously failed brachytherapy may prove particularly effective in achieving cure.

Complications

Performing cryosurgery in tissues that have been previously irradiated may be associated with increased tissue damage and more frequent complications. The same complications occur following cryosurgery either in the primary treatment or salvage settings; however, their frequency is higher with salvage cryosurgery. Reported complications include urethral sloughing, which is manifested by obstruction, urinary incontinence, perineal pain, rectal injury, and fistula formation, osteitis pubis, and erectile dysfunction. Lee et al reported that the risk of rectal fistula was 8.7% in patients who had been previously treated with radiation, compared with less than 0.5% in patients for whom cryosurgery was done as primary therapy.[33] Others confirmed a higher prevalence of prostate-related symptoms in patients undergoing salvage versus primary cryosurgery of the prostate.[34] The risk for urinary incontinence is increased in patients who undergo salvage cryosurgery and varies between 7% and 8% compared with 1.3% and 4% in patients in whom cryosurgery was performed as primary treatment.[24,28,35,36] Ensuring a positive temperature in the external sphincter during cryosurgery can reduce the incidence of urinary incontinence.[27] The risk for complications increases in patients with locally invasive or high Gleason grade tumors, presumably due to the need of more aggressive cryosurgery to achieve tumor control.[24] Similarly, we reported incontinence and urethral sloughing rates of 72% and 67%, respectively in a cohort of 150 patients in whom 90% had T3 to T4 tumors and/or Gleason scores of 8 to 10.[23] In six of these patients, major extirpative surgery was necessary to control chronic debilitating symptoms, including refractory hematuria, osteitis pubis, recto-urethral fistula, bladder outlet obstruction, and chronic rectal pain.[37] It is important to note that this high

complication rate was observed in patients whose treatment involved older equipment, including second-generation cryogenic probes, without the use of thermocouples. In order to maximize safety, we recommend using third-generation probes with judicious use of thermocouples particularly at Denonvilliers' fascia (to reduce the risk of rectal injury and fistula) as well as the external urinary sphincter (to reduce incontinence). Urethral protection is best achieved by the commercial designated warmer catheter, and its use is essential. The risk for urethral sloughing decreased significantly following the FDA approval of the designated warming catheter, and, consequently, the quality of life of patients who underwent salvage cryosurgery is better in contemporary series than in previous reports, and is comparable to that of patients undergoing primary cryosurgery.[34,38,39] Another feared complication is rectal fistula. In contemporary series, the incidence of this complication has been 1% to 3%.[22–26,34] Pelvic or rectal pain occurs in about 10% of the patients and typically subsides within 3 to 4 weeks. It is presumed that this is caused by cryogenic injury to sensory nerves. Ischemia of the rectal wall may be another possible cause, and topical nitrates have been used anecdotally to prevent the pain. Erectile dysfunction has been reported in 80% to 100% of the patients who underwent cryosurgery as primary treatment for prostate cancer with some improvement over time after the procedure.[27] In the salvage setting, erectile dysfunction is the rule, and can be expected to occur in almost all patients.

Salvage cryosurgery following previous cryosurgery

Radical prostatectomy aims to cure localized prostate cancer by en-bloc resection of the entire prostate gland, prostatic urethra, and seminal vesicles. Due to the multifocal nature of prostate cancer, there is no role for partial prostatectomy. Radical prostatectomy, therefore, provides one single surgical opportunity to cure the patient. Similarly, the cumulative lifetime tolerance to radiation limits the total dose that can safely be given without unacceptable morbidity. The maximal efficacy of radiation therapy is, therefore, achieved by delivering a maximally tolerated dose during one single radiation therapy course.

Conversely, cryosurgery is unique in that it can be repeated, if necessary, with no increased morbidity. Thus, this modality offers the patient a "second shot" to win the battle. Many of the series that report on cryosurgery as primary care for prostate cancer indicate that, in a subset of their patients, more than one cryosurgical session was necessary to achieve tumor control. As is the case with other circumstances of disease recurrence, the dilemma is whether the biochemical failure is caused by residual cancer that is confined to the prostate or represents metastatic disease. Because complete exposure of all prostate cells to two cycles of freezing to −40°C or below invariably results in necrosis and should lead to an undetectable PSA level, true localized cancer recurrence implies that such freezing conditions have not been achieved throughout the entire prostate.[40] Potential reasons of incomplete freezing include technical problems, the inability to include the entire prostate within the lethal isotherm without risking rectal injury, and the warming catheter that keeps a thin rim of viable prostatic tissue surrounding the urethra. A prostate biopsy may help to distinguish between a local source of PSA as viable glands within the prostate and extraprostatic disease. It has been our approach to perform an extensive (20-core) prostate biopsy in all patients with biochemical failure after cryosurgery. In the case that such biopsy demonstrates extensive coagulative necrosis with no viable glands, the PSA elevation should be attributed to extraprostatic sources, implying microscopic metastatic disease. When the biopsy shows viable glands, it supports the possibility of inadequate freezing. When the absolute PSA level is low (<2.0 ng/mL) and the PSA doubling time is long, localized disease can be assumed, and repeat cryosurgery can be reasonably elected. The chance of achieving a durable PSA response and of converting a positive biopsy to a negative one by repeat cryosurgery varies depending on patient selection. Overall, in patients with low-risk disease, there seems to be a 20% to 30% chance for a second cryosurgical ablation to achieve cancer control.[41–43] The risk for complications with repeated cryosurgery is equivalent to that of primary cryosurgery, although the occasional patients who remain potent after the first procedure are likely to lose erectile function following the salvage procedure.

Salvage cryosurgery following radical prostatectomy

A visible measurable target lesion into which cryogenic probes can be inserted is a prerequisite for cryosurgery performance. In the majority of patients who experience biochemical progression following radical prostatectomy, the disease is either outside the prostatic fossa or is only microscopic and cannot be treated by cryosurgery. In occasional patients, however, with histologically confirmed recurrence of prostate cancer and a measurable lesion at the anastomosis, salvage cryosurgery can be done. Cytron et al (Barzilai Medical Center, Israel) have performed salvage cryosurgery following radical prostatectomy on five patients (personal communication). In all patients, the target lesion was clearly visible by transrectal ultrasound, with a median volume of the treated lesions of 4.0 mL. A significant PSA decrease was observed in all patients after salvage cryosurgery. Undetectable PSA levels were achieved in three patients and were maintained for 2 years following the salvage procedure. Temporary urinary incontinence occurred following salvage cryosurgery; however, this resolved over the first 6 months. This probably represents the first series of salvage cryosurgery performed following initial radical prostatectomy. These preliminary results indicate that salvage cryosurgery may have a role in selected patients after failed radical prostatectomy and that this concept deserves further study.

Patient selection for salvage cryosurgery

Accomplishing cure by salvage cryosurgery depends on adequate technical performance of the procedure, state-of-the-art equipment, and appropriate patient selection. The best results can be achieved in patients with low-volume, low-grade disease that is confined to the prostate. Because the available staging methods are not accurate enough to identify the ideal candidates, some auxiliary parameters should be used. A low PSA level at the time of recurrence and a long doubling time (>12 months) have been associated with localized disease.[44,45] In addition, the grade and extent of extracapsular extension of cancer may be determined by staging biopsy with multiple cores. Magnetic resonance imaging may have a role in the detection of macroscopic extraprostatic tumor extension. Other important

considerations include prostate volume (effective cryosurgery is usually limited to 50 mL or less), adequate patient performance status, and absence of bladder outlet obstruction.

Salvage radiation therapy after failed cryosurgery

Occasional patients, who have recurrent disease following repeated cryosurgery and are believed to have localized disease benefit from salvage radiation therapy. Burton et al reported on 49 patients who received 63 Gy on average following biopsy-confirmed recurrence of prostate cancer after primary cryosurgery. The average pretreatment PSA was 2.4 ng/mL and a nadir PSA level below 1.0 ng/mL was achieved in 42 (86%) patients. With an average follow-up duration of 32 months the biochemical progression free survival was 60%.[46] Complete resolution of palpable lesion was observed in 4 of 6 patients in another series treated with salvage radiation therapy following primary cryosurgery.[47] Urethral strictures and proctitis were reported in both series, but the numbers are too small to permit comparison with radiation therapy series done as primary treatment.

Summary

Depending on the risk factors, patients with recurrent prostate cancer following primary therapy may have localized versus disseminated disease. In patients with localized cancer recurrence, salvage cryosurgery is a viable and effective treatment modality with efficacy comparable to that of salvage radical prostatectomy and a lower complication rate. Cryosurgery offers more flexibility in planning the treatment for prostate cancer by permitting repeated performance in the case of failure.

References

1. Stephenson RA. Population based prostate cancer trends in the PSA-era: data from the Surveillance, Epidemiology, and End Results (SEER) program. Monogr Urol 1998;19:1–19.
2. Newcomer LM, Stanford JL, Blumenstein BA, et al. Temporal trends in rates of prostate cancer: declining incidence of advanced stage disease, 1974 to 1994. J Urol 1997;158:1427–1430.
3. Moul JW. Prostate specific antigen only progression of prostate cancer. J Urol 2000;163:1632–1642.
4. Paulson DF. Impact of radical prostatectomy in the management of clinically localized prostate cancer. J Urol 1994;152:1826–1830.
5. Pound CR, Christens-Barry OW, Gurganus RT, et al. Digital rectal examinations and imaging studies are unnecessary in men with undetectable prostate specific antigen following radical prostatectomy. J Urol 1999;162:1337–1340.
6. Johnstone PA, McFarland JT, Riffenburgh RH, et al. Efficacy of digital rectal examination after radiotherapy for prostate cancer. J Urol 2001;166:1684–1687.
7. Kramer S, Gorich J, Gottfried HW, et al. Sensitivity of computed tomography in detecting local recurrence of prostatic carcinoma following radical prostatectomy. Br J Radiol 1997;70:995–999.
8. Silverman JM, Krebs TL. MR imaging evaluation with a transrectal surface coil of local recurrence of prostatic cancer in men who

have undergone radical prostatectomy. AJR Am J Roentgenol 1997;168:379–385.

9. Cher ML, Bianco FJ Jr, Lam JS, et al. Limited role of radionuclide bone scintigraphy in patients with prostate specific antigen elevations after radical prostatectomy. J Urol 1998;160:1387–1391.

10. Kahn D, Williams RD, Manyak MJ, et al. 111Indium - in the evaluation of patients with residual or recurrent prostate cancer after radical prostatectomy. The ProstaScint Study Group. J Urol 1998;159:2041–2046.

11. Kahn D, Williams RD, Haseman MK, et al. Radioimmunoscintigraphy with In-111 labeled capromab pendetide predicts prostate cancer response to salvage radiotherapy after failed radical prostatectomy. J Clin Oncol1998;16:284–289.

12. D'Amico AV, Cote K, Loffredo M, et al. Determinants of prostate cancer-specific survival after radiation therapy for patients with clinically localized prostate cancer. J Clin Oncol 2002;20:4567–4573.

13. Grossfeld GD, Stier DM, Flanders SC, et al. Use of second treatment following definitive local therapy for local prostate cancer: data from the CaPSURE database. J Urol 1998;160:1398–1404.

14. Zippe CD. Cryosurgery of the prostate technique and pitfalls. Urol Clin N Am 1996;23:147–163.

15. Rewcastle JC, Sandison GA, Hahn LJ, et al. A model for the time dependent thermal distribution within an iceball surrounding a cryoprobe. Med Phys 2001;28:1125–1137.

16. Gage AA, Baust J. Mechanisms of tissue injury in cryosurgery. Cryobiology 1998;37:171–186.

17. Jacob R, Hanlon AR, Horwitz EM, et al. The relationship of increasing radiotherapy dose to reduced distant metastases and mortality in men with prostate cancer. Cancer 2004;100:538–543.

18. Valicenti R, Lu J, Pielpich M, et al. Survival advantage from higher-dose radiation therapy for clinically localized prostate cancer treated on the Radiation Therapy Oncology Group trials. J Clin Oncol 2000;18:2740–2746.

19. Kuban DA, Thames HD, Levy LB, et al. Long-term multi-institutional analysis of stage T1-T2 prostate cancer treated with radiotherapy in the PSA era. Int J Radiation Oncol Biol Phys 2003;57:915–928.

20. Maartense S, Hermans J, Leer JW. Radiation therapy in localized prostate cancer: long-term results and late toxicity. Clin Oncol (Royal Col Radiol) 2000;12:222–228.

21. D`Amico AV. Radiation and hormonal therapy for locally advanced and clinically localized prostate cancer. Urology 2002;60:32–37.

22. Miller RJ, Cohen JK, Shuman B, et al. Percutaneous, transperineal cryosurgery of the prostate as salvage therapy for post radiation recurrence of adenocarcinoma. Cancer 1996;77:1510–1514.

23. Pisters LL, von Eschenbach AC, Scott SM, et al. The efficacy and complications of salvage cryotherapy of the prostate. J Urol 1997;157:921–925.

24. Chin JL, Pautler SE, Mouraviev V, et al. Results of salvage cryoablation of the prostate after radiation: identifying predictors of treatment failure and complications. J Urol 2001;165:1937–1942.

25. Chin JL, Touma N, Pautler SE, et al. Serial histopathology result of salvage cryoablation for prostate cancer after radiation failure. J Urol 2003;170:1199–1202.

26. De la Taille A, Hayek O, Benson MC, et al. Salvage cryotherapy for recurrent prostate cancer after radiation therapy: the Columbia experience. Urology 2000;55:79–84.

27. Han KR, Belldegrun AS. Third-generation cryosurgery for primary and recurrent prostate cancer. BJU international 2004;93:14–18.

28. Ghafar MA, Johnson CW, De la Taille A, et al. Salvage cryotherapy using an argon-based system for locally recurrent prostate cancer

after radiation therapy: the Columbia experience. J Urol 2001;166:1333–1338.

29. Bales GT, Williams MJ, Sinner M, et al. Short-term outcomes after cryosurgical ablation of the prostate in men with recurrent prostate carcinoma following radiation therapy. Urology 1995;46:676–680.

30. Izawa JI, Madsen LE, Scott SM, et al. Salvage cryotherapy for recurrent prostate cancer after radiotherapy: variables affecting patient outcome. J Clin Oncol 2002;20:2664–2761.

31. Leibovich BC, Zincke H, Blute ML, et al. Recurrent prostate cancer after radiation therapy: Salvage prostatectomy versus salvage cryosurgery. American Urological Association, 96th Annual Meeting. 2001;165:1595.

32. Cheng L, Sebo TJ, Slejak J, et al. Predictors of survival for prostate carcinoma patients treated with salvage radical prostatectomy after radiation therapy. Cancer 1998;83:2164–2171.

33. Lee F, Bahn DK, McHugh TA, et al. Cryosurgery of prostate cancer. Use of adjuvant hormonal therapy and temperature monitoring a one year follow-up. Anticancer Res 1997;17:1511–1516.

34. Anastasiadis AG, Sachdev R, Salomon L, et al. Comparison of health related quality of life and prostate associated symptoms after primary and salvage cryotherapy for prostate cancer. J Cancer Res Clin Oncol 2003;129:676–682.

35. Bahn DK, Lee F, Badalament R, et al. Targeted cryoablation of the prostate:7-year outcomes in the primary treatment of prostate cancer. Urology 2002;60:3–11.

36. Donnelly BJ, Saliken JC, Ernst DS, et al. Prospective trial of cryosurgical ablation of the prostate: 5-year results. Urology 2002;60:645–649.

37. Izawa JI, Ajam K, McGuire E, et al. Major surgery to manage definitively severe complications of salvage cryotherapy for prostate cancer, J Urol 2000;64:1978–1981.

38. Perrotte P, Litwin MS, McGuire EJ, et al. Quality of life after salvage cryotherapy: the impact of treatment parameters. J Urol 1999;162:398–402.

39. Robinson JW, Donnelly BJ, Saliken JC, et al. Quality of life and sexuality of men with prostate cancer 3 years after cryosurgery. Urology 2002;60:12–18.

40. Larson TR, Robertson DW, Corica A, et al. In vivo interstitial temperature mapping of the human prostate during cryosurgery with correlation to histopathologic outcomes. Urology 2000;55:547–552.

41. Cohen JK, Miller RJ, Rooker GM, et al. Cryosurgical ablation of the prostate: two year prostate specific antigen and biopsy results. Urology 1996;47:395–401.

42. Wong WS, Chinn DO, Chinn M, et al. Cryosurgery as the treatment of prostate carcinoma. Cancer 1997;79:963–974.

43. Koppie TM, Shinohara K, Grossfeld GD, et al. The efficacy of cryosurgical ablation of prostate cancer: The University of California San Francisco experience. J Urol 1999;162:427–432.

44. D'Amico AV, Cote K, Loffredo M, et al. Determinants of prostate cancer specific survival following radiation therapy during the prostate specific antigen era. J Urol 2003;170:S42–S46.

45. D'Amico AV, Moul JW, Carroll PR, et al. Surrogate end point for prostate cancer-specific mortality after radical prostatectomy or radiation therapy. J Natl Cancer Inst 2003;95:1376–1383.

46. Burton S, Brown DM, Colonias A, et al. Salvage radiotherapy for prostate cancer recurrence after cryosurgical ablation. Urology 2000;56:833–838.

47. McDonough MJ, Feldmeier JJ, Parsai I, et al. Salvage external beam radiotherapy for clinical failure after cryosurgery for prostate cancer. Int J Radiat Oncol Biol Phys 2001;51:624–627.

29

Neoadjuvant and adjuvant hormonal therapies for prostate cancer: data review and patient perspectives

William A See

Introduction

Hormonal therapy is being used increasingly in addition to primary therapies of curative intent, such as radiotherapy and radical prostatectomy, in patients with localized and locally advanced prostate cancer. The reason for the use of additional hormonal therapy is that a significant proportion of patients receiving these primary therapies alone will experience disease progression and may die from prostate cancer.

Improving overall survival remains the ultimate goal in the treatment of prostate cancer. However, other measurable endpoints in prostate cancer can also be relevant to treatment decisions, particularly, disease progression. Reducing the risk of disease progression is important for a number of reasons. Disease progression and concern about the risk of death from prostate cancer places a substantial emotional burden on patients and their families. There may also be serious clinical consequences for patients who experience disease progression, such as bone pain, spinal cord compression, pathologic fractures and urinary obstruction,[1] and the subsequent economic burden can be significant.[2] Whether considering disease progression or overall survival, a key question is whether additional hormonal therapy provides a positive balance between the benefits and risks of treatment. This balance is determined by the adverse effects of treatment relative to the beneficial effect on survival and quality of life. Regrettably few studies are able to provide insight into this risk:benefit ratio beyond the effect of treatment on progression or survival endpoints.

Options for patients receiving hormonal therapy in addition to their primary therapy include neoadjuvant hormonal therapy—short-term hormonal treatment used immediately before primary therapy—and adjuvant hormonal therapy—longer-term hormonal treatment given immediately after treatment of curative intent. The main aim of any additional hormonal therapy is usually to improve local control and overall survival compared with the primary therapy alone. Neoadjuvant hormonal therapy is also used to reduce the size of the prostate, with the intention of facilitating the primary therapy. For example, a reduction in prostate size before surgery or cryotherapy may reduce blood loss and operative difficulty. A reduction in prostate size before brachytherapy is intended to facilitate accurate seed implantation and allow a reduced radiation dose to be used. Similarly, neoadjuvant hormonal therapy given before external-beam radiotherapy may allow a smaller field size to be used.

Neoadjuvant or adjuvant hormonal therapies usually include luteinizing hormone-releasing hormone (LHRH) agonists, antiandrogens, or a combination of the two (combined androgen blockade [CAB]). Bilateral orchiectomy is also used occasionally.

Data from studies assessing additional hormonal therapies vary, in both quality and quantity, according to the different primary therapy modalities, hormonal therapies, and approaches (neoadjuvant or adjuvant) used. This chapter reviews the current role for neoadjuvant and adjuvant hormonal therapies in early prostate cancer and the supporting evidence. The focus is on published data relating to clinically important outcomes from prospective randomized controlled trials, subgroup analyses of such trials, and meta-analyses or systematic reviews of data from these studies. The level of evidence that supports the different treatment alternatives and the implications for patients and their urologists are discussed.

Primary therapy: radical prostatectomy

A number of patients treated with radical prostatectomy alone have a very low risk of disease progression and death from prostate cancer and, therefore, additional hormonal therapy has little or no role in their treatment. However, a significant proportion of patients with early stage prostate cancer treated with radical prostatectomy alone do subsequently experience disease progression, as a result of residual local disease or distant disease undetectable at diagnosis.

Several studies have investigated the clinical features that may help to predict disease progression following radical prostatectomy. A prospective, open-label trial in 1000 patients with localized (cT1–2) disease found that preoperative prostate-specific antigen (PSA) level, clinical stage, biopsy, postoperative Gleason score, extracapsular extension, seminal vesicle involvement, lymph node metastasis, and surgical margin status were all independent risk factors for metastatic progression (Figure 29.1).[3] Of the pretreatment characteristics examined, PSA level and Gleason score were the strongest predictive risk factors; for example, a pretreatment Gleason score of 8 to 10 was associated with a 42% risk of metastatic progression and an 18% risk of prostate cancer-related death within 10 years of radical prostatectomy.

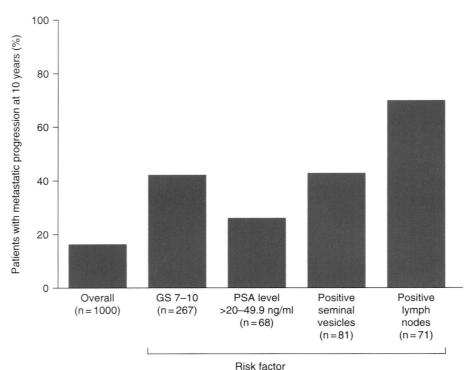

Figure 29.1
Ten-year risk of metastatic progression
following radical prostatectomy in
patients with localized (cT1–T2) prostate
cancer. (GS, Gleason score; PSA, prostate-
specific antigen.)

Reproduced with permission from Hull GW,
Rabbani F, Abbas F, Wheeler TM, Kattan MW,
Scardino PT. Cancer control with radical
prostatectomy alone in 1000 consecutive
patients. J Urol 2002;167:528–534.

The patient's risk profile is an important consideration when offering advice on treatment options; a key question is whether hormonal therapy can improve the prognosis of those patients identified as being at high risk of progression. To address this question, the following sections cover the evidence for neoadjuvant and adjuvant hormonal therapies in the surgical setting.

Is there a role for neoadjuvant hormonal therapy prior to radical prostatectomy?

A considerable number of randomized controlled trials of hormonal therapy neoadjuvant to radical prostatectomy have been conducted in patients with both localized and locally advanced prostate cancer. Overall, the available data do not show an improvement in clinical outcome with the use of neoadjuvant hormonal therapy prior to radical prostatectomy in terms of survival, disease progression, or postoperative morbidity. Indeed, the authors of one of these studies, using an LHRH agonist (triptorelin) as neoadjuvant hormonal therapy, concluded that 3 months of neoadjuvant hormonal therapy before radical prostatectomy offered no benefit to the patient and could not be recommended for routine clinical use.[4]

Of the studies conducted in this setting, some have only assessed characteristics such as tumor volume and surgical margin status,[5,6] while those with longer follow-up have also addressed PSA progression-free survival[4,7–13] (Table 29.1). The duration of these studies (longest follow-up median 7 years[4]) means that none of them is able to provide overall survival data.

In general, randomized controlled trials of neoadjuvant hormonal therapy in the surgical setting have demonstrated significant pathological down-staging of tumors, reduction in tumor volume,

and reduction in the proportion of patients with positive surgical margins compared with surgery alone. However, none demonstrated any significant improvement in PSA progression-free survival with neoadjuvant hormonal therapy compared with radical prostatectomy alone (see Table 29.1), although whether they were sufficiently powered to detect a difference was not always clear. Of the studies in Table 29.1 that did specify how they were powered, two were powered to detect differences in pathologic stage or surgical margin status[4,7] and only one was powered to detect a difference in terms of PSA progression.[10]

A subgroup analysis of 33 patients who had a baseline PSA level of more than 20 ng/mL, in a study assessing steroidal antiandrogen (cyproterone acetate [CPA]) neoadjuvant hormonal therapy in patients with clinically localized disease (median follow-up 6 years), identified a significant improvement in 7-year PSA progression-free survival compared with surgery alone (53% versus 35%; p = 0.015).[9] Prostate-specific antigen progression in this study was defined as a rise in PSA of more than 0.2 ng/mL on two consecutive occasions 4 weeks or more apart, or death from prostate cancer. However, given the lack of a significant difference in the overall population and the small number of patients analyzed, this result should be considered exploratory.

It seems contradictory that neoadjuvant hormonal therapy is associated with significant down-staging of tumors and a decrease in the rate of positive surgical margins but not an improvement in patient outcome. One possible reason for this is that hormonal deprivation leads to major histopathologic changes in the prostate, which may obscure evidence of residual tumor and result in the under-reporting of positive margins.[4,9,12] This reasoning is supported by a histologic study of androgen-ablated prostates, which showed that negative margins identified by hematoxylin–eosin staining may actually include residual tumor that can be detected by cytokeratin staining.[14] Incorrect information regarding margin status could have an adverse impact on treatment decisions following surgery, with consequent impairment of clinical outcomes.

To date, most studies have examined neoadjuvant hormonal therapy given for 3 months before radical prostatectomy; however, two randomized controlled trials have addressed whether longer periods of neoadjuvant hormonal therapy might lead to improved outcomes.

One study compared 3 and 6 months of CAB (bicalutamide plus goserelin) prior to radical prostatectomy in 431 men with localized or locally advanced (stage B or C) disease.[15] The results of this study showed that the additional 3 months of treatment improved the pathologic stage in patients with clinical stage C disease: organ-confined disease was seen in 32% and 63% of patients receiving 3 and 6 months of neoadjuvant hormonal therapy, respectively (p-value not given). However, similar improvements were not seen in patients with clinical stage B disease. The incidence of positive surgical margins following 3 or 6 months of neoadjuvant hormonal treatment was similar, irrespective of disease stage.

The second study compared 3 and 8 months of CAB (leuprorelin plus flutamide) in 547 men with localized (cT1c–2) disease.[16] Additional biochemical and pathologic regression of prostate tumors occurred between 3 and 8 months of neoadjuvant hormonal therapy, as demonstrated by significant increases in the numbers of patients with a preoperative PSA level of less than 0.1 ng/mL (43% versus 75% for 3 and 8 months, respectively; $p < 0.0001$) and decreases in the rates of positive surgical margins (23% versus 12% for 3 and 8 months, respectively; $p = 0.0106$).

Neither of these studies can offer the physician clear conclusions about the possible benefits of longer term neoadjuvant hormonal therapy in terms of PSA progression-free survival or overall survival, although this may be clarified with further follow-up.

Two systematic reviews of randomized controlled trials have assessed whether hormonal therapy neoadjuvant to radical prostatectomy offers any benefits in terms of reducing the difficulty of surgical dissection or surgical outcomes (e.g., operative time, blood loss, hospital stay, and postoperative complications).[17,18] Both reviews concluded there were no significant improvements in these parameters that would support the use of neoadjuvant hormonal therapy in this setting. The more recent review also found that neoadjuvant hormonal therapy might increase surgical difficulty and appears to increase post-operative patient morbidity as a consequence of the adverse effects of hormonal therapy in some patients.[18]

Is there a role for adjuvant hormonal therapy with radical prostatectomy?

Adjuvant hormonal therapy in the surgical setting has been studied in patients with localized and locally advanced prostate cancer; however, data from only a few randomized controlled trials are available at present.

Patients with localized prostate cancer

Only one randomized controlled trial currently provides data from patients with localized disease treated with hormonal therapy adjuvant to radical prostatectomy: the bicalutamide Early Prostate Cancer (EPC) program. Analyses of the subgroup of patients in this program with localized disease (T1–2, N0 or Nx, M0) who received radical prostatectomy (n = 2734) have been undertaken.[19] At a median

Table 29.1 Randomized controlled trials of 3 months' neoadjuvant hormonal therapy prior to radical prostatectomy compared with radical prostatectomy alone

Neoadjuvant hormonal therapy	Disease stage	No. patients randomized	Tumor volume	Patients with positive surgical margins	Follow-up, years	PSA progression-free survival
CAB (leuprorelin and CPA)[5]	cT1a–2b	183	Decreased in 31% of patients	39% vs 60% with RP alone (p = 0.01)	None	Not assessed
SAA (CPA)[7,9]	cT1b–2c	213	Decrease in mean volume from 42.8 cm³ to 32.9 cm³ (p = 0.0001)	27.7% vs 64.8% with RP alone (p = 0.001)	6 (median)	62.5% vs 66.4% with RP alone (p = NS)[a]
LHRH agonist (triptorelin)[4,8]	cT1b–3a	126	42% decrease in mean volume (from 36.9 cm³ to 19.6 cm³; p < 0.01)	23% vs 41% with RP alone (p = 0.013)	6.8 (median)	No difference (data not given; p = 0.588)[b]
CAB (leuprorelin and flutamide)[11,12]	cT2b	303	Decreased in 91% of patients	18% vs 48% with RP alone (p < 0.001)	5 (maximum)	64.8% vs 67.6% with RP alone (p = 0.663)[c]
CAB (goserelin and flutamide)[10,13]	cT2–3	402	Decrease in mean volume from 37.7 cm³ to 26.8 cm³ (p-value not given)	cT2 patients: 13% vs 37% with RP alone (p < 0.01) cT3 patients: 42% vs 61% with RP alone (p < 0.01)	4 (median)	74% vs 67% with RP alone (p = 0.18)[d]
CAB (leuprorelin and flutamide)[6]	B–C	161	Not given	7.8% vs 33.8% with RP alone (p < 0.001)	None	Not assessed

CAB, combined androgen blockade; CPA, cyproterone acetate; LHRH, luteinizing hormone-releasing hormone; NS, not significant; PSA, prostate-specific antigen; RP, radical prostatectomy; SAA, steroidal antiandrogen.

PSA progression-free survival defined as: [a]time from randomization to the first of two consecutive occurrences of PSA >0.2 ng/ml at least 24 weeks apart, or death from prostate cancer; [b]time to detection of PSA >0.5 ng/ml or death from prostate cancer; [c]time from surgery to detection of PSA >0.4 ng/mL; [d]time from surgery to the first of two subsequent occurrences of PSA >1 ng/mL, distant metastases or local recurrence (confirmed by biopsy).

5.4 years' follow-up, there was no statistically significant difference in risk of objective progression (defined as objective progression confirmed by bone scan, computed tomography/ultrasound/magnetic resonance imaging, or histologic evidence of distant metastases or death from any cause without progression) between patients treated with bicalutamide 150 mg/day as adjuvant hormonal therapy, compared with radical prostatectomy alone within 16 weeks of treatment (hazard ratio [HR] 0.93; 95% confidence intervals [CI] 0.72–1.20). This suggests no benefit from adjuvant bicalutamide therapy for this patient group. Survival data for patients who underwent radical prostatectomy in this study are currently immature, with only 8% deaths.[20]

Patients with locally advanced prostate cancer

The available data from patients with locally advanced disease show that treatment with an LHRH agonist (goserelin) or orchiectomy adjuvant to radical prostatectomy offers a survival benefit for patients with lymph node metastases (pN+, M0). In addition, in a large study of bicalutamide, adjuvant hormonal therapy with a non-steroidal antiandrogen has been shown to improve objective progression-free survival for patients with locally advanced disease, although overall survival data from this study are currently immature and a much smaller study of adjuvant flutamide treatment did not find a significant improvement in overall survival.

Messing et al compared immediate adjuvant with delayed hormonal therapy (with an LHRH agonist [goserelin] or orchiectomy) in 98 patients with clinically localized disease who were found to have lymph node metastases at surgery.[21,22] The most recent analysis, at a median follow-up of 10 years, showed that overall survival was significantly improved with immediate therapy compared with delayed hormonal therapy (72% versus 49%; p = 0.025).[22]

In another randomized controlled trial investigating 201 patients with locally advanced (T3–4) disease, treatment with an LHRH agonist (goserelin) adjuvant to radical prostatectomy resulted in a significant 25% advantage in terms of PSA progression-free survival (progression defined as PSA greater than 0.5 ng/mL or cytologic or histologic evidence of local or distant disease) compared with surgery alone (p < 0.05).[23] However, with a median follow-up of 5 years, overall survival data are not yet mature.

Analyses of the subgroup of patients with locally advanced disease (T3–4, any N, M0 or any T, N+, M0; n = 1719) who received radical prostatectomy in the EPC program show, at a median 5.4 years' follow-up, a significantly reduced risk of objective progression with bicalutamide 150 mg/day as adjuvant hormonal therapy, compared with radical prostatectomy alone (HR 0.71; 95% CI 0.57–0.89; p = 0.0034).[19] Current survival data for patients who underwent radical prostatectomy in this study are immature, with only 8% deaths.[20]

A smaller, open-label, randomized trial of another non-steroidal antiandrogen (flutamide) as adjuvant to radical prostatectomy has been conducted in 309 patients with locally advanced disease (pT3, N0).[24] At a median follow-up of 6.1 years, there was a significant improvement in PSA progression-free survival (progression defined as PSA >5 ng/mL; or >2 ng/mL on two occasions; or PSA >1 ng/mL on three occasions >3 months apart; or any clinical progression) with adjuvant hormonal therapy compared with radical prostatectomy alone (p = 0.0041). However, there was no statistically significant difference in overall survival between the two treatment groups (p = 0.92).

Comparative studies of neoadjuvant and adjuvant hormonal therapies with radical prostatectomy

To date there have been no studies of patients treated with radical prostatectomy that have directly compared outcomes with neoadjuvant and adjuvant hormonal therapy. It is unlikely that such comparative studies will be conducted as the current evidence suggests that, unlike adjuvant hormonal therapy, neoadjuvant hormonal therapy offers little benefit to patients treated with radical prostatectomy.

Primary therapy: external-beam radiotherapy

As in the surgical setting, a proportion of patients with early prostate cancer treated with external-beam radiotherapy are at low risk of disease progression and death from prostate cancer. However, the incidence of disease progression in patients treated with radiotherapy is higher than for patients treated with surgery, as radiotherapy is generally considered suitable for patients who present at a higher clinical stage than those who are usually treated surgically.

Analyses of pretreatment characteristics demonstrate that outcomes following conventional doses of external-beam radiotherapy vary considerably and tend to be poorer for patients with locally advanced disease. Meta-analysis of four Radiation Therapy Oncology Group (RTOG) randomized trials of radiotherapy identified four prognostic groups based on the following factors: Gleason score, T-stage, and pathologic lymph node status.[25] Of these factors, Gleason score was identified as the strongest predictor of progression. Patients in the highest risk grouping (T3, Nx, Gleason score 8–10; or N+, Gleason score 8–10) had a 36% risk of disease-specific death at 5 years (Figure 29.2).

A more recent analysis of 927 patients with clinically localized disease, for whom pretreatment PSA values were available, compared the predictive nature of this factor with those described above.[26] The analysis found that pretreatment PSA level is a significant, independent prognostic factor for overall survival, but is not as important as Gleason score or T-stage.

Once a patient's risk profile has been determined, it can be used in consultation with the patient to identify appropriate treatment options. As with patients treated surgically, the key question is whether hormonal therapy neoadjuvant or adjuvant to the primary therapy of curative intent can improve outcomes. To address this, the following sections cover the evidence for neoadjuvant and adjuvant hormonal therapies in patients receiving external-beam radiotherapy.

Is there a role for neoadjuvant hormonal therapy prior to external-beam radiotherapy?

A limited number of randomized controlled trials have examined neoadjuvant hormonal therapy prior to external-beam radiotherapy

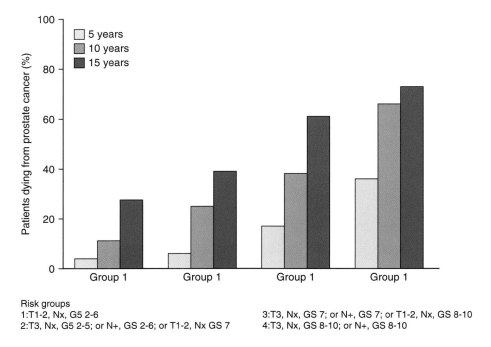

Figure 29.2

Risk of prostate cancer death following conventional dose external-beam radiotherapy in patients with localized or locally advanced prostate cancer (n = 1557). (GS, Gleason score.)

Reproduced with permission from Roach III M, Lu J, Pilepich MV, et al. Four prognostic groups predict long-term survival from prostate cancer following radiotherapy alone on Radiation Therapy Oncology Group clinical trials. Int J Radiat Oncol Biol Phys 2000;47:609–615.

in patients with localized or locally advanced disease. In these studies, the use of neoadjuvant hormonal therapy prior to external-beam radiotherapy reduced prostate volume and improved local control, progression-free survival, and disease-specific survival.

A large randomized controlled trial undertaken by the RTOG assessed neoadjuvant CAB (goserelin plus flutamide) given for 2 months prior to and 2 months during treatment with external-beam radiotherapy in 471 patients with localized or locally advanced (T2–4, N0 or N+ M0) disease.[27,28] Results at a median follow-up of 6.7 years showed a modest improvement in estimated 8-year clinical progression-free survival for patients receiving neoadjuvant hormonal therapy (33% versus 21% with radiotherapy alone; p = 0.004) and cause-specific mortality (23% versus 31% with radiotherapy alone; p = 0.05).[28] Subset analysis indicated that the beneficial effects specifically occurred in patients with a Gleason score of 2 to 6, for whom overall survival was significantly improved with neoadjuvant hormonal therapy compared with radiotherapy alone (70% versus 52%; p = 0.015). In patients with Gleason score 7 to 10 tumors, neoadjuvant hormonal therapy did not result in a statistically significant enhancement in either disease control or survival.

A smaller randomized controlled trial in 120 patients with localized or locally advanced (T2–4) prostate cancer compared local disease control with three different treatment regimens: external-beam radiotherapy alone; radiotherapy plus 3 months' neoadjuvant CAB (leuprorelin plus flutamide); and 3 months' neoadjuvant hormonal therapy plus adjuvant CAB for 6 months during and following radiotherapy.[29] The percentages of patients with positive biopsies at 24 months were 65% for external-beam radiotherapy alone, 28% for

radiotherapy plus neoadjuvant CAB, and 5% for neoadjuvant hormonal therapy plus adjuvant CAB during and following radiotherapy (p-values not given). Laverdière et al have also reported a similar study in 161 patients with localized or locally advanced (T2–3) disease with a median follow-up of 5 years.[30] In this report, estimated 7-year PSA progression-free survival rates (progression defined as two consecutive increases in PSA level with at least one value of 1.5 ng/mL) were 42% with radiotherapy alone, 66% with neoadjuvant hormonal therapy (p = 0.009 versus radiotherapy alone), and 69% with neoadjuvant plus adjuvant hormonal therapy (p = 0.003 versus radio-therapy alone; not significant versus neoadjuvant hormonal therapy).

Neoadjuvant CPA has also been studied in a randomized controlled trial of 298 men with locally advanced (stage B2-C) prostate cancer.[31] Cyproterone acetate was given for 12 weeks prior to radiotherapy and patients were monitored for the following 18 to 36 months. Neoadjuvant hormonal therapy significantly reduced prostate volume (p = 0.0016) and increased the number of patients free from clinical (71% versus 49%; p = 0.019) or biochemical (47% versus 22%; p = 0.0001) evidence of disease compared with radiotherapy alone.

The outcomes summarized above contrast with neoadjuvant hormonal therapy in the surgical setting, where no clinical benefit is observed. One possible reason for this difference is that the effects of androgen ablation and radiotherapy may be synergistic in activating apoptosis in prostate cancer cells. Consequently the use of neoadjuvant hormonal therapy in the radiotherapy setting may result in an increased level of prostate cancer cell death relative to either treatment alone.[32]

Is there a role for adjuvant hormonal therapy with external-beam radiotherapy?

A substantial amount of research has been conducted into hormonal therapy adjuvant to external-beam, conventional-dose radiotherapy, including a number of large randomized controlled trials in patients with localized or locally advanced prostate cancer (Table 29.2).[19,33–39] Data from these studies support the use of hormonal therapy adjuvant to external-beam radiotherapy in patients with locally advanced disease and those with high-risk localized disease.

Patients with localized prostate cancer

Two of the studies summarized in the next section included a small proportion of patients with localized disease in addition to those with locally advanced disease, but do not provide separate analyses of data from these patients. However, the bicalutamide EPC program does provide analysis of data from patients with localized disease treated with hormonal therapy adjuvant to radiotherapy.[19] Analysis of this subgroup of 1065 patients showed a small decrease in the risk of objective disease progression compared with radiotherapy alone (HR 0.80; 95% CI 0.62–1.03); however, this was not statistically significant, suggesting that bicalutamide 150 mg/day adjuvant to radiotherapy offers no clinical benefit in patients with localized disease. Currently, survival data for patients treated with radiotherapy in this study are immature, with 19% deaths.[40]

A recent randomized controlled trial has assessed the effect of 6 months CAB (leuprorelin or goserelin plus flutamide) adjuvant to radiotherapy in 206 patients with high-risk, clinically localized prostate cancer (PSA level ≥10 ng/mL, Gleason score ≥7 or radiographic evidence of extraprostatic disease).[33] At a median follow-up of 4.5 years overall survival was significantly higher for patients receiving adjuvant CAB, compared with radiotherapy alone, with 5-year estimates of survival of 88% and 78%, respectively (HR 2.07; 95% CI 1.02–4.20; p = 0.04).

Patients with locally advanced prostate cancer

Orchiectomy was studied as adjuvant hormonal therapy in a randomized controlled trial conducted in 91 patients with clinically localized (cT1–2 pN0; n = 37) or locally advanced (cT1–2 pN+ or cT3–4, any N; n = 54) prostate cancer.[39] After a median follow up of 9.3 years, there was a significant improvement in overall survival in patients who received adjuvant hormonal therapy compared with radiotherapy alone (62% versus 39%; p = 0.02); however, further subgroup analysis showed that the survival benefit was only significant for patients with lymph node metastases (p = 0.007).

An RTOG trial has examined long-term (indefinite duration) treatment with adjuvant LHRH agonist (goserelin) in 977 men with locally advanced disease (T1–2, N+ or T3, any N).[34–36] The most recent analysis of this study, at a median follow-up of 7.3 years, showed significant improvement in estimated 10-year overall survival with adjuvant hormonal therapy compared with radiotherapy alone (53% versus 38%; p < 0.0043).[36]

A European Organization for Research and Treatment of Cancer (EORTC) trial has also provided long-term follow-up data on the effect of an LHRH agonist (goserelin) adjuvant to radiotherapy in 415 men with high-risk localized (T1–2, Gleason score 3; 8% of the study population) or locally advanced (T3–4) tumors.[38,41] At a median follow-up of 5.5 years, 3 years' adjuvant hormonal therapy resulted in significant improvements in both 5-year disease-specific survival (94% versus 79%; p = 0.0001) and overall survival (78% versus 62%; p = 0.0002) compared with radiotherapy alone.

Analyses of the subgroup of patients with locally advanced disease who received radiotherapy in the bicalutamide EPC program have also been conducted.[19] At present, survival data for patients treated with radiotherapy in this study are immature, with 19% deaths.[40] However, at a median follow-up of 5.4 years, adjuvant bicalutamide 150 mg/day significantly decreased the risk of objective disease progression in the 305 patients with locally advanced disease by 42% compared with radiotherapy alone (HR 0.58; 95% CI 0.41–0.84; p = 0.00348).

Comparative studies of neoadjuvant and adjuvant hormonal therapies with external-beam radiotherapy

Relatively few studies have directly addressed whether neoadjuvant or adjuvant hormonal therapy offer the optimal outcome for a particular patient group. All such studies, however, have been undertaken in patients treated with external-beam radiotherapy as primary therapy. Overall, data from these studies provide no clear evidence as to whether neoadjuvant or adjuvant hormonal therapy provide superior benefits for patients receiving radiotherapy, although subgroup analyses suggest that patients in particular risk groups may have better outcomes with one type of hormonal therapy.

One RTOG randomized controlled trial has compared 4 months of hormonal therapy neoadjuvant or adjuvant to external-beam radiotherapy in 1323 patients with clinically localized disease, elevated PSA levels, and a 15% estimated risk of lymph node metastases.[42] At a median follow-up of 5 years, there was no significant difference between patients receiving neoadjuvant or adjuvant CAB with goserelin or leuprorelin plus flutamide in terms of 4-year PSA progression-free survival (52% with neoadjuvant versus 49% with adjuvant, p = 0.56; PSA progression defined as two consecutive PSA rises of ≥20% from baseline or of ≥0.3 ng/mL from a baseline of ≤1.5 ng/mL, local or metastatic progression, or death from any cause). However, in this study, patients received either whole pelvic or prostate only external-beam radiotherapy and for those patients who received whole-pelvic radiotherapy, there was a significant improvement in PSA progression-free survival with neoadjuvant compared with adjuvant hormonal therapy (60% versus 49%; p-value not given).

A second RTOG trial, in 1554 patients with locally advanced or high-risk localized (T2c–4) disease, addressed the effects of 2 years' treatment with an LHRH agonist (goserelin) adjuvant to radiotherapy plus neoadjuvant CAB (goserelin plus flutamide) compared with radiotherapy plus neoadjuvant CAB alone.[43] At a median follow-up of 5.8 years, this study found no significant difference in 5-year estimates of overall survival between the two patient groups (p = 0.73). However, an exploratory subset analysis showed that adjuvant hormonal therapy significantly improved overall survival for patients with Gleason score 8 to 10 tumors compared with neoadjuvant CAB and radiotherapy alone (81% versus 71%; p = 0.044).

Table 29.2 Randomised controlled trials of hormonal therapy adjuvant to external-beam radiotherapy compared with radiotherapy alone

Adjuvant hormonal therapy	Study	Disease stage	No. patients randomised	Treatment duration, years	Median follow-up, years	Progression-free survival	Overall survival
Orchiectomy	Granfors et al[39]	cT1–4, any N	91	Not applicable	9.3	69% vs 39% with RT alone (p = 0.005)[a]	62% vs 39% with RT alone (p = 0.02)
LHRH agonist (goserelin)	RTOG 85-31[34–36]	cT1–2, N+ or cT3, any N	977	Indefinite or until progression	7.3	Not given*	53% vs 38% with RT alone (p < 0.0043) [10-year estimate]
LHRH agonist (goserelin)	EORTC 22863[37,38]	cT1–2, Gleason grade 3 or cT3–4, any grade, N0–1	415	3 years	5.5	74% vs 40% with RT alone (p < 0.0001) [5-year estimate][b]	78% vs 62% with RT alone (p = 0.0002) [5-year estimate]
NSAA (bicalutamide)	EPC[19]	cT1b–2, N0/X cT3–4, any N or cT1b–2, N+	1065 305	≥2 years	5.4 (whole study)	HR 0.80; 95% CI 0.62, 1.03; p = 0.088[c] HR 0.58; 95% CI 0.41–0.84; p = 0.0035[c]	Survival data immature (19% deaths in RT group)
CAB (leuprorelin or goserelin plus flutamide)	D'Amico et al[33]	cT1b–2, PSA ≥ 10 ng/mL, GS ≥ 7	206	6 months	4.5	82% vs 57% with RT alone; HR 2.30; 95% CI 1.36–3.89; p = 0.002 (5-year estimate)[d]	88% vs 78% with RT alone; HR 2.07; 95% CI 1.02–4.20; p = 0.04 (5-year estimate)

*10-year estimates of local progression-free survival 77% vs 61% with RT alone, p<0.0001 and distant metastatic progression-free survival: 75% vs 61% with RT alone. Progression-free survival defined as: [a]time from randomization to the occurrence of clinically evident local tumor growth or bone or other distant metastases; [b]time to first clinical progression or death from any cause; [c]time from randomization to objective progression confirmed by bone scan, computed tomography/ultrasound/magnetic resonance imaging or histological evidence of distant metastases or death from any cause without progression; [d]time to initiation of salvage hormonal therapy.

CAB, combined androgen blockade; CI, confidence intervals; EPC, bicalutamide 150 mg early prostate cancer program; HR, hazard ratio; LHRH, luteinizing hormone-releasing hormone; NSAA, nonsteroidal antiandrogen; RT, external-beam radiotherapy.

A smaller study, in 325 patients with localized or locally advanced (T2–3) prostate cancer, compared 5 months of hormonal therapy neoadjuvant to and concomitant with external-beam radiotherapy with 10 months of hormonal therapy neoadjuvant, concomitant and adjuvant to radiotherapy.[30] This study found no significant difference between the two treatment groups in terms of 4-year PSA progression-free survival (65% versus 68% with 5 and 10 months' hormonal therapy, respectively; p = 0.55). Prostate-specific antigen progression was defined as two consecutive increases in PSA level, with at least one value of 1.5 ng/mL or more.

A meta-analysis of data from five RTOG randomized controlled trials, using the risk groups defined in Figure 29.2, investigated which patients are most likely to benefit from either neoadjuvant or adjuvant hormonal therapy.[44] This analysis found that, in group 2, benefit in terms of 8-year disease-specific survival was achieved with neoadjuvant CAB (goserelin and flutamide) for 2 months prior to, and for 2 months during, external-beam radiotherapy compared with radiotherapy alone (98% versus 83%; p = 0.003). Patients in groups 3 and 4 had an approximately 20% higher overall survival at 8 years with the addition of long-term adjuvant LHRH agonist (goserelin) following radiotherapy compared with radiotherapy alone (p ≤ 0.0004), while neoadjuvant hormonal therapy appeared to have no benefit in these risk groups.

Other primary therapies

Brachytherapy and cryotherapy are alternatives to radical prostatectomy and external-beam radiotherapy for patients with early prostate cancer. For patients receiving brachytherapy or cryotherapy, addition of hormonal therapy is an option for the same reasons as other primary therapies. However, no randomized controlled studies have been conducted in which patients received hormonal therapy neoadjuvant or adjuvant to either brachytherapy or cryotherapy. For this reason, only limited conclusions can be drawn about the benefits of adding hormonal therapy to either brachytherapy or cryotherapy.

For brachytherapy, some data are available from retrospective or observational studies of additional hormonal therapy. Most of these studies focus on neoadjuvant hormonal therapy because, as with other primary therapies, any reduction in prostate volume induced by the neoadjuvant hormonal therapy may facilitate brachytherapy. However, a recent literature review reported that there was little evidence to indicate that biochemical or clinical progression-free survival is improved by hormonal therapy either neoadjuvant or adjuvant to brachytherapy.[45] Moreover, this review suggested that use of hormonal therapy might lead to increased acute urinary morbidity and decreased erectile function.

There are no published studies assessing clinical outcomes with hormonal treatment neoadjuvant or adjuvant to cryotherapy. The literature is limited to a few observational studies that assessed hormonal therapy neoadjuvant to salvage cryotherapy.

Risk: benefit considerations

Decisions regarding additional hormonal therapy should be based on an informed discussion between patient and urologist, in the same

Table 29.3 Common adverse events associated with hormonal therapies

Hormonal therapy	Adverse event	Agent	Reported frequency (%)
LHRH agonists	Hot flushes	All	52–84[48–53]
	Loss of libido	All	73–85[48–53]
	Impotence	All	76–84[48–53]
Non-steroidal antiandrogens	Gynecomastia	Bicalutamide	37–66[54]
		Flutamide	21–80[54]
		Nilutamide	50[54]
	Breast pain	Bicalutamide	13–73[54]
		Flutamide	22–69[54]
		Nilutamide	Not reported
	Hot flushes	All	<10[54]
	Diarrhea	Flutamide	10–20[55]
		Bicalutamide	2–6[54,55]
		Nilutamide	2–4[55]
	Serious/fatal hepatotoxicity	Flutamide	[Estimated risk 3 per 10,000[56]]
		Bicalutamide	Rare[54]
		Nilutamide	Rare[54]
	Interstitial pneumonitis	Nilutamide	1–3.8[54]
		Bicalutamide	Rare[54]
		Flutamide	Rare[54]
	Delayed adaptation to darkness	Nilutamide	Unique to nilutamide: 11–50[54]
	Alcohol intolerance	Nilutamide	Unique to nilutamide: 4–17[54]
	Loss of libido/impotence	All	~33[54]
Steroidal antiandrogens	Cardiovascular events	CPA	9.5–11[54]
	Adverse changes in serum lipids	CPA	Decreased HDL cholesterol and increased VLDL triglyceride levels[54]
	Impotence	CPA	87–92[54]

CAB, combined androgen blockade; CPA, cyproterone acetate; HDL, high-density lipoprotein; LHRH, luteinizing hormone-releasing hormone; VLDL, very-low-density lipoprotein.

Table 29.4 Summary of evidence for neoadjuvant and adjuvant hormonal therapeutic approaches

Therapeutic approach	Disease stage	Strength of evidence*	Randomised controlled trials reviewed	Comments
Neoadjuvant to radical prostatectomy	Localized/locally advanced	—	Aus et al[4]; Prezioso et al[5]; Labrie et al[6]; Goldenberg et al[7]; Hugosson et al[8]; Klotz et al[9]; Schulman et al[10]; Soloway et al[11,12]; Witjes et al[13]	No overall survival data from randomized controlled trials; PSA progression-free survival data available from randomized controlled trials in patients with localized or locally advanced disease show no significant difference compared with radical prostatectomy alone; Studies of longer periods (>3 months) of neoadjuvant hormonal therapy required
Adjuvant to radical prostatectomy	Localized	–	Wirth et al[19]	Only randomized controlled study in patients with localized disease found no significant difference in risk of objective progression compared with radical prostatectomy alone; Further randomized controlled studies required
Adjuvant to radical prostatectomy	Locally advanced	+	Messing et al[21,22]; Prayer-Galetti et al[23]; Wirth et al[24]	Improvements in overall survival demonstrated in patients with N+, M0 disease; Improvements in PSA progression-free survival and risk of progression in T3–4 patients; Overall survival data in N0 patients and additional randomized controlled trials required
Neoadjuvant to external-beam radiotherapy	Localised/locally advanced	+/–	Pilepich et al[27,28]; Laverdière et al[29,30]; Porter et al[31]	Improvements in disease-free survival in patients with T2–4 disease; improved overall survival in patients with GS 2–6, but not GS 7–10, tumors; Improvements in PSA progression-free survival in patients with T2–3 and B2–C disease. Further overall survival data and additional randomized controlled trials required
Adjuvant to external-beam radiotherapy	Localized	+/–	D'Amico et al[33], Granfors et al[39]	Improvements in overall survival seen in a study of adjuvant orchiectomy, but these were confined to N+ patients; No significant difference in progression-free survival seen in a study of adjuvant non-steroidal antiandrogen therapy; Significant improvements in overall survival with adjuvant CAB in patients with high risk localized disease (PSA ≥ 10 ng/mL, GS ≥ 7 or radiographic evidence of extraprostatic disease); Further randomized controlled studies required to establish optimal duration of adjuvant hormonal therapy
Adjuvant to external-beam radiotherapy	Locally advanced	++	Wirth et al[19], Lawton et al[34], Pilepich et al[35,36], Bolla et al[38,41]	Improvements demonstrated in overall survival with an LHRH agonist (goserelin) and in risk of disease progression with a non-steroidal antiandrogen (bicalutamide); Studies required to clarify optimal duration of adjuvant hormonal therapy
Neoadjuvant to brachytherapy	Localized/locally advanced	–	No randomized controlled trials	Randomized controlled trials required
Adjuvant to brachytherapy	Localized/locally advanced	–	No randomized controlled trials	Randomized controlled trials required
Neoadjuvant to cryotherapy	Localised/locally advanced	–	No randomized controlled trials	Randomised controlled trials required
Adjuvant to cryotherapy	Localised/locally advanced	–	No randomized controlled trials	Randomised controlled trials required

*Summary of the strength of evidence for hormonal therapy in the setting described. ++, strong evidence of benefit (numerous large studies and consensus positive results); +, some evidence of benefit (limited overall survival data); +/–, mixed evidence (evidence of benefit in only certain patient groups) –, no strong supporting evidence (no randomized controlled trials or limited data suggesting no benefit); —, clear evidence of no benefit. GS, Gleason score; LHRH, luteinizing hormone-releasing hormone; PSA, prostate-specific antigen.

way as those relating to choice of primary therapy. Patients faced with a diagnosis of prostate cancer and a complex set of treatment options can experience strong emotional reactions, including depressive symptoms and feelings of overwhelming anxiety.[46] Their families can also be profoundly affected and may wish to have some input into treatment decisions. For example, a recent survey found that 88% of patients' partners reported an active involvement in the treatment decision-making process, with information gathering and emotional support as their primary roles.[47] The urologist guiding a patient through the treatment choices needs an understanding of the patient's, and their family's, concerns; the sources of information and support available to them; and the expectations they have. This will help to develop a positive patient–physician relationship and will contribute to a treatment decision the patient is happy with and, thus, more likely to adhere to.

While the focus of the preceding sections has been studies designed to determine the efficacy of hormonal therapy neoadjuvant or adjuvant to the primary therapy, there are a number of other important factors to consider when contemplating additional hormonal therapy. These include patient preference, age, life expectancy,

comorbid disease, and level of sexual and physical activity. Such factors, plus a patient's risk profile, will impact on decisions relating to both the choice of neoadjuvant or adjuvant hormonal therapy and the specific agent used.

The overall impact of a treatment regimen on a patient's quality of life needs careful consideration in the context of that individual's circumstances. Likewise, the tolerability profile of the specific agent or agents used for neoadjuvant or adjuvant hormonal therapy is important, and the differing adverse event profiles of LHRH agonists or antiandrogens and any between-agent differences within each class of treatment need to be considered (Table 29.3).[48–56] In the case of CAB, side effects of both agents may occur, with a consequent increase in the overall incidence of adverse effects, although with gynecomastia and breast pain, the combination of an LHRH agonist and an antiandrogen reduces the incidence of this adverse effect compared with antiandrogen therapy alone.[57] As well as forming part of the treatment decision-making process, clear communication of the possible side effects of treatments is important in promoting long-term adherence to the chosen treatment regimen.

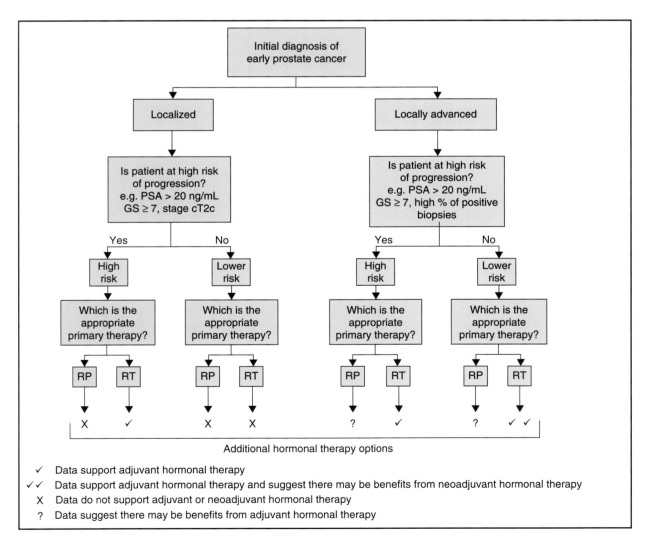

Figure 29.3
Flow diagram outlining the decision-making process for patients with early prostate cancer. (GS, Gleason score; PSA, prostate-specific antigen; RP, radical prostatectomy; RT, external-beam radiotherapy.)

Many of the studies outlined in this chapter show that some patients with early prostate cancer are at greater risk of a poorer outcome when primary treatment of curative intent is given alone. However, for those patients at low risk of progression, in the majority of cases, additional hormonal therapy is not advisable and these patients need to be counseled carefully about the potential benefit of neoadjuvant or adjuvant hormonal therapy compared with the impact of treatment on their quality of life.

Nomograms, which are designed to predict outcomes such as progression-free survival on the basis of a set of specific clinical parameters, are a helpful tool when assessing a patient's risk of progression. A variety of nomograms exist, not all of which have been validated; those developed by Partin et al and Kattan et al are among the better known.[58–61] When advising a patient about the balance between risks and benefits of a particular treatment, nomograms can provide useful additional input. The full complexity of the use and limitations of nomograms is discussed elsewhere in this book.

When weighing the potential risks and benefits of a treatment approach, an important part of the process is to examine the strength and quality of the evidence that supports the benefits provided by the therapy. Where fewer high-level data are available, or conclusions are not clear-cut, the decision may be weighted in favor of deferring hormonal therapy and thereby minimizing the risk of adverse events. Table 29.4 outlines the strength of data available for each therapeutic approach discussed in this chapter and highlights where additional research is needed to clarify the suitability of each treatment option.

Summary

The range of neoadjuvant and adjuvant hormonal therapeutic approaches that may delay disease progression and improve survival for prostate cancer patients is outlined in Figure 29.3. At present, there are no data to indicate that neoadjuvant hormonal therapy prior to radical prostatectomy offers benefit to patients with localized or locally advanced disease in terms of overall survival or delaying disease progression. Hormonal therapy adjuvant to radical prostatectomy is of benefit to patients with lymph node metastases (both in terms of progression and survival) and also appears to offer benefits in terms of delaying disease progression for other patients with locally advanced disease, but survival data are currently immature. For patients with T2 to T4, Gleason score 2 to 6 disease, the current data indicate that hormonal therapy neoadjuvant to external-beam radiotherapy may offer benefits. There is also evidence of benefit for patients with locally advanced or high-risk localized disease receiving hormonal therapy adjuvant to external-beam radiotherapy.

Ultimately, assessing where the balance lies between the potential benefits and the possible risks associated with neoadjuvant or adjuvant hormonal therapy is an individual process, unique to each patient and their urologist. Treatment decisions should be based on clinical evidence as well as the patient's disease status, personal circumstances, and preferences.

References

1. Smith JA Jr, Soloway MS, Young MJ. Complications of advanced prostate cancer. Urology 1999;54 (Suppl 6A):8–14.

2. Penson DF, Moul JW, Evans CP, et al. The economic burden of metastatic and prostate specific antigen progression in patients with prostate cancer: findings from a retrospective analysis of health plan data. J Urol 2004;171:2250–2254.

3. Hull GW, Rabbani F, Abbas F, et al. Cancer control with radical prostatectomy alone in 1,000 consecutive patients. J Urol 2002;167: 528–534.

4. Aus G, Abrahamsson P-A, Ahlgren G, et al. Three-month neoadjuvant hormonal therapy before radical prostatectomy: a 7-year follow-up of a randomized controlled trial. BJU Int 2002;90:561–566.

5. Prezioso D, Lotti T, Polito M, et al. Neoadjuvant hormone treatment with leuprolide acetate depot 3.75 mg and cyproterone acetate, before radical prostatectomy: a randomized study. Urol Int 2004;72:189–195.

6. Labrie F, Cusan L, Gomez J-L, et al. Neoadjuvant hormonal therapy: the Canadian experience. Urology 1997;49 (Suppl 3A): 56–64.

7. Goldenberg SL, Klotz LH, Srigley J, et al. Randomized, prospective, controlled study comparing radical prostatectomy alone and neoadjuvant androgen withdrawal in the treatment of localized prostate cancer. J Urol 1996;156:873–877.

8. Hugosson J, Abrahamsson PA, Ahlgren G, et al. The risk of malignancy in the surgical margin at radical prostatectomy reduced almost threefold in patients given neo-adjuvant hormone treatment. Eur Urol 1996;29:413–419.

9. Klotz LH, Goldenberg SL, Jewett MAS, et al. Long-term follow-up of a randomized trial of 0 versus 3 months of neoadjuvant androgen ablation before radical prostatectomy. J Urol 2003;170:791–794.

10. Schulman CC, Debruyne FMJ, Forster G, et al. 4-year follow-up results of a European prospective randomized study on neoadjuvant hormonal therapy prior to radical prostatectomy in T2-3N0M0 prostate cancer. Eur Urol 2000;38:706–713.

11. Soloway MS, Sharifi R, Wajsman Z, et al. Randomized prospective study comparing radical prostatectomy alone versus radical prostatectomy preceded by androgen blockade in clinical stage B2 (T2bNxM0) prostate cancer. J Urol 1995;154:424–428.

12. Soloway MS, Pareek K, Sharifi R, et al. Neoadjuvant androgen ablation before radical prostatectomy in cT2bNxMo prostate cancer: 5-year results. J Urol 2002;167:112–116.

13. Witjes WPJ, Schulman CC, Debruyne FMJ, for the European Study Group on Neoadjuvant Treatment of Prostate Cancer. Preliminary results of a prospective randomized study comparing radical prostatectomy versus radical prostatectomy associated with neoadjuvant hormonal combination therapy in T_{2-3} N_0 M_0 prostatic carcinoma. Urology 1997;49 (Suppl 3A):65–69.

14. Bazinet M, Zheng W, Begin LR, et al. Morphologic changes induced by neoadjuvant androgen ablation may result in underdetection of positive surgical margins and capsular involvement by prostatic adenocarcinoma. Urology 1997;49:721–725.

15. Bono AV, Pagano F, Montironi R, et al. Effect of complete androgen blockade on pathologic stage and resection margin status of prostate cancer: progress pathology report of the Italian PROSIT study. Urology 2001;57:117–121.

16. Gleave ME, Goldenberg SL, Chin JL, et al. Randomized comparative study of 3 versus 8-month neoadjuvant hormonal therapy before radical prostatectomy: biochemical and pathological effects. J Urol 2001;166:500–506.

17. Scolieri MJ, Altman A, Resnick MI. Neoadjuvant hormonal ablative therapy before radical prostatectomy: a review. Is it indicated? J Urol 2000;164:1465–1472.

18. Chun J, Pruthi RS. Is neoadjuvant hormonal therapy before radical prostatectomy indicated? Urol Int 2004;72:275–280.

19. Wirth M, See WA, McLeod DG, et al. Bicalutamide ("Casodex") 150 mg in addition to standard care in patients with localized or locally advanced prostate cancer: results from the second analysis of the Early

Prostate Cancer program at 5.4 years' median follow-up. J Urol 2004;172:1865–1870.

20. Wirth M, Iversen P, McLeod D et al. Bicalutamide ("Casodex") 150 mg as adjuvant to radical prostatectomy significantly increases progression-free survival in patients with early non-metastatic prostate cancer: analysis at a median follow-up of 5.4 years. Eur Urol Suppl 2004;3:48 [abstract 181].

21. Messing EM, Manola J, Sarosdy M, et al. Immediate hormonal therapy compared with observation after radical prostatectomy and pelvic lymphadenectomy in men with node-positive prostate cancer. N Engl J Med 1999;341:1781–1788.

22. Messing E, Manola J, Sarosdy M, et al. Immediate hormonal therapy compared with observation after radical prostatectomy and pelvic lymphadenectomy in men with node positive prostate cancer: results at 10 years of EST 3886. J Urol 2003;169:396 [abstract 1480].

23. Prayer-Galetti T, Zattoni F, Capizzi A, et al. Disease free survival in patients with pathological "C STAGE" prostate cancer at radical retropubic prostatectomy submitted to adjuvant hormonal treatment. Eur Urol 2000;38:504 [abstract 48].

24. Wirth MP, Weissbach L, Marx FJ, et al. Prospective randomized trial comparing flutamide as adjuvant treatment versus observation after radical prostatectomy for locally advanced, lymph node-negative prostate cancer. Eur Urol 2004;45:267–270.

25. Roach III M, Lu J, Pilepich MV, et al. Four prognostic groups predict long-term survival from prostate cancer following radiotherapy alone on Radiation Therapy Oncology Group clinical trials. Int J Radiat Oncol Biol Phys 2000;47:609–615.

26. Roach III M, Weinberg V, McLaughlin PW, et al. Serum prostate-specific antigen and survival after external beam radiotherapy for carcinoma of the prostate. Urology 2003;61:730–735.

27. Pilepich MV, Krall JM, Al-Sarraf M, et al. Androgen deprivation with radiation therapy compared with radiation therapy alone for locally advanced prostatic carcinoma: a randomized comparative trial of the Radiation Therapy Oncology Group. Urology 1995;45:616–623.

28. Pilepich MV, Winter K, John MJ, et al. Phase III Radiation Therapy Oncology Group (RTOG) trial 86-10 of androgen deprivation adjuvant to definitive radiotherapy in locally advanced carcinoma of the prostate. Int J Radiat Oncol Biol Phys 2001;50:1243–1252.

29. Laverdière J, Gomez JL, Cusan L, et al. Beneficial effect of combination hormonal therapy administered prior and following external beam radiation therapy in localized prostate cancer. Int J Radiat Oncol Biol Phys 1997;37:247–252.

30. Laverdière J, Nabid A, De Bedoya LD, et al. The efficacy and sequencing of a short course of androgen suppression on freedom from biochemical failure when administered with radiation therapy for T2-T3 prostate cancer. J Urol 2004;171:1137–1140.

31. Porter AT, Elhilali M, Manji M, et al. A phase III randomized trial to evaluate the efficacy of neoadjuvant therapy prior to curative radiotherapy in locally advanced prostate cancer patients. A Canadian Urologic Oncology Group study. Proc Am Soc Clin Oncol 1997;16:315a [abstract 1123].

32. Pollack A, Zagars GK, Kopplin S. Radiotherapy and androgen ablation for clinically localized high-risk prostate cancer. Int J Radiat Oncol Biol Phys 1995;32:13–20.

33. D'Amico AV, Manola J, Loffredo M, et al. 6-month androgen suppression plus radiation therapy vs radiation therapy alone for patients with clinically localized prostate cancer: a randomized controlled trial. JAMA 2004;292:821–827.

34. Lawton CA, Winter K, Murray K, et al. Updated results of the Phase III Radiation Therapy Oncology Group (RTOG) trial 85-31 evaluating the potential benefit of androgen suppression following standard radiation therapy for unfavorable prognosis carcinoma of the prostate. Int J Radiat Oncol Biol Phys 2001;49:937–946.

35. Pilepich MV, Caplan R, Byhardt RW, et al. Phase III trial of androgen suppression using goserelin in unfavorable-prognosis carcinoma of the prostate treated with definitive radiotherapy: report of Radiation Therapy Oncology Group protocol 85-31. J Clin Oncol 1997;15:1013–1021.

36. Pilepich MV, Winter K, Lawton C, et al. Androgen suppression adjuvant to radiotherapy in carcinoma of the prostate. Long-term results of phase III RTOG study 85-31. Int J Radiat Oncol Biol Phys 2003;57:S172 [abstract 82].

37. Bolla M, Gonzalez D, Warde P, et al. Improved survival in patients with locally advanced prostate cancer treated with radiotherapy and goserelin. N Engl J Med 1997;337:295–300.

38. Bolla M, Collette L, Blank L, et al. Long-term results with immediate androgen suppression and external irradiation in patients with locally advanced prostate cancer (an EORTC study): a phase III randomised trial. Lancet 2002;360:103–108.

39. Granfors T, Modig H, Damber J-E, et al. Combined orchiectomy and external radiotherapy versus radiotherapy alone for nonmetastatic prostate cancer with or without pelvic lymph node involvement: a prospective randomized study. J Urol 1998;159:2030–2034.

40. McLeod D, Iversen P, See W, et al. Bicalutamide ("Casodex") 150 mg as adjuvant to radiotherapy significantly improves progression-free survival in early non-metastatic prostate cancer: results from the bicalutamide Early Prostate Cancer programme after a median 5.4 years' follow-up. Eur Urol Suppl 2004;3:48 [abstract 182].

41. Bolla M, Gonzalez D, Kurth J, et al. Adjuvant hormonal therapy with goserelin improves survival in patients with locally advanced prostate cancer treated with radiotherapy. Results of phase III randomized trial of the EORTC Radiotherapy and Genito-urinary tract Cancer Cooperative Groups. Eur Urol 1998;33 (Suppl 1):135 [abstract 537].

42. Roach III M, DeSilvio M, Lawton C, et al. Phase III trial comparing whole-pelvic versus prostate-only radiotherapy and neoadjuvant versus adjuvant combined androgen suppression: Radiation Therapy Oncology Group 9413. J Clin Oncol 2003;21:1904–1911.

43. Hanks GE, Pajak TF, Porter A, et al. Phase III trial of long-term adjuvant androgen deprivation after neoadjuvant hormonal cytoreduction and radiotherapy in locally advanced carcinoma of the prostate: the Radiation Therapy Oncology Group Protocol 92-02. J Clin Oncol 2003;21:3972–3978.

44. Roach III M, Jiandong L, Pilepich MV, et al. Predicting long-term survival and the need for hormonal therapy: a meta-analysis of RTOG prostate cancer trials. Int J Radiat Oncol Biol Phys 2000;47:617–627.

45. Lee WR. The role of androgen deprivation therapy combined with prostate brachytherapy. Urology 2002;60:39–44.

46. Manne SL. Prostate cancer support and advocacy groups: their role for patients and family members. Semin Urol Oncol 2002;20:45–54.

47. Srirangam SJ, Pearson E, Grose C, et al. Partner's influence on patient preference for treatment in early prostate cancer. BJU Int 2003;92:365–369.

48. Heyns CF, Simonin MP, Grosgurin P, et al. Comparative efficacy of triptorelin pamoate and leuprolide acetate in men with advanced prostate cancer. BJU Int 2003;92:226–231.

49. Kaisary AV, Tyrrell CJ, Peeling WB, et al. on behalf of Study Group, Comparison of LHRH analogue (Zoladex) with orchiectomy in patients with metastatic prostatic carcinoma. Br J Urol 1991;67:502–508.

50. Parmar H, Edwards L, Phillips RH, et al. Orchiectomy versus long-acting D-Trp-6-LHRH in advanced prostatic cancer. Br J Urol 1987;59:248–254.

51. Vogelzang NJ, Chodak GW, Soloway MS, et al. Goserelin versus orchiectomy in the treatment of advanced prostate cancer: final results of a randomized trial. Urology 1995;46:220–226.

52. Suprefact® prescribing information, 2004.

53. Lupron Depot 3.75 mg package insert, 2004.

54. Fourcade R-O, McLeod D. Tolerability of antiandrogens in the treatment of prostate cancer. UroOncology 2004;4:5–13.

55. McLeod DG. Tolerability of nonsteroidal antiandrogens in the treatment of advanced prostate cancer. Oncologist 1997;2:18–27.

56. Wysowski DK, Fourcroy JL. Flutamide hepatotoxicity. J Urol 1996;155:209–212.

57. Kaisary AV. Compliance with hormonal treatment for prostate cancer. Br J Hosp Med 1996;55:359–366.

58. Kattan MW, Eastham JA, Stapleton AMF, et al. A preoperative nomogram for disease recurrence following radical prostatectomy for prostate cancer. J Natl Cancer Inst 1998;90:766–771.

59. Kattan MW, Wheeler TM, Scardino PT. Postoperative nomogram for disease recurrence after radical prostatectomy for prostate cancer. J Clin Oncol 1999;17:1499–1507.

60. Partin AW, Yoo J, Carter HB, et al. The use of prostate specific antigen, clinical stage and Gleason score to predict pathological stage in men with localized prostate cancer. J Urol 1993;150:110–114.

61. Partin AW, Mangold LA, Lamm DM, et al. Contemporary update of prostate cancer staging nomograms (Partin Tables) for the new millennium. Urology 2001;58:843–848.

30

The assessment and management of urinary incontinence in patients with prostate cancer

Jane Dawoodi, Zach S Dovey, Mark R Feneley

Introduction

Urinary incontinence is defined by the International Continence Society as the complaint of any involuntary leakage of urine,[1] where patients are unable to hold their own urine and consequently wet themselves. In men with prostate cancer, urinary incontinence may arise from treatment of early stage disease, but it is also common in advanced prostate cancer. The effects of aging, concomitant age-related conditions, and other treatable factors may aggravate loss of urinary control and impair lower urinary tract function. Incontinence causes considerable distress and debility with a major negative effect on quality of life, impacting patients and their families.[2]

The pathophysiology of urinary incontinence is often complex. Assessment demands careful and comprehensive evaluation of a patient's habits, performance status, comorbidity and age-related factors, pharmacotherapy, and previous iatrogenic interventions. As a rule every patient should have a careful history, physical examination, and basic laboratory investigations. Urinary infection and urinary retention must always be excluded or treated. Guided by a patient's presentation, investigations may include urine flow studies, ultrasound imaging, urodynamic testing, and cystoscopy. Once a full assessment has been made, a clear diagnosis can direct appropriate treatment, with close cooperation between urologic nurses and physicians.

Prostate cancer may cause incontinence through a variety of mechanisms. Tumor growth causes bladder outflow obstruction and may directly involve the bladder base, compromising normal detrusor and bladder neck function. Local invasion may compromise the integrity of the urinary sphincters and pelvic neurological pathways, and metastases may give rise to spinal cord and nerve root compression. The treatment of prostate cancer may also cause or contribute to urinary incontinence. Although incontinence is usually treatable, iatrogenic incontinence is sometimes feared more than prostate cancer itself, particularly when an excellent oncologic prognosis following treatment of early-stage disease can be anticipated.

For the purposes of this chapter, urinary incontinence associated with prostate cancer will be discussed first in relation to lower urinary tract pathophysiology (disease-associated incontinence), and then in relation to the effects of potentially curative treatment for localized disease (iatrogenic incontinence). Functional and pathologic conditions primarily affecting systems outside the lower urinary tract may also influence continence, lower urinary tract function, and related measures of quality of life, but their full consideration is beyond the scope of this chapter.

Disease-associated incontinence

Urinary continence is maintained by passive and active mechanisms acting on the bladder outlet and proximal urethra, coordinated with detrusor regulation of filling, storage, and voiding of urine. The pathophysiology of incontinence acquired in association with prostate cancer relates to variable abnormalities in components of the lower urinary tract and their integrated functionality, including sphincteric insufficiency, bladder outflow obstruction, and changes in detrusor function.

Urinary leakage, therefore, indicates underlying changes in lower urinary tract function and its control. Incontinence may occur as a result of urinary overflow with chronic urinary retention in those patients with or without prostate cancer. Leakage may also occur as a result of detrusor overactivity[2] when this overcomes existing continence mechanisms. Prostate cancer may compromise bladder neck and/or external sphincter function by direct invasion of these structures or their innervation. Structural changes in the bladder wall may arise from secondary effects of outflow obstruction, from invasion by prostate cancer itself, or from other intrinsic disease of the bladder including aging. By affecting bladder capacity, compliance, storage, sensation, and contraction, bladder dysfunction may compromise overall lower urinary tract function and continence, particularly where there is coexisting sphincteric dysfunction. The local effects of invasive prostate cancer may, therefore, contribute to many aspects of lower urinary tract dysfunction.

Overflow incontinence arises from chronic urinary retention and progressive deterioration in bladder emptying. Chronic retention may be low-pressure retention with low detrusor contractility, or high-pressure retention with high detrusor contractility. These conditions may develop insidiously, sometimes without the patient's awareness of voiding difficulty. High-pressure retention may present with nocturnal incontinence or impaired renal function, and is then usually associated with voiding symptoms. In patients with overflow incontinence and low-pressure urinary retention, incomplete bladder emptying is associated with detrusor underactivity or an acontractile detrusor, and when intravesical pressure exceeds maximum urethral pressure (such as on body movement), urine leakage occurs. Studies of outflow obstruction in the rat[3] and the pig,[4] confirming a deterioration in detrusor function, have demonstrated increasing residual urine volumes in association with impairment of voiding pressure, and increases in smooth muscle cell number and total detrusor collagen content. It is not clear why detrusor acontractility develops in some patients and detrusor overactivity in others. It is possible that there is an additional variable neurologic element.

Parys et al[5] found that 73% of their patients with chronic urinary retention demonstrated a sensory suprasacral abnormality with intact sacral reflex pathways. They proposed this as an adaptive mechanism in higher neurological centers to bladder outflow obstruction that results in low-pressure retention and renal protection.

Urinary incontinence may occur in association with detrusor overactivity. In men with prostate cancer, this generally develops secondary to bladder outflow obstruction, but it may be acquired independently with aging. The pathophysiology of detrusor overactivity due to outflow obstruction is the same for prostate cancer as for benign prostatic hyperplasia or any other cause of bladder outflow obstruction.[6] About 75% to 80% of men with prostatic obstruction develop detrusor overactivity and irritative bladder symptoms, including urinary frequency, urgency, nocturia, and urge incontinence.[6] There are quite marked ultrastructural changes that occur in conjunction with this, including collagenous infiltration of detrusor smooth muscle bundles combined with smooth muscle hypertrophy.[7,8] There is also a reduction in acetylcholine-positive nerve profiles in association with an increase in the ratio of abnormal to normal myoneural junctions,[8] both of which is in keeping with a muscular denervation response to the increase in bladder pressure. These changes may be caused by repeated episodes of detrusor ischemia that have been demonstrated in bladder outflow obstruction,[9] and they lend support to the belief that detrusor overactivity results from a post-junctional hypersensitivity phenomenon due to denervation.[10,11] Overactivity in other transmitter systems, such as non-cholinergic activation via purinergic receptors, has also been suggested as an etiological factor.[12] Studies have shown that relief of obstruction restores detrusor stability in about three quarters of patients; in the remaining quarter, it persists.[13]

Iatrogenic incontinence

Iatrogenic incontinence refers to incontinence that arises as a direct result of medical intervention or treatment. Primary treatment modalities for clinically localized prostate cancer include radical prostatectomy, external-beam radiotherapy, and brachytherapy. Cryotherapy is emerging as an alternative treatment option but tends to be reserved for patients with locally advanced cancer or those with recurrent disease after radiotherapy. The incidence and pathophysiology of incontinence following each of these treatments will be considered separately. Transurethral resection of the prostate (TURP) may sometimes cause or contribute to incontinence, and will be considered within the following sections.

Radical prostatectomy

Radical prostatectomy is undertaken as curative therapy for men with localized prostate cancer. By removing the whole prostate, the bladder neck and prostatic smooth muscle mechanisms that normally contribute to continence are lost. Following removal of the urethral catheter after surgery, some degree of immediate incontinence may be anticipated. In the majority of patients, this will be followed by gradual improvement in urinary control and continence. Nocturnal incontinence tends to resolve first, before daytime stress incontinence. Continence on standing from sitting tends to be reestablished last, and retraining contributes considerably to full recovery. In most patients, continence will continue to improve

during the first 2 years after surgery. Persistent and troublesome incontinence beyond 2 years is unusual (see below), but may have a significant impact on the individual's quality of life.[14]

Post-prostatectomy incontinence is usually associated with an incompetent urethral closure mechanism. The clinician should be aware, however, that anastomotic stricture, detrusor dysfunction, or reduced bladder compliance may also contribute to the clinical picture.[15] Detrusor overactivity may have been present preoperatively (see above) or may result from bladder denervation injury acquired at the time of surgery. Functional recovery of continence that generally follows radical prostatectomy implies significant reversibility in the immediate postoperative dysfunction. Alongside resolution of neuropraxia and neuromuscular inactivity, healing, tissue repair, and regeneration may contribute to the function of remaining continence mechanisms. Factors that may promote their functional recovery include the vascularization, innervation, and viability of remaining normal tissues; potential for revascularization, re-innervation, functional tissue regeneration (particularly sphincteric), and mechanisms for compensatory neurologic control are currently poorly understood but may be important in the early postoperative period. Conversely, fibrosis, apoptosis, and ischemia may adversely affect recovery. Similar healing processes may influence recovery of erectile function. The importance of surgical technique and experience for functional recovery has been emphasized by Walsh in his description of the "anatomic radical retropubic prostatectomy"[16] (see Chapter 80).

Operative injury to the rhabdosphincter or its nerve supply is probably the most common factor in post-prostatectomy incontinence.[17] Continence following radical prostatectomy requires a functional distal urinary sphincter, and both active and passive mechanisms contribute to sphincteric competence. Components responsible for passive continence include opposing urethral mucosa for assuring a watertight seal, and fibroelastic and smooth muscle tissue within the wall of the urethra and the rhabdosphincter. The puborectalis part of the levator ani is responsive to sudden rises in intra-abdominal pressure, thereby also contributing to continence. Fibrosis or rigidity of the membranous urethra may compromise mucosal apposition and sphincteric function. Anastomotic stricture associated with sphincteric deficiency must be excluded. On clinical and urodynamic assessment of 88 patients with post prostatectomy incontinence, Groutz et al[18] reported that in 88% intrinsic sphincter deficiency was the cause. One third of men with sphincteric deficiency were associated with detrusor overactivity, whereas isolated detrusor overactivity was present in only 6%; another 6% had outflow obstruction associated with stricture. Other authors have suggested that impaired posterior urethral sensation may contribute to postoperative incontinence by preventing the afferent loop of a guarding reflex of the periurethral striated sphincter.[19]

Reports of incidence for incontinence vary widely in the literature due to differences in definition, method of patient assessment (by physicians, patient questionnaires, or third parties), variations in surgical technique and length of follow-up.[20] Depending on the definition of incontinence (including the wearing of pads), reported prevalence rates after 1 year range from 8%[21] to 69%.[22] Predicting patients who are at risk has also proved problematic. Age is certainly a factor and a number of studies have shown that men over the age of 70 years are more likely to develop urinary incontinence postoperatively.[23,24] The continence index developed by Marsh and Lepor[25] attributes a score based on a clinical assessment of continence, bladder distention volume at the time of urine leakage, and the ability of the patient to stop and start the urinary stream. This score, measured by a clinician at the time of catheter removal post radical prostatectomy, has been shown to be valuable in predicting men who will regain continence and those in whom urinary incontinence will remain permanent. They suggest those men with low scores (a negative indication) should start treatment and biofeedback early in the postoperative period to facilitate recovery.

Surgical factors that contribute to long-term continence rates include meticulous operative technique in preserving the external striated sphincter mechanism, operative experience, and case selection. For individual cases where oncologic control will not be compromised, bilateral preservation of the neurovascular bundles (supplying the membranous urethra as well as penile corpora) may contribute to higher continence rates.[21,26] This effect, however, decreases with increasing age.[27] Employing two pubo-urethral suspension stitches may also contribute to postoperative continence and, by increasing the Valsalva leak point pressure, may reduce the severity of incontinence if it occurs.[28] Bladder neck preservation does not improve the long-term recovery of continence, but in those patients who will be continent, their recovery has been shown to be quicker.[29] The choice of either the perineal or retropubic route has not been shown to effect postoperative urinary incontinence rates.[30] Laparoscopic or robotic radical prostatectomy allows precise construction of the urethrovesical anastomosis in the hands of surgeons who are skilled and experienced in these techniques, and continence may be acquired quickly following (generally earlier) catheter removal. Overall, long-term continence rates appear to be comparable between different surgical approaches.[31]

External-beam radiotherapy

External-beam radiotherapy provides an alternative primary treatment for clinically localized prostate cancer that leaves irradiated prostate and sphincter mechanisms in situ. Side effects may be early (within the first 6 months of treatment) or late (acquired months or years later). In the early post-treatment period, urinary side effects relate to inflammation and may induce a transient clinical syndrome of acute cystitis, with or without prostatitis, including urgency and sometimes urge incontinence. There have been reported incidences from 70% to 90% for mild, 20% to 45% for moderate and 1% to 4% for severe reactions.[32–34] Acute side effects are expected to settle in 4 to 6 weeks, and they are dependent on the volume of tissue treated (pelvis or prostate) as well as radiation dose. Late complications are associated with ongoing chronic inflammation and tissue fibrosis with sequelae that may include chronic cystitis, bladder ulcer, urethral stricture, urinary urgency, incontinence, and impotence. In this late situation, incontinence can arise from a variety of mechanisms: overflow incontinence associated with a fibrotic shrunken bladder, stress incontinence with sphincteric insufficiency, urgency with detrusor overactivity and combinations of these. The incidence of late urinary complications is believed to be dose-dependent and reported in 5% to 12% of cases.[35,36] The overall incidence of urinary incontinence after radiotherapy has been reported as between 1.3% and 7%.[37,38] Patients are at higher risk of urinary incontinence if they have undergone previous TURP, especially if this is performed after radiotherapy.[27] Interestingly, radiotherapy for biochemical failure after radical prostatectomy does not increase the risk of urinary incontinence,[39] but salvage prostatectomy after radiation therapy can have a very high incontinence rate, with reports of as many as 58% to 64% of patients affected.[40,41]

Brachytherapy

In suitable patients, prostate brachytherapy is emerging as an alternative to radical prostatectomy and external-beam radiotherapy for clinically localized prostate cancer.[42] Side effects relate to intervention that manipulates the prostate and leaves it in situ, including prostatitis, urethritis, retention, stricture, and irritative voiding symptoms. Reported rates of urinary incontinence vary from 0% to 6%,[43–51] but, again, interpretation is difficult owing to variations in data collection and dosimetry.

Previous TURP is often considered a contraindication to brachytherapy, and may increase substantially the risk of incontinence, but with recent developments in brachytherapy technique, the risk of damage to sphincter function may be minimized (see Chapter 82). Previous studies where urinary incontinence was not used as a specific end-point have suggested there may be a relationship between urethral morbidity and urethral dose.[52–55] Other reports have suggested the risk of incontinence is increased by combined external-beam radiotherapy and brachytherapy, affecting as many as 41% of patients at 4 years.[56] More recently, McElveen et al[42] demonstrated that high urethral doses and pre-implant (International-Prostate Symptom Score) I-PSS are predictive factors for the development of urinary incontinence, which in their patients was a mild form of stress incontinence. They recommended limiting the urethral dose to as close to the prescription dose as possible and selecting patients with an I-PSS less than 15.

Cryotherapy

Cryosurgery has gained some favor since the mid-1990s as local treatment after failure of primary radiation therapy for prostate cancer or for locally advanced clinical stage disease. Incidence rates for urinary incontinence vary depending on definition and technology, with reported rates around 5% for primary cryosurgery, and 10% for secondary salvage cryosurgery.[57] The risk may be increased in those patients who have previously had TURP.[57] Since urethral-warming catheters have been introduced, the incidence of stress incontinence has declined. Thermocouples allow the temperature around the sphincter to be monitored and maintained at a healthy level throughout the procedure. Urethral fistula should be a rare complication with third-generation cryo-therapy delivering a precisely controlled freeze zone and real time monitoring.

Clinical assessment

On the basis of a medical history, incontinence can be described as stress, urge, or mixed—unfortunately, these descriptions do not necessarily correlate with underlying pathophysiology and urodynamic findings. Patients with overflow incontinence tend to complain of complete loss of bladder sensation with repeated, and at times constant, dribbling of urine with no significant urinary stream or volume. Enuresis may raise suspicion of high-pressure chronic retention with overflow. The history will also identify previous interventions and management strategies that may have significant bearing on etiology and further treatment.

Urgency is an almost irresistible desire to pass urine because of fear of wetting oneself or pain. It is usually sudden in onset, felt in the perineum or suprapubic region, and is not the same as the normal sensation of bladder fullness. Sometimes it may be associated with incontinence if the patient is unable to relieve himself. The presence of urgency resulting in incontinence is strongly linked with detrusor overactivity. In some cases, if the patient has lost awareness of bladder sensation, detrusor overactivity will cause incontinence and leakage without any discomfort. Other symptoms that complete the urge syndrome include frequency (voiding more than once every 2 hours or more than 7 times a day) and nocturia when the desire to pass urine wakes the patient.[58]

With stress incontinence, urine leakage occurs on coughing or with other physical efforts associated with a rise in intra-abdominal pressure. Importantly, there may be concomitant detrusor overactivity (so called "mixed incontinence") that may complicate the clinical picture. Under these circumstances it is imperative that the clinical assessment includes urodynamic investigation and anastomotic stricture is excluded (see below).

Physical signs are not a major part of the clinical picture, but a complete examination should be undertaken in all patients. There may be systemic signs of urinary tract infection or uremia. The bladder may be palpable with urinary retention, but, in some situations, retention can be difficult to detect clinically. Spinal cord compression may be suspected from neurologic examination of the lower limbs. Digital rectal examination (DRE) will assess the extent of local cancer spread. Examination will also contribute to the assessment of a patient's overall health and fitness, an important consideration when planning future treatment.

Initial investigations will be guided by the medical history and examination findings. Urinary tract infection is not only commonly associated with incontinence, but may aggravate it and should be treated. Urine culture will identify infecting organisms and provide antibiotic sensitivities. Ultrasound scans can assess or exclude urinary retention, incomplete bladder emptying, and hydronephrosis. Renal function and prostate specific antigen profile may need to be monitored in particular cases. Pain or dysuria in the absence of infection may require further assessment with imaging (such as computed tomography [CT] or magnetic resonance imaging [MRI]) and cystoscopy.

Uroflow studies showing poor flow in spite of adequate voided volumes suggest underlying bladder outflow obstruction (including the possibility of anastomotic stricture) or detrusor acontractility. An acontractile detrusor may be associated with chronic retention, and it may be due to longstanding bladder outflow obstruction or surgical denervation injury. Where the diagnosis is uncertain and would influence treatment, or a trial of therapy has been unsuccessful, urodynamic assessment is imperative.[18,59] Cystometry may establish the pathophysiology of bladder filling, storage, and emptying.[60] Video-urodynamic studies may demonstrate incontinence and pressure-flow dynamics, and characterise the underlying pathophysiology.

Management of urinary incontinence in men with prostate cancer requires assessment of both sphincteric and detrusor components. Sphincteric insufficiency may coexist with detrusor overactivity, and it may conceal instability where the functional capacity of the bladder is compromised by incontinence; this may also apply during urodynamic assessment. Stress incontinence generally implies a degree of sphincteric insufficiency that may reflect disease or iatrogenic factors. Transurethral resection of the prostate involves resection of the bladder neck mechanism contributing to continence, along with prostate tissue that provides passive resistance to urine flow. Radical prostatectomy, radiotherapy, and TURP may also contribute specifically to weakness of the external striated sphincter.

The number of pads used per day gives a rather unreliable idea of degree of incontinence and its impact on the individual. It is sometimes helpful for the patient to complete a fluid intake/voiding/incontinence diary for a period of days and weigh pads daily. A quality-of-life questionnaire can be used to assess and monitor individual patients.

Treatment

Interventions for incontinence include general advice and conservative measures, with pharmacotherapy and surgery reserved for appropriately selected patients. Attention to fluid intake, diet, and voiding habit may be sufficient for some patients, or will at least reduce extraneous exacerbating factors. Conservative interventions including physiotherapy, bladder retraining, biofeedback, and electrical stimulation can be beneficial alone or in combination with pharmacotherapy. Surgical options are usually reserved for cases in which these measures have failed and troublesome incontinence persists beyond a period necessary for improvement.

Urinary infection should be treated with appropriate antibiotics. Infection must be excluded before invasive urologic investigations or procedures. Urinary retention should also be treated according to its etiology and circumstances. Both infection and retention may exacerbate other causes of incontinence.

Conservative measures

Patients with urinary incontinence may benefit from advice on fluid and dietary intake, identifying those factors that aggravate incontinence due to diuretic effects, bladder irritation, or bowel disturbance. Generally, one and a half liters per day are sufficient for hydration and an adequate urine output. Moderate quantities of tea, coffee, and soft drinks have mild diuretic and irritative effects on the bladder that can be avoided. Specific additives that can be avoided include caffeine and artificial sweeteners. Spicy foods and excessive alcohol consumption should be avoided and a regular bowel habit maintained. Pharmacotherapy for unrelated conditions may aggravate incontinence through effects on lower urinary tract pathophysiology and warrant review. Many of these considerations and other conservative approaches (below) are used in post radical prostatectomy rehabilitation, to be discussed later in this chapter.

For patients with urge incontinence, bladder retraining is a useful initial approach and is often undertaken by continence nurse specialists. Frequency–volume charting gives a starting point for the training, and the patient will have a base line of how frequently he is passing urine (Figure 30.1). The aim is for the patient to suppress the urge to void in order to expand functional bladder capacity, improve the volumes held, and increase continence. Additional pelvic floor exercises may also be helpful.[61] Anticholinergics can be used as a "crutch" until the patient has made some progress with retraining, after which the drug therapy can be discontinued.

Other conservative interventions include electrical stimulation, delivered via a rectal probe or perineal surface electrodes, and may both increase the contractility of the pelvic floor muscles and inhibit detrusor overactivity.[20] There have been studies proposing effective treatment of overflow incontinence outside the context of prostate cancer with electrical stimulation.[62] Other modalities that may be helpful in particular circumstances include hypnotherapy[63] and acupuncture.[64]

For incontinent patients with prostate cancer in whom continence cannot be restored, penile compression devices, urinary

Continence

Frequency – volume chart

Name: _____   Week commencing: _____

☐ In the blank column please record with (i) a tick each time you pass urine, or(ii) an "IE" for each incontinent episode.

▨ In the shaded column please record the amount and type of fluid intake e.g. cup/tea, glass/juice etc.

	Sunday		Monday		Tuesday		Wednesday		Thursday		Friday		Saturday	
6am														
7am														
8am														
9am														
10am														
11am														
Midday														
1pm														
2pm														
3pm														
4pm														
5pm														
6pm														
7pm														
8pm														
9pm														
10pm														
11pm														
Midnight														
1am														
2am														
3am														
4am														
Total														

Figure 30.1
Frequency–volume and continence chart: patients are asked to document fluid intake (including time, volume, and type of beverage), voided urine (time and volume), and episodes of incontinence (if any). This enables the patient and their advisor to relate the voiding pattern to fluid intake, and measures total daily volumes taken and voided over several days.

collection devices, or absorbent pads can be used provided there is not a significant degree of retention.[65] There may be concerns, however, with safety of long-term penile clamp usage. In refractory cases, an indwelling urethral catheter may become unavoidable, particularly where there is otherwise significant retention or renal function is compromised by bladder outflow obstruction. Pelvic tumors including prostate cancer relatively contraindicate suprapubic catheter placement, particularly when local disease is extensive or uncontrolled. Difficulties may arise in relation to their placement and ongoing-care; and a permanent tract can become a conduit for tumor invasion.

Pharmacotherapy

Pharmacotherapy targeting specific mechanisms of lower urinary tract function may contribute to urinary continence and bladder control, either alone or in combination with other conservative or surgical interventions. For instance, sphincter tone may be increased by alpha-adrenergic agonists (e.g., imipramine, pseudoephedrine, and phenylpropanolamine). Such drugs have been shown to improve mild stress incontinence, but cardiovascular side effects can limit their use. Imipramine also has some potentially beneficial anticholinergic activity, acting also in the bladder.

Anticholinergic pharmacotherapy with muscarinic antagonists is the first-line medical treatment for detrusor instability. There are a number of different anticholinergics available each with different efficacy and pharmacokinetics (oxybutinin, tolterodine, trospium). New compounds are being developed, such as solifenacin and darifenacin,[66] that are more selective, theoretically limiting the side effect profile (dry mouth, constipation, and blurred vision). These drugs, in spite of sometimes adverse effects on bladder emptying, surprisingly rarely precipitate urinary retention. It is important to try different anticholinergics and controlled release preparations in individual patients, as their suitability will vary according to efficacy and side effects profile.

Alpha-blockers (e.g. alfuzosin, tamsulosin, terazosin, and doxazosin) relax the smooth muscle fibers of bladder neck and prostatic smooth muscle. These drugs improve lower urinary tract symptoms and quality of life in men with symptomatic benign prostatic hyperplasia, but in men with prostate cancer whose prostate remains in situ, they have an extremely limited role. They have no role after radical prostatectomy, by which the target tissues are removed, and indeed this class of drugs should be avoided (for instance as treatment for unrelated conditions such as hypertension), owing to their pharmacological action that relaxes sphincteric smooth muscle.

Channel transurethral resection of the prostate

Urinary retention, symptomatic bladder outflow obstruction and symptomatic detrusor acontractility may be relieved by channel TURP in men with prostate cancer who have not had radical prostatectomy. Particular care should be exercised in those patients with detrusor overactivity, as relieving obstruction can exacerbate symptoms of detrusor overactivity, especially urgency and urge incontinence. Coexisting sphincter weakness will increase this tendency, and some previously continent patients can be rendered incontinent. Channel TURP restores the lumen of the prostatic urethra and may be performed (with the patient's prior consent) after diagnostic cystoscopy and bimanual examination. It is a palliative procedure that does not attempt complete resection of the tumor bulk. Prostatic stents (e.g., Prostakath, Prostacoil, and Memotherm permanent prostatic stent systems) represent alternatives to channel TURP with advantages over indwelling catheters and repeated TURP procedures. They can also remain in situ if further radiotherapy is required.[67-69]

Post radical prostatectomy rehabilitation

Since sphincter function usually recovers following radical prostatectomy, physiotherapy, bladder retraining, and pharmacotherapy are mainstays of early postoperative rehabilitation. These approaches have been introduced in the above discussion. Electrical pelvic floor stimulation and biofeedback techniques may also be considered for individual patients. Conservative and supportive measures remain important during the phase of functional recovery[70]; these include attention to good skin care, fluid intake (both content and volume), diet, bowel function, and pharmacotherapy. Penile compression devices and condom catheters must be avoided in post-radical prostatectomy patients to facilitate restoration of pelvic floor, sphincter musculature, and reflexes necessary for urinary control and continence.

Stress incontinence may be considerably improved by pelvic floor (Kegal) exercises. These exercises help to strengthen the voluntary urinary sphincter and pelvic floor; bladder control may also improve. They should be practiced every day, and it is important that an individual program for each patient is developed. Both slow and fast contractions should be performed, and this should involve not holding the pelvic floor muscles for more than 10 seconds. It is also important to teach "the knack" (when a pelvic floor contraction is encouraged during an increase in intra-abdominal pressure, for example, with sneezing or coughing). The best positions for patients to be in for performing these exercises are lying on their back with their knees bent up or sitting on a chair with the knees apart. The exercises can then be taught in two parts. First the patient should learn to tighten the anus as though trying to control flatus or diarrhea and second he should imagine trying to stop the flow of urine midstream. This can be taught by suggesting the patient looks in a mirror, whilst standing, to see the base of the penis move nearer to the abdomen and the testicles rise. The patient is then taught to tighten these muscles and hold on, for example, for the count of five, then gently let go and repeat this series of contractions five times. He should also do 20 short sharp contractions once a day. This involves tightening the pelvic floor and immediately letting go. Pelvic floor exercises may be taught prior to radical prostatectomy, and this may facilitate an individual's appreciation of pelvic floor and sphincter control; studies have suggested this may contribute to earlier achievement of continence, but is unlikely to influence persistent or severe incontinence.[71]

Other techniques may be used in conjunction with pelvic floor exercises to improve an individual's exercise technique and stimulate normal pelvic floor function. Biofeedback can be achieved with a small anal probe or skin surface electrodes and either visual display or audio equipment to register pelvic floor activity.[72-74] Specifically, it may promote control and strength of the levator ani muscle. Electrical stimulation may also be used to stimulate the pelvic floor with either an anal probe or surface electrodes.[19,75,76]

If conservative approaches fail the treatment options include collagen injection therapy, implantation of an artificial urinary sphincter, or a bulbourethral sling procedure. Collagen injection therapy tends to give short-term success in 20% to 62% of patients,[77-80] may require repeated injections and is most effective in milder forms of stress incontinence.[16] A study of over 250 patients with over 2 years follow-up showed 20% were dry and 39% were significantly improved with a mean number of injections of 4.4 (range 1–11).[81] Patients with milder incontinence (less than 6 pads/day) had much higher success rates, but often four injections were required for cure. Cespedes[82] also emphasized that more than four treatments may be worthwhile, using injections of 2.5 to 7.5 mL to avoid mucosal ulceration, not less than 1 month apart. Attempts to inject collagen in an antegrade fashion on the basis of better visualization have not yielded significantly better results,[83] and collagen injection is known to be less effective in patients who have a bladder neck contracture or who have undergone radiation, cryotherapy, or bladder neck incision.[16] Collagen injections should be reserved for patients with mild stress incontinence who have failed conservative treatment and who would not be suitable for an artificial sphincter. Allergy to collagen should be ruled out by a prior skin test.

Artificial urinary sphincter placement offers the best opportunity for cure in suitable patients with persistent and troublesome incontinence, with 90% achieving a socially adequate degree of continence, and 30% to 50% achieving dryness.[84,85] A periurethral cuff inserted around the bulbar urethra maintains continence and, when the patient chooses to pass urine, he applies pressure to a pump placed in the scrotum to shift fluid out of the cuff into a reservoir. The cuff opens, the patient voids, the cuff then re-fills with fluid and continence is regained[16] (Figure 30.2). The revision rate after insertion is of the order of one-third, and between 4.5% and 23% will require removal of prosthesis within 10 years due to infection.[86] In the context of previous radiotherapy reports are conflicting; some studies have suggested the continence rate is lower (66%),[87] whereas others have found the outcomes to be similar.[88] In view of these success rates, some urologists would recommend using the artificial sphincter as first line treatment for post-prostatectomy incontinence.[16] Management of incontinence with an artificial sphincter may, however, be complicated by coexisting anastomotic stricture (see below).

The bulbourethral sling procedure is emerging as a third surgical treatment option, originally proposed by Clemens in 1976.[89] There are a number of variations on the technique, but generally a sling is placed transperineally around the bulbar urethra and fixed to the medial aspect of the descending pubic rami using titanium bone screws[90] (Figure 30.3). Sling tension is adjusted intraoperatively in relation to urethral and leak-point pressure. Although initial reports were guarded and perineal discomfort was a persistent complication, more recently reports have been favorably compared to artificial sphincters, with up to 67% of patients becoming pad free and 92% showing some improvement.[90]

The management of post-prostatectomy incontinence may be complicated by coexisting anastomotic stricture. The management of anastomotic stricture depends upon lower urinary tract function and factors that include stricture length and caliber; detailed discussion is beyond the scope of this chapter. Surgical interventions include dilatation, optical incision, or transurethral resection; and patients may be required to carry out regular clean intermittent self-catheterization to prevent recurrence. Continence may improve or recover following treatment of stricture depending on detrusor and sphincter function. In those patients with persistent incontinence,

artificial sphincter placement should be deferred until further recovery of sphincter function is unlikely and the anastomosis is sufficiently healthy and mature that further intervention and intermittent catheterization are not required. In some circumstances where there is a recurrent contracture, an artificial sphincter can be combined with a urethral stent for symptomatic improvement.[91] In severe cases, urethral obliteration by fibrosis may be permitted to restore continence where an alternative continent conduit can be established surgically for intermittent catheterization. A long-term catheter is an undesirable alternative, with its inevitable complications, and ileal loop urinary diversion is a very last resort. Surgical interventions for incontinence other than those for anastomotic stricture and overflow incontinence should generally be deferred for at least 1 year and usually longer to allow sufficient opportunity for functional recovery and healing processes to mature.

Quality of life

Clinicians must appreciate the impact of urinary incontinence, uncontrolled urinary leakage, and urinary wetness for the patient and his family, including their potential effects on quality of life, lifestyle, social behavior, and employment. Studies have repeatedly confirmed that a physician's estimation of urinary incontinence is more favorable than that of the patient.[20,92] The impact on quality of life is measurable and can be substantial. Poor communication by healthcare professionals also adversely affects quality of life, particularly in the early post-treatment period.[93,94] The concept of urinary "bother" has also developed, referring to the annoyance and interference caused by the impairment in lower urinary tract function. Bother may not, however, correlate with the degree of incontinence.[95] Despite observations showing that use of pads is greater and urinary leak after treatment is more common with radical prostatectomy than radiation,[92,96] most patients are satisfied with their treatment decision with no significant difference in bother score between treatments.[95] Attending support groups, and meeting patients with similar experience may encourage individuals, and improve their understanding and access to local resources, and some will in time become active in helping others through similar experiences. Psychological adjustment by patients, and the possibility of changing attitudes with time and experience contribute to the complexity of the relationship between medical decision-making,

A
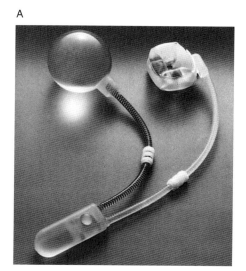

B
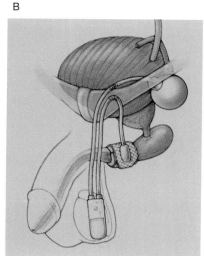

Figure. 30.2
A, AMS 800 Artificial Urinary Sphincter™ (American Medical Systems, MN, USA) device for stress urinary incontinence due to sphincter weakness, including inflatable cuff, pump chamber, and reservoir. B, Drawing showing placement of AMS 800 artificial urinary sphincter with inflatable cuff around bulbar urethra, pump chamber in scrotum, and reservoir in preperitoneal space.

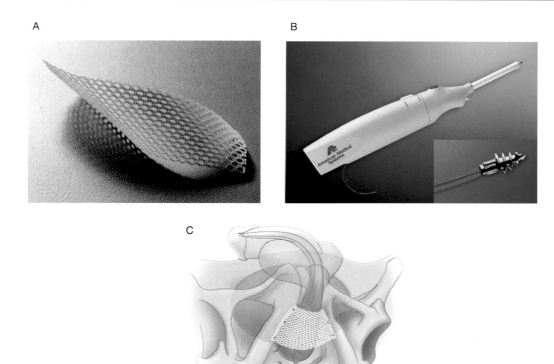

Figure 30.3
Invance™ (American Medical Systems, MN, USA) male urethral sling system for minimally invasive treatment of stress urinary incontinence. *A,* Intemesh™ biocompatible silicone-coated multifilament polyester knitted weave mesh allowing for tissue ingrowth. *B,* Screw inserter and 5 mm self-tapping screw (inset). *C,* Drawing showing mesh in position, anchored with six bone screws inserted into inferior aspect of pubic rami.

urinary incontinence, quality of life and bother. These issues are addressed in detail in Chapters 61, 69, and 70.

Summary

Urinary incontinence is extremely debilitating to patients with prostate cancer. When associated with advanced-stage disease, management can become extremely difficult, particularly after conservative, pharmacologic, and surgical methods become ineffective or inappropriate. In such circumstances, attention to hygiene, skin care, and infection is mandatory, and devices to control urinary drainage such as a penile clamp, convene, or long-term catheterization must be considered according to an individual patient's needs and circumstances.

Fortunately, long-term iatrogenic incontinence is uncommon. With effective treatment strategies and growing numbers of patients having treatment for early-stage disease, iatrogenic incontinence may be a significant problem for individual patients, and faced increasingly by urologists. Incontinence may be due to overflow, detrusor overactivity, incompetent urethral closure, stricture, or a combination of these factors. It is manifest clinically as overflow incontinence, urge or stress or mixed incontinence, and, rarely, continuous incontinence. In the face of such varied underlying pathophysiology, the use of urodynamic assessment should not be underestimated, particularly in those patients with unexplained or persistent refractory incontinence. Patient communication and

education should be emphasized and can have a direct positive influence on patient quality of life. Conservative management includes medical treatment, advice about diet and fluid intake, physiotherapy techniques such as pelvic floor exercises, and bladder retraining. Biofeedback, electrical stimulation, and other specific or supervised interventions may contribute to functional recovery in individual patients. Supportive measures such as skin care and use of absorbent pads are important in all patients, whereas a penile clamp or convene should be avoided during post-prostatectomy rehabilitation and advised only according to individual circumstances. Surgical options for persistent post-radical prostatectomy incontinence include collagen injections, bulbourethral sling procedure, placement of an artificial sphincter, and occasionally complex urologic reconstruction. Urinary incontinence following treatment of early stage prostate cancer is overall an uncommon complication that can usually be treated or managed effectively according to the underlying pathophysiology and individual patient factors.

References

1.   Abrams P, Cardiozo L, et al. The standardisation of terminology of lower urinary tract function report from the Standardisation Sub-Committee of the International Continence Society. Neuro Urodyn 2002;21:167–178.
2.   Herr HW. Quality of life of incontinent men after radical prostatectomy. J Urol 1994;151:652–654.

3. Parys BT, Machin DG, Woolfenden KA, et al. Chronic urinary retention – a sensory problem? BJU 1988;62:546–549.

4. Nielsen KK, Andersen CB, Petersen LK, et al. Morphological, stereological and biochemical analysis of the mini-pig urinary bladder after chronic outflow obstruction and after recovery from obstruction. Neurourol Urodyn 1996;15:167.

5. Saito M, Ohmura M, Kondo A. Effects of long term partial outflow obstruction on bladder function in the rat. Neurol Urodyn 1996;15:157–165.

6. Chapple C, Turner-Warwick R. Bladder outflow obstruction in the male. In AR Mundy, TP Stephenson, AJ Wein (eds): Urodynamics: Principles, practice and application. Churchill Livingstone. 1984, pp 233–257.

7. Gosling JA, Dixon JS. Structure of trabeculated detrusor smooth muscle in cases of prostatic hypertrophy. Urologia Internationalis 1980;35:351–355.

8. Tse V, Wills E, Szonyi G, et al. The application of ultrastructural studies in the diagnosis of bladder dysfunction in a clinical setting. J Urol 2000;163:535–539.

9. Greenland JE, Brading AF. The effect of bladder outflow obstruction on detrusor blood flow changes during the voiding cycle in conscious pigs. J Urol 2001;165:245–248.

10. Andersson KE. Changes in bladder tone during filling: Pharmacological aspects. Scand J Urol Nephrol Suppl 1999;201:67–72.

11. Sibley GN. The pathophysiological response of the detrusor muscle to experimental bladder outflow obstruction in the pig. BJU 1987;60:332–336.

12. Andersson, KE. Overactive bladder – pharmacological aspects. Scand J Urol Nephrol Suppl 2002;210:72–81.

13. Turner-Warwick R. Observations on the function and dysfunction of the sphincter and detrusor mechanisms. Urol Clin N Am 1979;6:13–30.

14. Fowler FJ, Barry MJ, Lu-Yao G, et al. Effect of radical prostatectomy on patient quality of life: results from a Medicare survey. Urology 1995;45:1007–1013.

15. MacDiarmid SA. Incontinence after radical prostatectomy: pathophysiology and management. Curr Urol Rep 2001;2:209–213.

16. Walsh PC. Anatomic radical retropubic prostatectomy. In Walsh PC, Retik AB, Vaughan ED, Wein AJ (eds): Campbell's Urology, 8th ed. Philadelphia: WB Saunders, 2002.

17. Feneley MR, Walsh PC. Incontinence after radical prostatectomy. Lancet 1999;353:2091–2092.

18. Groutz A, Blaivas JG, Chaikin DC, et al. The pathophysiology of post-radical prostatectomy incontinence: a clinical and video urodynamics study. J Urol 2000;163:1767–1770.

19. John H, Sullivan MP, Bangerter U, et al. Effect of radical prostatectomy on sensory threshold and pressure transmission. J Urol 2000;163:1761–1766.

20. Grise P, Thurman S. Urinary incontinence following treatment of localised prostate cancer. Cancer Control 2001;8:532–539.

21. Catalona WJ, Carvalhal GF, Mager DE, et al. Potency, continence and complication rates in 1870 consecutive radical retropubic prostatectomies. J Urol 1999;162:433–438.

22. Bates TS, Wright MP, Gillat DA. Prevalence and impact of incontinence and impotence following total prostatectomy assessed anonymously by the ICS-male questionnaire. Eur Urol 1998;33:165–169.

23. Eastham JA, Kattan MW, Rogers E, et al. Risk factors for urinary incontinence after radical prostatectomy. J Urol 1996;156:1707–1713.

24. Stanford JL, Feng Z, Hamilton AS, et al. Urinary and sexual function after radical prostatectomy for clinically localised prostate cancer: the Prostate cancer outcomes study. JAMA 2000;283:354–360.

25. Marsh DW, Lepor H. Predicting continence following radical prostatectomy. Curr Urol Rep 2001;2:248–252.

26. O'Donnell PD, Finan BF. Continence following nerve sparing prostatectomy. J Urol 1989;142:1227–1229.

27. Smith JA. Outcome after radical prostatectomy depends on surgical technique but not approach. Curr Urol Rep 2002;3:179–181.

28. Campenni MA, Harmon JD, Ginsberg PC, et al. Improved Continence after radical retropubic prostatectomy using two pubo-urethral suspension stitches. Urol Int 2002;68:109–112.

29. Selli C, De Antoni P, Moro U, et al. Role of bladder neck preservation in urinary incontinence following radical retropubic prostatectomy. Scand J Urol Nephrol 2004;38:32–37.

30. Gray M, Petroni GR, Theodorescu D. Urinary function after radical prostatectomy: a comparison of retropubic and perineal approaches. Urology 1999;53:881–891.

31. Herrel SD, Smith JA. Laparoscopic and robotic radical prostatectomy: what are the real advantages? BJU Int 2005;95:3–4.

32. Duncan W, Warde P, Catton CN, et al. Carcinoma of the prostate: results of radical radiotherapy, 1970–1985. Int J Radiat Oncol Biol Phys 1993;26:203–210.

33. Amdur RJ, Parsons JT, Fitzgerald LT, et al. Adenocarcinoma of the prostate treated with external beam radiation therapy: 5 year minimum follow up. Radiother Oncol 1990;18:235–246.

34. Mithal NP, Hoskin PJ. External beam radiotherapy for carcinoma of the prostate: a retrospective study. Clin Oncol1993;5:297–301.

35. Schellhammer PF, El-Mahdi AM. Pelvic complications after definitive treatment of prostate cancer by interstitial or external beam radiation. Urology 1983;21:451–457.

36. Lawton CA, Won M, Pilepich MV, et al. Long-term treatment sequelae following external beam irradiation for adenocarcinoma of the prostate: analysis of RTOG studies 7506 and 7706. Int J Radiat Oncol Biol Phys 1991;21:935–939.

37. Griffiths TR, Neal DE. Localised prostate cancer: early intervention or expectant therapy? J R Soc Med 1997;90:665–669.

38. Lee WR, Schultheiss TE, Hanlon AL, et al. Urinary Incontinence following external beam radiotherapy for clinically localised prostate cancer. Urology 1996;48:95–99.

39. Van Cangh PJ, Richard F, Lorge F, et al. Adjuvant radiation therapy does not cause urinary incontinence after radical prostatectomy: results of a prospective randomised study. J Urol 1998;159:164–166.

40. Pontes JE, Montie J, Klein E. Salvage surgery for radiation failure in prostate cancer. Cancer 1993;71:976–980.

41. Rogers E, Ohori M, Kassabian VS. Salvage radical prostatectomy: outcome measured by serum prostate specific antigen levels. J Urol 1995;153:104–110.

42. McElveen TL, Waterman FM, Kim H, et al. Factors predicting for urinary incontinence after prostate brachytherapy. Int J Radiat Oncol Biol Phys 2004;59:1395–1404.

43. Ragde H, Blasko JC, Grimm PD, et al. Brachytherapy for clinically localised prostate cancer: results at 7 and 8 year follow up. Semin Surg Oncol 1997;13:438–443.

44. Ragde H, Elgamal AA, Snow PB, et al. Ten year disease free survival after transperineal sonography guided iodine 125 brachytherapy with or without 45 gray external beam irradiation in the treatment of patients with clinically localised, low to high Gleason grade prostate carcinoma. Cancer 1998;83:989–1001.

45. Talcott JA, Clark JA, Starck PC, et al. Long term treatment related complications of brachytherapy for early prostate cancer. A survey of patients previously treated. J Urol 2001;166:494–499.

46. Gelblum DY, Potters L, Ashley R, et al. Urinary morbidity following ultrasound guided transperineal prostate seed implantation. Int J Radiat Oncol Biol Phys 1999;45:59–67.

47. Kaye KW, Olsen DJ, Payne JT. Detailed preliminary analysis of 125 iodine implantation for localised prostate cancer using the percutaneous approach. J Urol 1995;153:1020–1025.

48. Brown D, Colonias A, Miller R, et al. Urinary morbidity with a modified peripheral loading technique of transperineal 125 I prostate implantation. Int J Radiat Oncol Biol Phys 2000;47:353–360.

49. Stokes SH, Real JD, Adams PW, et al. Transperineal ultrasound guided radioactive seed implantation for organ confined carcinoma of the prostate. Int J Radiat Oncol Biol Phys 1997;37:337–341.

50. Benoit RM, Naslund M, Cohen JL. Complications after prostate brachytherapy in the medicare population. Urology 2000;55:91–96.

51. Wallner K, Lee H, Wasserman S, et al. Low risk of urinary incontinence following prostate brachytherapy in patients with prior transurethral prostate resection. Int J Radiat Oncol Biol Phys 1997;37:565–569.

52. Desai J, Stock RG, Stone NN, et al. Acute urinary morbidity following I 125 interstitial implantation of the prostate gland. Radiat Oncol Investig 1998;6:135–141.

53. Wallner K, Roy J, Harrison L. Dosimetry guidelines to minimise urethral and rectal morbidity following transperineal I 125 prostate brachytherapy. Int J Radiat Oncol Biol Phys 1995;32:465–471.

54. Merrick GS, Butler WM, Tollenaar BG, et al. The dosimetry of prostate brachytherapy-induced urethral strictures. Int J Radiat Oncol Biol Phys 2002;52:461–468.

55. Zelefsky MJ, Yamada Y, Marion C, et al. Improved conformality and decreased toxicity with intraoperative computer-optimised transperineal ultrasound guided prostate brachytherapy. Int J Radiat Oncol Biol Phys 2003;55:956–963.

56. Joly F, Brune D, Couette JE, et al. Health-related quality of life and sequelae in patients treated with brachytherapy and external beam irradiation for localised prostate cancer. Ann Oncol 1998;9:751–757.

57. Ahmed S, Davies J. Managing the complications of prostate cryosurgery. BJU Int 2005;95:480–481

58. Stephenson T, Mundy AR. The urge syndrome. In AR Mundy, TP Stephenson, AJ Wein (eds): Urodynamics: Principles, practice and application. Churchill Livingston, 1984.

59. Leach GE, Trockman B, Wong A, et al. Post-prostatectomy incontinence: urodynamic findings and treatment outcomes. J Urol 1996;155:1256–1259.

60. Abrams P. Urodynamics, 2nd ed. Springer, 1997.

61. Frewem WM. The management of urgency and frequency of micturition. BJU 1980;52:367–369.

62. Moore KN. Treatment of urinary incontinence in men with electrical stimulation: is practice evidence based? J Wound Ostomy Continence Nurse 2000;27:20–31.

63. Freeman RM, Baxby K. Hypnotherapy for incontinence caused by the unstable detrusor. Br Med J 1982;284:1831–1834.

64. Philp T, Shar PRJ, Worth PHL. Acupuncture in the treatment of bladder instability. BJU 1988;61:490–493.

65. Richardson DA. Overflow incontinence and urinary retention. Clin Obstet Gynecol 1990;33:378–381.

66. Kershen RT, Hsieh M. Preview of new drugs for overactive bladder and incontinence: darifenacin, solifenacin, trospium, and duloxetine. Curr Urol Rep 2004;5:359–367.

67. Aridogan IA, Yachia D. Relief of bladder outlet obstruction caused by prostate cancer using a long term urethral stent (Prostacoil), In Yachia D, Paterson PJ (eds). Stenting in the Urinary System. 2004, pp 435–439.

68. Gottfried HW. Permanent prostatic stent in the management of obstructive prostate cancer in high risk patients. In Yachia D, Paterson PJ (eds). Stenting in the Urinary System. 2004, pp 439–445.

69. Gez E, Cederbaum M. External Irradiation for prostate cancer in patients with urethral stents. In Yachia D, Paterson PJ (eds). Stenting in the Urinary system. 2004, pp 445–453.

70. Hunter KF, Moore KN, Cody DJ, et al. Conservative management for postprostatectomy urinary incontinence. Cochrane Database Syst Rev. 2004:CD001843.

71. Parekh AR, Feng MI, Kirages D, et al. The role of pelvic floor exercises on post-prostatectomy incontinence. J Urol 2003;170:130–133.

72. Jackson J, Emerson L, Johnston B, et al. Biofeedback: a noninvasive treatment for incontinence after radical prostatectomy. Urol Nurs 1996;16:50–54.

73. Bales GT, Gerber GS, Minor TX, et al. Effect of preoperative biofeedback/pelvic floor training on continence in men undergoing radical prostatectomy. Urology 2000;56:627–630.

74. Franke JJ, Gilbert WB, Grier J, et al. Early post-prostatectomy pelvic floor biofeedback. J Urol 2000;163:191–193.

75. Wille S, Sobottka A, Heidenreich A, et al. Pelvic floor exercises, electrical stimulation and biofeedback after radical prostatectomy: results of a prospective randomized trial. J Urol 2003;170:490–493.

76. Moore KN, Griffiths D, Hughton A. Urinary incontinence after radical prostatectomy: a randomized controlled trial comparing pelvic muscle exercises with or without electrical stimulation. BJU Int 1999;83:57–65.

77. Faerber GJ, Richardson TD. Long term results of transurethral collagen injection in men with intrinsic sphincter deficiency. J Endourol 1997;11:273–277.

78. Cummings JM, Boullier JA, Parra RO. Transurethral collagen injection in the therapy of post radical prostatectomy stress incontinence. J Urol 1996;155:1011–1013.

79. Cespedes RD, O'Connell HE, McGuire EJ. Collagen injection therapy for the treatment of male urinary incontinence. J Urol 1996;155:1458A.

80. Politano VA, Stanisic TH, Jennings CE, et al. Transurethral polytef injection for post-prostatectomy urinary incontinence. A urodynamic and fluoroscopic point of view [Surgical therapy of urinary incontinence in the male]. A bladder behavior clinic for post prostatectomy patients. Br J Urol 1992;69:26–28.

81. Bevan-Thomas R, Wesley OL, Cespedes RD, et al. Long term follow up of periurethral collagen injection for male intrinsic deficiency. J Urol 1999;166:257.

82. Cespedes RD. Collagen injection or artificial sphincter for post-prostatectomy incontinence. Urology 1999;55:5–7.

83. Wainstein MA, Klutke CG. Antegrade techniques of collagen injection for post-prostatectomy stress urinary incontinence: the Washington University experience. World J Urol 1997;15:310–315.

84. Marks JL, Light JK. Management of urinary incontinence after prostatectomy with the artificial urinary sphincter. J Urol 1989;142:145–1461.

85. Fishman IJ, Shabsigh R, Scott FB. Experience with the artificial sphincter AS800 in 148 patients. J Urol 1989;141:307.

86. Venn SN, Greenwell TJ, Mundy AR. The long term outcome of artificial urinary sphincters. J Urol 2000;164:702–707.

87. Manunta A, Guille F, Patard JJ et al. Artificial sphincter insertion after radiotherapy: is it worthwhile? BJU Int 2000;85:490.

88. Gomha MA, Boone TB. Artificial urinary sphincter for post-prostatectomy incontinence in men who had prior radiotherapy: a risk and outcome analysis. J Urol 2002;167:591–596.

89. Clemens JQ, Bushman W, Schaeffer AJ. Questionnaire based results of the bulbourethral sling procedure. J Urol 1999;162:1972–1976.

90. Ullrich NFE, Comiter CV. The male sling for stress urinary incontinence: 24 month follow up with questionnaire based assessment. J Urol 2004;172:207–209.

91. Elliot DS, Boone TB. Combined stent and artificial urinary sphincter for management of severe recurrent bladder neck contracture and stress incontinence after prostatectomy: a long term evaluation. J Urol 2001;165:413–415.

92. McCammon KA, Kolm P, Main B, et al. Comparative quality of life analysis after radical prostatectomy or external beam radiation for localised prostate cancer. Urology 1999;54:509–516.

93. Moore KN, Estey A. The early postoperative concerns of men after radical prostatectomy. J Adv Nurs 1999;29:1121–1129.

94. Brockopp DY, Hayko D, Davenport W, et al. Personal control and the needs for hope and information among adults diagnosed with cancer. Cancer Nurs 1989;12:112–116.

95. Moul JW, Mooneyhan RM, Kao TC, et al. Preoperative and operative factors to predict incontinence, impotence and stricture after radical prostatectomy. Prostate Cancer Prostatic Dis 1998;1:242–249.

96. Shrader-Bogen CL, Kjellberg JL, McPherson CP, et al. Quality of life and treatment outcomes: prostate carcinoma patients' perspectives after prostatectomy or radiation therapy, Cancer 1997;79:1977–1986.

31

Rehabilitation of sexual function following definitive treatment of local prostate cancer

Francesco Montorsi, Alberto Briganti, Andrea Salonia, Patrizio Rigatti

Introduction

Radical prostatectomy is an increasingly used therapeutic option for patients with clinically localized prostate cancer and a life expectancy of at least 10 years.[1] The pioneering work by Walsh and Donker[2] significantly contributed to the understanding of the surgical anatomy of the prostate and posed the bases for the subsequent development of the anatomic radical prostatectomy technique, i.e., a surgical approach aimed at completely excising the prostate providing optimal cancer control while maintaining the integrity of the anatomic structures devoted to the functions of urinary continence and sexual potency.[3–5] Since the initial reports on this technique, an increasing number of studies have reported very satisfactory postoperative rates of urinary continence, while the preservation of erectile function after surgery has clearly been shown to be a major challenge for most urologists.[6–8] This finding contributed to the development of an increasing interest in the elucidation of the pathophysiology of postoperative erectile dysfunction (ED) and on its potential prophylaxis and treatment.[9,10] Furthermore ED after radical prostatectomy shows a profound effect on quality of life (QoL). Indeed, it has been shown that more than 70% of patients who had undergone radical retropubic prostatectomy had a moderately or severely affected QoL because of their postoperative ED, when investigated.[11] Moreover, although the International Index of Erectile Function (IIEF)[12] has been widely accepted as a validated instrument to assess ED, it has it has been demonstrated that different definitions of potency after surgery yield different results when applied to the same patients in the same time. This underlines the observation that sexual function entails more than penile erection as the classic definition of potency firm enough for intercourse in fact demonstrated variable agreement.[13]

Patient selection

The anatomic nerve-sparing approach to the prostate is considered for patients with clinically localized prostate cancer. Patients with clinical stages T1 and T2, as defined following digital rectal examination and/or transrectal ultrasonography of the prostate, are the best candidates. As clinical stage is often correlated to both prostate-specific antigen (PSA) values and the biopsy Gleason sum, it has

been suggested that a nerve-sparing approach may be considered in patients with PSA less than 10 ng/mL and a Gleason sum of 7 or less.[14]

Patients being considered for a nerve-sparing radical prostatectomy should be potent prior to the procedure. This is of major importance as patients who report some degree of ED or patients who use phosphodiesterase type 5 inhibitors (PDE5Is) prior to the procedure are more likely to develop severe ED after the procedure itself.[15] The use of validated questionnaires such as the IIEF[12] may facilitate the diagnosis of preoperative ED during the initial patient assessment. This questionnaire assesses various domains of male sexuality, including erectile and ejaculatory function, orgasm, desire, and intercourse satisfaction, and by reviewing the results of this patient self-assessment interesting baseline information are always obtained. Morphology of the corpora cavernosa deteriorates with aging, and this may be correlated with the high prevalence of ED seen in the aging men.[16] Rates of recovery of erectile function after a nerve-sparing radical prostatectomy are inversely correlated with the patient's age, i.e., best postoperative potency rates are obtained in the younger patient population, and it seems reasonable to consider patients of 65 years of age or less as candidates for a nerve-sparing procedure.[3] Patient age seems to be one of the most important factors for the recovery of sexual potency also after unilateral nerve sparing surgery. Indeed, in a group of 46 patients who received unilateral nerve-sparing radical retropubic prostatectomy, 14 (30.4%) regained full potency after surgery and, in the vast majority of them, recovery occurred within a period of 18 months. Of these patients, those aged less than 60 years reported the highest rate of recovery of potency, sufficient for vaginal penetration, after a mean of 13 months after surgery.[17] Comorbid conditions seem also to affect the recovery of spontaneous erections postoperatively as they may impact on the baseline penile hemodynamics. Therefore, a concomitant diagnosis of diabetes mellitus, hypertension, ischemic heart disease, hypercholesterolemia, or history of cigarette smoking identified at the time of the preoperative patient assessment should be taken into account as a potential negative predictive factor for potency recovery after surgery.[15] Although a higher prostate volume could be associated with higher intraoperative bleeding, it does not seem to influence postoperative potency rate.[18,19] Nevertheless, body weight does not seem to be related with the feasibility of a nerve-sparing approach, even in clinically obese patients.[19]

Surgical technique

In suitable candidates, radical excision of the prostate should be performed with the objective of achieving total cancer control (i.e., removing all cancer present in the prostatic tissue), while maintaining the integrity of the anatomic structures on which urinary continence and erectile function are based (i.e., the corpora cavernosa receive the innervation responsible for erections through the cavernosal nerves which branch out from the pelvic plexus). This latter structure is located adjacent to the tip of the seminal vesicles on the anterolateral wall of the rectum and may be damaged during radical prostatectomy. The cavernous nerves course adjacent to small vessels forming the so-called neurovascular bundle along the posterolateral margin of the prostate, bilaterally, and are located between the visceral layer of the endopelvic fascia and the prostatic fascia. The neurovascular bundles are located at the 5 and 7 o'clock positions at the level of the membranous urethra and, after piercing the urogenital diaphragm, they enter the corpora cavernosa where they innervate the smooth muscle cells of the penile vessel walls and sinusoids.[20]

Based on the better understanding of the surgical anatomy of the prostate, Walsh has clearly described the technique of anatomic radical prostatectomy in a step-by-step fashion.[20] The use of a frontal xenon light and of magnifying loupes significantly improves vision during the procedure, and I feel that this armamentarium should be always used when performing nerve-sparing radical prostatectomies. Some crucial surgical steps deserve particular attention. Following pelvic lymphadenectomy, the endopelvic fascia is incised to allow the dissection of the prostatic apex. Care should be taken to ligate small branches of pudendal vessels, which are located just underneath the endopelvic fascia in the area of the prostatic apex; cautery should not be used to secure these vessels in order to avoid damage to pudendal nerve branches also located there. Ligation of the Santorini's plexus is a fundamental step in the procedure as it must guarantee perfect hemostasis in order to obtain the best visualization of the surgical field during the excision of the prostate. Walsh has suggested ligation of the Santorini's plexus distally first, with its subsequent division with scissors; control of the proximal stump of the venous plexus is then achieved with a V-shaped suture, which avoids a central retraction of the neurovascular bundles, thus facilitating the nerve sparing procedure. After controlling and dividing the Santorini's plexus, the visceral layer of the endopelvic fascia should be bluntly incised on the lateral side of the prostate to allow for the gentle lateral displacement of the neurovascular bundles, which is achieved with the use of small sponge sticks. If this maneuver is performed correctly, the neurovascular bundles become clearly visible along their entire course from the membranous urethra and the seminal vesicles in most patients. It is of mandatory importance to avoid the use of the cautery during every step of the prostatic excision as this can facilitate a definitive damage of the neurovascular bundles. As the pelvic plexus is located adjacent to the posterolateral tips of the seminal vesicles, particular care should be taken while excising them. The possible advantage of partially excising of the seminal vesicles to reduce the risk of damaging the pelvic plexus has been reported.[21] Hemostasis must be accurate, and this is usually obtained with small-sized clips. When pelvic hematomas occur, it is advisable to drain them surgically as the fibrosis occurring after the slow spontaneous resolution of any blood collection significantly lengthens the duration of cavernosal neuropraxia. Reviewing the videotapes of one's own nerve-sparing radical prostatectomies and comparing the surgical technique with the results seen in terms of margins status, urinary continence, and erectile function may be of significant importance, as it allows to identify the parts of the operation that are at higher risks for surgical errors from the surgeon.[22]

Pathophysiology of erectile dysfunction following nerve sparing radical prostatectomy

Patients undergoing nerve-sparing radical prostatectomy often experience impairment of erections in the early postoperative period. This has been related to the development of neuropraxia, which is believed to be caused by some damage to the cavernosal nerves that inevitably occurs during the excision of the prostate, even in the hands of most experienced surgeons. Absence of early postoperative erections is associated with poor corporeal oxygenation, which may facilitate the development of corporeal fibrosis, ultimately leading to veno-occlusive dysfunction.[23] Recently, the role of apoptosis has been considered in the pathophysiology of post-prostatectomy ED. Apoptosis, or programmed cell death, is essential for the normal development of multicellular organism as well as for physiologic cell turnover. Morphologically this phenomenon is characterized by chromatin condensation, membrane blebbing, and cell volume loss. In the penis, chronic hypoxia and denervation have been shown to stimulate apoptosis: it is possible that cellular apoptosis leads to increased deposition of connective tissue, which may finally lead to a decrease in penile distensibility.[24–27] Recently, User et al[28] have elegantly elucidated the role of apoptosis in the pathophysiology of post-prostatectomy ED in the rat model. Post-pubertal rats were randomized to bilateral or unilateral cavernous nerve transection versus a sham operation. At different time intervals following the procedure, penile wet weight, DNA content, and protein content were measured. Tissue sections of the penis were stained for apoptosis, and the apoptotic index was calculated. Finally, staining for endothelial and smooth muscle cells was done to identify the apoptotic cell line. Wet weight of the denervated penises was significantly decreased after bilateral cavernous neurotomy, while unilateral cavernous neurotomy allowed much greater preservation of penile weight. DNA content was also significantly reduced in bilaterally denervated penises, while no difference was found between unilaterally denervated penises and controls. Bilateral cavernous neurotomy induced significant apoptosis, which peaked on postoperative day 2. In addition, it was found that most apoptotic cells were located just beneath the tunica albuginea of the corpus cavernosum, i.e., the anatomical area where the subtunical venular plexus is located. Finally, the authors found that apoptotic cells were smooth muscle cells and not endothelial cells. The subsequent hypothesis suggested by the authors was that the bilateral injury to the cavernous nerves may induce significant apoptosis of smooth muscle cells, particularly in the subtunical area, thus causing an abnormality of the veno-occlusive mechanism of the corpus cavernosum. Apoptosis seems to play a role also in the genesis of ED seen in the aging population (which is clearly of crucial importance in the radical prostatectomy patient group) as it has been shown that antiapoptotic genes and proteins are expressed in young rats but not in aging rats.[24] These findings on apoptosis following radical prostatectomy confirm the known fact that most patients reporting postoperative ED develop massive corporeal venous leaks in the long term.[29] However, a reduction of the arterial inflow to the corpora cavernosa in patients with post-prostatectomy ED has been reported by several authors as a significant etiological cofactor.[30,31]

In conclusion, the postoperative combination of reduced penile arterial inflow and excessive venous outflow due to the apoptosis-induced damage of the veno-occlusive mechanism leads to reduced oxygen transport and increased production of transforming growth factor-β. This subsequently causes significant tissue damage, i.e., increased corporeal fibrosis, which not only is at the root of the known penile hemodynamic abnormality but also is probably causing the postoperative decrease of penile length, recently reported in an interesting study.[32]

Pharmacologic prophylaxis and treatment of postoperative erectile dysfunction

Prophylaxis

The better understanding of pathophysiology of post-prostatectomy ED, including the concept of tissue damage induced by poor corporeal oxygenation, paved the way for the application of pharmacologic regimens aimed at improving early postoperative corporeal blood filling. Montorsi et al[33] showed that by using intracorporeal injections of alprostadil early after a bilateral nerve-sparing radical prostatectomy the rate of recovery of spontaneous erections was significantly higher than observation alone. In the author's experience, alprostadil injection therapy should be started as soon as possible after the procedure, usually at the end of the first postoperative month. The initial dose is alprostadil 5 μg. Patients should be instructed to use injections 2 or 3 times per week in order to obtain penile tumescence; injections are not necessarily associated with sexual intercourse, but it is clear that if the patient desires, he may be able to resume satisfactory sexual intercourse with penetration as soon as he is able to identify the correct dosing of the drug. Brock et al[34] have also shown that the continuous use of intracavernous alprostadil injection therapy was able to significantly improve penile hemodynamics and the return of spontaneous erections (either partial or total) in patients with arteriogenic ED, thus confirming a potential curative role of this therapeutic modality in selected patients. The early postoperative use of intracavernosal injection therapy may exert also a significant psychological role. Commonly, after a nerve sparing radical prostatectomy with the slow return of spontaneous erections, a dysfunctional sexual dynamic may develop in couples. The patient withdraws sexually as he is increasingly discouraged with his lack of erectile function, which is a constant reminder of his cancer. The female partner, relieved that the patient has survived the surgery, may be satisfied with his companionship and is not anxious to upset him by making sexual overtures that may frustrate him. Successful intracorporeal injection therapy early after radical prostatectomy may contribute to breaking this negative cycle.[15]

The advent of PDE5Is in the treatment of ED has clearly revolutionized the management of this medical condition. This class of agents acts within the smooth muscle cell by inhibiting the enzyme phosphodiesterase type 5, which naturally degrades cyclic guanosine monophosphate (cGMP) an intracellular nucleotide which acts as second messenger in the process smooth muscle cell relaxation. The cascade of intracellular events that leads to the relaxation of the smooth muscle cell is initiated by the release of nitric oxide, which follows sexual stimulation. Both intracorporeal cavernous nerve terminals and endothelium release nitric oxide, which as a gas diffuses into the smooth muscle cells and activates the enzyme guanylate cyclase, which ultimately catalyzes the reaction from guanosine triphosphate (GTP) to cGMP. Increased levels of cGMP lead to the activation of cGMP-specific protein kinases that activate further intracellular events leading to the final reduction of intracellular calcium—this being associated with smooth muscle cell relaxation. At present, sildenafil, tadalafil, and vardenafil are approved for clinical use in the European Union and have been utilized also to treat post-prostatectomy ED. The rationale for the use of these drugs as prophylaxics is not yet well understood. The basic concept would be to administer a PDE5I at bedtime in order to facilitate the occurrence of nocturnal erections, which are believed to have a natural protective role on the baseline function of the corpora cavernosa. Montorsi et al showed that when sildenafil citrate 100 mg is administered at bedtime in patients with ED of various etiologies, the overall quality of nocturnal erections as recorded with the RigiScan device is significantly better than those obtained after the administration of placebo.[35] Padma-Nathan et al[36] recently reported on the prospective administration of sildenafil 50 and 100 mg versus placebo, daily and at bedtime, in patients undergoing bilateral nerve sparing radical prostatectomy who were potent preoperatively. Four weeks after surgery, patients were randomized to sildenafil or placebo which were administered for 36 weeks. Eight weeks after discontinuation of treatment, erectile function was assessed with the question "Over the past 4 weeks, have your erections been good enough for satisfactory sexual activity?" and by IIEF and nocturnal penile tumescence assessments. Responders were defined as those having a combined score of 8 or more for IIEF questions 3 and 4, and a positive response to the above question. Twenty seven percent of the patients receiving sildenafil were responders (i.e., demonstrated a return of spontaneous normal erectile function) compared with 4% in the placebo group ($P = 0.0156$). Postoperative nocturnal penile tumescence (NPT) assessments were supportive. I believe that in the hands of experienced surgeons, a 27% overall rate of return to normal erectile function after a bilateral nerve-sparing procedure is far from being impressive but the important message from this study is that daily bedtime administration of sildenafil 50 or 100 mg after this procedure should be able to improve every surgeon's baseline results. Although similar data are not available yet for tadalafil and vardenafil, I believe there is no reason not to expect similar findings with these drugs. In practical terms, I feel that the need for postoperative prophylactic therapy should be discussed with the patient when counseling him about radical prostatectomy as one of the treatment options for prostate cancer. Patients must also have the chance to guide their choice by being informed of the pharmacologic approaches needed to recover a normal postoperative erectile function.

Treatment

Phosphodiesterase type 5 inhibitors

Phosphodiesterase type 5 inhibitors have acquired an established role in the treatment of post-prostatectomy ED. As the mechanism of action of this class of drugs implies the presence of nitric oxide within the corporeal smooth muscle cells, only patients undergoing a nerve-sparing procedure should be expected to respond to these agents. Sildenafil is the drug that has been studied more extensively in this patient subgroup as it has been on the market worldwide since 1998. In general terms, it is now known that sildenafil gives the best results in young patients (those less than 60-years-old responding the best), in patients treated with a bilateral nerve-sparing procedure, and in patients who show some degree of spontaneous postoperative erectile function. Sildenafil is usually administered at the largest available dose, although it is common experience to have post-prostatectomy patients responding to the 25 and 50 mg doses. Typically the response to sildenafil has been shown to improve with time after the procedure: best results are seen from 12 to 24 months postoperatively.[5,37–41] Unfortunately, no data from multicenter, randomized, placebo controlled trials assessing sildenafil in patients undergoing nerve-sparing radical prostatectomy are available to date. It has been suggested that the early postoperative prophylactic administration of alprostadil injections allowed a subsequent better response rate for sildenafil, with lower doses of the drug being necessary.[42] Raina et al recently reported the long-term results of sildenafil use in patients affected by ED after radical prostatectomy.[43] This study enrolled 91 patients stratified according to the type of nerve-sparing procedure they had undergone: bilateral nerve sparing (n = 53), unilateral nerve sparing (n = 12) and non-nerve-sparing (n = 26) radical retropubic prostatectomy. All patients, at least 3 months after surgery, were prescribed sildenafil with the starting dose of 50 mg, which was titrated up to 100 mg in cases with unsatisfactory responses. At the 12-month assessment, performed by completion of Sexual Health Inventory of men (SHIM) and Erectile Dysfunction Inventory for Treatment Satisfaction (EDITS) questionnaires, 48 out of the 91 patients enrolled (52.7%) reported successful vaginal intercourse. This percentage increased to 71.7% (38 out of 53) if only those who had had the bilateral nerve-sparing approach were considered. Moreover, at the 3-year follow-up assessment, 31 out of 43 (72%) patients who returned the questionnaires were still using sildenafil for sexual intercourse, with a variable degree of partial erections. Interestingly, when the responses were stratified according to the neurovascular bundle status, the magnitude of improvement in SHIM score over time was greater in the bilateral nerve-sparing group than unilateral nerve-sparing and non-nerve-sparing groups. This data suggests how the vast majority of the patients affected by ED after radical prostatectomy who initially respond to sildenafil continue to do so and are satisfied with the treatment regimen. Furthermore, early use of high-dose sildenafil after radical prostatectomy seems to be associated with preservation of smooth muscle content within human corpora cavernosa. Indeed, Schwartz et al enrolled 40 potent patients affected by localized prostate cancer who underwent radical retropubic prostatectomy at a single institution and were subsequently treated either with daily sildenafil 50 mg (group 1) or 100 mg (group 2) for 6 months starting from the day of catheter removal.[44] Patients underwent percutaneous penile biopsy both preoperatively (under general anesthesia prior to surgical incision) and 6 moths after surgery (using local anesthesia). Interestingly, while in group 1 there was no statistically significant difference change in the mean intracavernosal smooth muscle content between the preoperative and postoperative measurements (51.1% and 52.6%, respectively), in group 2 a statistically significant increase in mean smooth muscle content after surgery (42.8% versus 56.8%; $P < 0.05$) was found. Therefore, although it remains unclear how the chronic administration of sildenafil could increase the intracavernosal smooth muscle content after surgery, daily high-dose administration of PDE5Is may be a key factor in the cavernosal smooth muscle preservation, thus reinforcing the idea of the clinical application of sexual pharmacologic prophylaxis after surgery.

Vardenafil has been tested in patients treated with ED following a unilateral or bilateral nerve-sparing prostatectomy in a multicenter, prospective, placebo-controlled, randomized study done in the US

and Canada. This was a 12-week parallel-arm study comparing placebo to vardenafil 10 and 20 mg. In this study, sildenafil failures were excluded. Seventy-one percent and 60% of patients treated with a bilateral nerve-sparing procedure reported an improvement of erectile function following the administration of vardenafil 20 mg and 10 mg, respectively. A positive answer to SEP question 2 ("Were you able to insert your penis into your partner's vagina?") was seen in 47% and 48% of patients using vardenafil 10 and 20 mg, respectively. A positive answer to the more challenging SEP question 3 ("Did your erections last long enough to have successful intercourse?") was seen in 37% and 34% of patients using vardenafil 10 and 20 mg, respectively[45]

Tadalafil was also evaluated in a large multicenter trial conducted in Europe and in the US involving patients with ED following a bilateral nerve sparing procedure. Seventy-one percent of patients treated with tadalafil 20 mg reported the improvement of their erectile function compared with 24% of those treated with placebo ($P < 0.001$). The erectile function domain score of the IIEF was significantly higher after treatment with tadalafil 20 mg compared with placebo, and this difference was clinically significant (21.0 versus 15.2; $P < 0.001$).[12] Tadalafil 20 mg allowed a 52% rate of successful intercourse attempts, which was significantly higher than the 26% obtained with a placebo ($P < 0.001$).[46]

The adverse event profile of the three PDE5Is was very similar in this patient population, and I feel that discontinuation from treatment with one of the PDE5Is is usually caused by lack of efficacy, while tolerability is overall more than satisfactory. There is a necessity to obtain comparative data between the three drugs in terms of efficacy, safety, tolerability, and overall patient preference also in this challenging patient population . Well-designed head-to-head trials are ongoing at present, and this information will become available soon.

Other medical treatments

Patients either who do not respond to or who cannot use PDE5Is are typical candidates for second-line pharmacologic treatments, which currently include the intraurethral and the intracorporeal administration of alprostadil. The most recent information on the use of intraurethral alprostadil use suggests that its combination with oral sildenafil may salvage a significant proportion of sildenafil failures.[47,48] Intracorporeal injection therapy with alprostadil is effective in the majority of post-prostatectomy patients, regardless of the status of their cavernosal nerves (Figure 30.1). Recently, Gontero et al have shown that the best clinical and hemodynamic response with alprostadil injection therapy is seen 1 month after the procedure, but that the attrition rate for this approach is high when it is started early after surgery. They proposed that, in order to optimize long-term success with intracavernous injections of alprostadil, this treatment should be started 3 months after surgery.[49] In my experience, the use of alprostadil monotherapy should be matched against the use of the combination of alprostadil, papaverine, and phentolamine mesilate. Patients treated with the three-drug combination obtain very high response rates, and report penile pain, the typical adverse event related to alprostadil, only rarely.[50] The major disadvantage of the use of the three-drug combination is caused by its non-availability on the market, which obliges the urologist to prepare the solution and then distribute it to the patient. This off-label use requires the approval of the Ethics Committee of the hospital and a signed informed consent from the patient. In a retrospective study conducted by Raina et al, 102 patients using intracorporeal injections for ED following radical prostatectomy, were assessed by

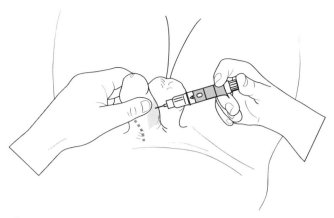

Figure 31.1
The intracavernosal injection of alprostadil is usually effective regardless of the status of the cavernosal nerves.

means of preoperative and postoperative SHIM administration a mean of 4 ± 2.2 years after surgery.[51] Of these 102 patients, 40 had a bilateral nerve-sparing, 19 a unilateral nerve-sparing, and 43 a non-nerve-sparing procedure. Injection therapy, based on use of either PGE1 alone (10 or 20 µg/mL in normal saline; 61%) or high-dose (20 µg/mL PGE1 + 1 µg/mL phentolamine + 30 µg/mL papaverine; 19%) or low-dose (5.88 µg/mL PGE1 + 0.59 µg/mL phentolamine + 17.65 µg/mL papaverine) (20%) triple therapy, was started a mean of 9 months (range: 6–12) after surgical procedure. Overall, 68% (69/102) of the patients achieved and maintained an erection sufficient for sexual intercourse and 48% (49/102) of the patients continued a long-term therapy. This excellent long-term efficacy, despite the type of the intracavernosal compound used, has also been associated with a high compliance that reached up to 70% of patients. Although no statistically significant differences have been reported between the three-drug formulations, no mention has been made by the authors regarding eventual differences in local or systemic side effects.

Cavernous nerve reconstruction

Cavernous nerve reconstruction has generated great interest recently for preserving erectile function after radical prostatectomy. The interest is guided by the premise that nerve grafts provide a scaffold for autonomic nerve regrowth and reconnection with targets that mediate erectile function. Original preclinical studies by Quinlan et al[52] and Ball et al[53] using the genitofemoral nerve as a replacement for resected cavernous nerves in rats introduced the possibility of interposition nerve grafting for the recovery of erectile function after injury of the penile innervation. The surgical application was extended to the human level in the context of radical prostatectomy initially by Walsh who used the genitofemoral nerve as an autologous nerve graft[54] and subsequently by Kim et al[55] who applied the sural nerve as a conduit.

Kim et al described definite promise for cavernous nerve interposition grafting based on their success.[55–60] Among several reports by this group, they described their extended experience involving 28 men undergoing bilateral sural nerve grafting at radical prostatectomy (with a mean follow up of 23 months), of whom 6 of 23 (26%) men completing IIEF questionnaires had spontaneous, medically unassisted erections sufficient for sexual intercourse and an IIEF erectile function domain score of 20.[56] Their inclusion of

4 additional men whose partial erections were enhanced sufficiently to allow sexual intercourse using sildenafil resulted in an overall potency rate of 43% (10 of 23).[56] They also identified the benefit of unilateral sural nerve grafting based on a 78% erectile function rate with this treatment (compared with the 30% rate without grafting), which approximated the level of recovery observed in their hands for men having undergone bilateral nerve-sparing surgery (79%).[55,56]

Other groups have also described their early experiences with sural nerve grafting after radical prostatectomy. Anastasiadis et al described 4 of 12 (33%) men who achieved spontaneous erections sufficient for intercourse based on an IIEF erectile function domain score of 20 (with a mean follow up of 16 months) after unilateral nerve grafting (including one man recovering erections who required bilateral cavernous nerve excision).[61] Chang et al determined that 18 of 30 (60%) patients who underwent bilateral autologous sural nerve grafting achieved spontaneous erectile ability and 13 of these 30 (43%) were able to have intercourse (with a mean follow-up of 23 months).[62]

The evolution of the procedure has related to the application of a variety of technical modifications. One such modification is the use of electrical stimulation to confirm the function and location of the recipient nerve.[58–62] Additional recommendations include the use of microsurgical instruments and loupe magnification, and attention to such procedural details as maintenance of hemostasis within the surgical field and completion of grafting without tension. The feasibility of sural nerve grafting by a laparoscopic approach has also been demonstrated.[63]

Before assigning the fundamental utility of cavernous nerve interposition grafting as for any innovation, the procedure must withstand a critical process of evaluation. Clearly, advantages of sural nerve grafting include the autogenous basis for the nerve conduit, which confers biocompatibility without apparent immunogenicity, as well as support from earlier demonstrations that autonomic nerve replacement grafting succeeds.[64–66] The reportedly negligible functional compromise or consequence from the donor site also represents a favorable consideration. However, concerns persist along the primary grounds that the procedure may be technically impracticable and infrequently useful. The first consideration relates to the difficulty in identifying and performing grafting in humans in which the cavernous nerve is contained within a heterogeneous structure of nerve fibers and blood vessels, unlike the rat in which the cavernous nerve is easily identifiable as a large, discrete cable-like structure. Of greater concern is the issue that the majority of candidates for radical prostatectomy in the modern era of early prostate cancer detection are likely to be satisfactorily treated with nerve-sparing techniques that do not compromise the intent of cancer control. On this basis, the widespread applicability of this procedure may be questioned. Quite likely, the candidate selected for nerve grafting will have high-stage disease that is associated with a low probability of sexual function recovery after surgery and likely will require adjuvant therapy, further reducing the likelihood of the graft preserving erectile function.[54] A fair statement at this time may well be that this innovation requires further investigation, particularly through clinical trials, before establishing its optimal role.

Conclusions

Radical prostatectomy is an increasingly performed procedure in patients with prostate cancer. As the mean age of this patient subgroup is progressively declining due to the advent of prostate cancer screening programs, the demand for optimal postoperative quality of life is becoming more important. Erectile function can be preserved in patients undergoing a nerve sparing radical prostatectomy provided that the patient is rigorously selected prior to surgery and that an anatomic radical prostatectomy following the most modern templates is precisely performed. Pharmacologic prophylaxis, either with oral or intracavernosal drugs, may potentially have a significantly expanding role in the future strategies aimed at preserving postoperative erectile function. The advent of the on demand use of PDE5Is has clearly improved the overall postoperative potency rate also in this challenging subgroups of patients. Future management avenues including cavernous nerve reconstruction and neuroprotection strategies are based on interesting rationales but need to undergo the test of time.

References

1. Holmberg L, Bill-Axelson A, Helgesen, et al. A randomised trial comparing radical prostatectomy with watchful waiting in early prostate cancer. N Engl J Med 200;2347:781–789.
2. Walsh PC, Donker PJ. Impotence following radical prostatectomy: insight into etiology and prevention. J Urol 1982;128:492–497.
3. Walsh PC, Marschke P, Ricker D, et al. Patient-reported urinary continence and sexual function after anatomic radical prostatectomy. Urology 2000;55:58–61.
4. Walsh PC. Radical prostatectomy for localized prostate cancer provides durable cancer control with excellent quality of life: a structured debate. J Urol 2000;163:1802–1807.
5. Rabbani F, Stapleton AM, Kattan MW, et al. Factors predicting recovery of erections after radical prostatectomy. J Urol 2000;164:1929–1934.
6. Stanford JL, Feng Z, Hamilton AS, et al. Urinary and sexual function after radical prostatectomy for clinically localized prostate cancer: The Prostate Cancer Outcomes Study. JAMA 2000;283:354–360.
7. Mulcahy JJ. Erectile function after radical prostatectomy. Semin Urol Oncol, 2000;18:71–75.
8. Lepor H. Practical considerations in radical retropubic prostatectomy. Urol Clin North Am 2003;30:363–368.
9. Montorsi F, Salonia A, Zanoni M, et al. Counselling the patient with prostate cancer about treatment-related erectile dysfunction. Curr Opin Urol 2001;11:611–617.
10. Meuleman EJ, Mulders PF. Erectile function after radical prostatectomy: a review. Eur Urol 2003;43:95–101.
11. Meyer JP, Gillat DA, Lockyer R, et al. The effect of erectile dysfunction on the qulity of life of men after radical prostatectomy. BJU Int 2003;92:929–931.
12. Rosen RC, Cappelleri JC, Gendrano N 3rd. The International Index of Erectile Function (IIEF): a state-of-the-science review. Int J Impot Res 2002;14:226–244.
13. Krupski TL, Saigal CS, Litwin MS. Variation in continence and potency by definition. J Urol 2003;170:1291–1294.
14. Aus G, Abbou CC, Pacik D, et al. Guidelines on prostate cancer. EAU Guidelines, 2005 (in Press).
15. McCullough AR. Prevention and management of erectile dysfunction following radical prostatectomy. Urol Clin North Am 2001;28:613–627.
16. Wespes E. Erectile dysfunction in the ageing man. Curr Opin Urol 2000;10:625–628.
17. Van der Aa F, Joniau S, De Ridder D, et al. Potency after unilateral nerve sparing surgery: a report on functional and oncological results of unilateral nerve sparing surgery. Pros Can Pros Dis 2003;6:61–65.
18. Foley CL, Bott SRJ, Parkinson MC, et al. A large prostate at radical retropubic prostatectomy does not adversely affect cancer control, continence or potency rate. BJU Int 2003;92:370–374.
19. Hsu EI, Hong EK, Lepor H. Influence of body weight and prostate volume on intraoperative, perioperative and postoperative outcomes after radical prostatectomy. Urology 2003;61.601–606.
20. Walsh PC. Anatomic radical retropubic prostatectomy. In: Walsh PC, Retik AB, Vaughan ED Jr, Wein AJ (eds): Campbell's Urology, 8th ed. Philadelphia: WB Saunders, 2002, pp 3107–3129.
21. Sanda MG, Dunn R, Wei JT, et al. Sexual function recovery after prostatectomy based on quantified pre-prostatectomy sexual function and use of nerve-sparing and seminal-vesicle-sparing surgical technique. J Urol 2003;4(Suppl):181.
22. Walsh PC, Marschke P, Ricker D et al. Use of intraoperative video documentation to improve sexual function after radical retropubic prostatectomy. Urology 2000;55:62–67.
23. Moreland RB. Is there a role of hypoxemia in penile fibrosis: a viewpoint presented to the Society for the Study of Impotence. Int J Impotence Res 1998;10:113–120.
24. Yamanaka M, Shirai M, Shiina H, et al. Loss of anti-apoptotic genes in aging rat crura. J Urol 2002;168:2296–2300.
25. Yao KS, Clayton M, O'Dwyer PJ. Apoptosis in human adenocarcinoma HT29 cells induced by exposure to hypoxia. J Natl Cancer Inst 1995;158:656–659.
26. Chung WS, Park YY, Kwon SW. The impact of aging on penile hemodynamics in normal responders to pharmacological injection: a Doppler sonographic study. J Urol 1997;157:2129–2131.
27. Klein LT, Miller MI, Buttyan R, et al. Apoptosis in the rat penis after penile denervation. J Urol 1997;158:626–630.
28. User HM, Hairston JH, Zelner DJ, et al. Penile weight and cell subtype specific changes in a post-radical prostatectomy model of erectile dysfunction. J Urol 2003;169:1175–1179.
29. De Luca V, Pescatori ES, Taher B, et al. Damage to the erectile function following radical pelvic surgery: prevalence of veno-occlusive dysfunction. Eur Urol 1996;29:36–40.
30. Mulhall JP, Slovick R, Hotaling J, et al. Erectile dysfunction after radical prostatectomy:hemodynamic profiles and their correlation with the recovery of erectile function. J Urol 2002;167:1371–1375.
31. Mulhall JP, Graydon RJ. The hemodynamics of erectile dysfunction following nerve-sparing radical retropubic prostatectomy. Int J Impot Res 1996;8:91–94.
32. Savoie M, Kim SS, Soloway MS. A prospective study measuring penile length in men treated with radical prostatectomy for prostate cancer. J Urol 2003;169:1462–1464.
33. Montorsi F, Guazzoni G, Strambi LF, et al. Recovery of spontaneous erectile function after nerve-sparing radical retropubic prostatectomy with and without early intracavernous injections of alprostadil: results of a prospective, randomised trial. J Urol 1997;158:1408–1410.
34. Brock G, Tu LM, Linet OI. Return of spontaneous erection during long-term intracavernosal alprostadil (Caverject) treatment. Urology 2001;57:536–541.
35. Montorsi F, Maga T, Strambi LF, et al. Sildenafil taken at bedtime significantly increases nocturnal erections: results of a placebo-controlled study. Urology 2000;20;56:906–911.
36. Padma-Nathan E, McCullough AR, Giuliano F, et al. Postoperative nightly administration of sildenafil citrate significantly improves the return of normal spontaneous erectile function after bilateral nerve-sparing radical prostatectomy. J Urol 2003;4(Suppl):375.
37. Zippe CD, Jhaveri FM, Klein EA, et al. Role of Viagra after radical prostatectomy. Urology 2000;55:241–245.
38. Lowentritt BH, Scardino PT, Miles BJ, et al. Sildenafil citrate after radical retropubic prostatectomy. J Urol 1999;162:1614–1617.
39. Hong EK, Lepor H, McCullough AR. Time dependent patient satisfaction with sildenafil for erectile dysfunction (ED) after nerve-sparing radical retropubic prostatectomy (RRP). Int J Impot Res1999;11 Suppl 1:S15–22.
40. Feng MI, Huang S, Kaptein J, et al. Effect of sildenafil citrate on post-radical prostatectomy erectile dysfunction. J Urol 2000;164:1935–1938.
41. Blander DS, Sanchez-Ortiz RF, Wein AJ, et al. Efficacy of sildenafil in erectile dysfunction after radical prostatectomy. Int J Impot Res. 2000;12:165–168.
42. Montorsi F, Salonia A, Barbieri L, et al. The subsequent use of I.C. alprostadil and oral sildenafil is more efficacious than sildenafil alone in nerve sparing radical prostatectomy. J. Urol 2002;167:279 [abstract 1098].

43. Raina R, Lakin MM, Agarwal A, et al. Long-term effect of sildenafil citrate on erectile dysfunction after radical prostatectomy: 3-year follow-up. Urology 2003;62:110–115.

44. Scwartz EJ, Wong P, Graydon J. Sildenafil preserves intracorporeal smooth muscle after radical retropubis prostatectomy. J Urol 2004;171:771–774.

45. Brock G, Nehra A, Lipshultz LI, et al. Safety and efficacy of vardenafil for the treatment of men with erectile dysfunction after radical retropubic prostatectomy. J Urol 2003;170:1278–1283.

46. Montorsi F, Nathan HP, McCullough A, et al. Tadalafil in the treatment of erectile dysfunction following bilateral nerve sparing radical retropubic prostatectomy: a randomized, double-blind, placebo controlled trial. J Urol 2004;172:1036–1041.

47. Nehra A, Blute ML, Barrett DM, et al. Rationale for combination therapy of intraurethral prostaglandin E1 and sildenafil in the salvage of erectile dysfunction patients desiring noninvasive therapy. Int J Impot Res 2002;14 Suppl 1:S38–42.

48. Raina R, Oder M, Afarwal A, et al. Combination therapy: muse enhances sexual satisfaction in sildenafil citrate failures following radical prostatectomy (RP). J Urol 2003;4(Suppl):354.

49. Gontero P, Fontana F, Bagnasacco A, et al. Is there an optimal time for intracavernous prostaglandin E1 rehabilitation following nonnerve sparing radical prostatectomy? Results from a hemodynamic prospective study. J Urol 2003;169:2166–2169.

50. Montorsi F, Guazzoni G, Bergamaschi F, et al. Effectiveness and safety of multidrug intracavernous therapy for vasculogenic impotence. Urology 1993;42:554–558.

51. Raina R, Lakin MM, Thukral M, et al. Long-term efficacy and compliance of intracorporeal (ICI) injection for erectile dysfunction following radical prostatectomy: SHIM (IIEF-5) analysis. Int J Impot Res 2003;15:318–322.

52. Quinlan DM, Nelson RJ, Walsh PC. Cavernous nerve grafts restore erectile function in denervated rats. J Urol 1991;145:380–383.

53. Ball RA, Richie JP, Vickers MA Jr. Microsurgical nerve graft repair of the ablated cavernosal nerves in the rat. J Surg Res 1992;53:280–286.

54. Walsh PC. Nerve grafts are rarely necessary and are unlikely to improve sexual function in men undergoing anatomic radical prostatectomy. Urology 2001;57:1020–1024.

55. Kim ED, Scardino PT, Hampel O, et al. Interposition of sural nerve restores function of cavernous nerves resected during radical prostatectomy. J Urol 1999;161:188–192.

56. Kim ED, Scardino PT, Kadmon D, et al. Interposition sural nerve grafting during radical retropubic prostatectomy. Urology 2001;57:211–216.

57. Kim ED, Nath R, Kadmon D, et al. Bilateral nerve graft during radical retropubic prostatectomy: 1-year followup. J Urol 2001;165:1950–1956.

58. Scardino PT, Kim ED. Rationale for and results of nerve grafting during radical prostatectomy. Urology 2001;57:1016–1019.

59. Kim ED, Nath R, Slawin KM, et al. Bilateral nerve grafting during radical retropubic prostatectomy: extended follow-up. Urology 2001;58:983–987.

60. Canto EI, Nath RK, Slawin KM. Cavermap-assisted sural nerve interposition graft during radical prostatectomy. Urol Clin North Am 2001;28:839–848.

61. Anastasiadis AG, Benson MC, Rosenwasser MP, et al. Cavernous nerve graft reconstruction during radical prostatectomy or radical cystectomy: safe and technically feasible. Prostate Cancer Prostatic Dis 2003;6:56–60.

62. Chang DW, Wood CG, Krol, SS, et al. Cavernous nerve reconstruction to preserve erectile function following non-nerve-sparing radical retropubic prostatectomy: a prospective study. Plast Reconstr Surg 2003;111:1174–1181.

63. Turk IA, Deger S, Morgan WR, et al. Sural nerve graft during laparoscopic radical prostatectomy. Initial experience. Urol Oncol 2002;7:191–194.

64. Hammerschlag PE. Facial reanimation with jump interpositional graft hypoglossal facial anastomosis and hypoglossal facial anastomosis: evolution in management of facial paralysis. Larynogoscope 1999;109:1–23.

65. Hogikyan ND, Johns MM, Kileny PR, et al. Motion-specific laryngeal reinnervation using muscle-nerve-muscle neurotization. Ann Otol Rhinol Laryngol 2001;110:801–810.

66. Golub DM, Kheinman FB, Novikov II, et al. Reinnervation of internal organs and vessels by the neuropexy technic. Arkh Anat Gistol Embriol 1979;76:5–16.

32

The limitations of evidence-based comparisons of treatment for localized prostate cancer

Lars Ellison

Introduction

The primary goal of evidence-based medicine (EBM) is the rapid and efficient diffusion of new medical findings in order to effect rational changes in clinical practice patterns. To achieve this goal, analytic techniques for EBM rely heavily on the use of standard measures of patient outcome. For many disease states, reliance on patient outcome measures is not an impediment: for example, viral load counts and low-density lipoproteins (LDL) levels are effective outcome measures in human immunodeficiency virus (HIV) infection and cardiac disease, respectively.

However, measures of outcome for patients with localized prostate cancer are not standardized: there is no agreement on the use of prostate-specific antigen (PSA) as a biomarker, nor is there an accepted gold standard for the measurement of quality-of-life issues. In this chapter, I argue that the failure of the prostate cancer research community to identify standard endpoints for reporting treatment outcomes has resulted in a heterogeneous literature that defies the application of EMB techniques to comparisons of treatment for localized prostate cancer. Until such time as standard endpoints are agreed upon the development of best practice guidelines for treatment of localized prostate cancer using EBM will remain highly problematic.

Background

The challenge of translating bench research to bedside patient care has always been difficult. Often the findings of basic science require multiple refinements prior to the development of meaningful and practical clinical applications. Since the end of World War II and the sudden expansion of medical funding in the United States, the guiding principal of medical practice has been the integration of detailed understanding of pathophysiology combined with "expert" interpretation regarding the best methods for treatment.[1] This marriage of scientific method and opinion thus form the nexus at which the practice of medicine becomes an "Art."

Expert opinion is intended to provide objective and informed practice recommendations. The strengths of this approach are self-evident. Experts tend to have a strong basic science background and, therefore, work at the interface between bench research and clinical application. Their broad knowledge as thought leaders gives them unique perspective regarding the relative value of new findings. In addition, these same individuals often are involved with key regulatory, policy and research funding decisions.

The problem with reliance of this form of analysis is that it is subject to a number of significant biases that, in the estimation of many, far outweigh the relative benefits.[2] The primary concern is that opinion may not represent the full spectrum of data. Often, these thought pieces reflect an aspect of the research agenda of the author and may not incorporate the findings of other lines of inquiry. The resulting unstructured analysis of the literature is subject to both intentional and unintentional omissions.[3] Second, not every important clinical observation has an *a priori* set of basic science findings. What is more, at times the underlying basic science may stand in stark contrast to the observed outcomes at the clinical level. While this may seem obvious, it is just this type of discordance that is subject to omission in an opinion-based system. When studies contradict basic science, or stand alone as observation, they tend to receive minimal attention.[4]

Evidence-based medicine concepts

It is from these criticisms of "expert opinion" that the competing concept of "evidence-based medicine" was born. In the late 1980s, individuals at Macallister University began to discuss the limitations of developing medical practice patterns in the face of an ever-increasing volume of scientific findings.[5] The primary concern was that the rapid expansion of medical literature was far outpacing the rate of change in medical practice. As a result of this expansion, it became necessary to develop systems for analyzing the quality of studies reported, and then rank ordering and aggregating data when possible.[6] While the concepts of meta-analysis and structured literature reviews had been described previously, these have served as the cornerstones for this new movement.

The accepted definition of EBM is "the explicit, judicious and conscientious use of current best evidence from health care research in decisions about the care of individuals and populations."[5] To achieve this end, three broad elements from the principals of clinical epidemiology arise for grading studies. First, the research question must be clearly identified and must address a clinically relevant issue. Unfortunately, for many peer reviewed journals this most basic of premises is not rigorously upheld.[7] Second, the study design must be concise, reproducible, and free of inherent biases. Many studies suffer from failure to use validated quality-of-life instruments or standard clinical endpoints. Third, the study population must resemble the usual clinical population. Highly selected subgroups modify treatment effect and result in blunted outcomes when applied to the general population. Finally, the outcomes measured must be relevant to patients. While biochemical measures may appease patient's anxiety, ultimately, the hard outcomes of morbidity and mortality are what drive patient adherence and compliance.

Rank ordering the importance of studies is the second step in this process. One particularly appealing ranking system is that used by the American Society of Clinical Oncology (ASCO).[8] Within this hierarchy, the randomized trial retains its position as the gold standard for study design. However, combining the data from multiple comparable studies in a scientific manner, the meta-analysis provides greater accuracy for point estimates of true clinical effect. Interestingly, it is important to note that committee reports and expert opinion hold a ranking below that of a clinical case series. This serves as a rather scathing indictment of what has traditionally been considered the preeminent method of disseminating new recommendations for clinical practice.

As the 1990s progressed, the EBM concept became the driving force behind efforts to take the lessons from published studies and, where appropriate, implement the findings into usual practice. The guiding principal is that scientific observations should define best practices. This necessitates that the system of evaluating studies for scientific and clinical merit is reliable and reproducible. On the surface, this appears as a perfectly reasonable application of sound epidemiologic and applied research analysis of study design and outcome.

Fluid endpoints are the failure of prostate cancer research

Prostate cancer is clearly a disease that has significant associated morbidity and mortality. There is mounting evidence that active treatment has beneficial effect on survival.[9] However, the indolent course of the disease means that survival, the one true hard outcome, requires years of observation.[10] Consequently, even large well-designed studies suffer from low event rates, loss of participants, and confounding medical conditions.

In order to circumvent this limitation, there has been a long and to date fruitless search for surrogate primary endpoints.[11–17] Prostate-specific antigen has been the obvious primary target of this search. The correlation with long-term survival and trends in PSA after definitive local therapy is weak at best. To be sure, recent findings regarding PSA velocity hold promise as prognostic indicators for specific subgroups of prostate cancer patients.[18] Indeed, the failure to predict recurrence has provided quality-of-life advocates fertile ground for active commentary regarding the relative value of the available primary treatments. The net result has been a slow but steady transition of the debate regarding the value of these treatments from that of "cancer control" and "survival" to that of preservation of "quality of life."

The primary failure of prostate cancer research is the absence of accepted standards for assessing and reporting outcomes after definitive therapy. It appears that the success of population-based prostate cancer screening has served as the primary driver in reductions in prostate cancer mortality since the mid-1990s. While the screening issue has not been without debate, the actual practice of screening when performed is relatively uniform, with set protocols prompting further evaluation of the patient. However, once initial treatment has been delivered, broad consensus on follow-up intervals and thresholds for definition of cancer control are lacking. This

disconnect is a function of the failure of the radiation therapists and urologists to identify common biochemical trends shared by the competing treatment modalities.

Health-related quality of life (HRQOL) has also suffered from a lack of consensus of definitions. This is, in large part, due to the limitations of previously available instruments. As more accurate instruments have been developed, application of these to ever larger cohorts of men have been attempted.[19] To date, studies have been primarily limited to single institutions.[20]

I would argue that the inability to identify standard methods for assessing patient outcome has precluded prostate cancer from the benefits of widespread application of EBM analysis. Essentially, there is minimal capacity for comparisons of different treatments (radical prostatectomy [RP], external-beam radiotherapy [EBRT], and brachytherapy) because the various stakeholders have been incapable of agreeing on standard reporting schemes of patient outcomes.

Urology

The plausibility that PSA is a biochemical surrogate for disease status after initial treatment of prostate cancer is in large part based on the observed performance of PSA as a screening tool. This argument is supported by multiple observational studies that have correlated the changes in serum concentration of PSA after RP with subsequent patient outcomes (local recurrence, development of metastases, and disease-specific mortality).

Partin et al reported a retrospective review of PSA trends in 955 men treated with RP over a 10-year period (1982–1991).[21] Of those men whose PSA became detectable, 28% developed evidence of local or metastatic disease. In addition, when stratified by postoperative year of failure, men with detectable PSA within the first year had significantly higher rates of progression than men with detectible PSA found after the first year.

The threshold for the definition of "detectible PSA" has been examined by a number of authors.[22,23] While a consensus on the critical absolute serum concentration of "detectible" PSA has not been reached (<0.1 ng/mL versus 0.2 ng/mL versus 0.4ng/mL), it has been accepted that the postoperative level should be very low and remain as such.

A rising PSA is accepted as a poor prognostic sign. Pound analyzed 1997 men treated with RP between 1982 and 1997.[24] In this case series 15% of men developed a rising PSA. Of these 304 men, the median time to metastasis was 8 years. The median survival from the time of the development of distant metastasis was 5 years. Furthermore, the authors identified time of biochemical recurrence, pathologic grade (Gleason score), and PSA doubling time as predictors of progression to metastatic disease.

The net result is that there are as many competing surveillance strategies as "thought leaders." As a result, the heterogeneity of study design precludes systematic aggregation of data and EBM-type generation of best practice guidelines.

Radiation oncology

In contrast to single institution reports and competing proposed criteria for cancer control in the urologic literature, the American Society for Therapeutic Radiology and Oncology (ASTRO) convened a consensus panel to develop a set of criteria for patients treated with radiation therapy for prostate cancer.[25] The report outlined the salient characteristics of PSA and a set of guidelines for post-treatment surveillance. Among the guiding principals were two key concepts. First, that post-treatment PSA nadir should be used in place of an absolute serum threshold. Second, that time of failure should be determined from backdating a sequentially rising PSA. The guidelines were intended to unify management within radiation oncology, and to set standards for reporting outcomes. Since the publication of the ASTRO criteria, a number of studies have critically appraised and offered refinement to the guidelines.

Reports in the radiation therapy literature have generally provided evidence that early trends in PSA using the ASTRO criteria predict general measures of disease control. Horwitz reported correlation between biochemical failure and 5-year actuarial distant metastasis-free survival, disease-free survival, cause-specific survival, and local control.[26] Despite the short follow-up, the authors determined that ASTRO defined biochemical failure appropriately predicted clinical outcome at 5 years. Following on this study, Shipley conducted a pooled analysis of 1765 men with clinically localized disease, treated at six different institutions between 1988 and 1995.[27] Using the ASTRO criteria, the PSA failure rate for a subset of men whose presentation PSA was less than 10 ng/mL was 22% at 5 years and 27% at 7 years.

More recently, others have suggested that PSA velocity may be a better predictor than consecutive rises, and alternatively that the threshold nadir of 1.0 ng/mL may provide better discrimination of probability of progression.[28]

ASTRO criteria applied to surgery cohorts

A number of researchers have attempted to apply the ASTRO criteria to post-RP patients. D'Amico reported trends in PSA failure using the ASTRO criteria as applied to a pooled two-institution data set of surgery, eternal-beam radiotherapy, and brachytherapy patients.[11] Relative risks of PSA failure by treatment modality and pretreatment risk groups were reported. Amling applied ASTRO criteria to RP patients.[29] While the analysis suggested a higher threshold for the definition of PSA recurrence might be more appropriate, they found the radiation therapy standard provided poor accounting of disease progression.

The definition of cancer control is critical. The absence of an accurate and broadly applicable yardstick for the assessment of prostate cancer treatment is a major problem. Urologists have attempted to use PSA thresholds as critical indicators of cancer control. Radiation therapists have applied PSA trends as the defining characteristics of cancer control. Either approach in isolation has significant limitations and biases one treatment over the other. Ultimately, the goal of a biochemical definition of cancer control is to guide appropriate initiation of adjuvant therapy. Currently, a single definition of cancer control does not exist. As long as there are heterogeneous definitions of cancer control, accurate evidence-based comparisons of treatments for localized prostate cancer will not be possible.

Health-related quality-of-life instruments

While a single definition of cancer control has remained elusive, health-service researchers have begun to standardize the measure-

ment of the known complications associated with the treatment of localized prostate cancer (e.g., urinary incontinence and impotence). The quality-of-life field has moved from simple studies measuring cross-sectional or retrospective HRQOL after treatment, to elegant longitudinal prospective models. Along with increased sophistication of study design, the instruments for measurement of quality of life have improved.

With the introduction of the University of California Los Angeles Prostate Cancer Index (UCLA-PCI), assessment of prostate cancer-specific HRQOL took a significant leap forward.[19] Prior instruments incorporated crude measures of general urinary and sexual function and were intended for use in men with advanced prostate cancer. The UCLA-PCI has been recently modified.[20] The new Expanded Prostate Cancer Index (EPIC) allows for accurate discrimination between the domains of urinary incontinence and irritative symptoms. In addition, the instrument quantifies the impact of hematuria, provides an expanded assessment of bowel function, and measures the impact of hormone ablation. These are critical domains when comparing the effects of surgery versus those of radiation therapy.

Application of the EPIC instrument to a retrospective cohort of patients treated either with RP or brachytherapy from a single institution was recently reported.[30] The results suggest that 1 year after treatment, brachytherapy patients have preponderance of irritative urinary symptoms, whereas surgery patients are more likely to have problems with urinary incontinence. In addition, the impact of hormonal symptoms on HRQOL appears much greater than previously appreciated.

It has been assumed that RP, EBRT, and brachytherapy each have an associated constellation of potential complications. The development and acceptance of a single instrument for measuring HRQOL is an important contribution. Application of such an instrument in a multi-institutional and multi-treatment longitudinal setting would provide robust benchmark data to which future trials data could be compared.

Conclusion

Prostate cancer is an important medical condition that has fallen victim to the tradition model of medical education in the United States. "Expert opinion" has failed to identify common standard endpoints to measure the performance of the various initial treatments for localized disease. The result is a heterogeneous body of literature that in large part does not lend itself to analysis using evidence-based measures. What is more, there is no will on the part of the treating stakeholders (urologists and radiation therapists) to accept that true equipoise exists regarding radical surgery and radiation therapy. The failures of the SPIRIT Trial to achieve recruitment goals, and my own personal experience attempting to initiate a cohort study comparing high-volume treatment centers underscores these barriers to change.

If prostate cancer patients are to benefit from rapid acceptance and diffusion of important clinically relevant medical advances, the treating community must first identify standard and well-defined outcome measures for biochemical cancer control as well as HRQOL. These standards must become the core of prostate cancer clinical trials. Additionally, the editors of major medical journals must embrace these as minimum standards to manuscripts entering into the peer review process. Until this happens EBM will remain an outsider to the debates that surround the treatment of localized prostate cancer.

References

1. Haynes RB. What kind of evidence is it that Evidence-Based Medicine advocates want health care providers and consumers to pay attention to? BMC Health Serv Res 2002;2:3.

2. Woolf SH, Grol R, Hutchinson A, et al. Clinical guidelines: potential benefits, limitations, and harms of clinical guidelines. BMJ 1999;318:527–30.

3. Haynes RB, Wilczynski NL. Optimal search strategies for retrieving scientifically strong studies of diagnosis from Medline: analytical survey. BMJ 2004;328:1040.

4. Bornstein BH, Emler AC. Rationality in medical decision making: a review of the literature on doctors' decision-making biases. J Eval Clin Pract 2001;7:97–107.

5. Haynes RB. Evidence-based medicine and healthcare: advancing the practice. Singapore Med J 2004;45:407–409.

6. Upshur RE. Seven characteristics of medical evidence. J Eval Clin Pract 2000;6:93–97.

7. Seigel D. Clinical trials, epidemiology, and public confidence. Stat Med 2003;22:3419–3425.

8. Smith TJ, Somerfield MR. The ASCO experience with evidence-based clinical practice guidelines. Oncology (Huntingt) 1997;11:223–227.

9. Johansson JE, Andren O, Andersson SO, et al. Natural history of early, localized prostate cancer. JAMA 2004;291:2713–2719.

10. Neugut AI, Grann VR. Waiting time in prostate cancer. JAMA 2004;291:2757–2758.

11. D'Amico AV, Desjardin A, Chung A, et al. Assessment of outcome prediction models for patients with localized prostate carcinoma managed with radical prostatectomy or external beam radiation therapy. Cancer 1998;82:1887–1896.

12. de Reijke TM, Collette L. EORTC prostate cancer trials: what have we learnt? Crit Rev Oncol Hematol 2002;43:159–165.

13. Eisenberger M, Partin A. Progress toward identifying aggressive prostate cancer. N Engl J Med 2004;351:180–181.

14. Lieberman R, Nelson WG, Sakr WA, et al. Executive Summary of the National Cancer Institute Workshop: Highlights and recommendations. Urology 2001;57:4–27.

15. Scher HI, Mazumdar M, Kelly WK. Clinical trials in relapsed prostate cancer: defining the target. J Natl Cancer Inst 1996;88:1623–1634.

16. Schroder FH, Kranse R, Barbet N, et al. Prostate-specific antigen: A surrogate endpoint for screening new agents against prostate cancer? Prostate 2000;42:107–115.

17. Woolf SH, Rothemich SF. Screening for prostate cancer: the roles of science, policy, and opinion in determining what is best for patients. Annu Rev Med 1999;50:207–221.

18. D'Amico AV, Moul JW, Carroll PR, et al. Surrogate end point for prostate cancer-specific mortality after radical prostatectomy or radiation therapy. J Natl Cancer Inst 2003;95:1376–1383.

19. Litwin MS, Hays RD, Fink A, et al. The UCLA Prostate Cancer Index: development, reliability, and validity of a health-related quality of life measure. Med Care 1998;36:1002–1012.

20. Wei JT, Dunn RL, Litwin MS, et al. Development and validation of the expanded prostate cancer index composite (EPIC) for comprehensive assessment of health-related quality of life in men with prostate cancer. Urology 2000;56:899–905.

21. Partin AW, Pound CR, Clemens JQ, et al. Serum PSA after anatomic radical prostatectomy. The Johns Hopkins experience after 10 years. Urol Clin North Am 1993;20:713–725.

22. Patel A, Dorey F, Franklin J, et al. Recurrence patterns after radical retropubic prostatectomy: clinical usefulness of prostate specific antigen doubling times and log slope prostate specific antigen. J Urol 1997;158:1441–1445.

23. Zincke H, Oesterling JE, Blute ML, et al. Long-term (15 years) results after radical prostatectomy for clinically localized (stage T2c or lower) prostate cancer. J Urol 1994;152:1850–1857.

24. Pound CR, Partin AW, Eisenberger MA, et al. Natural history of progression after PSA elevation following radical prostatectomy. JAMA 1999;281:1591–1597.

25. Consensus statement: guidelines for PSA following radiation therapy. American Society for Therapeutic Radiology and Oncology Consensus Panel. Int J Radiat Oncol Biol Phys 1997;37:1035–1041.

26. Horwitz EM, Vicini FA, Ziaja EL, et al. The correlation between the ASTRO Consensus Panel definition of biochemical failure and clinical outcome for patients with prostate cancer treated with external beam irradiation. American Society of Therapeutic Radiology and Oncology. Int J Radiat Oncol Biol Phys 1998;41:267–272.

27. Shipley WU, Thames HD, Sandler HM, et al. Radiation therapy for clinically localized prostate cancer: a multi-institutional pooled analysis. JAMA 1999;281:1598–1604.

28. Critz FA, Williams WH, Holladay CT, et al. Post-treatment PSA < or = 0.2 ng/mL defines disease freedom after radiotherapy for prostate cancer using modern techniques. Urology 1999;54:968–971.

29. Amling CL, Bergstrath EJ, Blute ML, et al. Defining prostate specific antigen progression after radical prostatectomy: what is the most appropriate cut point? J Urol 2001;165:1146–1151.

30. Wei JT, Dunn RL, Sandler HM, et al. Comprehensive comparison of health-related quality of life after contemporary therapies for localized prostate cancer. J Clin Oncol 2002;20:557–566.

33

Reflections on prostate cancer: personal experiences of two urologic oncologists

Paul H Lange, Paul F Schellhammer

Introduction

This chapter aims to enhance urologists' understanding of certain subjective events surrounding radical prostatectomy. We both had radical prostatectomies several years ago and were emotionally, and in one case practically, involved in each other's surgical process (Paul H Lange (PHL) performed the radical prostatectomy on Paul F Schellhammer (PFS)). We are urologists whose practical and academic interests (and accomplishments) have principally centered on prostate cancer. Also, we have been close friends for many years and thus have had frequent occasions to reflect on and discuss many facets of prostate cancer in relation to our own experiences. We will individually describe the experiences surrounding our diagnoses, surgeries, and subsequent events, using them as discussion points for academic commentaries. Finally, we will present our mutual insights about these experiences. While this effort is highly personal, for a variety of reasons we have chosen to say very little about the sexual aspects of our experiences other than to state that the outcome has been satisfactory to both of us: PHL had a bilateral nerve-sparing prostatectomy and has no problem, and PFS had a unilateral nerve-sparing prostatectomy and uses some assistance. In the realm of sexual performance and urinary function, satisfactory post-treatment outcomes are very much predicated on pretreatment knowledge and expectations. In brief, we both were very much aware of what we were getting into and were very satisfied with the quality of life afterwards. The key word is "awareness." Unrealistic expectations that life will not be altered after treatment can lead to a dissatisfied patient.

Reflections of PHL

Though we had known of each other early in our academic careers, the friendship between PFS and I deepened over events involving prostate cancer in my family. Briefly, my father-in-law, who lived in the Norfolk area, had a transurethral resection of the prostate (TURP) for benign disease carried out by PFS's partner, Charles Devine. When Charles retired, PFS took over my father-in-law's routine care, and we then began to communicate regularly about that care. Several years later I got a letter from PFS apologizing that my father-in-law, now 82 years old, had been given a PSA blood test by mistake. I was informed that his PSA level was 20 ng/ml, and, because I had by then started speaking and publishing on the use of PSA,[1]

PFS asked for my advice. Of course, we did not then appreciate the importance of a PSA of 20 ng/ml and, while healthy, my father-in-law was 82! I do remember enquiring of some of my urologic oncology friends, and particularly remember one very famous one who looked at me as if I were crazy to even contemplate following up on the PSA. So I advised (and PFS agreed) that nothing be done or even followed, and I thwarted off the confusions of my wife and my extended family about why I was not concerned, if PSA was so important and prostate cancer so serious. PFS did confirm that my father-in-law's digital rectal examination (DGE) was unremarkable for a post-TURP patient.

Over the next 2 years my father-in-law watched his brother-in-law and two of his close golfing partners die from prostate cancer. During this time I tried to educate him about length and lead-time biases over diagnosis and so forth. He was very intelligent but had a business man "bottom line" personality at heart. He kept asking, given that prostate cancer was a possibility, didn't I want to diagnose and possibly treat it, especially since his mother was still alive at 102. Finally, PFS and I acquiesced, got a PSA, which now was 30 ng/ml, caved in to a biopsy in this benign feeling gland, and got a diagnosis of grade 4/3 prostate cancer. His staging studies were negative. My father-in-law had recently lost his wife, was uninterested in sexual activity, and was adamant about beginning therapy, which was hormone ablation. This therapy lasted for 13 years, his PSA remained undetectable, and he had no serious obvious complications from the therapy. He died recently of cardiac failure at 97 years. My wife's family (and my father-in-law when he was alive) were incredulous that anyone would say that this aggressive approach to diagnosis and therapy did not extend his life, and I must admit that I am hard pressed to deny their position.

During this time, PFS and I used this management dilemma and my yearly visits to the Norfolk area to visit family to deepen our relationship and conversations about prostate cancer in general. Little did we suspect that later in our acquaintance this subject would become more personally important.

PFS Perspective

As the urologist to whom PHL's family looked for counseling and care, I shared the misgivings of "attacking" prostate cancer in an asymptomatic octogenarian. When treatment was begun and the PSA level plummeted to and remained undetectable, the patient's anxiety and apprehension vanished, and his energy seemed primed at each visit, which yielded a normal DRE and an undetectable PSA level.

I was providing medicine that was certainly good for his soul and wellbeing, regardless of how operative it was in extending survival. I also achieved a somewhat heroic status as a healer and was so recognized at the large family reunions I was fortunate to attend. As physicians we are privileged to enjoy this respect but must be cautious not to become enamored and entitled by it.

Radical prostatectomy

I was involved in the early elucidation of the clinical value of serum PSA,[1] and I first measured my own PSA when I was in my early 40s in 1984 as part of these experimental efforts. The level was 0.7 ng/ml. I was reassured; that value was considered normal. Of course, today we have a different perspective. For example, in the Prostate Cancer Prevention Trial (PCPT), as many as 15% of men with a PSA level less than 4 ng/ml over a 7-year period were found to have prostate cancer, and 5% of these cancers were found when the PSA was less than 0.5 ng/ml. Also, some of these cancers in the PCPT controls were of intermediate or high grade.[2] It is now known that the median PSA level for a 40-year old is less than 0.7 ng/ml.[3] Indeed, the draft of the new National Comprehensive Cancer Network (NCCN) clinical care pathway for prostate cancer diagnosis is hotly debated as it proposes to measure PSAs at age 40 in all men, and if this is greater than 0.6 ng/ml, for yearly PSAs and DREs to be performed, and for biopsies to be taken if the PSA or DRE becomes "suspicious."[4] Conversely, Stamey, who brought PSA to the attention of the general medical community over 20 years ago by correlating serum PSA levels with tumor volume,[5] now claims that levels between 2 and 10 ng/ml are attributed primarily to benign hyperplasia and are not related to cancer.[6]

Over the years I regularly determined my PSA value and noted that very gradually, and in a somewhat "saw tooth" fashion, the values rose. When it "hit" 3.0 ng/ml, I remember reassuring myself that the slope was less than 0.75 ng/ml, which according to Carter et al[7] was a good sign. Then, about 2 years later, it was 3.7 ng/ml—still a reassuring velocity. However, by then there was talk from my good friend Bill Catalona about lowering the normal cut-off to 2.5 ng/ml,[8] and because my prostate was small (I had yearly DREs that were normal), suggesting a worrisome PSA density, I somewhat whimsically decided to have a biopsy, confidently expecting it to be negative for the above reasons and because there was no prostate cancer in my very large family of primary relatives. The sextant biopsy was preformed by my colleague Bill Ellis somewhat secretly (only he, my nurse, and our main prostate pathologist Larry True knew). I also remember remarking that the biopsy was not as uncomfortable as a sigmoidoscopy but that local anesthesia (then not given or studied) might be very useful here (especially if more than six biopsies were taken). That prediction was based on my observations years before when we conducted our trial of TURPs under local anesthesia.[9] I was shocked when pathologic analysis revealed 1 mm of Gleason 5 (it would be the ubiquitous 6 now) on the left side in one of six cores.

What to do? I pondered, reread the literature, reflected especially on watch and wait, and flirted with denial. I even called my friend Martin Gleave who was leading the neoadjuvant androgen ablation trial in Canada,[10] obfuscating the problem by stating that "I had a patient who wanted to know about….," and asked what the pathologic no-tumor (P₀) rate was after 8 months of hormone therapy. When he told me it was less than 10%, I abandoned the escapist solution of going on hormone therapy for 8 months (keeping up a tan and a strict diet to avert suspicion) and then getting periodic PSAs and biopsies to delay or infinitely postpone aggressive treatment.

Finally, I decided to have a second biopsy and again 1 mm of Gleason 5 was found in about the same place. That was it! I wanted to be treated despite all my scholastic ruminations about watch and wait, length and lead-time biases, and the turtles and birds.[11] Deciding what treatment I should have was not a problem. However, contemplating my treatment choice did highlight my intellectual realization that despite my surgical orientation and practice, the relative value of surgery versus radiation therapy regarding quality of life and survival is unknown, and I remember feeling ashamed that it was not, and gaining more sympathy for the layman patient who has to decide amidst this intellectual and entrepreneurial confusion.

Surgery was my only option for several reasons. First, if I had had radiation therapy, the opprobrium from my colleagues would have been too much. However, John Blasko later commented that if I had gotten radiation therapy, I would have received many speaking invitations and honorariums for radiation oncology meetings. He also said that in similar circumstances he, for the same reasons of loyalty to his procedure and profession, could hardly have considered surgery and would have had the "seed" option. More seriously, with my experience I had little fear of the surgery, and with my personality I just wanted to know what was in there and to get the problem behind me if possible. This, I have come to realize, is the main legitimate reason for a surgical choice and is what I seek to hear from those of my patients who chose surgery.

I was surprised by the amount of trepidation I experienced. I thought that with all my experience I would embrace this necessity with aplomb. I was wrong. With my cancer parameters, I feared impotence and incontinence, not diminished survival. This was despite the realization that most of my patients did very well on those scores. "When it's you, it's different" now had a more poignant meaning.

Who was going to do my surgery was not a very difficult problem once analyzed. I realized that going somewhere else to "keep it quiet" would be impossible. Also, I knew that my associate Bill Ellis did the operation pretty much as I did (so it seemed almost like fulfilling a cocky surgeon's dream of using a mirror), and I trusted him. He agreed to do it and did a wonderful job under what must have been some significant pressure. I realized that the comfortable and very personal sense of trust and reassurance of "home ground," in addition to expertise, were more important elements than I had heretofore acknowledged.

While awaiting surgery, I was running an errand and passed an alternative medicine store which I had passed many times before. I must admit I had been very vocal in my criticism of alternative medicine approaches, believing that medicine needed to defend its hard-won evidence-based position. Yet, I entered the store and was enthralled with all the optimistic advertisements and comforting labels with pictures of fruit and such on the bottles of pills. Before I knew it, I walked out with two bottles (one was selenium and the other I forget). When I realized what I had done, I had a good laugh at myself, and never used them. However, the weekend before my surgery I thought I was getting a cold. The prospect of having to reschedule was overwhelming. Thus, I literally snuck into a drug store and bought a bottle of Echinacea. I did not get a cold and I had my surgery. I began to wonder about Echinacea's validity and then had to laugh at myself once again when the randomized study on Echinacea's effectiveness for preventing colds was announced 6 months later and was negative.[12] However, I realized that empowering the patient to do something for himself, even if through the use of yet unproven remedies, has merit. Also, I realized that medicine must determine better ways to retain the placebo effect without lying to the patient, and to teach these to future practitioners in a more systematic way. Finally, it reinforced a lesson that I had gleaned years before from my association with Michael Milken; namely, waiting for 100% proof is not a good way to make business decisions and possibly not scientific ones when it comes to prostate cancer.[13]

The recovery was relatively easy: pain was manageable, the catheter was more bothersome than I had imagined, and the only real surprise was the degree of fatigue that I experienced over a 3- to 4-week period. This was not from blood loss (I lost very little), but something else hard to define. Yet I was playing tennis at 4 weeks, though with less effectiveness than usual. I look forward to a scientific analysis of laparoscopic radical prostatectomy in that regard; I suspect the fatigue factor will be much less.

My pathology was good (vida infra) and the catheter was removed at 2 weeks. Its discomfort has pushed me to try to shorten that period even further in most of my patients. For 3 weeks I was not continent and I was very unhappy. Like any good Northern European Lutheran, I feared the worst. I did learn that once accepted, pads, at least temporarily, are not that odious. Thereafter, I gained continence quickly. I am now firmly ensconced in the continent group by any definition. Yet I am not as continent as I was before surgery. Though I use no pads or such, there are times when I do leak a little though almost never to the point of social embarrassment; these times include such events as the need to pass flatus, an overly full bladder precipitated by coffee, sexual anticipation, more than my usual alcoholic intake, or when extremely fatigued. Yet leakage with these events is unpredictable and rare. I have now begun to question my heretofore continent patients in ways I never did before and found similar though never quite the same stories. Of course, when I queried them why they had not told me this before, it was because I never asked. I have come to believe that almost no post-radical prostatectomy patient is totally continent and that current quality-of-life questionnaires need further refinement. Furthermore, there are more physiologic factors related to continence in this context then we realize, and these factors have little to do with how the radical prostatectomy is performed and/or how the patient heals. For years now I have told my patients that they can generally expect social continence but I cannot promise that they will be "trampoline dry."

My PSA has remained undetectable for over 6 years now, emotionally I have dismissed prostate cancer as a worry, and I admit to neglecting getting my PSA in a timely fashion. Yet initially and even now, waiting for the PSAs to come back gives me some anxiety.

I am almost glad I had this experience with prostate cancer. In ways that are hard to articulate, I think it has made me a better urologist when it comes to dealing with patients with the disease. I listen more; I am more empathetic; I have better insight into the morbidities of the surgery and yet more confidence that surgery offers a very good therapeutic solution. As an academic surgeon scientist, I have a greater sense of purpose in conducting and administrating research on prostate cancer. I have often been asked "would I do it again; would I have surgery if I were not a urologist; would I have more seriously considered watch and wait with a Gleason 6, 1-mm cancer?" One academic urologist who has made many contributions to prostate cancer, even expounded that I should not have had a biopsy. Also, if I had been so unwise as to have a biopsy, he explained, I should not have had the surgery even if I had known what my surgical pathology revealed; namely, 1 cm^3 of low-grade cancer with negative margins. He furthered explained that: 1) theoretically by half life considerations, it would have taken almost 20 to 30 years to reach "lethal" volumes; and 2) I could have at least waited another 10 years. No way! Taking a chance on the surgery was infinitely less fearsome than taking a chance on cancer theory. Besides, I won: no real morbidities, I am probably cured, and it has made me a better servant in the fight against this disease.

Reflections of PFS

When PHL was approached concerning this chapter, I could not resist. We have known each other for 30 years. As described above, the cementing of our friendship and prostate cancer relationship was originally based on the fact that PHL's father-in-law, who resided in my city, had prostate cancer, and was a patient. On his visits East, our mutual interest—prostate cancer—was often a subject of discussion and became even more so after PHL's diagnosis and surgery in 1999, and my diagnosis and surgery by him in 2000. We often concluded our discussions with the promise that we needed to write a book or at least a chapter on the subject. PHL, ever energetic, did write that book—Prostate Cancer for Dummies[14]—and when the opportunity for this chapter arose, he kindly asked me to participate.

In writing of my personal experience, I recognize two important principles. First, you cannot place yourself in another's shoes when walking a decision pathway since each individual processes and acts on information based on certain genetic predispositions and environmental conditioning. Even the closest of biologic and environmental human experiments, identical twins, will not process and react identically on each and every issue. I am married to an identical twin and can testify to this. Second, the ability of an individual to conclusively state his decisions relative to a hypothetical event, in this case the diagnosis and treatment of prostate cancer, might find that position quite altered when confronted with the reality of the diagnosis. To use a military analogy, there is a huge difference between boot camp and the battlefield, or a sporting analogy, between the practice and playing field.

I had started Proscar in 1998 due to urinary symptoms. A PSA in 2000 was 2.5 ng/ml (corrected to 5.0 ng/ml), which represented a significant rise from my prior levels. That I had prostate cancer was intuitively very clear to me. My annual PSA readings, beginning at age 50, had been very stable at 2.0 to 2.5 ng/ml between 1990 and 1998 (a cardiac event [see below] interfered with my 1999 annual draw). I was very content with these PSA levels, but they have since been shown to be associated with a five-fold increase in cancer risk.[15] Furthermore, at age 50 to 60, a PSA of greater than 0.7 ng/ml when compared to a PSA less than 0.7 ng/ml is associated with a 3.5-fold increase in risk for prostate cancer by age 70.[3] The PCPT has demonstrated a 23% incidence of prostate cancer at PSA levels between 2 and 3 ng/ml.[2] A PSA of 5.0 ng/ml was abnormal by any standard for a 60-year old.

Several strategies materialized in my mind. I decided I would have numerous biopsies (about 25) initially, not the then routine 6, to avoid repeat sessions to clarify the etiology of the PSA elevation. I did not want to come back to the biopsy scenario again and again. I presumed a Gleason 3 + 3 cancer since it was the grade most commonly found among patients with a diagnosis in this PSA range and which I diagnose on almost a daily basis.

Radical prostatectomy

What treatment approach? As a surgeon, I was viscerally inclined to surgery, although intellectually, I could not identify radiation by either interstitial implant of external beam as any less effective. I was also attracted to a definitive pathology report. I put erectile dysfunction and incontinence in perspective and had the advantage of first-hand knowledge of intervention that could soften their impact. Having been to France to observe a new laparoscopic approach and being adventurous in nature, I considered this option for the anticipated 3 + 3 low-risk cancer. The biopsy session was uneventful and I was correct in my first hunch—prostate cancer was found. Only 3 (all unilateral) of the 25 cores were positive, and I was certainly pleased that I had chosen the multiple biopsy approach. Fewer cores might have missed the cancer. However, my second hunch, that the cancer would be scored Gleason 3 + 3 was incorrect. All biopsies had predominant pattern 4. Bone and CT scan were normal. I put aside the adventure of a laparoscopic procedure for the tried and true open prostatectomy. Should I have the operation in my home hospital by my partner or take the "monkey off the locals back" and go elsewhere? I consulted with my good friend, PHL, who had had a prostatectomy, and we had operated together. He kindly agreed to do the surgery. I traveled to the University of Washington. The Gleason pattern influenced my attitude of weighing surgical side effects with benefits. My focus was on benefit (life centered) and the risk of urinary and sexual dysfunction became very secondary. This contrasts with PHL's primary concern about side effects when dealing with focal 3 + 3 cancer. I did not favor unilateral nerve-sparing on the biopsy-negative side, unless, at surgery, all circumstances (prostate size, adherence, consistency, ease of dissection) permitted it. A radical retropubic prostatectomy with pelvic node dissection was performed by PHL. The pathology report brought the good news of absence of lymph node involvement, a unilateral pT2 lesion with negative margins. The Gleason pattern 4 + 3 was confirmed but also with some Gleason 5 tertiary pattern. Gleason 4 + 3 + 5 has been plotted on the biochemical no evidence of disease (NED) curve and very much parallels the 4 + 4 curve.[16] A second pathologic opinion by an expert labeled the tumor as 4 + 5 with tertiary 3. Histopathology can be subjective! Also my 2-year course of Proscar may have caused a grading artifact. At least this is one of the explanations used to reconcile the PCPT results.[17]

We decided initially against adjuvant radiotherapy. However, a year after surgery, PSA "creep" began and the menu of uncertainty addressing salvage strategies was brought to my table. Anticipating a PSA failure, I had obtained frequent PSA assays and watched them rise through 0.1 and 0.2. When my PSA exceeded 0.2 ng/ml on two occasions (0.27 and 0.34) I chose to initiate external beam radiation therapy to the prostate bed with neoadjuvant and adjuvant androgen deprivation for 6 months. Androgen deprivation was a choice based on extrapolation of the studies aimed at primary therapy and the apparent synergistic or at least additive benefit of androgen deprivation when combined with radiation. It has been reported with salvage protocols as well.[18] While salvage radiation likely achieves better results with increasing time interval from surgery to PSA rise, and a lower Gleason sum cancer, the potential of a 5-year biochemical control, when initiated "early" (i.e. a PSA <1.0 ng/ml or even 0.6 ng/ml) is quite reasonable for a salvage therapy.[19] The opportunity for a "second chance," whether 10% or substantially more, was very attractive.

Now, two and a half years after restoration of my testosterone level, I anticipate each periodic PSA check with apprehension. I find myself scheduling the blood draw after important events like weddings, holidays, and family visits, so as not to risk blunting the joie de vie associated with these events. I am well, modifying the pace of life, and now appreciate more the interesting future that prostate cancer presents—a cancer that is chronic, that mimics life with its slow and steady attrition but, thankfully, permits rather extended life with good quality. However, the blessing and curse of PSA, especially the latter, can not be underestimated. Even in the elderly male, for whom life-expectancy is limited, the knowledge that a particular process is measurable and that increases, however small, indicate disease activity focuses attention almost exclusively on that disease to the extent that other more debilitating and life-threatening issues are relegated to secondary importance or ignored completely. The

ticking clock, regardless of how slow the tick, still is an audible and repetitive reminder of the limitations of life. Yes, we all are subject to the ticking clock, but there is something quite powerful in seeing its face as cancer and envisioning a disabling terminus.

A brief comment regarding urinary function and bother is applicable here. The return of continence was prolonged in part due to a psoas abscess and the vesicle irritation that it produced. Briefly, I began experiencing some mild intermittent right leg pain and toe numbness about 12 days after surgery, which was not very bothersome until I experienced fever and chills 6 weeks after surgery. A CT diagnosed a psoas abscess, which was percutaneously drained and all problems quickly resolved.

I have achieved a very satisfactory continence status which requires one small pad (a liner) daily; I could indeed get by many days without protection but the uncertainty of leaking with a sudden cough, sneeze or positional change, especially at day's end, make protection insurance wise. I agree with PHL that return to the state described as "trampoline dry" is probably quite rare post-prostatectomy, and relying on a patient interview to assess and report perfect continence is a trap for the unwary urologist. When my surgeon asks me if I am continent, I respond with a strong "yes." Only if specifically asked and coached to a detailed description will I state the exact situation and do this to provide academic information and not to describe bother or displeasure. However, I am not perfectly continent and, if I had been promised so as a patient, I would feel disappointed.

PHL Comments

I was of course flattered when PFS asked me to do his surgery. Being a professional, the surgery was not particularly stressful for me or my team and it went very well in all respects. I was very aggressive on the side of his cancer with the lymphadenectomy; no wider surgical margin was technically possible, and on the other side, I reflected on PFS's wishes but saved the nerves nonetheless. I was very happy with the procedure as we closed and while he recuperated at my house. I was pleased that the margins were negative and that there was no cancer on the unilateral nerve-sparing side.

However, after surgery I took every event in PFS's recovery and clinical course very personally. I have never had a patient with a psoas abscess postoperatively and cannot think of a surgical cause for this one. Yet this result and the rising PSA continue to elicit that irrational response: I could have done better. I would want it no other way; for him and in fact for all our patients.

Further reflections by PFS

Approximately 2 years prior to the diagnosis of prostate cancer, I experienced an event which, like prostate cancer, only even more so, comprises the rite of passage for the aging male. Sudden crushing chest pain brought me to my knees. Fortunately, it occurred at home rather than in a hotel room, car, or airplane. A prompt angioplasty and stent corrected the obstruction of the left anterior descending coronary artery. There are several reasons for mentioning this event. Prior to transfer from the emergency room to the angio suite, the cardiologist outlined for me a four-arm clinical trial for which he advised my participation. The trial randomized to angioplasty ± stent with anticoagulation A or B. I am sure every individual addresses instant information and decisions differently. I am also certain that most individuals, myself included, would ask the consenting physician, in this circumstance, "do you think this is a good idea and should I participate?" In this urgent situation, an affirmative from the physician invariably results in consent to the proposed trial. And so I consented. I can only contrast this process with the laborious explanations, interactions, and reviews with patients and significant others that was required to inform and encourage patients to consider the SPIRIT trial. This trial was initiated by the American College of Surgeons Oncology Group in the US and Canada and was a randomized trial between brachytherapy and radical prostatectomy for low-risk disease. Both PHL and I spent many months in helping getting this trial started, but we were ultimately unsuccessful (see below). The deck is certainly stacked, at least in this situation, in favor of a cardiology intervention trial versus a prostate cancer intervention trial. This was so despite the fact that both arms of the prostate trial had a proven track record of success, whereas the cardiology trial was constructed to measure the unknown of adding a new stent procedure to angioplasty. The trial playing field is overwhelmingly tipped in favor of cardiology intervention based on urgency and ultimate "at the mercy of the MD and situation" status of a cardiac event.

Another reason for mentioning this cardiac event is to compare the visceral response and emotion associated with the diagnosis of cardiac disease and prostate cancer. After my coronary occlusion, during and after rehabilitation (parenthetically the rehabilitation experience in the company of fellow patients cemented the concept that group interaction is good for both body and soul, and supports participation in post-prostate cancer treatment support groups), my mindset was one of establishing a program of understanding of and cooperation with my heart. Through diet modifications, exercise, and other strategies, I committed to a partnership for mutual recovery. This was satisfying and comforting to implement. My reactions generated by a prostate cancer diagnosis were totally different. A sense of betrayal and hostility toward the betraying organ were overpowering and were followed by a committed investment to destroy it by whatever means.

The emerging field of psychoneuroimmunology or mind–body interaction lends support to a relationship between mental attitude and physical recovery. Prayer and meditation tend to relax the mind and body, offset stress, and exert many positive influences. They are receiving more attention and study.[20,21] As we learn more about these disciplines or approaches, it becomes evident that responses to therapy, in addition to the application of the traditional modalities of allopathic medicine, depend on the patient's state of mind. The astute diagnostician William Osler recognized this interaction when he stated that it was more important to know about the patient who had the disease than about the disease the patient had. I therefore concur with PHL's comments about exploiting the placebo effect.

Final reflections and conclusion (PHL and PFS)

Although much has already been written about personal reactions to the events surrounding radical prostatectomy, we hope our accounts have been interesting if not informative, perhaps because they were experienced by men who have had long careers treating prostate cancer. In reflecting on our individual and somewhat different situations and reactions, we find several common themes that deserve reemphasis.

Fear

We were both surprised at the degree of fear we felt despite our familiarity with the disease and its management. The objects of this fear are of course survival, suffering, loss of control, and the morbidities of incontinence and impotence. We experienced them in different proportions, but we were both humbled by their disruptive power.

Uncertainty

Of course, one cause of fear is the uncertainty surrounding the relative effectiveness of the various local treatments. We were both ashamed that our specialty had not worked harder to remedy this deficiency. In fact, we were heavily involved in launching the so-called SPIRIT Trial—a randomized comparison of brachytherapy versus radical prostatectomy for low-risk prostate cancer. We were sobered by the difficulties we had in randomizing these men but learned many things about how to do it, primarily from the Canadians who were actually quite successful. However, in the US we found meager support both among radiotherapists and surgeons for this effort. The trial was eventually dropped by the National Cancer Institute. There was of course great skepticism initially about its feasibility; PFS has already commented on why such trials are particularly difficult, but the greatest barrier was the lack of will and lack of culture in urology to do difficult randomized clinical trials. We believe this lack does not exist as much among practitioners of other cancers and in other diseases. In our opinion this must change if urology is to maintain its place as a leader in prostate cancer management.

Quality of life

Urinary, sexual, and bowel function can be impacted substantially by local therapies. Much has already been written about this subject. However, how an individual patient will react to this alteration will depend on two factors, namely the degree of alteration and the patient's attitude towards it. We believe that there is a general underestimation and reporting of the impact of side effects. The resilience of the human spirit generates an attitude to deal with dysfunction. In this setting physicians need to be wary that they do not become overconfident in their ability to return the patient to his preoperative state. There are some patients for whom this assurance can have a devastating effect postoperatively because of unrealistic expectations.

We have several particular observations about incontinence. First, wearing pads is not as bad as we anticipated once we got used to it. It could be that familiarizing men to wearing them before the surgery may have merit despite its negative connotations. Also, continence after radical prostatectomy is relative and rarely absolutely achieved. Thus, the current quality-of-life surveys may need modification, especially regarding mild incontinence. We believe the use of so-called safety pads, such as "panty liners," should be included in the assessments. This is because most pads can absorb as much as 60 ml with the wearer never really feeling wet, while liners can tolerate little more than a few drops. In our view acceptable continence after radical prostatectomy is no pads or just one liner a day, since the difference between these groups regarding continence is small (or even nonexistent) while "one pad" can cover many different degrees of incontinence, almost all of which are "limiting."

Also, it appears that the precipitating events surrounding what causes mild incontinent episodes vary greatly between men, and often it is not the usual events associated with stress incontinence such as lifting and straining. Some men leak upon wiping after defecation, others do not; some with significant alcohol intake, but not everyone; some with sexual foreplay or just mental anticipation; many but not all when passing flatus. We believe this suggests that men differ significantly in some neurologic aspects of continence, and we need to better understand these differences if we are to continue to strive to understand and improve continence after radical prostatectomy.

Alternative/complementary/ integrative medicine and patient control

We both learned the power of the complementary/integrative medicine movement. We must work harder to legitimately interface with that world and develop better ways to empower patients to participate substantially in their disease management. If nothing else, the placebo effect must not be labeled as a nefarious phenomenon, but exploited honestly to the patients benefit.

PSA Anxiety

Of course, PSA anxiety varies among patients and with the severity of disease, but it exists in almost all. This burden is mostly unavoidable and an acceptable price for the value of PSA monitoring, but perhaps it can be lessened by giving the patient more control over when he has the test and more importantly how he gets the result. Waiting for a doctor or nurse to call or return a call produces stress. Perhaps some web-based system allowing more patient control could be developed. Undoubtedly, there are other methods in other areas besides PSA anxiety and alternative/complementary medicine whereby the patient can have more control over the experiences surrounding surgery.

PSA Recurrence

The options for treating PSA failure carry as much or even more uncertainty than those involved with the discussion of primary therapy. The patient recognizes that, with failure of primary therapy, there is diminishing likelihood of cure, and his apprehension is heightened. Practitioners should make every effort to couch their explanations and directions with a sense of assurance and hope. To do otherwise would risk the patient's emotional state and compound the negative impact of recurrent disease.

As previously implied, both of us are in retrospect thankful we had this experience because it has made us more empathetic in many ways, some of which are hard to convey. We are certainly more effective (and we think more even handed) at initial orientation. We are better listeners. Also, we both have developed more effective ways of relating to patients during their management. We appreciate more the need to provide hope, to develop trust, and to encourage a sense of control. Finally, we have become more passionate about facilitating progress in prostate cancer diagnosis and cure.

References

1. Ercole CJ, Lange PH, Mathisen M, et al. Prostatic specific antigen and prostatic acid phosphatase in the monitoring and staging of patients with prostatic cancer. J Urol 1987;138:1181–1184.
2. Thompson IM, Goodman PJ, Tangen CM, et al. The influence of finasteride on the development of prostate cancer. N Engl J Med 2003;349:215–224.
3. Fang J, Metter EJ, Landis P, et al. Low level of prostate specific antigen predict long-term risk of prostate cancer: results from the Baltimore Longitudinal Study Aging. Urology 2001;58:411–426.
4. National Comprehensive Cancer Network (NCCN). Clinical Practice Guidelines in Oncology. Prostate Cancer Early Detection, vol 1, 2004. www.nccn.org
5. Stamey TA, Yang N, Hay AR, et al. Prostate-specific antigen as a serum marker for adenocarcinoma of the prostate. N Engl J Med 1987;317:909–916.
6. Stamey TA, Caldwell M, McNeal JE, et al. The prostate specific antigen era in the United States is over for prostate cancer: what happened in the last 20 years? J Urol 2004;172:1297–1301.
7. Carter HB, Pearson JD, Metter EJ, et al. Longitudinal evaluation of prostate-specific antigen levels in men with and without prostate disease. JAMA 1992;267:2215–2220.
8. Krumholtz JS, Carvalhal GF, Ramos CG, et al. Prostate-specific antigen cutoff of 2.6 ng/ml for prostate cancer screening is associated with favorable pathologic tumor features. Urology 2002;60:469–474.
9. Sinha B, Haikel G, Lange PH, et al. Transurethral resection of the prostate with local anesthesia in 100 patients. J Urol 1986;135:719–721.
10. Gleave ME, Goldenberg SL, Chin JL, et al. Randomized comparative study of 3 versus 8-month neoadjuvant hormonal therapy before radical prostatectomy: biochemical and pathological effects. J Urol 2001;166:500–506, discussion 506–597.
11. Lange PH. Future studies in localized prostate cancer. What should we think? What can we do? J Urol 1994;152:1932–1938.
12. Taylor JA, Weber W, Standish L, et al. Efficacy and safety of Echinacea in treating upper respiratory tract infections in children: a randomized controlled trial. JAMA 2003;290:2824–2830.
13. Daniels C. Beating cancer: the man who changed medicine. Fortune Mag 2004;150:90–112.
14. Lange PH, Adamec C. Prostate Cancer for Dummies. New York: Wiley Publishing, 2003.
15. Gann PH, Hennekens CH, Stampfer MJ. A prospective evaluation of plasma prostate-specific antigen for detection of prostatic cancer. JAMA 2004;172:1297–1301.
16. Pan CC, Potter S, Partin AW, et al. The prognostic significance of tertiary Gleason patterns of higher grade in radical prostatectomy specimens: a proposal to modify the Gleason grading system. Am J Surg Path 2000;24:563–569.
17. Thompson IM, Goodman PH, Tangen CM, et al. The influence of finateride on the development of prostate cancer. N Engl J Med 2003;349:215–224.
18. Jani AB, Sokoloff M, Shalhav A, et al. Androgen ablation adjuvant to postprostatectomy radiotherapy: complication-adjusted number needed to treat analysis. Urology 2004;64:976–981.
19. Stephenson AJ, Shariat SF, Zelefski MJ, et al. Salvage radiotherapy for recurrent prostate cancer after radical prostatectomy. JAMA 2004;291:1325–1332.
20. Holland JC, Lewis S. The Human Side of Cancer. New York: Harper Collins Publishers, 2000.
21. Dossey L. Healing Words: The Power of Prayer and the Practice of Medicine. New York: Harper Collins Publishers, 1993.

34

Coping with a diagnosis of prostate cancer: the patient and family perspective

Brian Wells

Introduction

Prostate cancer kills men from all socioeconomic groups, races, and cultures. Some are retired, others are at the peak of their careers, usually with wives/partners and often with (sometimes young) children.

The prostate remains something of a mystery to the public, although general awareness is being raised by organized campaigns, celebrity cases reported by the media, and the enhanced profile of "men's wellness" generally, although it still falls a long way behind that of women.

A diagnosis of prostate cancer, no matter how it is revealed and presented, is likely to have a profound emotional effect on the patient and his family, as well as others in close contact, such as work colleagues. This should be remembered and treated in an appropriate context, which will vary according to the age, nationality, culture, and resources of the patient, as well as the healthcare systems available. Few of these systems are well equipped to deal comprehensively, rapidly, and effectively with the myriad of potential problems that may arise. There is much ignorance and confusion about prostate cancer, and the overall experience can be traumatic or relatively trouble free.

Relevant factors include:

- Prostate cancer is only found in men ("manhood" issues, responsibilities, etc).
- TNM stage of the disease.
- Lifestyle of the family (this can be complicated).
- Philosophical, spiritual/religious, and other values involved.
- Family system and dynamics (there may be 20 years of "baggage" between husband and wife, or the relationship may be "healthy" and highly supportive).
- "What goes on" at home and at work (this is often difficult for clinicians to appreciate when patients are seen in hospitals and clinics).
- Previous family experience of illness, doctors, and treatments.

Example cases

Case 1

Patient X is a 57-year-old managing director of a company that employs 70 staff in northern England. He has been married for 30 years and has three mature children who have left home. A routine annual visit to his family doctor reveals an asymptomatic prostate-specific antigen (PSA) of 6 ng/ml with an unremarkable digital rectal examination (DRE). He is referred to a local urologist who organizes a transrectal ultrasonography (TRUS) biopsy, which he finds uncomfortable and "messy" to say the least. He waits for the results, is told that he has a Gleason score of 7, adenocarcinoma of the prostate, and is referred for an MRI and bone scan. At this point he tells his wife and children. Again, they wait for results and are told that "the tumor seems to be localized" and that if he has appropriate treatment, there is a "good chance of complete cure."

His wife (an intelligent former nurse) has talked to friends, explored the Internet, and begun to reach a stage of "information overload." She worries about her anxious husband, treatment options, side effects, and what the future holds, but both are relieved that he is unlikely to die of prostate cancer.

Neither feels inspired by the urologist who has an abrupt manner and seems too busy. Despite assurances that a radical prostatectomy is likely to lead to cure, the couple remains concerned about possible complications.

Their 25-year-old son phones a friend whose father is a cardiologist in Los Angeles. The friend reports back that, compared to radical prostatectomy, brachytherapy is "far more popular on the west coast," has a similar success rate, is less invasive, and is unlikely to cause incontinence or erectile dysfunction. However, should the disease recur (15–20% chance), further radiotherapy will not be an option, and surgery will be virtually excluded due to tissue damage caused by the radioactive seeds. Various transatlantic phone calls take place; patient X and his supportive wife visit a total of five "experts" (they have a health insurance scheme that allows for some flexibility) and talk to former patients who share their experiences.

Eight weeks after the diagnosis has been presented, they opt for a radical prostatectomy in London, under the care of a surgical team that has been recommended as "the best," and in which they have confidence. Another 8 weeks postop, patient X returns to work, but feels tired, irritable, and bored with the problems presented to him, and over the ensuing 6 months arranges to take early retirement.

Two years later (having required a dilatation 3 months postop), his PSA is unreadable. He and his wife have developed an intimacy that is deeper than previously (including adequate erectile function with the aid of PD5 inhibitors). They travel, enjoy mutual interests, exercise together, and the family, which now includes two grandchildren, look back on the entire process as having been traumatic but subsequently life-enhancing. Patient X is determined to "give something back." He makes regular donations to prostate-related charities and declares himself available to share his experiences with other patients, either by telephone or in a group setting.

Case 2

Patient Y is a 47-year-old Islamic international businessman from the Lebanon. He has three wives, is deeply religious, and wishes to have more children. His active sexual life is of great importance and he is distraught at having been diagnosed with prostate cancer at so young an age. After consulting a multitude of professionals in various countries, he eventually decides to visit a sperm bank and opts for brachytherapy. He keeps his diagnosis a secret from everyone (including his wives who are baffled by the sudden use of condoms) because he is concerned that the stigma of "cancer" will be used to his disadvantage by business competitors.

Four months post-treatment he begins to experience erectile dysfunction and becomes depressed. This leads to a short admission at a psychiatric facility where he improves, following culturally sensitive counseling and antidepressant pharmacotherapy. He remains under the care of an Arabic-speaking psychiatrist, and 1-year post-brachytherapy is considering in vitro fertilization (IVF) with one of his wives.

Case 3

Patient Z is a 64-year-old alcoholic divorcee, living alone in Ohio, having previously served in Vietnam. His three adult children all live in different cities and the family tries to get together, complete with grandchildren, at Thanksgiving and Christmas. Over a 3-year period, he becomes aware of worsening symptoms. His local Veterans Administration hospital finds a PSA in excess of 300 ng/ml with secondary tumors in the lower spine. Hormone therapy is commenced and after 3 months a concomitant 8-week course of external beam radiotherapy is undertaken. Subsequently, when family members call on the phone, he is usually drunk, sometimes aggressively minimizing his loneliness and the extent of his bone pain. The family is by now used to "Dad's alcoholism" and unpredictable nature. All members have been affected by his drinking over the previous 30 years. Feelings are mixed, and support is offered in a variable and sometimes ambivalent manner by family members who have problems of their own; one being divorced, another following a "recovery" program resulting from his own addiction to drugs and alcohol, consequences of which included an 18-month jail sentence.

The patient and family journey

These three examples serve to illustrate a tip of the emotional icebergs that can accompany prostate cancer. "Emotional language" is often difficult to articulate, as emotions are experiential, and sometimes difficult to describe. Some patients and family members are "psychologically sophisticated" and can express feelings more comprehensively than others. Cultures vary in the manner that emotions are expressed and just as some patients have higher and lower thresholds to physical pain, the same is true for emotional pain.

Many adverse life events (deaths, robberies, accidents, etc.) lead to a *grief reaction*. It can be helpful for the patient and his family to be aware of the psychological components of this often subconscious series of defences. Not only is it healthy to progress through these phases, it is important in order to survive traumatic experiences. The phases are not necessarily in strict order, or of the same intensity, but are likely to be experienced by the patient and his significant others at various stages of "the journey":[1]

- Denial.
- Anger (often displaced).
- Bargaining (if only the doctors knew more).
- Depression (rarely requires psychiatric treatment in this context).
- Acceptance.

Prostate cancer, if diagnosed early, is highly treatable with a good prognosis. The patient journey, however, will vary according to:

- Patient and family confidence in their healthcare professionals (families are often more distressed than the index patient).
- "Mid-life" issues (awareness of mortality, financial stability, activities, and interests other than work, etc.).
- Appointment schedules (sometimes complicated), poor communication, sitting in waiting rooms, delayed results, attitudes and personalities of staff (including secretaries).
- Sensitivity of staff to potentially traumatic procedures such as TRUS biopsies (which can produce negative results despite a rising PSA).
- Postoperative care in the short-, medium-, and long-term.
- Feelings of "violation" (manhood having been affected, etc.).
- Competent advice regarding catheters, bladder control, future erectile dysfunction, etc.

Conflicting advice, "anti-doctor" attitudes found on websites and "chat rooms," as well as a need for greater research clarity, can make decision-making difficult (See Chapter 2). "Fuzzy indicators," such as PSA results, can confuse. Professional competition, financial incentives, and an overall absence of culturally-sensitive under-standing and support from within the profession, can lead patients and families to feel isolated. Some institutions offer emotional help by making use of volunteers and "survivors of cancer" (support groups, etc). However, professional supervision and guidance in this area is generally lacking. While relatively few patients and families require the services of a psychiatrist, basic counseling skills do involve an element of training.

As technology advances, research results appear, and professionals become increasingly skilled with new equipment, there are good reasons for future optimism.

At the time of writing, it is interesting for a psychiatrist to witness the professional and political conflicts that currently surround the diagnosis and management of prostate cancer. Controversy over routine PSA testing, watchful waiting (active surveillance) versus curative treatments, and passionate debate on future quality of life issues, make prostate cancer a rich source of technical, scientific, and emotional material.

Reference

1.   Kubler Ross E. On Death and Dying 1970 Collier Paperbacks.

Section 3

Treatment of locally advanced and metastatic prostate cancer

35

Androgen deprivation for the treatment of prostate cancer: general principles

David G McLeod, Albaha Barqawi

Historical background

Hormonal manipulation for the treatment of prostate disease dates back more than 100 years. However, little was known of the effect of sex hormones on the initiation and progression of prostate cancer until the late 1930s. In 1941, Huggins and Hodges at the University of Chicago presented their Nobel prize-winning paper in which they demonstrated that, due to the dependence of the normal prostate gland on sex hormones for growth, either surgical castration or treatment with diethylstilbestrol (DES) had significant therapeutic implications for men with prostate cancer.[1] This discovery marked the beginning of modern hormonal manipulation in men with prostate cancer.

Since the 1940s, hormonal manipulation has been the mainstay of the systemic treatment of advanced prostate cancer. In the 1940s, estrogen treatments, primarily DES, became the primary alternative to orchiectomy. In the 1960s, trials initiated by the Veterans Administration Co-operative Urological Research Group (VACURG) found no statistically significant differences in median and in 2-, 5-, and 10-year survival rates in patients either receiving DES or undergoing orchiectomy.[2,3] A later review of three VACURG trials concluded that the use of either DES or orchiectomy provided a significant survival benefit in patients with locally advanced non-metastatic prostate cancer.[4] However, estrogen therapy fell out of favor due to the increased risk of cardiovascular death after treatment with 5 mg/day DES in these studies. In addition, a more recent study showed that daily treatment with 3 mg DES as the primary hormonal therapy for stage D2 prostate cancer caused more serious cardiovascular or thromboembolic complications than occurred with the antiandrogen flutamide.[5]

A parenteral route of administration for estrogen therapy has been suggested as a way to minimize cardiovascular adverse events by avoiding the first-pass effect in the liver, thereby minimizing over-production of coagulation factor VII.[6–8] However, in trials conducted to date, parenteral estrogens have not been shown to offer a survival advantage.[9] In a small study, Henriksson et al found that intramuscular injections of polyestradiol phosphate had clinical effects comparable with bilateral orchiectomy.[10] Although parenteral estrogens have been shown to be inferior to androgen blockade using luteinizing hormone-releasing hormone (LHRH) agonists, a recent large randomized study from Sweden reported that current parenteral estrogen therapy and complete androgen blockade using an LHRH agonist with an antiandrogen had comparable efficacy in terms of overall survival and cardiovascular safety.[11] Compared with LHRH agonists, synthetic estrogens have been shown to reduce testosterone production from extratesticular sites and to achieve a greater reduction in serum testosterone.[12]

In 1977, Schally won the Nobel Prize for Medicine and Physiology for his extensive research in hypothalamic regulatory hormones, including the isolation and synthesis of LHRH.[13] The emergence of synthetic LHRH agonists following the pioneering work by Schally and his colleagues led to the most dramatic changes in hormonal treatment of prostate cancer since the work of Huggins and Hodges.[14] The discovery of LHRH, which was well known by the mid-1980s,[15] marked the beginning of a new era in the manipulation of hormones in prostate cancer patients, and the use of LHRH agonists has become standard therapy for the treatment of metastatic prostate cancer. In their systematic meta-analysis of the literature, Seidenfeld et al found no difference in survival after either LHRH-agonist therapy or orchiectomy.[16] Nevertheless, LHRH-agonist therapy gained in popularity, primarily due to greater patient acceptance and tolerance of this medical approach compared with surgical castration.

Luteinizing hormone-releasing hormone agonist therapy greatly reduces testosterone levels.[17] Although less than 50 ng/dL is usually considered a castrate level of testosterone, the National Comprehensive Cancer Network has provisionally recommended setting a lower testosterone threshold (i.e., <20 ng/dL) to match the effect of orchiectomy.[18] This lower testosterone level can be achieved by an LHRH agonist alone or by combined androgen blockade. The latter approach utilizes an LHRH agonist to block testicular production of testosterone in combination with a nonsteroidal antiandrogen (e.g., flutamide, bicalutamide, or nilutamide) to achieve maximal binding of circulating adrenal androgens at the cellular level.[19]

Nonsteroidal antiandrogens can also be used as monotherapy in some patients. Monotherapy with flutamide or bicalutamide has been show to have a palliative effect on symptoms while preserving libido and sexual potency.[20] However, the American Society of Clinical Oncology recommends that monotherapy using steroidal antiandrogens, such as cyproterone acetate, not be offered to patients.[21] A number of trials have compared the outcome of using a combined total androgen blockade versus monotherapy with an LHRH agonist. In their meta-analysis, Samson et al found no statistical difference in long-term survival between patients receiving monotherapy and those receiving combined therapy.[22] In order for patients to make an informed decision about therapy, they must be fully informed about the cost and toxicity of combined hormonal treatment versus its marginal additional survival benefit. Nevertheless, combined androgen blockade should be considered in all men with spinal bony metastasis or in whom there is a high risk of voiding dysfunction in order to counteract the initial flare phenomenon[23] (i.e., the transitory rise in testosterone levels following treatment with an LHRH agonist). It is important to recognize that the risk of experiencing a testosterone flare effect is not totally eliminated with combined androgen blockade; close clinical observation of symptoms is warranted.

Recent evidence supports the role of LHRH antagonists (e.g., abarelix and ganirelix) in the treatment of prostate cancer and the benefit of applying hormonal manipulation in the early stages of disease.[24] Use of abarelix has been shown to result in rapid medical castration without a testosterone surge, thereby avoiding the initial testosterone flare observed with LHRH agonists.[25] However, any potential advantages associated with LHRH antagonist therapy have not yet been shown to extend survival.[26]

Mechanism of action and regulation of prostate hormone-sensitive cell growth

Effect of testosterone

Testosterone, which is essential for the growth and differentiation of prostate cells and for the development and function of the prostate, is regulated by androgen activity.[27] In the male, testosterone is secreted primarily from the Leydig cells in the testis. In addition, the adrenals produce inactive testosterone precursors, including dehydroepiandrosterone (DHEA) and androstenedione, which can be converted to active testosterone both in the prostate and in most peripheral tissues. The adrenal glands are the source of approximately 10% of total testosterone, which contributes to intraprostatic dihydrotestosterone (DHT).

The enzyme 5α-reductase acts to convert testosterone to the more potent DHT in the prostate. Therefore, testosterone acts as both a hormone and a prohormone, exerting its action via the intracellular androgen receptor (AR), a ligand-dependent transcription activator. Testosterone is also converted to an estrogen in tissues that have a high level of aromatase via the estrogen receptor (ER). Numerous in-vitro studies have shown a synergistic activation of the ligand-independent AR by various growth factors and cytokines in the presence of smaller amounts of androgens.[28,29] The role of these observations in the long-term effect of hormonal treatment on prostate cancer remains unclear.

The hypothalamic-pituitary-testicular axis is responsible for the primary regulation of testosterone production by way of a negative feedback mechanism that is based on the release of LHRH from the pituitary gland under the influence of gonadotropin-releasing hormone from the hypothalamus (Figure 35.1). Agonists of LHRH suppress synthesis of endogenous testicular gonadotropin, and the chronic administration of LHRH agonists causes a hypogonadal condition, with suppression of luteinizing hormone and follicle-stimulating hormone levels. Thompson et al found that the testosterone flare phenomenon occurred in 11% of 765 patients within the first 1 to 2 weeks of LHRH agonist therapy.[30] The flare phenomenon may manifest as severe hot flashes and voiding dysfunction. In addition, there is concern about cord compression and ureteral obstruction in patients with widely disseminated metastases.

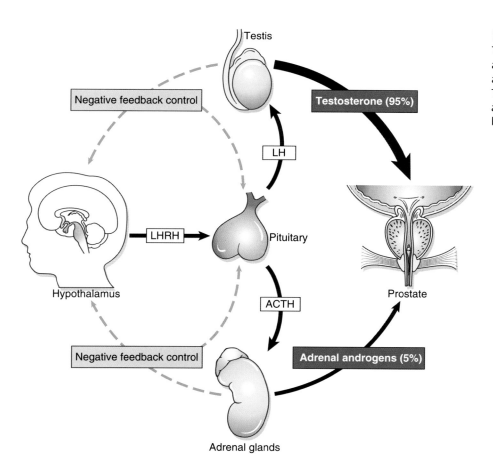

Figure. 35.1
The hypothalamic-pituitary-testicular axis is responsible for around 95% of androgen stimulus to the prostate. The remaining 5% stems from the adrenal glands and can be blocked by antiandrogens.

Effect of hormonal deprivation on apoptosis

Most prostate cancers are a heterogeneous mixture of androgen-dependent and -independent cell colonies at the time of diagnosis. Castration has been shown to promote an extensive apoptotic response both in normal prostate cells[31] and in androgen-dependent tumor cells.[32] In the early stages of the malignant transformation of prostate cancer, hormonal deprivation appears to have a reduction in or to lose its effect on the apoptotic response in androgen-independent cells in 80% of cases[33]; however, the effect is seen primarily in the reduction of cell proliferation rather than in an apoptotic response. Since most of these cells retain their molecular factors and mechanisms for apoptosis, they represent a potential target for new chemotherapeutic regimens currently under investigation.

It has been postulated that some androgen-dependent cells can evolve during therapy, transforming into androgen-independent cells. Although the mechanisms underlying this transformation are still poorly understood, it has been suggested that Bcl2, a suppressor of apoptosis, may play a pivotal role.[34] Some researchers are exploring the idea that androgen-dependent cancer cells that are sensitive to apoptosis may predominate in patients on androgen-deprivation therapy who maintain undetectable levels of prostate-specific antigen (PSA) for a prolonged period (i.e., >1 year). This subset of patients can receive the most benefit from intermittent hormonal manipulation.[35] To date, no prospective randomized trials have supported the use of intermittent LHRH agonist therapy in all patients with prostate cancer.

Treatment of early prostate cancer

Rationale for the use of hormone therapy: a brief overview

Although the long-term benefit of hormone deprivation in advanced prostate cancer has been well established in clinical practice, the use of hormonal manipulation in early prostate cancer is still controversial. Numerous studies have shown a significant reduction in positive margin rates after prolonged neoadjuvant hormonal treatment before radical prostatectomy.[36] However, neoadjuvant therapy did not reduce PSA recurrence in these studies.[37] A study conducted by Messing et al showed a significant improvement in survival in patients with node-positive prostate cancer who received immediate hormonal therapy after radical prostatectomy and pelvic lymphadenectomy.[38] In addition, a therapeutic advantage was reported for the use of adjunctive (i.e., during or immediately following) and neoadjuvant androgen deprivation with radiation therapy.[39,40]

Nomograms and artificial neural network programs have been developed in an effort to identify those patients who will achieve a survival benefit from early hormonal treatment. These programs define predictors of poor outcome in a subgroup of patients with specific predictors (e.g., Gleason score, initial PSA, and clinical stage).[41] However, the optimal initiation time, duration, and continuity of hormonal manipulation in early prostate cancer remains unknown. Prostate-specific antigen doubling time appears to be the best basis for recommending early hormonal treatment; for example, it is advisable to start hormonal therapy as early as possible in men with a short PSA doubling time (i.e., <3 months). Although the effect of hormone therapy on long-term overall survival and PSA-free progression is still undetermined in early prostate cancer, this approach appears to offer the best advantage in the group of men at high risk based on Gleason score, extent of the tumor, and pretreatment initial PSA velocity.

Duration of androgen deprivation in conjunction with primary therapy

Most patients diagnosed with clinically localized prostate cancer receive a recommendation for either surgery or radiation as primary treatment, and fewer patients are currently being put on a regimen of close observation, or "watchful waiting." Studies have shown that neoadjuvant androgen therapy dramatically reduces the rate of local recurrence after tumor excision. In a phase III randomized trial, the rate of PSA recurrence and positive margin were significantly reduced in patients treated intramuscularly with leuprolide 7.5 mg/month and oral flutamide 250 mg t.i.d for 3 or 8 months before radical prostatectomy.[42] In another study, patients who received neoadjuvant therapy for more than 3 months prior to surgery showed a significant reduction in the incidence of biochemical failure.[43] Numerous randomized trials have addressed the impact of using short-term (i.e., 4 months) versus long-term (i.e., 2 or more years) androgen deprivation with radiation therapy.[44–46] In patients with clinical stage T3 to T4 disease, cancer-specific survival was no better when the patient received 4 months of hormonal treatment than with no adjuvant hormonal therapy. Although patients receiving 2 years of hormonal therapy had better cancer-specific survival at 5 years than patients receiving 4 months of therapy, overall survival was similar in both groups. Longer term hormonal manipulation was better than no treatment at 2 years and with lifelong treatment. It is interesting to note that overall survival was comparable between patients who received either 2 years or 4 months of hormonal treatment. However, it is important to wait until the cancer-specific survival-benefit results are known before judging short-term treatment to be beneficial. Today, the standard of practice in men with clinically advanced local prostate cancer remains long-term (i.e., 2–3 years) hormonal therapy in conjunction with radiation therapy.[40]

Side effects to be aware of prior to initiating hormonal therapy

As studies continue to provide evidence supporting the use of androgen deprivation early in the management of prostate cancer, the toxicity associated with this treatment has become more of an issue. Table 35.1 lists the side effects most often associated with hormonal therapy.[47–54] Loss of libido, impotence, and erectile dysfunction are well recognized side effects of androgen deprivation.[55] Other side effects, including fatigue, hot flashes, muscle wasting, cognitive problems, and gynecomastia, can affect a patient's quality of life.[56] The metabolic changes resulting from hormonal therapy are associated with significant morbidity; they adversely affect the lipid profile and can result in anemia, osteoporosis, and liver toxicity.

Table 35.1 Incidence of adverse events associated with androgen deprivation therapy

Adverse events	Frequency (%)
Fatigue[47]	14
Hot flashes	50–80
Erectile dysfunction	50–100
Decline in cognitive function[48,49]	0–50
Bone fracture[50,51]	6–9
Anemia[52]	81
Gynecomastia[53]	16
Increase in liver function test[54] *	22

*Antiandrogen therapy

Hot flashes, which are the most common symptom associated with androgen deprivation, are due to an alteration in the thermoregulatory center of the hypothalamus in response to an increase in catecholamine production following the positive feedback resulting from a lack of testosterone. Patients who find hot flashes to be intolerable may be treated with selective serotonin (5-hydroxytryptamine) reuptake inhibitors (e.g., venlafaxine).[57] These agents provide more effective treatment than estrogen preparations, megestrol acetate, DES, and soy supplements that are commonly used to control hot flashes in these patients.

The lack of testosterone following androgen deprivation therapy has been linked to muscle wasting and a net increase in body weight, primarily due to increased fat deposition.[58] These changes may have a profound effect on a patient's lipid profile and may theoretically increase the risk of cardiovascular complications. Currently, the use of LHRH agonists has not been linked to these complications in controlled studies. Nevertheless, since high doses of antiandrogens have been associated with increased mortality, clinicians should use caution when prescribing these drugs, particularly in high-risk patients. Long-term (i.e., >6 months) treatment with androgen deprivation therapy may be associated with impairments in memory, attention, and executive functions.[48] In contrast, Salminen et al found no such impairment in cognitive functions in a small cohort of 25 men after up to 12 months of androgen deprivation.[49] Further randomized controlled trials addressing the issue of side effects after long-term androgen deprivation are needed. Meanwhile, patients should be made aware of the risks associated with hormone therapy when treatment options are discussed in the early stage of their disease.

Downregulation of both the production and activity of nitric oxide is another side effect of androgen deprivation.[59] In addition, the effects of surgical or radiation treatment on the neurovascular conduction pathways can also affect symptoms. Therefore, the efficacy of sexual health-enhancing medications prescribed for these patients can vary from no effect to a return to satisfactory sexual intercourse.

Bone fractures—especially osteoporotic fractures of the hip and spine—are associated with significant morbidity and mortality (i.e., 20% mortality at 1 year after an osteoporotic hip fracture[60]), particularly in older men. Stepan et al first reported the association between castration in prostate cancer patients and a progressive loss of bone mineral density leading to fractures.[61] Increasing evidence has recently confirmed the effects of androgen deprivation on bone loss[62] and osteoporosis.[63] Prostate cancer patients with no apparent bone metastasis who were on androgen deprivation therapy are reported to have had a two-fold increase in fracture rate (after adjusting for

age and preexisting osteoporosis).[64] African-American men and individuals with a high body mass index appear to be protected against skeletal fractures associated with androgen suppression.[65] All men who receive androgen deprivation therapy should be counseled about following a regular exercise regimen, using vitamin D and calcium supplements, and making other lifestyle changes to reduce their risk of osteoporosis. Various bisphosphonates have also been recommended as prophylactic agents in men receiving antiandrogen deprivation therapy for extended time periods.

Liver toxicity, including rising transaminase levels, has been associated mainly with antiandrogen therapy (i.e., flutamide).[54,66] There have also been sporadic reports in the literature linking liver necrosis and severe hepatitis to hormonal manipulation with antiandrogens.[67] Other less common side effects associated with androgen deprivation therapy include hair loss, dry eyes, depression, and vertigo.

Conclusions

Many questions about the use of androgen deprivation in early prostate cancer as yet remain unanswered. Should monotherapy or combined androgen blockade be used? What is the role of androgen deprivation as either neoadjuvant or adjuvant therapy? What effects do the adverse events associated with hormone therapy have on the quality of life of these patients? Only large, well-designed, randomized, controlled trials can provide the answers to these important questions.

References

1. Huggins C, Hodges CV. Studies on prostatic cancer, 1. The effect of castration, of estrogen and of androgen injection of serum phosphatases in metastatic carcinoma of the prostate. Cancer Res 1941;1:293–297.
2. The Veterans Administration Co-operative Urological Research Group. Treatment and survival of patients with cancer of the prostate. Surg Gynecol Obstet 1967;124:1011–1017.
3. Jordan WP Jr, Blackard CE, Byar DP. Reconsideration of orchiectomy in the treatment of advanced prostatic carcinoma. South Med J 1977;70:1411–1413.
4. Byar DP, Corle DK. Hormone therapy for prostate cancer: Results of the Veterans Administration Cooperative Urological Research Group studies. NCI Monogr 1988;7:165–170.
5. Chang A, Yeap B, Davis T, et al, Double-blind, randomized study of primary hormonal treatment of stage D2 prostate carcinoma: flutamide versus diethylstilbestrol. J Clin Oncol 1996;14:2250–2257.
6. Henriksson P, Blomback M, Bratt G, et al. Effects of oestrogen therapy and orchidectomy on coagulation and prostanoid synthesis in patients with prostatic cancer. Med Oncol Tumor Pharmacother 1989;6:219–225.
7. Carlstrom K, Collste L, Eriksson A, et al, A comparison of androgen status in patients with prostatic cancer treated with oral and/or parenteral estrogens or by orchidectomy. Prostate 1989;2:177–182.
8. von Schoultz B, Carlstrom K, Collste L, et al. Estrogen therapy and liver function—metabolic effects of oral and parenteral administration. Prostate 1989;14:389–395.
9. Mikkola AK, Ruutu ML, Aro JL, et al. Parenteral polyoestradiol phosphate vs orchidectomy in the treatment of advanced prostatic cancer. Efficacy and cardiovascular complications: a 2-year follow-up report of a national, prospective prostatic cancer study, Finnprostate Group. Br J Urol 1998;82:63–68.

10. Henriksson P, Carlstrom K, Pousette A, et al. Time for revival of estrogens in the treatment of advanced prostatic carcinoma? Pharmacokinetics, and endocrine and clinical effects, of a parenteral estrogen regimen. Prostate 1999;40:76–82.

11. Hedlund PO, Henriksson P. Parenteral estrogen versus total androgen ablation in the treatment of advanced prostate carcinoma: effects on overall survival and cardiovascular mortality. The Scandinavian Prostatic Cancer Group (SPCG)-5 Trial Study. Urology 2000;55:328–333.

12. Kitahara S, Yoshida K, Ishizaka K, et al. Stronger suppression of serum testosterone and FSH levels by a synthetic estrogen than by castration or an LH-RH agonist. Endocr J 1997;44:527–532.

13. Schally AV. Aspects of hypothalamic regulation of the pituitary gland with major emphasis on its implications for the control of reproductive processes, Nobel Lecture, December 8, 1977, http://nobelprize.org/medicine/laureates/1977/schally-lecture.html

14. Schally AV, Redding TW, Comaru-Schally AM. Inhibition of prostate tumors by agonistic and antagonistic analogs of LH-RH. Prostate 1983;4:545–552.

15. Smith JA Jr, Glode LM, Wettlaufer JN, et al. Clinical effects of gonadotropin-releasing hormone analogue in metastatic carcinoma of prostate. Urology 1985;25:106–114.

16. Seidenfeld J, Samson DJ, Hasselblad V, et al. Single-therapy androgen suppression in men with advanced prostate cancer: a systematic review and meta-analysis, Ann Intern Med 2000;132:566–577.

17. Limonta P, Montagnani Marelli M, et al. LHRH analogues as anticancer agents: pituitary and extrapituitary sites of action. Expert Opin Investig Drugs 2001;10:709–720.

18. Oefelein MG, Feng A, Scolieri MJ, et al. Reassessment of the definition of castrate levels of testosterone: implications for clinical decision making. Urology 2000;56:1021–1024.

19. Crawford ED, Eisenberger MA, McLeod DG, et al. A controlled trial of leuprolide with and without flutamide in prostatic carcinoma. N Engl J Med 1989;321:419–424.

20. Boccon-Gibod L. Are non-steroidal anti-androgens appropriate as monotherapy in advanced prostate cancer? Eur Urol 1998;33:159–164.

21. Loblaw DA, Mendelson DS, Talcott JA, et al. American Society of Clinical Oncology recommendations for the initial hormonal management of androgen-sensitive metastatic, recurrent, or progressive prostate cancer. J Clin Oncol 2004;22:2927–2941.

22. Samson DJ, Seidenfeld J, Schmitt B, et al. Systematic review and meta-analysis of monotherapy compared with combined androgen blockade for patients with advanced prostate carcinoma. Cancer 2002;95:361–376.

23. Altwein JE, Complete androgen blockade versus monotherapy. Urologe A 1998;37:149–152 [Article in German].

24. Stricker HJ. Luteinizing hormone-releasing hormone antagonists in prostate cancer. Urology 2001;58 (2 Suppl 1):24–27.

25. Trachtenberg J, Gittleman M, Steidle C, et al. A phase 3, multicenter, open label, randomized study of abarelix versus leuprolide plus daily antiandrogen in men with prostate cancer. J Urol 2002;167:1670–1674.

26. Weckermann D, Harzmann R. Hormone therapy in prostate cancer: LHRH antagonists versus LHRH analogues. Eur Urol 2004;46:279–284.

27. Mooradian AD, Morley JE, Korenman SG. Biological actions of androgens. Endocr Rev 1987;8:1–28.

28. Huang ZQ, Li J, Wong J. AR possesses an intrinsic hormone-independent transcriptional activity. Mol Endocrinol 2002;16:924–937.

29. Dai J, Shen R, Sumitomo M, et al. Synergistic activation of the androgen receptor by bombesin and low-dose androgen. Clin Cancer Res 2002;8:2399–2405.

30. Thompson IM, Zeidman EJ, Rodriguez FR. Sudden death due to disease flare with luteinizing hormone-releasing hormone agonist therapy for carcinoma of the prostate. J Urol 1990;144:1479–1480.

31. English HF, Kyprianou N, Isaacs JT. Relationship between DNA fragmentation and apoptosis in the programmed cell death in the rat prostate following castration. Prostate 1989;15:233–250.

32. Isaacs JT, Lundmo PI, Berges R, et al. Androgen regulation of programmed death of normal and malignant prostatic cells. J Androl 1992;13:457–464.

33. Murphy WM, Soloway MS, Barrows GH. Pathologic changes associated with androgen deprivation therapy for prostate cancer. Cancer 1991;68:821-828.

34. Tang DG, Porter AT. Target to apoptosis: a hopeful weapon for prostate cancer. Prostate 1997;32:284–293.

35. Strum SB, Scholz MC, McDermed JE. Intermittent androgen deprivation in prostate cancer patients: factors predictive of prolonged time off therapy. Oncologist 2000;5:45–52.

36. Kollermann J, Caprano J, Budde A, et al. Follow-up of nondetectable prostate carcinoma (pT0) after prolonged PSA-monitored neoadjuvant hormonal therapy followed by radical prostatectomy. Urology 2003;62:476–480.

37. Gleave ME, La Bianca SE, Goldenberg SL, et al. Long-term neoadjuvant hormone therapy prior to radical prostatectomy: evaluation of risk for biochemical recurrence at 5-year follow-up. Urology 2000;56:289–294.

38. Messing EM, Manola J, Sarosdy M, et al. Immediate hormonal therapy compared with observation after radical prostatectomy and pelvic lymphadenectomy in men with node-positive prostate cancer. N Engl J Med 1999;341:1781–1788.

39. Pilepich MV, Caplan R, Byhardt RW, et al. Phase III trial of androgen suppression using goserelin in unfavorable-prognosis carcinoma of the prostate treated with definitive radiotherapy: report of Radiation Therapy Oncology Group Protocol 85-31. J Clin Oncol 1997;15:1013–1021.

40. Bolla M, Gonzalez D, Warde P, et al. Improved survival in patients with locally advanced prostate cancer treated with radiotherapy and goserelin. N Engl J Med 1997;337:295–300.

41. Crawford ED. Early versus late hormonal therapy: debating the issues. Urology 2003;61(2 Suppl 1):8–13.

42. Gleave ME, Goldenberg SL, Chin JL, et al. Randomized comparative study of 3 versus 8-month neoadjuvant hormonal therapy before radical prostatectomy: biochemical and pathological effects. J Urol 2001;166:500-506; discussion 506–507.

43. Meyer F, Bairati I, Bedard C, et al. Duration of neoadjuvant androgen deprivation therapy before radical prostatectomy and disease-free survival in men with prostate cancer. Urology 2001;58 (2 Suppl 1):71–77.

44. Hanks GE, Pajak TF, Porter A, et al. Phase III trial of long-term adjuvant androgen deprivation after neoadjuvant hormonal cytoreduction and radiotherapy in locally advanced carcinoma of the prostate: the Radiation Therapy Oncology Group Protocol 92-02. J Clin Oncol 2003;21:3972–3978.

45. Bolla M, Collette L, Blank L, et al. Long-term results with immediate androgen suppression and external irradiation in patients with locally advanced prostate cancer (an EORTC study): a phase III randomised trial. Lancet 2002;360:103–106.

46. Shipley WU, Lu JD, Pilepich MV, et al. Effect of a short course of neoadjuvant hormonal therapy on the response to subsequent androgen suppression in prostate cancer patients with relapse after radiotherapy: a secondary analysis of the randomized protocol RTOG 86-10. Int J Radiat Oncol Biol Phys 2002;54:1302–1310.

47. Stone P, Hardy J, Huddart R, et al. Fatigue in patients with prostate cancer receiving hormone therapy. Eur J Cancer 2000;36:1134–1141.

48. Green HJ, Pakenham KI, Headley BC, et al. Altered cognitive function in men treated for prostate cancer with luteinizing hormone-releasing hormone analogues and cyproterone acetate: a randomized controlled trial, BJU Int 2002;90:427–432.

49. Salminen E, Portin R, Korpela J, et al. Androgen deprivation and cognition in prostate cancer. Br J Cancer 2003;89:971–976.

50. Hatano T, Oishi Y, Furuta A, et al. Incidence of bone fracture in patients receiving luteinizing hormone-releasing hormone agonists for prostate cancer. BJU Int 2000;86:449–452.

51. Townsend MF, Sanders WH, Northway RO, et al. Bone fractures associated with luteinizing hormone-releasing hormone agonists used in the treatment of prostate carcinoma. Cancer 1997;79:545–550.

52. Asbell SO, Leon SA, Tester WJ, et al. Development of anemia and recovery in prostate cancer patients treated with combined androgen blockade and radiotherapy. Prostate 1996;29:243–248.

53. Rizzo M, Mazzei T, Mini E, et al. Leuprorelin acetate depot in advanced prostatic cancer: a phase II multicentre trial. J Int Med Res 1990;18 (Suppl 1):114–125.

54. Rosenthal SA, Linstadt DE, Leibenhaut MH, et al, Flutamide-associated liver toxicity during treatment with total androgen suppression and radiation therapy for prostate cancer, Radiology 1996;199:451–455.

55. Bokhour BG, Clark JA, Inui TS, et al. Sexuality after treatment for early prostate cancer: exploring the meanings of "erectile dysfunction." J Gen Intern Med 2001;16:649–655.

56. Basaria S, Lieb J 2nd, Tang AM, et al. Long-term effects of androgen deprivation therapy in prostate cancer patients. Clin Endocrinol (Oxf) 2002;56:779–786.

57. Loprinzi CL, Pisansky TM, Fonseca R, et al. Pilot evaluation of venlafaxine hydrochloride for the therapy of hot flashes in cancer survivors. J Clin Oncol 1998;16:2377–2381.

58. Tayek JA, Heber D, Byerley LO, Steiner B, Rajfer J, et al. Nutritional and metabolic effects of gonadotropin-releasing hormone agonist treatment for prostate cancer. Metabolism 1990;39:1314–1319.

59. Baba K, Yajima M, Carrier S, et al. Effect of testosterone on the number of NADPH diaphorase-stained nerve fibers in the rat corpus cavernosum and dorsal nerve. Urology 2000;56:533–538.

60. Osteoporosis Prevention, Diagnosis, and Therapy. NIH Consensus Statement. March 27-29, 2000;17:1-45. Available at http://consensus.nih.gov/cons/111/111_statement.pdf. Accessed 08-04.

61. Stepan JJ, Lachman M, Zverina J, et al. Castrated men exhibit bone loss: effect of calcitonin treatment on biochemical indices of bone remodeling. J Clin Endocrinol Metab 1989;69:523–527.

62. Diamond T, Campbell J, Bryant C, et al. The effect of combined androgen blockade on bone turnover and bone mineral densities in men treated for prostate carcinoma: longitudinal evaluation and response to intermittent cyclic etidronate therapy. Cancer 1998;83:1561–1566.

63. Daniell HW, Dunn SR, Ferguson DW, et al. Progressive osteoporosis during androgen deprivation therapy for prostate cancer. J Urol 2000;163:181–186.

64. Melton LJ 3rd, Alothman KI, Khosla S, Achenbach SJ, Oberg AL, Zincke H. Fracture risk following bilateral orchiectomy. J Urol 2003;169:1747–1750.

65. Oefelein MG, Ricchuiti V, Conrad W, et al. Skeletal fracture associated with androgen suppression induced osteoporosis: the clinical incidence and risk factors for patients with prostate cancer. J Urol 2001;166:1724–1728.

66. Gomez JL, Dupont A, Cusan L, et al. Incidence of liver toxicity associated with the use of flutamide in prostate cancer patients. Am J Med 1992;92:465–470.

67. Crownover RL, Holland J, Chen A, et al. Flutamide-induced liver toxicity including fatal hepatic necrosis. Int J Radiat Oncol Biol Phys 1996;34:911–915.

36

Hormonal therapy for prostate cancer: optimization and timing

David Kirk

Introduction

Hormone therapy is an effective treatment for prostate cancer and continues to have a key role in the management of the disease.[1] It is the only initial systemic treatment available for the man with advanced disease. Despite prostate-specific antigen (PSA) testing, many men still have incurable disease at diagnosis, and failure of curative treatment is often seen as an indication for hormonal treatment.[2] Disease presenting at an advanced stage where hormonal treatment is the only option continues to be common in many countries. Paradoxically, there may well now be more men who are candidates for hormonal treatment than ever before. There is also considerable interest in exploring the merits of adjuvant treatment[3] (Chapter 29)[CN]—the urologic equivalent of tamoxifen in breast cancer.

The effect of hormonal therapy on survival continues to be debated. However, doubts about the value of immediate versus deferred treatment are not confined to survival issues alone. With earlier diagnosis, many could be on treatment for many years. There is an increasing awareness of the toxicity of hormonal therapy, which has to be balanced against any benefits. The decision when to start therapy and which treatment to use depends on the balance of benefit and risk.

Clinical trials

Although trials in prostate cancer are dealt with in Chapters 29 and 93 and other chapters in this book, some important issues are relevant here.

1. Meaningful data can only come from randomized trials, analyzed on an intention to treat basis. Due to potential bias "statistical significance" from nonrandomized data is meaningless—the difference may be significant, but not necessarily for the reason being investigated.
2. Demonstration of equivalence between two treatment strategies requires substantially more patients than are included in most trials. Although a difference with $P > 0.05$ may not be significant in the statistical sense, it should *not* be concluded that there is *not* a difference. It often means simply that insufficient numbers have been included to rule out the *possibility* of chance. Also, statistical significance does not always equate with clinical significance.
3. In assessing survival differences, "snapshots" of data can be misleading. Even where survival curves show a highly significant difference, the difference in numbers alive at any one point is often small. Also, absolute numbers surviving on a particular date will include patients who have been in the study for varying lengths of time.
4. An issue of particular importance, and regularly discussed in prostate cancer, is the relationship between disease-specific versus overall survival. Interventions that reduce or delay mortality from prostate cancer are often perceived not to affect overall survival. In the Medical Research Council (MRC) study PR03, comparing immediate versus deferred hormonal treatment, current survival curves (Figure 36.1) confirm that the highly significant improvement in disease-specific survival in those treated immediately in earlier reports[4] persists. However, although overall survival is longer in those treated immediately, the difference is not significant. This apparent discrepancy is a familiar finding, and was also seen in the recently published Scandinavian Radical Prostatectomy Study.[5] In both instances, it has been concluded that the intervention, be it early hormone treatment or radical prostatectomy does not increase the patient's life span. This is an example of the erroneous assumption that, although there was a difference in overall survival, because it was not significant (i.e., $P > 0.05$) there was actually *no* difference.

Survival in men with prostate cancer

Prostate cancer occurs in an elderly population, who will experience co-morbidity, and as they get older have a reducing life expectation (Tables 36.1 and 36.2). The actual proportion of men surviving is the product of life expectation and prostate cancer survival. Even where survival from prostate cancer is similar, as men get older, fewer will survive because of comorbid deaths. Therefore, an intervention which will significantly extend prostate cancer survival will clearly improve the survival of a group of 60-year-olds but will have a negligible effect on that of men in their 80s. It is this effect of age and comorbidity that reduces the statistical significance of overall survival—the coincidental deaths diluting any overall benefit from improved prostate cancer survival.

If an intervention improving prostate cancer survival was genuinely associated with an unchanged overall mortality then that intervention should be associated with a treatment-related mortality.

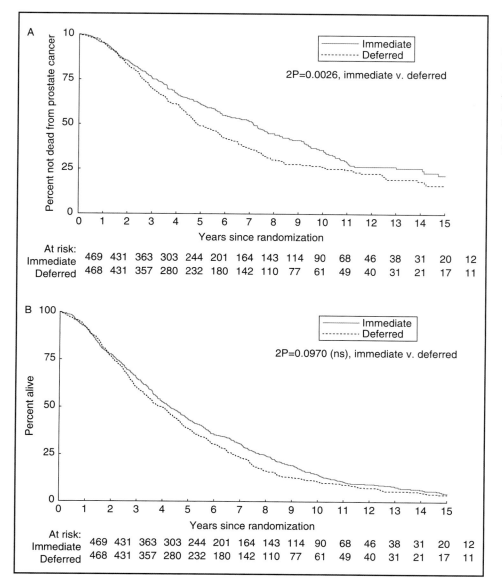

Figure 36.1
Medical Research Council (MRC) trial of immediate versus deferred hormone treatment—survival curves for all patients, by randomization group. *A*, Disease-specific survival. Time to death from prostate cancer, showing statistical significance. *B*, Overall survival. Time to death from any cause, not significant.

Table 36.1 Cause specific versus overall survival; overall survival is the product of the 10 year mortality from prostate cancer and the age related survival for other causes of death

Age	Expected 10-year survival, %	Prostate cancer survival, %	Overall survival, %
60	75	60	45
70	50	60	30
80	25	60	15

Table 36.2 Effect of treatment which reduces prostate cancer mortality from 40% to 28%, related to age

Age (years)	Expected 10 year survival, %	Prostate cancer survival, %	Overall survival, %
60	75	72 vs 60	54 vs 45
70	50	72 vs 60	36 vs 30
80	25	72 vs 60	18 vs 15

This was indeed the case in patients treated with estrogens, due to an increased risk of cardiovascular death,[6] but no such effect is apparent in trials using orchiectomy or luteinizing hormone releasing hormone (LHRH) analogs (unpublished meta-analysis), nor is such an effect apparent in MRC PR03 (see Figure 36.2). In comments on the Scandinavian Radical Prostatectomy study[5] it has been stated "there was no difference in overall mortality",[7] but there *was* a difference, numerically almost the same as the difference in prostate cancer survival (there was one postoperative death). It was

not statistically significant because of "dilution" by deaths from other causes, but it was a difference none the less.

In other words, improved survival from prostate cancer should be seen as a bonus on top of the patients' other risks of dying, but one which will only be realized by a small proportion of men in their 80s. The real issue is whether sufficient men will benefit to justify the intervention, something which may well apply in men with age and comorbidity that severely reduces life expectation.

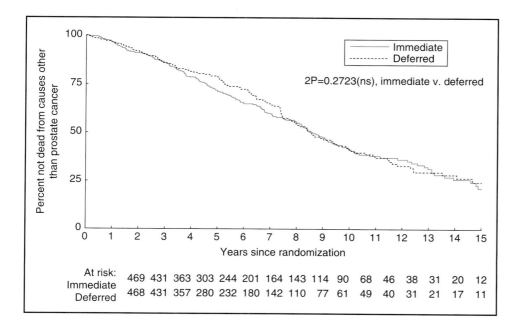

Figure 36.2
Medical Research Council (MRC) trial of immediate versus deferred hormone treatment—survival curves for all patients, by randomization group. Time to death from causes other than prostate cancer. No excess deaths apparent in the immediate group.

Table 36.3 Medical Research Council (MRC) PR03, comparison of immediate versus deferred hormone treatment in advanced prostate cancer–current status (2004)

	Immediate, n (%)	Deferred, n (%)
Entered	469	469
No with follow-up data	469	468
Died	446 (95.1)	449 (95.9)
Patients with metastases	126/130 (96.9)	130/131 (99.2)

Immediate versus deferred treatment

The issue of immediate versus deferred treatment has been discussed since the inception of hormonal therapy.[8] The results of MRC trial PR03, first published in 1996,[4] which demonstrated a disease-specific survival benefit from immediate treatment, have been contro-versial. The main concern[9] was that there were a number of patients who apparently died from prostate cancer without treatment. The number was not as great as initially reported, and the suggestion that failure to treat these patients explained the difference does not stand up to analysis.[10] This was an example of the misuse of the "snapshot," as, even if their survival had been increased by treatment, it is likely they still would have died before that date.

The current status of MRC PR03 is indicated in Table 36.3. Since the majority of patients have now died, the data is mature and unlikely to change significantly in future. From other studies, including those of adjuvant hormone treatment in patients receiving radiotherapy,[11] a consistent pattern is emerging that hormonal treatment improves survival in advanced prostate cancer. The issue of survival should finally be resolved by a meta-analysis of all studies involving immediate versus deferred treatment, although this is awaiting the outcome of an EORTC study.

Other benefits from hormone treatment

In 1996, results from PR03 demonstrated a reduction in complications in those treated immediately. Although in many cases, the complications, particularly spinal cord compression, occurred in the deferred treatment group after treatment had already been started for another unrelated cause, it did seem likely that, as the data matured, these complications would appear more frequently in the immediate treatment group, who would "catch up." Except for the incidence of ureteric obstruction, this does not seem to have happened (Table 36.4), and suggests that tumor progression, taking place during the period for which treatment is deferred, may not be fully reversible. Clearly, the reduction in these events has clear quality-of-life benefits, albeit for a minority of patients, to set against the disadvantages of hormone therapy.

Androgen deprivation—the disadvantages

Hormonal therapy conventionally involves androgen deprivation, whether achieved by orchiectomy or use of LHRH analogs. Reduction in serum testosterone has a number of adverse effects. In addition to the immediate problems with sexual dysfunction[12] and hot flushes,[13] in the medium term, patients experience weight increase and loss of muscle mass.[14] Patients can become anemic, and recently, it has been recognized that there can also be a loss of cognitive function.[15] Perhaps the most serious problem is osteoporosis,[16] with an increased incidence of pathologic fractures not due to metastases; most significant, in view of the trend towards earlier use of hormonal treatment, is its relation to duration of treatment.

The principle trials of immediate versus deferred treatment did not have access to modern quality-of-life measurements. Thus, a recent study by Gardiner et al[17] is of particular importance. This small, randomized study, has shown a clear loss of quality of life up

Table 36.4 Medical Research Council (MRC) PR03 incidence of complications (all patients by randomization group)

Complication	Results in 1996		Results in 2004	
	Immediate, n	Deferred, n	Immediate, n	Deferred, n
Spinal cord compression	9	23	10	24
Pathologic fracture	11	21	14	22
Extraskeletal metastases	37	55	47	63
Ureteric obstruction	33	55	50	65
Transurethral resection of the prostate*	65	141	88	152
(*>6/52 after entry)				
Number of patients reported with pain from metastases				
Number died from prostate cancer	–	–	249	295
Number with pain	–	–	138	223

Table 36.5 Hormone therapies: effects on luteinizing hormone releasing hormone (LHRH), luteinizing hormone (LH), follicle stimulating hormone (FSH), and testosterone

Therapy	LHRH	LH	FSH	Testosterone
Orchiectomy	↑	↑	↑	↓
LHRH analog	↑	↓	↓	↓
Cyproterone acetate	↓	↓	↓	↓R
Nonsteroidal antiandrogen	↓ or →	↑ or →	↓ or →	↑ or →
Estrogens	↓	↓	↓	↓R

R = testosterone replaced by non androgen steroid hormone.

to 1 year after starting treatment. However, patients for whom this period represents a significant portion of their survival will probably have had a mandatory indication for treatment with symptomatic disease. In others with longer expectation of survival, later benefits from delay in progression might compensate for the earlier loss of quality of life. This study does give pause for thought before commencing hormonal treatment in those for whom the benefits are unproven, and the results should be introduced into the discussion of treatment options with the patient. There will be some for whom short-term quality of life is more important than maximum longevity.

Choice of treatment

Whereas once the only choice available was between orchiectomy and estrogen treatment, there are now several options. These produce different endocrine changes (Table 36.5), which influence their potential side effects, and possibly their relative efficacy.

It is generally accepted that LHRH analogs are equivalent therapeutically to earlier methods of hormone treatment—but is this really the case? The clinical trials on which this is based[18–22] involved from 80 to less than 300 patients—too small a number to conclusively exclude a difference that might be clinically significant. In these studies, the survival curves were far from coincident, and, again, an assumption of equivalence was made because the differences did not reach clinical significance. The large randomized trial

necessary to prove this point will never be done, so likely equivalence in efficacy must be accepted. However, the possibility that testosterone may not have been suppressed to castrate levels should be considered if a patient does not respond to LHRH analog treatment as expected

Orchiectomy versus luteinizing hormone releasing hormone analog treatment

Accepting the therapeutic equivalence of orchiectomy and luteinizing hormone releasing hormone analog treatment, the decision as to which to use relates to the practical and other consequences of the treatment. Orchiectomy involves an operation and potential surgical complications. Whether "castration" produces the psychological problems often assumed is less clear. Most urologists will do a subcapsular orchiectomy, which reduces the size of the testis rather than removing it. There are clear advantages in terms of compliance, and, although the procedure is irreversible, there must be few occasions when this will matter. Luteinizing hormone releasing hormone analogs have the problem of tumor flare,[23] and most users will recommend flare prevention with an antiandrogen. The need for continuing injections may, over a long period, cancel out the disadvantage of an operation, and occasional drug idiosyncrasies can occur. In practice, although in the author's practice a few patients do opt for orchiectomy, LHRH analog treatment is the current standard, whether as monotherapy or as part of a combined regime.

Reducing morbidity from hormone treatment

Deferred treatment is essentially a strategy to reduce morbidity. If deferment involved no loss of therapeutic benefit, there would be no issue. If earlier treatment does improve survival, a complex equation emerges. Perhaps some of the concern about quality of life ignores the fact that throughout medicine, and especially in oncology, there is always a price to pay, both in terms of potential side effects and of cost. Why should prostate cancer be different? Unlike chemotherapy, which produces severe short-term complications but is given for a defined period, hormonal therapy is an ongoing treatment for which the risk of significant toxicity increases with time. Hormonal therapy is a form of disease control, not a cure, and, until we can elucidate the problem of hormone refractory relapse, will ultimately fail. Add to this the fact that many men will not die from prostate cancer and a picture emerges which, for example, contrasts strongly with the treatment of testicular cancer in young men.

Alternatively, to maximize any survival advantage, there are alternative strategies to reduce toxicity of treatment, some of which are discussed in other chapters of this book.

The use of other drugs

There is some evidence that nonsteroidal antiandrogens may have less toxicity.[24] Bicalutamide 150 mg/day, licensed for use as monotherapy in locally advanced disease, may be appropriate for selected patients and can be discussed as an alternative option. Were it not for cardiovascular toxicity, estrogens would have much to commend them.[25] Toxicity could be reduced either by use in low dosage combined with aspirin, or by parenteral administration avoiding the initial metabolism in the liver, believed to be the source of the toxicity. The depot injection estrodurin was used in a Scandinavian study,[26] which demonstrated equivalent efficacy. However, the number of cardiovascular adverse events was increased and although there was no excess in cardiovascular mortality, this may have been the result of the small numbers involved.

Other regimens

Particularly in early disease (i.e., PSA relapse after radical treatment) there is interest in drug escalation,[27] perhaps commencing with a 5α-reductase inhibitor, then an antiandrogen, with the medical or surgical castration only as relapse occurs. This approach is probably not appropriate in advanced disease. Intermittent therapy is discussed in detail in another chapter. It may not only reduce the impact of toxicity but also delay the onset of hormone-refractory disease.[28] Complications might be preempted by therapy such as bisphosphonate treatment, which, although principally to modify the develop-ment of metastatic disease, may also help prevent osteoporosis.[29]

Combined androgen blockade

If this book had been written in the mid-1990s, it would certainly have contained a whole chapter devoted to combination treatment with androgen deprivation (be it orchiectomy or LHRH analog) and antiandrogens. Although the Prostate Cancer Trialist's Collaborative Group's second meta-analysis published in 2000[30] did show a statistically significant survival benefit, this was small, and generally seems not to be thought clinically worthwhile. Certainly in the UK, after over a decade of intense investigation, interest in routine use of combined androgen blockade as primary hormone treatment has waned. In patients in whom there has been a good response to primary monotherapy with androgen deprivation, addition of an antiandrogen may produce a further response,[31] and the author's practice is to start an LHRH analog for patients relapsing on antiandrogen monotherapy.

Hormonal treatment in 2006

There seems a general consensus that treatment is indicated on diagnosis of M1 disease. Deferred treatment is likely to be needed early, and these are the patients most at risk from serious complications like spinal cord compression. Trial data on survival after deferred treatment is inconclusive, and is likely to remain so, partly because treatment is delayed for such a short time (Peto, personal communication). In most cases, an LHRH analog will be indicated, although the need for a speedy effect makes disease presenting with actual or impending spinal cord compression an indication for orchiectomy.[32]

In locally advanced disease, although the debate about immediate versus deferred treatment continues, the following points can be made:

- Hormone treatment does have an impact on advanced prostate cancer.
- Immediate treatment may reduce, not simply delay, significant complications.
- Disease progression during deferred period may not be completely reversible.
- Disease-specific survival is improved.
- The lack of statistically significant overall survival benefit in individual trials may simply reflect the expected mortality from other diseases in men surviving longer from prostate cancer.
- Even if a reduction in prostate cancer mortality is at the expense of an increase in deaths from other causes, it might be better to die from a myocardial infarct than from prostate cancer.

However, although in M0 disease, immediate treatment seems to improve local and distant disease control and may produce a survival advantage, this has to be balanced against the risk of toxicity in what may be a prolonged period of treatment. In practice, each patient has to be considered individually and should be involved himself in the decision. His age, health, and aspirations are all important. Deferred treatment remains an option in many, selected patients, but the patient's compliance is essential, with careful follow-up and responding to rapid PSA rises, which may be the best indicator of aggressive disease, with prompt treatment. The balance in this equation changes as the stage of the disease reduces and the length of time for which treatment is likely to continue increases. Failure of curative treatment is dealt with elsewhere in this book. Although there is randomized study suggesting survival benefit from hormone treatment in patients with node positive disease,[33] it should be interpreted with caution because of its small size. The adverse implications of early initiation of hormonal treatment must be carefully considered until the benefits of treatment at this stage of the disease become clearer.

References

1. Rabbini F, Gleave ME. Treatment of metastatic prostate cancer: endocrine therapy. In: Hamdy FC, Basler JW, Neal DE, Catalona WJ (eds): Management of Urologic Malignancies. Edinburgh: Churchill Livingstone, 2002, pp 210–226.
2. Davis NB, Jani AB, Vogelzang NJ. Selecting a treatment. Urol Clin N Am 2003;30:403–414.
3. See WA. Wirth MP, Mcleod DG, et al, Bicalutamide as immediate therapy either alone or as adjuvant to standard care of patients with localised or locally advanced prostate cancer: first analysis of the early prostate cancer program. J Urol 2002;168:429–435.
4. Medical Research Council Prostate Cancer Working Party Investigators Group. Immediate versus deferred treatment for advanced prostatic cancer: initial results of the Medical Research Council Trial. Brit J Urol 1997;79:235–246.

5. Holmberg L, Bill-Axelson A, Helgesen F, et al. A randomised trial comparing radical prostatectomy with watchful waiting in early prostate cancer. New Eng J Med 2002;347:781–789.

6. Byar DP. The Veterans Administration Cooperative Research Group's studies of cancer of the prostate. Cancer 1973;32:1126–1130.

7. Kirby RS, Fitzpatrick JM. Radical prostatectomy or watchful waiting? Br J Urol International 2003;91:5.

8. Nesbit RM, Baum WC. Endocrine control of prostatic cancer. Clinical survey of 1818 cases. JAMA 1950;143:1317–1320.

9. Schröder FH. Endocrine treatment of prostate cancer – recent developments and the future. Part 1: maximal androgen blockade. Early vs delayed endocrine treatment and side effects. Br J Urol Intl 1999;83:161–170.

10. Kirk D. Medical Research Council immediate versus deferred treatment study; patients dying without treatment. Br J Urol 1998;81:31.

11. Bolla M, Gonzalez D, Warde P, et al. Improved survival in patients with locally advanced prostate cancer treated with radiotherapy and goserelin. N Engl J Med 1997;337:295–300.

12. Ellis WJ, Grayhack JT, Sexual function in aging males after orchiectomy and estrogen therapy. J Urol 1963;89:895–899.

13. Radlmier A, Bormacher K, Neumann F. Hot flushes: mechanism and prevention. Prog Clin Biol Res 1990;359:131–140.

14. Morley JE, Kaiser FE, Hajjar R, Perr HM III. Testosterone and frailty. Clin Geriat Med 1997;13:655–695.

15. Gardiner RA, Green H, Yaxley J, et al. Cognition and hormonal manipulation in prostate cancer. Br J Urol Intl 2000;86:218–219.

16. Daniell HW. Osteoporosis after orchiectomy for prostate cancer. J Urol 1997;157:439–444.

17. Green HJ, Pakenham KI, Headley, BC, et al. Quality of life compared during pharmacological treatments and clinical monitoring for non-localised prostate cancer: a randomised controlled trial. Br J Urol Intl 2004;93:975–979.

18. Mahler C. Is disease flare a problem? Cancer 1993;72:3799–3802.

19. Soloway MS, et al. Zoladex versus orchiectomy in treatment of advanced prostate cancer: a randomised trial. Urology 1991;37:46–51.

20. Kaisary AV, Tyrell CJ, Peeling WB, et al on behalf of Study Group. Comparison of LHRH analogue (Zoladex) with orchiectomy in patients with metastatic prostate cancer. Br J Urol 1991;67:502–508.

21. Botto H, Richard F, Mathieu F, Camey M. Decapeptyl in the treatment of metastatic prostatic cancer. Comparative study with pulpectomy. In Liss AR: Prostate Cancer, Part A: Research, Endocrine Treatment, and Histopathology. 1987, pp 199–296.

22. The Leuprolide Study Group. Leuprolide vs diethylstilbestrol for metastatic prostate cancer. N Eng J Med 1984;311:1281–1286.

23. Mahler C. Is disease flare a problem? Cancer 1993;72:3799–3802.

24. Anderson J. The role of antiandrogen monotherapy in the treatment of prostate cancer. Br J Urol Intl 2003;91:455–61.

25. Bishop MC, Experience with low-dose oestrogen in the treatment of advanced prostate cancer: a personal view. Br J Urol 1996;78:921–928.

26. Hedlund PO, Ala-Opas M, Brekkan E, et al. Parenteral estrogen versus combined androgen deprivation in the treatment of metastatic prostate cancer. Scand J Urol Nephrol 2002;36:405–413.

27. Fleshner NE, Trachtenberg J. Sequential androgen blockade: a biological study in the inhibition of prostatic growth. J Urol 1992;148:1928–1931.

28. Goldenberg SL, Bruchovsky N, Gleave ME, et al. Intermittent androgen suppression in the treatment of prostate cancer: a preliminary report. Urology 1995;45:839–844.

29. Ernst DS. The role of bisphosphonates in prostate cancer. In: Bangma CH, Newling DWW (eds): Prostate and renal cancer, benign prostatic hyperplasia, erectile dysfunction and basic research an update. New York: Parthenon, 2003, pp 414–420.

30. Prostate Cancer Trialists' Collaborative Group. Maximum androgen blockade in advanced prostate cancer: an overview of the randomised trials. Lancet 2000;355:1491–1498.

31. Fujikawa, Matsui Y, Fukuzawa S, Takeuchi H. Prostate-specific antigen levels and clinical response to flutamide as a second hormone therapy for hormone-refractory prostate carcinoma. Eur Urol 2000;37:218–222.

32. Basler JW, Werschman J. Prostate cancer: management of sequelae, voiding dysfunction and renal failure In Hamdy FC, Basler JW, Neal DE, Catalona WJ (eds): Management of Urologic Malignancies Edinburgh Churchill Livingstone, 2002, pp 261–269.

33. Messing E, Manola J, Sarosdy M, et al. Immediate hormonal therapy vs observation for node positive prostate cancer following radical prostatectomy and pelvic lymphadenectomy. N Engl J Med 1999;314:1781–1788.

37

Controversies in hormone treatment for prostate cancer

Mario A Eisenberger

Introduction

For several decades, it has been well known that the growth and differentiation of prostate cancer cells is to a great extent under hormonal control.[1,2] Circulating testosterone (T) is converted to dihydrotestosterone (DHT) by the enzyme 5α-reductase. Dihydrotestosterone will bind to intracellular androgen receptor (AR) and subsequently induce intra nuclear transcriptional activity.[1] The AR is also activated by other androgens including T and adrenal androgens, which are converted peripherally to T or DHT.[3] Androgen deprivation for prostate cancer focuses primarily in maneuvers that will reduce circulating testosterone to levels around or below castrate levels (<50 ng/mL). Gonadal androgen deprivation is the standard therapeutic approach. It triggers the induction of a swift apoptotic cascade resulting in irreversible changes in the genomic DNA and, clinically, it represents one of the most effective systemic palliative treatments known for solid tumors in man.[1,3]

The biology of the AR has been the focus of significant attention over the past several years. Transcriptional activity of the AR can be induced by ligand dependent and ligand independent mechanisms as well as coactivators. Undoubtedly, the molecular and functional status of the AR play an important role in the endocrine dependence of prostate cancer and over the past years has also been focus of various therapeutic interventions.[4]

While androgen deprivation treatment for prostate cancer has been extensively applied in the clinic for many years, there are important remaining controversies regarding its optimal use. The focus of this chapter is not to review in any major detail the different approaches currently in clinical practice, but to highlight the background of some of the unresolved controversies associated with endocrine treatment for prostate cancer.

Optimal timing for androgen ablation: the immediate versus deferred treatment controversy

At the present time there is a general consensus that immediate hormonal therapy improves the quality of life of patients with *metastatic disease* despite the fact that survival is not clearly better than treatment deferred until time of progression. The Veterans Administration Cooperative Research Group (VACURG) conducted important studies in patients with various stages of prostate cancer.[5–7] These studies have made a significant impact on various current issues related to endocrine treatment for this disease even though they were conducted approximately 4 decades ago. In VACURG study 1, patients with stage D2 and stage C were randomized to receive initial treatment with bilateral orchiectomy plus either placebo or 5 mg/day diethylstilbestrol (DES), or 5 mg/day DES alone, or a placebo alone. The data suggested that patients randomized to the placebo arm and subsequently crossed over to one of the three other study arms at the time of disease progression had a comparable survival to those randomized to initial treatment on the remaining three arms.[5,6] These data prompted the controversy that immediate androgen deprivation treatment for patients with metastatic disease was not associated with a survival benefit compared with treatment at the time of disease progression. While treatment with 5 mg/day DES was associated with comparable death rates due to prostate cancer as bilateral orchiectomy, there was a significant increase in deaths due to cardiovascular complications attributed to the use of DES. A subsequent study, VACURG study 2, was designed to evaluate the safety of different doses of DES (5.0, 1.0, or 0.2 mg/day) compared with a placebo initially. The final results of VACURG study 2, indicated that 1.0 mg/day was as effective as 5 mg/day DES in terms of deaths due to prostate cancer; however, there was a significant decrease in the incidence of severe and potentially fatal cardiovascular complications on the 1.0 mg/day arm. Both 5 mg/day and 1.0 mg/day DES had a lower incidence of deaths due to prostate cancer compared with a dose of 0.2 mg/day of DES or placebo. Unlike VACURG study 1, several patients on the placebo arm never received any treatment at the time of progression, and so study 2 is not perceived as an adequate test of the immediate versus deferred treatment question. Furthermore, VACURG study 2 was designed primarily to address the safety issue.

Several years later, the Medical Research Council (MRC) evaluated the survival of men receiving immediate treatment versus deferred treatment (at the time of progression) in patients with metastatic (M+; 434 patients) and nonmetastatic (M0; 500 patients) disease.[8,9] In the 434 patients with M+ disease there was no significant difference in prostate cancer-specific survival, however, the incidence of pathologic fractures, epidural cord compression, and renal failure was significantly lower in those receiving immediate treatment. While in the M0 group, the proportion of deaths due to prostate cancer was substantially lower in those receiving immediate treatment, a substantial number of patients randomized to deferred treatment never received any treatment at all. In the MRC studies, the criteria for initiating treatment on the deferred group was left at the discretion of the primary general physician. Despite the severe methodologic shortcomings of these studies, which prevent definitive recommendations regarding survival advantages for immediate treatment, the choice of immediate treatment for patients with M+ disease or locally advanced disease (M0) disease is primarily aimed at the reduction of severe disease related morbidity. An overview analysis conducted by the agency for Health Care Policy and Research (AHCPR) evaluating various aspect on hormonal therapy for prostate cancer concluded that the survival benefits of early hormonal therapy were not statistically significant with a combined hazard ratio of 0.914.

Adjuvant and concomitant androgen suppression with radiation and surgery in patients with clinically localized prostate cancer

There is a growing amount of information on combined approaches employing hormonal therapy with concomitant radiation therapy for patients with palpable primary tumors. In one of the first studies reported by Pilepich et al[12] (RTOG 8531) patients with high-risk disease (M0) or with local recurrence after surgery were randomized to receive external-beam radiation therapy (EBRT) with or without permanent gonadal (medical or surgical) suppression. With a median follow-up of 13 years,[12] there was a statistically significant survival advantage for those receiving radiation plus permanent hormonal therapy. Of concern is that over the entire follow-up period of this study, the methodology used to evaluate patients and document progression changed significantly during the lifetime of the study. Furthermore no information regarding initiation of deferred treatment is available at this time. At the time of initiation of study (1985), the RTOG investigators did not count with the availability of PSA tests, which only became widely utilized much later during the conduct of the study. Two subsequent studies, RTOG 8610 and RTOG 9202,[10,11] have demonstrated a survival advantage for hormonal therapy on subsets only. RTOG 8610 demonstrated that a short course of 4 months adjuvant/neoadjuvant hormonal therapy is adequate for low-risk patients, whereas a 2-year hormonal therapy is effective in prolonging survival in high-risk patients on RTOG 9202. EORTC 22863 (Bolla et al) which included mostly high-risk patients, demonstrated that a 3-year androgen deprivation treatment plus EBRT was superior to EBRT alone in terms of local control, clinical and biochemical disease-free survival, and overall survival. Ongoing trials in the US are likely to provide additional information to support routine use of ADT plus radiation therapy in patients with palpable, clinically localized prostate cancer. Of importance is that none of these studies were designed to address the question of immediate versus deferred hormonal therapy. The primary hypothesis in these trials involves the biologic interaction between radiation and androgen deprivation, however, given the known effects of androgen deprivation in delaying the onset of distant metastatic disease, survival remains the key endpoint of clinical trials. Most North American studies (all except RTOG 8531) have only shown a survival benefit in subsets thus far, but despite this most physicians recommend a combined approach to patients with palpable primary tumors who are candidates for EBRT. It is hope that the ongoing RTOG studies will shed more light on the optimal duration of ADT on these patients and further characterized short- and long-term toxicities.

The Eastern Cooperative Oncology Group carried out a randomized prospective analysis of immediate hormonal therapy compared with observation in men following radical prostatectomy who had positive lymph nodes.[14] Ninety-eight men were randomized to either immediate hormonal ablation or followed until disease progression. After a median of 7.1 years of follow-up there was a significant difference in survival favoring immediate therapy. This result is rather surprising because there was a fairly large difference in survival within a relatively short period of observation. In this study, cancer-specific survival in the observation group was 78% at 5 years. This is quite low compared with the rate of 91% in two contemporary series of patients with microscopic nodal metastasis who were treated with radical prostatectomy alone.[15–17] Furthermore, a series from the Mayo Clinic series, which represents the largest retrospective series with a nonrandomized control arm of patients and almost 3 decades of follow-up, found that the survival advantage in favor of immediate androgen deprivation was limited to DNA diploid tumors and did not become apparent until after 10 years.[16] Indeed, in that study of 790 men with lymph node-positive disease who underwent radical prostatectomy, androgen ablation therapy had no effect on cause-specific survival in nondiploid tumors. In the 57 men with diploid tumors who were followed for 10 years, there was also no significant difference in survival. At 15 years there were 14 patients with diploid tumors, 12 of whom received early hormonal therapy and 2 who did not. It is only in this small group where there was a statistical difference in survival ($83.2 \pm 4.1\%$ versus $48.5 \pm 13\%$). Thus, this finding is based on 14 patients out of 790 node positive men. Why is this ECOG study so different from the others? In an editorial, that accompanied the paper, a concern was raised that this study never realized its projected goal of 240 patients.[18] This is important because the outcome of patients with nodal metastasis is extremely variable and can be affected by a number of known and possibly unknown prognostic factors. Such effects on the outcome of trials can be minimized by randomization, but this ECOG trial was relatively small and might have been affected by imbalances of factors that had not been identified at the time the study began. The fact that 50% of the men in the deferred arm had progressed at 5 years and 22% were dead supports the argument that the control arm (deferred treatment) in the ECOG study most likely represented a high-risk group of patients composed of many high-grade tumors. These observations stress the importance of patient selection factors in the outcome of relatively small clinical studies in the adjuvant setting and highlight the complexities involved in the interpretation of results.

Another treatment explored in early stage prostate cancer is the use on antiandrogens as single agent. The most extensively developed drug in this setting is bicalutamide. Data in patients with metastatic disease suggest that bicalutamide (50 and 150 mg/day) as monotherapy is inferior to bilateral orchiectomy in prospective randomized trials.[19,20] The data in patients without metastasis is too preliminary for definitive conclusions. One large international placebo controlled study evaluated the adjuvant role of 150 mg/day of bicalutamide in high-risk patients treated with radical prostatectomy and radiotherapy or no treatment (watchful waiting). With a relatively short follow-up time, a statistically significant difference in progression was observed in favor of bicalutamide, treatment was unblinded and the study was terminated. Toxicity (gynecomastia, gastrointestinal) was significant and because of the early unblinding of treatment, survival data may not be reliable. More recent evaluation ,with a median follow-up of 5.4 years, there were 25% of deaths on the bicalutamide arm compared with 20% on placebo (hazard ratio [HR] 1.2; 95% confidence interval [CI] 1.0–1.5).[1]

Complete androgen blockade

While there is extensive data supporting a heterogeneity of cell populations with regard to androgen dependence[21,22] (androgen-dependent and -independent cell clones), it is increasingly recognized that the AR[3,4] albeit molecularly and functionally altered, continues to influence the progression of prostate cancer even after gonadal ablation. Transcriptional activity of the AR can be induced by ligand-dependent and ligand-independent mechanisms as well as coactivators. One of the earliest hypotheses focusing on a combined approach of gonadal androgen suppression and a blockade of AR, was promoted by Labrie et al[22,23] over 20 years ago. These authors suggested that following gonadal ablation prostate cancer cells continued a clinically significant hormone dependent tumor growth primarily due to the effects of androgens of adrenal origin. To neutralize the effects of adrenal androgens, a combined use of surgical or medical castration with a nonsteroidal antiandrogen was proposed and this approach was promoted as complete androgen blockade (CAB).[22] The concept generated a vigorous response from the urologic community in the world. A total of 27 prospectively randomized clinical trials involving more than 8000 patients were conducted to compare the efficacy of surgical or medical castration alone (monotherapy) to almost every possible combination of castration and antiandrogens. The first published large-scale prospectively randomized clinical trial was the NCI sponsored INT-0036, published by Crawford et al in 1989.[25] Six hundred and seventeen patients with stage D2 disease were randomly assigned to receive daily subcutaneous injections (1 mg/day) of leuprolide acetate plus flutamide versus leuprolide and placebo. The median overall survival with CAB and monotherapy was 35 and 29 months respectively (2 sided, p = 0.03). A number of factors, not directly related to the CAB concept, could not be excluded as alternative reasons for the outcome observations of INT-0036. One prevalent argument was that the difference in outcome could have been a result of the neutralizing effects of the antiandrogen on the flare phenomenon associated with leuprolide treatment alone. Indeed on NCI INT-0036, it was evident during the first 12 weeks of treatment that patients randomized to the CAB arm had a more favorable trend in the directions of pain control, performance status, and serum acid phosphatase. The second explanation related to possible compliance problems with the daily injections, which could result in inadequate testicular suppression, and consequently favor those receiving leuprolide with flutamide. In view of these two unresolved issues, a confirmatory trial employing surgical castration as the underlying method of gonadal ablation was subsequently conducted under the auspices of the National Cancer Institute (NCI INT-0105). NCI INT-0105 was a prospectively randomized, double-blinded, placebo-controlled trial comparing bilateral orchiectomy with and without flutamide in 1387 patients with stage D2 prostate cancer.[26] With a median follow-up time of approximately 50 months and with 70% deaths occurring at the time of the final analysis INT-0105 failed to confirm the initial findings of INT-0036. The median survival of patients on the CAB arm was 33 months compared with 30 months on the orchiectomy arm, which was not statistically significant (2 sided stratified, p = 0.14; HR, 0.91; 95% CI 0.81–1.01).[26] The Australian multicenter trial reported by Zalcberg et al[27] compared bilateral orchiectomy plus flutamide versus bilateral orchiectomy and placebo. This trial accrued 222 patients and was reported with a relatively short follow-up time. Interestingly, the Kaplan–Meier estimates of median survival favored the orchiectomy arm (31 and 23 months respectively) although the difference was not statistically significant (p = 0.21).

The second positive trial was reported by Dijkman et al[28] on a multinational prospectively randomized placebo-controlled study comparing orchiectomy plus nilutamide with orchiectomy alone. The results of this trial demonstrated a small but significant difference in median survival (27.3 versus 23.6 months, p = 0.032), observed after 8.5 years follow-up, in favor of the CAB regimen. Crawford et al subsequently reported the results of a prospective trial comparing the combination of leuprolide acetate plus nilutamide or leuprolide alone, which demonstrated no difference in survival.[29]

The third positive trial was conducted by the European Organization for Research and Treatment of Cancer (EORTC study 30853) comparing goserelin plus flutamide to bilateral orchiectomy in 327 patients mostly with stage D2 disease (M1 disease). EORTC 30853 demonstrated a 7 months difference in median overall survival (p = 0.04) in favor of the CAB arm.[30] The Danish Prostatic Cancer Group (DAPROCA) conducted a virtually identical study, with the same treatment arms and approximately the same number of patients. This study was completed around the same time as EORTC 30853 and showed a longer overall survival in favor of the monotherapy arm although the difference was not statistically significant.[31] The DAPROCA and EORTC-30853 trials had comparable populations and study parameters. A combined analysis of both studies performed to enhance the power of comparisons did not show a significant survival difference.

In 1995, the Prostate Cancer Trialists' Collaborative Group (PCTCG)[32] reported on the first meta-analysis that was conducted as a measure to increase the statistical power of the observations of individual trials. Their report included data from 22 randomized trials comparing CAB to gonadal ablation alone in 5710 patients, which showed a 2.1% difference in mortality in favor of CAB treatment (6.4% reduction in annual odds of death, which is not statistically significant). The results were not influenced by the type antiandrogens (flutamide, nilutamide, or CPA) or the method of gonadal ablation.

The Agency for Health Care Policy and Research (AHCPR) published on the internet (*http://www.ahcpr.gov/clinic/index.html# evidence*—AHCPR report No.99-E012) the result of a comprehensive meta analysis based on all published CAB studies, which found no difference in 2-year survival rates (HR, 0.970; 95% CI 0.866–1.087). Only 10 of 27 trials reported both 2- and 5-year survival figures and in these 10 trials the preliminary results suggested a minimal 5-year survival difference in favor of CAB, which was considered of questionable clinical significance (HR, 0.871; 95% CI 0.805–0.9887). Quality of life was prospectively evaluated in patients undergoing CAB treatment on NCI INT-0105 in a companion study reported by Moinpour et al.[33] Patients on the CAB arm reported of a higher frequency of diarrhea and worsening of emotional functioning. It was concluded that the quality-of-life benefit resulting from orchiectomy in metastatic prostate cancer patients appeared to be offset by the addition of flutamide, primarily because of an increased incidence of adverse effects.

The lack of confirmatory results in trials of comparable design suggests that the most compelling explanation for the occasionally positive trial is that the overall CAB treatment effect size is indeed small (or perhaps minimal) and of questionable clinical significance.[34] The role of antiandrogens as second line treatment options for patients who demonstrate evidence of progression after gonadal ablation alone deserves further evaluation. The extensive clinical and laboratory investigation evolving from the initial reports on CAB have placed emphasis on AR biology research and added a new dimension on the consideration that progression after initial castration represents evidence of hormone resistance.

References

1. Miyamoto H, Messing EM, Chang C. Androgen deprivation therapy for prostate cancer. Current status and future prospects. Prostate 2004;61:324–331.

2. Huggins C, Hodges CV. Studies on prostate cancer: effect of castration, of estrogen and of androgen injection on serum acid phosphatase in metastatic carcinoma of the prostate. Cancer Res 1941;1:293–297.

3. Feldman BJ, Feldman D. The development of androgen independent prostate cancer. Nature Rev Cancer 2001;1:34–45.

4. Gelman EP. Molecular Biology of the androgen receptor. J Clin Oncol 2002;20:3001–3015.

5. Byar DP. The Veterans Administration Cooperative Urological Research Groups studies of cancer of the prostate. Cancer 1973;32:1126–1130.

6. Veterans Administration Cooperative Urological Research Group. Factors in the prognosis of carcinoma of the prostate: A cooperative study. J Urol 1968;100:59–65.

7. Walsh PC, DeWeese T, Eisenberger MA. A structured debate: Immediate versus deferred androgen suppression in prostate cancer: evidence for deferred treatment. J Urol 2001;166:508–516.

8. Immediate versus deferred treatment for advanced prostatic cancer: initial results of the Medical Research Council. Prostate Cancer Working Party Investigators Group. Br J Urol 1997;79:235–246.

9. AHCPR report No. 99-E012. http://www.ahcpr.gov/clinic/index.html.

10. Pilepich MV, Caplan R, Byhardt RW, et al. Phase III trial of androgen suppression using goserelin in unfavorable-prognosis carcinoma of the prostate treated with definitive radiotherapy: report of Radiation Therapy Oncology Group Protocol 8531. J Clin Oncol 1997;15:1013–1021.

11. Pilepich MV, Winter K, John MJ, et al. Phase III radiation therapy oncology group (RTOG) study 8610 of androgen deprivation adjuvant to definitive radiation in locally advanced carcinoma of the prostate. Int J Rad Oncol Biol Phys 2001;50:1243–1252.

12. Pilepich MV, Winter K, Lawton RE. Phase III trial of androgen suppression adjuvant to definitive radiotherapy. Long term results of RTOG 8531. Proc ASCO 22 2003;381:1530 [abstract].

13. Bolla M, Gonzalez D, Warde P, et al. Improved survival in patients with locally advanced prostate cancer treated with radiotherapy and goserelin. N Engl J Med 1997;337:295–300.

14. Messing EM, Manola J, Sarosdy M, et al. Immediate hormonal therapy compared with observation after radical prostatectomy and pelvic lymphadenectomy in men with node-positive prostate cancer. N Engl J Med 1999;341:1781–1788.

15. deKernion JB, Neuwirth H, Stein A, et al. Prognosis of patients with stage D1 prostate cancer following radical prostatectomy with and without early endocrine therapy. J Urol 1990;144:700–703.

16. Sgrignoli AR, Walsh PC, Steinberg GD, et al. Prognostic factors in men with stage D1 prostate cancer: identification of patients less likely to have prolonged survival after radical prostatectomy. J Urol 1994;152:1077–1081.

17. Cheng L, Bergstralh E J, Cheville JC, et al. Cancer volume of lymph node metastasis predicts progression in prostate cancer. Am J Surg Pathol 1998;22:1491–1500.

18. Eisenberger MA, Walsh PC. Early androgen deprivation for prostate cancer? N Engl J Med 1999;341:1837–1838.

19. Tyrrel CJ, Kaisary AV, Iversen P, et al. A randomized comparison of casodex 150-mg monotherapy versus castration in the treatment of metastatic and locally advanced prostate cancer. Eur Urol 1998;33:447–456.

20. Iversen P, Tyrrell CJ, Karisary AV, et al. Casodex (bicalutamide) 150 mg monotherapy compared with castration in patients with previously untreated nonmetastatic prostate cancer: results from two multicenter randomized trials at a median follow-up of 4 years. Urology 1998; 51:389.

21. DeMarzo A, Nelson WG, Isaacs WB, et al. Pathological and molecular aspects of prostate cancer. Lancet 2003;361:955–964.

22. Craft N, Sawyers CL. Mechanistics concepts in androgen- dependence of prostate cancer. Cancer Metastasis Rev 1998;17;421–427.

23. Labrie F, Veillux R, Fournier A. Low androgen levels induce the development of androgen-hypersensitive cell clones shionogi mouse mammary carcinoma cells in culture. J Natl Cancer Inst 1988;80: 1138–1147.

24. Labrie F, Dupont A, Belanger A, et al. Combination therapy with flutamide and castration (LHRH agonists or orchiectomy) in advanced prostatic cancer: a marked improvement in response and survival. J Steroid Biochem 1985;23:833–841.

25. Crawford ED, Eisenberger MA, Mcleod DG, et al. A controlled trial of leuprolide with and without flutamide in prostatic carcinoma. N Eng J Med 1989;321:419–424.

26. Eisenberger MA, Blumenstein BA, Crawford ED, et al. A randomized and double-blind comparison of bilateral orchiectomy with or without flutamide for the treatment of patients with stage D2 prostate cancer: Results of NCI Intergroup Study 0105. N Eng J Med 1998;339:1036–1042.

27. Zalcberg JR, Raghhaven D, Marshall V, et al. Bilateral orchidectomy and flutamide versus orchidectomy alone in newly diagnosed patients with metastatic carcinoma of the prostate: an Australian multicentre trial. Br J Urol 1996;77:865–869.

28. Dijkman GA, Fernandez del Moral P, Debruyne FMJ, et al. Improved subjective response to orchiectomy plus nilutamide in comparison to orchiectomy plus placebo in metastatic prostate cancer. Eur Urol 1995;27:196–201.

29. Crawford ED, Kasimis BS, Gandara D, et al. A randomized controlled clinical trial of leuprolide and anandron vs. leuprolide and placebo for advanced prostate cancer. Proc Annu Meet Am Soc Clin Oncol 1990;9:A523.

30. Denis LJ, Keuppens F, Smith PH, et al. Maximal androgen blockade: final analysis of EORTC phase III trial 30853. Eur Urol 1998;33:144–151.

31. Iversen P, Ramussen F, Klarskov P, et al. Long-term results of Danish Prostatic Cancer Group Trial 86: Goserelin acetate plus flutamide versus orchiectomy in advanced prostate cancer. Cancer 1993;72:3851–3854.

32. Prostate Cancer Trialists Collaborative Group: Maximum androgen blockade in advanced prostate cancer: an overview of 22 randomized trials with 3283 deaths in 5710 patients. Lancet 1995;346:265–269.

33. Moinpour CM, Savage MJ, Troxel A, et al. Quality of life in advanced prostate cancer: Results of a randomized therapeutic trial. J Natl Cancer Inst 1998;90:1537–1544.

34. Laufer M, Denmeade S, Sinibaldi V, et al. Complete Androgen Blockade for Prostate Cancer. What went wrong? J Urol 2000;164:3–9.

38

Androgen deprivation therapy: the future

Marc B Garnick, Camille Motta

Introduction

Defining the future of androgen deprivation therapy (ADT) for prostate cancer can be best addressed by briefly reviewing the multitude of established uses, and then by evaluating the emerging utilities of hormonal therapy, which are not yet standard of practice. Box 38.1 presents an overview, with references, of existing and emerging uses of hormonal therapies in prostate cancer. Examples of the former include the use of ADT in patients with metastatic disease (N+, M+); use as a neoadjuvant and adjuvant therapy prior to, during, or after definitive radiation therapy; to downsize prostate gland volume prior to either external-beam radiation therapy (XRT) or brachytherapy. Emerging uses include ADT as an adjunct in the adjuvant setting for patients who have undergone radical prostatectomy and are found to harbor unfavorable pathologic characteristics (e.g., pT2 and pT3 with unfavorable histologies); use of hormonal therapies for those with a biochemical relapse following definitive therapy (so called rising prostate-specific antigen [PSA] following definitive therapy); use of ADT for intermittent hormonal therapy; use of ADT for primary therapy of clinically localized prostate cancer; use of sequences of hormonal therapies, either alone or in combination, in a sequential fashion such as "step-up" therapy; the use of therapies that induce androgen deprivation, either alone or in combination with cytotoxic chemotherapy for those with androgen independent prostate cancer; use of ADT, alone or in combination with cytotoxic chemotherapy for regionally advanced prostate cancer (e.g., cT3 or pT3 or greater) or those with intermediate or high risk characteristics (e.g., those with a ≤50% biochemical 5-year disease-free survival following definitive localized treatment).

While this list is probably not exhaustive, it does represent the vast majority of uses of hormonal therapy in current usage throughout the world. These uses—both established and emerging—utilize commercially available hormonal agents that induce states of actual or functional androgen deficiency, and represent luteinizing hormone releasing hormone (LHRH) agonists; steroidal and nonsteroidal antiandrogens; progestational agents; estrogenic compounds; the recently introduced class of gonadotropin releasing hormone (GnRH) antagonists; and surgical removal (bilateral orchiectomy) of the main source of androgenic steroids.

Under development are a variety of additional compounds, including other LHRH analogs (both agonists and antagonists) and other classes of novel inhibitors of proliferation (that include both endocrine and non-endocrine mechanisms) that are being evaluated as both first- and second-line therapies for prostate cancer. As these therapies and usage patterns change, the potential for differing side effects also emerges. One example is bone mineral density loss associated with prolonged androgen deprivation therapies,[1,2]

which can now be partially addressed with newer generation of bisphosphonates, zoledronic acid, in particular.[3,4] Another is the recent recognition that ADTs may be associated with non-thrombotic cardiovascular effects, such as prolongation of the electrocardiographic QT interval.[5] Thus, as the treatment programs that involve ADT evolve, the clinician will need to be aware of a spectrum of additional effects associated with these new treatments. Finally, the emergence of prostate cancers that have become "hormonally refractory" or androgen independent poses serious scientific and clinical challenges. Understanding the mechanisms underlying the transition to this more refractory state should help provide new directions in designing better and more targeted therapies.

Hormonal therapy for prostate cancer

The use of ADT, also called hormonal therapy, endocrine therapy, castration therapy (either medical or surgical), or simply hormones, has for the past 65 years been the mainstay in the systemic management of advanced prostate cancer. Initially identified by the late Dr Charles Huggins,[6-8] the fundamental premise identified nearly 7 decades ago is that prostate cancer is under the tropic influence of the male hormones, including, but not limited to, testosterone and dihydrotestosterone. Indeed, under the influence of exogenous androgen administration, prostate cancer grows, and with this growth patients may experience worsening symptoms associated with proliferating cancer cells.[9] Conversely, the removal of androgenic sources, either by surgical removal of the testicles, a main source of androgens, or by medically abrogating the production of androgen via interruption of the hypothalamic-pituitary-gonadal axis, results in improvement in the signs and symptoms of a substantial proportion of patients.

Up until the more widespread introduction of the prostatic fraction of acid phosphatase, the majority of men who received ADT were those with extensive regional disease, leading to urinary obstruction, hydronephrosis, and pelvic adenopathy; or those with frank metastatic disease, in which patients presented with osseous disease, weight loss, anemia, and a generalized decrease in overall performance status. Thus, this population of patients who did not enjoy the advantage of earlier diagnosis of prostate cancer by currently available biochemical methods of diagnosis was identified later in the course of their disease. The use of ADT in these settings did lead to the palliation of both the signs and symptoms of disease

Box 38.1 Existing and emerging uses of hormonal therapy in prostate cancer

Existing
- Metastatic disease D_1, D_2, N+, M+; advanced stages T3, T4[27,48]
- Neoadjuvant—prior to surgery[19,49–51]
- Neoadjuvant—prior to radiotherapy[55,56]
- Adjuvant—post-external-beam radiation therapy for locally advanced prostate cancer[13,64]
- Neoadjuvant + adjuvant to external-beam radiation therapy[66]
- Prostate gland volume reduction[68–70]
- Sequential androgen blockade (anti-androgen + 5α-reductase inhibitor)[71–75]

Emerging
- Adjuvant—post-radical prostatectomy for unfavorable pathologic characteristics (seminal vesicle invasion and lymph node disease)[14,17]
- Adjuvant—post-radical prostatectomy in localized disease[21,52–54]
- Intermittent hormonal therapy[57–63]
- Androgen-independent prostate cancer alone or in combination with chemotherapy[43,65]
- Regionally advanced prostate cancer alone or in combination with chemotherapy[67]
- Rising prostate-specific antigen post definitive therapy; biochemical relapse[42]
- Primary therapy of local prostate cancer[76,77]

advancement. Although the Veteran's Administration Cooperative Urological Research Group (VACURG) did study either single or combinations of hormonal therapies in earlier stage patients, the standard of practice usually dictated the use of ADT in more advanced patient populations.[10–12]

Since the 1980s, a series of clinical investigations has evaluated a multidisciplinary approach to prostate cancer. In addition, the introduction and widespread use of PSA-based methods of prostate cancer diagnosis has led to an ongoing dialog on the definition of the optimal treatment program that could include the disciplines of surgery, radiation, and systemic medical management. This chapter will evaluate the emerging uses of these combination approaches and discuss further strategies in which the role of ADT emerges as an integral part of both the regional and systemic management of patients with prostate cancer. With these novel uses of ADT, in which patients may be exposed to lowered testosterone for years, a new set of side effects have emerged, again requiring a deeper knowledge of the multitude actions of androgens on various tissues. This chapter will review some of these new adverse drug effects.

Emerging uses

Neoadjuvant and adjuvant hormonal therapy

The uses of neoadjuvant or adjuvant hormonal therapy have been well covered in other chapters of this book. Several key studies, however, are worth emphasizing, as they may serve to chart the future of subsequent strategies that incorporate hormonal therapy into overall treatment programs.

Adjuvant hormonal therapy

One randomized trial of 415 patients with locally advanced prostate cancer (T1/T2 tumors of World Health Organization [WHO] grade 3 or T3/T4, N0/N1, M0 tumors) found that XRT combined with an analog of LHRH for 3 years (XRT + HT) conferred an improved 5-year disease-free survival over XRT alone of 74% versus 40% ($P = 0.0001$), as well as improved 5-year overall survival of 78% versus 62% ($P = 0.0002$); and a 5-year disease specific survival of 94% versus 79%.[13]

Another study of 98 men treated with radical prostatectomy and pelvic lymphadenectomy and nodal metastases were randomly assigned to receive immediate ADT (goserelin or bilateral orchiectomy) or no ADT. Both groups were followed until disease progression. After a median follow-up of 7.1 years, 7 of 47 in the ADT group had died, compared with 18 of 51 men in the control (no ADT) group ($P = 0.02$). The cause of death was prostate cancer in 3 ADT patients compared with 16 controls ($P < 0.01$).[14] This conclusion was recently validated by a new central pathology slide review, and evaluation and reassessment of Gleason scores. Revised results are in keeping with those published earlier. In addition to overall survival at median of 11.9 years follow-up, the advantages of immediate hormone therapy versus observation/delayed therapy include disease-specific survival (85% versus 51%), recurrence-free survival (62% versus 24%), and PSA progression-free survival (55% versus 14%).[15]

These two studies serve as the basis for combining hormonal therapy with either radiation therapy for men with both localized and regionally advanced prostate cancer, or radical prostatatectomy for men with nodal metastases. The first study evaluated the effect of 3 years of hormonal therapy and demonstrated that long-term adjuvant hormonal therapy is critical to improving survival, and the second study evaluated the utilization of immediate ADT. Anecdotally, many men do not tolerate such long-term androgen suppression well, and clinicians often treat with ADT for shorter periods of time.

A more recent study has evaluated the use of 6 months of ADT following 70 Gy 3D-conformal radiation therapy and suggested an overall survival advantage when added to patients with clinically localized prostate cancer treated with 3D-conformal radiation therapy.[16] These three studies serve as a basis for consideration of the timing, schedule, and duration of ADT associated with localized treatments in future trials.

Other less well-controlled studies also suggest advantages when ADT is added to localized treatments. A recent review of prospective randomized studies and of clinical information on stage pT3b cancer from a large single-institution prostate cancer database shows that early adjuvant hormonal therapy after radical prostatectomy has a significant impact on time to progression and causes specific survival in patients with seminal vesicle invasion and limited lymph node disease.[17]

Neoadjuvant therapy—how long shall we treat patients in the future?

There have been several recent investigations into the optimal treatment time for neoadjuvant hormonal therapy in an attempt to determine if longer is better. This remains an issue to be resolved in the future.

A recent Canadian study[18] evaluated the effect of 3 months versus 8 months of neoadjuvant hormonal therapy before conventional dose radiotherapy (RT) on disease-free survival using PSA and biopsies as end points for clinically localized prostate cancer. Three hundred seventy-eight men were randomized to either 3 or 8 months of flutamide and goserelin before conventional-dose RT (66 Gy) at four participating centers. The actuarial freedom from failure rate (biochemical by American Society for Therapeutic Radiology and Oncology definition), local or distant, for the 3-month versus 8-month arms at 3 years was 66% versus 68% and by 5 years was 61% versus 62%, respectively ($P = 0.36$). No statistically significant difference was noted in the types of failure between the two arms (crude final status): biochemical, 22.2% versus 22.3%; local, 10.2% versus 6.5%; and distant, 3.4% versus 4.4% ($P = 0.61$). A suggestion of improvement was found in the 8-month arm for disease-free survival at 5 years for high-risk patients (39% versus 52%) but did not achieve statistical significance. Results suggest that a longer period of neoadjuvant hormonal therapy before standard-dose RT does not appear to confer a benefit in terms of disease-free survival or to alter failure patterns. A suggested benefit was noted with a longer period of hormonal therapy for high-risk patients.

A prospective phase III trial[19] compared 8-month with 3-month neoadjuvant hormonal therapy prior to radical prostatectomy to determine reduction of PSA recurrence rates. Five hundred forty-seven men with organ-confined prostate cancer received either 7.5 mg leuprolide (i.m.) monthly and 250 mg flutamide (p.o.) 3 times/day for 3 months or for 8 months before radical prostatectomy. Mean serum PSA decreased 98% to 0.12 ng/mL after 3 months, with a further 57% to 0.052 ng/mL from 3 to 8 months. Prostate gland volume decreased by 37% from a mean of 40.6 to 25.4 cm³ after 3-month neoadjuvant hormonal therapy ($P = 0.0001$) and a further 13% to 22.2 cm³ after 8 months ($P = 0.03$). Five hundred men underwent radical prostatectomy. Positive margin rates were significantly lower in the 8-month than in the 3-month group (12% versus 23%, respectively; $P = 0.0106$). Since there appears to be ongoing regression, both biochemical and pathologic, of the prostate tumor that occurs between month 3 and month 8 of neoadjuvant therapy, results suggests that the optimal duration of neoadjuvant hormonal therapy is longer than 3 months. Additional patient follow-up is needed to determine whether longer therapy alters PSA recurrence rates.

Antiandrogen monotherapy following treatment of clinically localized prostate cancer

Because of complications associated with conventional ADT—loss of potency, libido, bone mineral density loss, and vasomotor hot flashes—several programs have addressed the utility of nonsteroidal, anti-androgen monotherapy, such as bicalutamide, to be administered as an adjunct to definitive localized therapies in an attempt to improve overall survival and progression-free survival. While preliminary results of these studies using 50 mg/day bicalutamide[20] were encouraging in prolonging disease free survival, and led to the marketing approval outside of the United States, when given to locally advanced patients at 150 mg/day (three times the conventional dose of 50 mg/day), although similar survival outcome to castration was observed, toxicity was also found, consisting of breast pain and gynecomastia, at times irreversible.[21–23]

Further analyses demonstrated an overall survival disadvantage of antiandrogen monotherapy when compared with placebo. At 5-year follow-up, a trend was noted for an increase in the number of deaths in patients with localized prostate cancer receiving bicalutamide (Casodex) 150 mg compared with patients who received placebo (196 [25.2%] deaths versus 174 [20.5%] deaths.) This finding precipitated its removal from marketing authorization as a treatment for localized prostate cancer in Canada, the UK, and several other European countries.[24,25] The US FDA never granted marketing approval for this type of monotherapy.

Novel hormonal agents

Gonadotropin releasing hormone antagonists

Gonadotropin releasing hormone is a natural decapeptide. The synthetic GnRH antagonist decapeptide has five or more amino-acid substitutions; modifications involving position 6 hinder cleavage by serum proteases; substitutions at positions 2 and 3 affect gonadotropin release; and changes at positions 1, 6, and 10 affect receptor binding. In contrast to the LHRH agonists, GnRH antagonists bind immediately and competitively to GnRH receptors in the pituitary gland. Luteinizing hormone concentrations are reduced (51–84%) and follicle-stimulating hormone (FSH) concentrations are lessened (17–42%) within 8 to 24 hours following the first dose. The competitive blocking of the GnRH receptor results in a rapid, reversible decrease in LH, FSH, and testosterone, without any flare. Also, when GnRH antagonist therapy is stopped, a more rapid recovery of pituitary-gonadal function is possible.[26] Figure 38.1 portrays this mechanism of action.

Recently, the US FDA has approved abarelix for injectable suspension for the management of a subset of patients with advanced symptomatic prostate cancer in whom LHRH agonists are not appropriate and who refuse treatment with surgical castration. Abarelix is the first GnRH antagonist decapeptide formulated in a

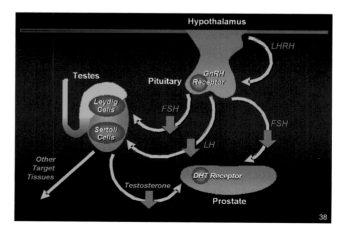

Figure 38.1
Mechanism of action of gonadotropin-releasing hormone antagonist, abarelix. (DHT, dihydrotestosterone; FSH, follicle-stimulating hormone; GnRH, gonadotropin-releasing hormone; LHRH, luteinizing hormone releasing hormone.)

depot suspension indicated for prostate cancer. Other GnRH anatagonists (cetrorelix, ganirelix) are approved for shorter term administration for use in women for in-vitro fertilization.

Effects of abarelix in advanced symptomatic prostate cancer patients

An open label, uncontrolled study[27] of abarelix was conducted in 72 evaluable men with advanced symptomatic prostate cancer who were at risk for clinical exacerbation ("clinical flare") if treated with an LHRH agonist. This study defined the approved patient population for use with of abarelix. The objective was to demonstrate that such patients could avoid surgical castration through at least 12 weeks of treatment. Patients were enrolled with bone pain from prostate cancer skeletal metastases; an enlarged prostate gland or pelvic mass causing bladder neck outlet obstruction; retroperitoneal adenopathy with ureteral obstruction; impending neurologic compromise from spinal, spinal cord, or epidural metastases. All patients were able to avoid the requirement for surgical castration throughout the study. Although

the study was not designed to assess specific clinical outcomes, outcomes consistent with the expected benefits of castration and avoidance of adverse consequences of clinical flare were observed, and included relief of bladder outlet and ureteral obstruction; decreased bone pain and need for narcotic analgesics; avoidance of neurologic compromise, including spinal cord compression in those with vertebral or epidural metastases.

Investigational therapies with novel hormonal mechanisms of action being studied for prostate cancer

Table 38.1 lists other hormonal therapies recently introduced or under development for prostate cancer.

Table 38.1 Hormonal therapies recently introduced or under development for prostate cancer[78,79]

Name	Mechanism of action	Route of admin	Phase	Notes	Refs
SARMs	Selective androgen receptor modulators	A-p.o.	Preclinical		80,81
Abiraterone acetate*	C17-20 Lyase inhibitor; Steroid synthesis inhibitor	A-p.o.	I (W)		28,29
Leuprolide inhalation	LHRH agonist	Inhaled 1×day	I (W)		82
NBI-42902	GnRH antagonist, 2nd generation	A-p.o.	I (USA)		
Izonsteride	5-alpha reductase inhibitor	p.o.	I (US)		83
Leuprorelin implant	LHRH agonist	Implant 4–6 mo. Depot	II (W)		84
Degarelix	GnRH antagonist	various	II (W)		85,86
D-63153	GnRH antagonist	P-i.m.	II (W)		87
Leupromaxx	LHRH agonist	P-varies 24 day & 84 day form.	II (W)	Extended release ProMaxx System	
Phenoxodiol*	Apoptosis stimulant; mitosis inhibitor; signal transduction pathway inhibitor	P-i.v. A-p.o.	II (W)		33
Teverelix LA	GnRH antagonist	P-s.c	IIa	Immed rel. & Sustained Rel.	88
Cetrorelix	GnRH antagonist	P-s.c	II	Already launched for other indications	89
Avorelin	LHRH agonist	P-s.c	II	6 month depot	90
Osaterone acetate (TZP 4238)	Androgen antagonist Steroidal antiandrogen	A-p.o.	II		91
PCK 3145 (PSP 94)	Apoptosis stimulant	i.v.	II (UK)	For AIPC	92,93
Tesmilifene (DPPE)	Estrogen antagonist; Intracellular histamine antagonist	P-i.v.	II (US & Can)	For AIPC combined with other drugs	34–37,94
Toremifene	Selective estrogen receptor modulator	A-p.o.	III	For AIPC	95,96
DN-101 (calcitriol)*	Vitamin D receptor agonist	A-p.o.	III (W)	For AIPC combined w/docetaxel	38–41
Vapreotide (RC-160)	Somatostatin (SST) analog Growth hormone antagonist	P-s.c P-i.v.	III	Also for AIPC	97–99
Histrelin (hydrogel implant)	LHRH agonist	P-s.c. 12 month depot (implant)	III (Can)		100,101
Atrasenten*	Endothelin A receptor antagonist	A-p.o.	III (USA)	For AIPC	46,47
Plenaxis*	GnRH antagonist	P-i.m.	IV	Launched 11/2003	27;45;102–104

*Discussed in this chapter.
AIPC, androgen-independent prostate cancer; GnRH, gonadotropin-releasing hormone; LHRH, luteinizing hormone releasing hormone. Phase: W, World; US, USA; Can, Canada. Rte Admin: A, alimentary; P, parenteral; i.m., intramuscular; i.v., intravenous; p.o., by mouth; s.c., subcutaneous.

For hormonally-sensitive prostate cancer

Abiraterone acetate

Abiraterone acetate (CB7630) is a new compound that shows potential in the treatment of cancer and other hormonally-responsive, testosterone-related diseases. It is an orally active inhibitor (structurally related to ketoconazole) of the steroidal enzyme 17α-hydroxylase/C17,20-lyase, a cytochrome p450 complex that is involved in testosterone production (Figure 38.2). In preclinical studies, abiraterone has demonstrated the ability to selectively inhibit the target enzyme, resulting in inhibition of testosterone production in both the adrenals and the testes. In phase I trials, abiraterone was administered to 26 patients with prostate cancer. These clinical studies demonstrated that the compound: 1) at a single oral dose of 800 mg, can successfully suppress testosterone levels to the castrate range; 2) can suppress testosterone produced by both the testes and the adrenals; 3) is well tolerated and non-toxic. This is the first report of the use of a specific 17α-hydroxylase[17,20] lyase inhibitor in humans. However, this level of testosterone suppression to the castrate range may not be sustained in all patients due to compensatory hypersecretion of luteinizing hormone. Adrenocortical suppression may necessitate concomitant treatment with replacement glucorticoid.[28,29] Abiraterone acetate is currently under development as a second-line hormonal therapy for prostate cancer for patients who are refractory to first-line treatment with an LHRH agonist/antagonist and antiandrogen therapy.

Phenoxodiol

Phenoxodiol belongs to a new class of anticancer drugs known as multiple signal transduction regulators (MSTRs) that show promise in the treatment of solid cancers, including prostate and breast, and benign prostatic hyperplasia. Phenoxodiol is the lead compound in a series of synthetic phenolic hormone analogues. Phenolic hormones are naturally occurring compounds produced in the human body from isoflavones in food.[30] Phenoxodiol is an effective inhibitor of three key enzymes involved in signal transduction processes; topoisomerase II, epidermal growth factor tyrosine kinase, and sphingosine kinase (primary target). It inhibits antiapoptotic proteins (c-FLIP and XIAP) and increases proapoptotic proteins (BAX). These MSTRs work by inducing programmed cell death in cancer cells (apoptosis), with little or no effect on normal cells.

In animal studies, phenoxodiol significantly inhibited the growth of transplanted human prostate tumors at nontoxic doses by induction of apoptosis and inhibition of cell division. Phenoxodiol caused cancer cells to differentiate into normal cells and inhibited growth of human leukemia, melanoma, breast, prostate, and bowel cancer cell cultures.[31,32] In phase Ib/IIa clinical trials with hormone-refractory prostate cancer patients, interim results show that two patients treated with the two highest dosages (200 and 400 mg) showed stabilization of their PSA levels after 3 months of therapy, while six (50%) showed a decrease in PSA levels. Two of these six responders showed a decline in PSA levels of greater than 75%.[33] Phenoxodiol is being developed as a monotherapy for early-stage and late-stage hormone-refractory prostate cancer patients, and as a combination therapy where it acts to enhance the efficacy of chemotherapeutic agents in chemosensitive patients and to restore sensitivity to those drugs in chemoresistant patients.

For hormone-refractory cancer

Tesmilifene

An intracellular histamine antagonist, tesmilifene (also known as DPPE), is being developed as a chemopotentiator for the treatment of malignant solid tumors. The compound is cytotoxic to tumor cells and cytoprotective to the gut and to normal bone marrow progenitor cells. Research suggests that it is able to augment the in-vivo antitumor activity of numerous cytotoxic drugs routinely used in the treatment of many types of cancers, such as doxorubicin, cyclophosphamide, fluorouracil, cisplatin, and mito-xantrone.[34,35] It has been shown to increase the cytotoxicity of fluorouracil and daunorubicin in cancer cell lines; and has increased the antitumour effects of doxorubicin and daunorubicin in mice.

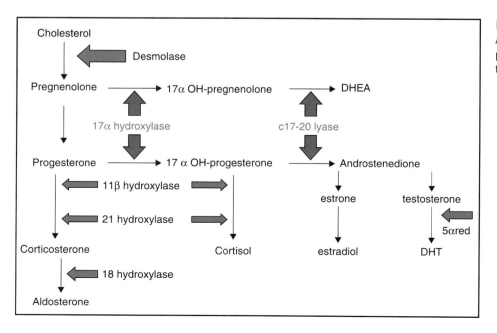

Figure 38.2
Abiraterone acetate; steroid synthesis pathway. (DHEA, dehydroepiandrosterone; DHT, dihydrotestosterone.

The results of a study investigating the efficacy of tesmilifene plus cyclophosphamide in 20 patients with metastatic prostate cancer refractory to hormonal therapy have been reported. Tesmilifene and cyclophosphamide were both administered by i.v. infusion. Treatment was given for as long as the patient was deemed to benefit. Five of seven patients (71%) with measurable soft tissue disease had a partial remission. Three of 16 (19%) with assessable bone disease responded, one with complete remission and two partial remission. Nine of 18 (50%) with an elevated serum level of PSA had more than a 50% decrease. Eleven of 13 (85%) with bone pain had partial or complete resolution of this symptom; the PSA level and bone scan improved in six and two of these subjects, respectively.[36]

In a phase II trial in hormone-refractory prostate cancer, patients received mitoxantrone, prednisone, and tesmilifene, with mitoxantrone delivered during the last 20 min. Sixty-eight percent had both improved pain and reduced analgesia, 50% PSA reduction was seen in 13 patients (50%) and 75% PSA reduction in 11 patients (42%). Toxicity was the same as for mitoxantrone alone, except for three cases of transient hallucinations. Median survival was 18 months, and 38% survived more than 2 years[37]

Calcitriol

DN-101 contains high amounts of calcitriol (1,25 dihydroxycholecalciferol) a naturally occurring hormone and the biologically active form of vitamin D. In high doses, calcitriol is synergistic with many commonly used chemotherapeutic agents, producing antitumor activity as measured in laboratory and animal models. Until recently, the clinical use of calcitriol as an anticancer therapy has been limited by elevations in serum calcium (hypercalcemia) at doses thought to be required for antitumor activity. Available technology has overcome this problem and enables high-dose administration of calcitriol. Although the key physiologic function of calcitriol is maintenance of calcium homeostasis, it has potent growth inhibitory (antiproliferative) activities in multiple cancer cell lines and animal models of cancer (e.g., prostate, breast, colon, head and neck, lymphoma, and myeloma). Preclinical data indicate that transient high plasma levels are sufficient to effect antitumor activity in animals. Additionally, calcitriol is synergistic with many commonly used chemotherapeutic agents, such as taxanes, platinums, dexamethasone, mitoxantrone, and doxorubicin. While the exact mechanism for this synergy is not known, calcitriol has been shown in preclinical models to improve or restore the apoptosis pathway and cause cell cycle arrest during cell division. The pretreatment of a tumor with calcitriol and subsequent administration of a cytotoxin is hypothesized to significantly increase the proportion of cell kill via these mechanisms. In a phase II study, 22 prostate cancer patients, who had a recurrence as evidenced by a rising PSA level despite definitive local therapy and who had not yet received hormonal therapy for recurrent disease, were treated with commercially available calcitriol on a high-dose pulse administration schedule. Patients received calcitriol until a four-fold increase in PSA or other evidence of disease progression was obtained. After a median treatment duration of 10 months, this therapy appeared to be well tolerated. No hypercalcemia or kidney stones were seen. Mild elevations in liver blood tests and mild anemia were the most common toxicities seen, and no severe toxicities related to the drug were reported. In an open-label phase II study of androgen-independent prostate cancer patients, the combination of weekly high doses of commercially available calcitriol and docetaxel (Taxotere) appeared active as measured by declines in PSA levels and tumor shrinkage. Of the 37 patients who received the combination treatment, 81% had a

confirmed PSA reduction of 50% or more as compared to 36%–45% of patients in comparable previous studies of docetaxel alone. The PSA responses in this study persisted for a longer period of time (11.4 months) compared with patients who received docetaxel alone in other studies (5 months). Toxicity in this study was similar to toxicity seen in patients in other studies who received docetaxel alone. The most common severe toxicities in this study were lowering of the white blood cell counts and elevations in blood glucose.[38–41]

Abarelix

Two clinical studies were conducted to evaluate the clinical efficacy of abarelix in hormone-refractory prostate cancer patients and to measure its effect on serum FSH levels. For the two studies, patients were identified as nonresponsive to hormonal therapy based on either disease progression during LHRH agonist therapy or progression after orchiectomy. The objective of the first study (n = 16)[42] was to determine the efficacy of abarelix in patients with androgen-independent prostate cancer progressing after orchiectomy and to measure its effect on serum FSH. Although none of the patients met the criteria for PSA response (50% reduction confirmed 4 weeks later), five patients experienced confirmed reductions in the PSA level ranging from 9.3% to 31.8% and six patients remained stable without PSA progression or other signs of disease progression. All patients had a decline in their FSH concentration. The mean FSH concentration declined from 45.1 IU/L to 5.3 IU/L after 4 weeks and to 5.6 IU/L after 8 weeks. The FSH concentration remained suppressed after 20 weeks (mean 3.6 IU/L).

The second study[43] elaborated on the clinical efficacy of abarelix in patients (n = 20) with androgen-independent prostate cancer and measured its effect on serum FSH and testosterone. No patients met the criteria for PSA response (50% reduction confirmed 4 weeks later), although two patients remained stable without PSA progression or other signs of disease progression. Median time to progression was 8 weeks. Mean serum FSH decreased by more than 50% from a baseline of 5.7 IU/L and remained suppressed throughout the observation period. Mean serum testosterone did not change after 4 and 8 weeks of therapy and remained in the anorchid range.

Since preclinical data[44] suggests that FSH may be an independent growth factor for hormone-refractory prostate cancers, it follows that potent suppressors of FSH may prove to be effective therapies for androgen-independent prostate cancers. Published clinical data demonstrates that LHRH agonist therapy results in only partial suppression of FSH levels in prostate cancer patients, while abarelix, a GnRH antagonist, has been shown to promptly and substantially reduce FSH to levels lower than LHRH agonists.[45]

Atrasentan

Atrasentan belongs to a class of oral drugs that block the activity of endothelin, a protein normally produced in the body that can stimulate the growth and spread of cancer cells. Both endothelin and its receptor are found in various cancers including prostate, non-small cell lung, colorectal, breast, and renal. There are two endothelin receptors, ETA and ETB. The ETA receptor, selectively targeted by atrasentan, appears to be important in prostate cancer progression.

Atrasentan was studied in two randomized, controlled phase II trials with a total population of 1097 hormone refractory prostate cancer patients. Patients were randomized to atrasentan or to placebo. Analyzed separately, the two studies demonstrated a trend toward delayed time to progression, but the difference was not statistically significant. The smaller of the two trials involved 288 patients. An analysis limited to 244 evaluable patients showed that the 10 mg dose of altrasentan significantly prolonged time to progression compared with placebo.[46]

Analysis of data from the phase III trials of hormone-refractory patients showed that atrasentan demonstrated statistically significant improvements in mean change of PSA levels versus placebo (175 ng/mL versus 257 ng/mL; $P = 0.045$); development of bone pain as an adverse event (24% versus 34%; $P = 0.003$); and improvements in mean change of biochemical markers of skeletal progression, although there was not a statistically significant improvement in time to disease progression.[47]

Emerging adverse events associated with hormonal therapy

Complications of ADT include those that primarily affect the patient's quality of life, such as hot flashes, fatigue, weight gain, dry eyes, mood swings, muscle weakness, balance problems, insomnia, decreased libido, and impotence, as well as those that are associated with significant morbidity such as decrease in bone mineral density, cognitive dysfunction, and changes in lipid profiles.[105] Some side effects are associated with patient morbidity and mortality, such as anemia, blood glucose changes, liver enzyme changes, rare but potentially fatal hepatoxicity, and cardiac failure.[106,107] Box 38.2 outlines some recently reported adverse events associated with hormonal therapies, which are elaborated on briefly here.

Bone mineral density loss

Several reports have indicated a decrease in bone mineral density (BMD) in patients undergoing androgen deprivation therapy.[108,109] Since duration of treatment may lead to progressive bone loss,[110] it is prudent to investigate bone mineral density and the prediction of bone loss in patients undergoing continuing hormonal therapy.

There have been several recent studies that elucidate the nature of biochemical markers that are precursors of bone mineral loss. Biochemical markers represent the enzymes and skeletal component released into the circulating blood during bone formation or resorption. One study[1] elucidated the increase in biochemical markers during ADT as a reflection of the increase in the bone turnover rate and decrease in BMD. In 60 men with prostate cancer (19 men received LHRH agonist therapy and 41 did not) and 197 healthy controls of similar age, BMD, biochemical markers of bone turnover, and body composition were assessed. Bone mass density was assessed by dual

***

Box 38.2 Novel adverse events associated with hormonal therapies

- Decrease in bone mineral density / osteoporosis[1,2,108,109,126]
- Elongation of QT interval[5,114]
- Anemia[116,127]
- Cognitive dysfunction[120,121,128]
- Interstitial pneumonitis[123,124,129]

***

energy X-ray absorptiometry and ultrasound. Biochemical markers of bone turnover included markers of bone resorption (urinary N-telopeptide) and bone formation markers (bone-specific alkaline phosphatase and osteocalcin). Body composition (total body fat and lean body mass) was assessed by dual energy X-ray absorptiometry. Significantly lower BMD was found at the lateral spine, total hip, and forearm in men receiving LHRH agonist therapy compared with those with prostate cancer who did not. Significant differences were also seen at the total body, finger, and calcaneus. The BMD values in eugonadal men with prostate cancer and healthy controls were similar.

Markers of bone resorption (urinary N-telopeptide) and bone formation (bone-specific alkaline phosphatase) were elevated in men receiving LHRH agonist therapy compared with those in eugonadal men with prostate cancer. Men receiving LHRH agonist therapy also had a higher percent total body fat (29 ± 5% versus 25 ± 5%; $P < 0.01$) and lower percent lean body weight (71 ± 5% versus 75 ± 5%; $P < 0.01$) compared with eugonadal men with prostate cancer. The study concluded that men with prostate cancer receiving ADT have a significant decrease in bone mass and increase in bone turnover, thus placing them at increased risk of fracture.

Another study[2] used carboxy-terminal pro-peptide of human type I procollagen (PIPC) and pyridinoline cross-linked carboxy-terminal telopeptide of type I collagen (ICTP) as serum biochemical markers of bone metabolism; the former is released into the blood serving as a marker of the formation of type I collagen, a marker of bone formation, and the latter is released into the blood during degradation of type I collagen and thus serves as a marker of bone resorption. These specific markers were measured in 27 consecutive patients with prostate cancer without bone metastasis. The results showed that after 2 years of treatment, there was a statistically significant lowering of BMD from values measured immediately before the start of treatment. Immediately after start of treatment, ICTP began to increase and was significantly greater after 6 months of treatment. Immediately after the start of treatment, PICP showed a rise and after 6 months it was greater than before treatment, although this was not a statistically significant difference. Because a lowering of BMD was accompanied by changes in the markers of bone metabolism, the decrease in BMD can be attributed to the effects of hormonal therapy rather than being aging-related. Because PICP began to increase slightly later than ICTP increased, this suggests that LHRH agonists stimulate bone formation to compensate for lower bone mass and indicates a coupling between bone resorption and formation. Consequently, PICP and ICTP values might be predictors of bone loss in patients undergoing ADT.

Bisphosponates, particularly zoledronic acid, have been shown to increase bone mass in men undergoing ADT and is now an additional option that can provide benefits to patients with prostate cancer throughout the course of their disease. Zoledronic acid is the only bisphosphonate that has demonstrated efficacy in reducing objectively measurable skeletal complications in patients with bone metastases secondary to prostate cancer and appears to have potent activities against osteoclasts, which affect bone integrity.[3,4,111] Recently, however, spontaneous reports of osteonecrosis of the jaw, occurring mainly in cancer patients, has caused the manufacturer of zoledronic acid to revise its product labeling to include mention of this adverse reaction.

QT interval prolongation

Since the mid-1990s, the single most common cause of the withdrawal or restriction of the use of drugs that have already been marketed has been the prolongation of the electrocardiographic QT interval associated with polymorphic ventricular tachycardia, or torsade de pointes, which can be fatal.[112,113] An association between hormonal therapy for prostate cancer and QT prolongation was demonstrated in three studies involving a total of 376 patients receiving initial hormonal treatment for prostate cancer.[5,114] In a trial comparing abarelix with goserelin plus bicalutamide,[115] QT intervals were evaluated prospectively at baseline and on days 84 and 336. In trials comparing abarelix to leuprolide monotherapy[102] and abarelix to leuprolide plus bicalutamide,[104] QT intervals were evaluated retrospectively at baseline and on day 169. The mean QT interval increased in all treatment groups, but the magnitude of the increase differed among the various hormonal therapies. With goserelin plus bicalutamide, baseline QT interval averaged 402 ms and increased by an average of 18 ms, which was significantly greater than the 13 ms increase from the 407 ms baseline mean in the abarelix group ($P = 0.018$). Baseline QT interval averaged 413 ms in patients treated with leuprolide monotherapy and increased by 21 ms. Patients treated with leuprolide plus bicalutamide had a mean baseline QT interval of 417 ms which increased by 9 ms. No patient developed torsades de pointes or ventricular tachycardia during the studies.

Anemia

The incidence and severity of anemia in patients on complete androgen blockade (CAB) was examined in a study of 142 patients receiving CAB.[116] Up to 90% of patients experienced at least a 10% decline in hemoglobin levels and in 13% of patients, hemoglobin declined by 25% or more. The anemia, occurring routinely in men receiving CAB, was characterized as normochromic, normocytic, and temporally-related to the initiation of androgen blockade, usually resolving after CAB is discontinued. This study led to the recommendation that patients receiving CAB undergo hematological testing at baseline, 1 to 2 months after initiating CAB, and periodically thereafter.

Cognitive dysfunction

There is considerable evidence suggesting that gonadal steroid hormones play an important role in the modulation of mood and cognitive function in women and in men. This has been physically observed in subjects taking LHRH agonists with or without estradiol replacement or progesterone replacement who have undergone positron-emission tomography scans during neuropsychological tests.[117] For women suffering from endometriosis, while LHRH agonists reduce the extent of the endometrial lesions and the occurrence of pelvic pain associated with the disease, agonists have been associated with physical and psychiatric side effects. Results of a prospective, double-blind placebo-controlled study and an open label trial indicate that depressive mood symptoms increase in women treated with LHRH agonist therapy for endometriosis.[118] There are case reports in the literature of women of reproductive age with no prior psychiatric history who were treated with a LHRH agonist for endometriosis. These women developed symptoms consistent with various psychiatric disorders, including panic disorder and major depression with and without psychotic features.[119]

Androgen suppression monotherapy for prostate cancer was found to be potentially associated with impaired memory, attention, and executive functions. Eighty-two men with extraprostatic prostate cancer were randomly assigned to receive either continuous leuprorelin, goserelin (both LHRH analogs), cyproterone acetate (a steroidal antiandrogen), or close clinical monitoring. These patients underwent cognitive assessments at baseline and before starting treatment, and then 6 months later. Compared with the baseline assessments, men receiving androgen suppression monotherapy performed worse in two of 12 tests of attention and memory; 24 of 50 men randomized to active treatment and assessed 6 months later had a clinically significant decline in one or more cognitive tests but not one patient randomized to close monitoring showed a decline in any test performance.[120,121]

Interstitial pneumonitis

Pulmonary toxicities have been linked to treatment with antiandrogens, especially nilutamide, as is reflected in a black-box warning on its FDA-approved labeling. Interstitial pneumonitis has been reported in 2% of patients in controlled clinical trials in patients exposed to nilutamide. A small study in Japanese subjects showed that 8 of 47 patients (17%) developed interstitial pneumonitis. Reports of interstitial changes including pulmonary fibrosis that led to hospitalization and death have been reported rarely postmarketing. Symptoms included exertional dyspnea, cough, chest pain, and fever.[122] A class effect has been suggested, after a review of 3-years worth of records in the US FDA's adverse event reporting database.[123] All cases of pneumonitis associated with bicalutamide, flutamide, and nilutamide that were reported between 1998 and 2000 were reviewed. Pneumonitis occurred in 12 patients receiving bicalutamide, 16 patients receiving flutamide, and 50 patients receiving nilutamide at a median of 7.5, 5, and 8 weeks of treatment. Deaths were reported from pulmonary toxicities in all three therapies. A note of caution, however, that incidence rates should not be calculated from spontaneously reported data because of extensive underreporting; fewer than 10% of serious reactions are reported to the FDA.[124]

Immediate onset systemic allergic reactions

The use of abarelix is accompanied by a black box warning indicating that immediate-onset systemic allergic reactions (occurring within 30 minutes of dosing), were observed in 1.1% of patients (15 of 1397) dosed with abarelix in clinical trials. Fourteen of these developed symptoms within 8 minutes of injection. Seven of the 15 experienced transient hypotension or syncope, representing 0.5% of all patients. The incidence was higher in patients with advanced symptomatic prostate cancer. The product label[125] further states that patients should be observed for at least 30 minutes after each injection of abarelix and that supportive measures such as leg elevation, oxygen, i.v. fluids, antihistamines, corticosteroids, and epinephrine (alone or in combination) should be employed if an allergic reaction occurs. Prescribing of abarelix will require adherence to a risk management plan that includes both a signed physician and patient attestation confirming that the risks and benefits of using abarelix are understood.

Summary

This chapter has reviewed new hormonal therapies with their different mechanisms of action. As these therapies emerge, the following unanswered questions remain, which should be the subject of future research:

- What should be the role of neoadjuvant hormonal therapy?
  1. Which patients?
  2. Which therapies?
  3. How long should they be used?
- What should be the role of adjuvant hormonal therapy?
  1. Which patients?
  2. For which pathologic characteristics?
  3. What stages?
  4. How long should they be used?
- What is the role of hormonal therapy in patients with pathologically advanced features?
- How can we improve our understanding of the resistance to existing hormonal therapies in the hormone-refractory patient?
- Should hormonal therapy be used alone or in combination with chemotherapy?
- Can we induce second- or third-line response with novel therapies?
- What constitutes the optimal management for newly emerging adverse events associated with hormonal therapies?

Disclosure

Dr Garnick is an officer of Praecis Pharmaceuticals Incorporated, from which he derives a salary and is a shareholder. Dr Motta is an employee of Praecis, from which she derives a salary and is a shareholder. Praecis markets Plenaxis® (abarelix for injectable suspension) for prostate cancer, which is mentioned in this chapter.

References

1. Stoch SA, Parker RA, Chen L, et al. Bone loss in men with prostate cancer treated with gonadotropin-releasing hormone agonists. J Clin Endocrinol Metab 2001;86:2787–2791.
2. Miyaji Y, Saika T, Yamamoto Y, et al. Effects of gonadotropin-releasing hormone agonists on bone metabolism markers and bone mineral density in patients with prostate cancer. Urology 2004;64:128–131.
3. Smith MR, Eastham J, Gleason DM, et al. Randomized controlled trial of zoledronic acid to prevent bone loss in men receiving androgen deprivation therapy for nonmetastatic prostate cancer. J Urol 2003;169:2008–2012.
4. Saad F, Schulman CC. Role of bisphosphonates in prostate cancer. Eur Urol 2004;45:26–34.
5. Garnick MB, Pratt C, Campion M, et al. Increase in the electrocardiographic QTc interval in med with prostate cancer undergoing androgen deprivation therapy: results of three randomized controlled clinical studies [abstract]. European Association of Urology 19th Congress, Vienna, Austria March 24-27, 2004. 3-24-2004.
6. Huggins C, Hodges CV. Studies on prostate cancer I. The effect of castration, of estrogen and of androgen injection on serum phosphatases in metastatic carcinoma of the prostate. Cancer Res 1941;1:293–297.
7. Huggins C, Stevens RE, Jr., Hodges CV. Studies on prostatic cancer. II. The effects of castration on advanced carcinoma of the prostate gland. Arch Surg 1941;43:209–223.
8. Huggins C, Scott WW, Hodges CV. Studies on prostatic cancer. III. The effects of fever, of desoxycorticosterone and of estrogen on clinical patients with metastatic carcinoma. J Urol 1941;46:997–1006.
9. Fowler JE Jr, Whitmore WF Jr. The response of metastatic adenocarcinoma of the prostate to exogenous testosterone. J Urol 1981;126:372–375.
10. Bailar JC III, Byar DP. Estrogen treatment for cancer of the prostate. Early results with 3 doses of diethylstilbestrol and placebo. Cancer 1970;26:257–261.
11. Byar DP. Proceedings: The Veterans Administration Cooperative Urological Research Group's studies of cancer of the prostate. Cancer 1973;32:1126–1130.
12. Veterans Administration Cooperative Urological Research Group. Treatment and survival of patients with cancer of the prostate. The Veterans Administration Co-operative Urological Research Group. Surg Gynecol Obstet 1967;124:1011–1017.
13. Bolla M, Collette L, Blank L, et al. Long-term results with immediate androgen suppression and external irradiation in patients with locally advanced prostate cancer (an EORTC study): a phase III randomised trial. Lancet 2002;360:103–106.
14. Messing EM, Manola J, Sarosdy M, et al. Immediate hormonal therapy compared with observation after radical prostatectomy and pelvic lymphadenectomy in men with node-positive prostate cancer. N Engl J Med 1999;341:1781–1788.
15. Messing EM, Manola J, Yao J, et al. Immediate vs delayed hormonal therapy (HT) in patients with nodal positive (N+) prostate cancer who had undergone radical prostatectomy (RP) + pelvic lymphadenectomy (LND): results of central pathology review (CPR);[abstract #1455]. Annual Meeting of the American Urological Association, San Francisco, CA. 5-11-2004.
16. D'Amico AV, Manola J, Loffredo M, et al. 6-month androgen suppression plus radiation therapy vs radiation therapy alone for patients with clinically localized prostate cancer: a randomized controlled trial. JAMA 2004;292:821–827.
17. Zincke H, Lau W, Bergstralh E, et al. Role of early adjuvant hormonal therapy after radical prostatectomy for prostate cancer. J Urol 2001;166:2208–2215.
18. Crook J, Ludgate C, Malone S, et al. Report of a multicenter Canadian phase III randomized trial of 3 months vs. 8 months neoadjuvant androgen deprivation before standard-dose radiotherapy for clinically localized prostate cancer. Int J Radiat Oncol Biol Phys 2004;60:15–23.
19. Gleave ME, Goldenberg SL, Chin JL, et al. Randomized comparative study of 3 versus 8-month neoadjuvant hormonal therapy before radical prostatectomy: biochemical and pathological effects. J Urol 2001;166:500–506.
20. Chodak G, Sharifi R, Kasimis B, et al. Single-agent therapy with bicalutamide: a comparison with medical or surgical castration in the treatment of advanced prostate carcinoma. Urology 1995;46:849–855.
21. Kolvenbag GJ, Iversen P, Newling DW. Antiandrogen monotherapy: a new form of treatment for patients with prostate cancer. Urology 2001;58:16–23.
22. Iversen P. Bicalutamide monotherapy for early stage prostate cancer: an update. J Urol 2003;170:S48–S52.
23. Iversen P, Tyrrell CJ, Kaisary AV, et al. Bicalutamide monotherapy compared with castration in patients with nonmetastatic locally advanced prostate cancer: 6.3 years of followup. J Urol 2000;164:1579–1582.
24. Duff G. Casodex 150 mg (Bicalutamide): no longer indicated for treatment of localised prostate cancer; Broadcast to Directors of Public Health of PCTs. London, UK: Dept of Public Health, Committee on Safety of Medicines. Posted at http://www.info.doh.gov.uk/doh/embroadcast.nsf/. Ref CEM/CMO/2003/15. 10-28-2003.
25. Health Canada MHPD. Accelerated deaths in localized prostate cancer patients: Health Canada has withdrawn its approval for Casodex 150 mg for early (localized) prostate cancer. Ottawa, Canada: Health Canada. Available at http://www.hc-sc.gc.ca/hpfb-dgpsa/tpd-dpt/casodex_prof_e.html. 8-26-2003.
26. Weckermann D, Harzmann R. Hormone Therapy in Prostate Cancer: LHRH Antagonists versus LHRH Analogues. Eur Urol 2004;46:279–284.

27. Koch M, Steidle C, Brosman S, et al. An open-label study of abarelix in men with symptomatic prostate cancer at risk of treatment with LHRH agonists. Urology 2003;62:877–882.

28. Barrie SE, Potter GA, et al. Pharmacology of novel steroidal inhibitors of cytochrome P450(17 alpha) (17 alpha-hydroxylase/C17-20 lyase). J Steroid Biochem Mol Biol 1994;50:267–273.

29. O'Donnell A, Judson I, Dowsett M, et al. Hormonal impact of the 17alpha-hydroxylase/C(17,20) lyase inhibitor abiraterone acetate (CB7630) in patients with prostate cancer. Br J Cancer 2004;90:2317–2325.

30. Kelly GE, Husband AJ. Flavonoid compounds in the prevention and treatment of prostate cancer. Methods Mol Med 2003;81:377–394.

31. Constantinou AI, Mehta R, Husband A. Phenoxodiol, a novel isoflavone derivative, inhibits dimethylbenz[a]anthracene (DMBA)-induced mammary carcinogenesis in female Sprague-Dawley rats. Eur J Cancer 2003;39:1012–1018.

32. Constantinou AI, Husband A. Phenoxodiol (2H-1-benzopyran-7-0,1,3-(4-hydroxyphenyl)), a novel isoflavone derivative, inhibits DNA topoisomerase II by stabilizing the cleavable complex. Anticancer Res 2002;22:2581–2585.

33. Kelly G, Edwards M. Interim results of a phase Ib/IIa study of oral phenoxodiol in patients with late-stage, hormone-refractory prostate cancer. 95th Annual Meeting of the American Association for Cancer Research: Late Breaker Abstracts 2004;103–104.

34. Brandes LJ, Bracken SP. The intracellular histamine antagonist, N,N-diethyl-2-[4-(phenylmethyl)phenoxy] ethamine.HCL, may potentiate doxorubicin in the treatment of metastatic breast cancer: Results of a pilot study. Breast Cancer Res Treat 1998;49:61–68.

35. Brandes LJ, LaBella FS, Warrington RC. Increased therapeutic index of antineoplastic drugs in combination with intracellular histamine antagonists. J Natl Cancer Inst 1991;83:1329–1336.

36. Brandes LJ, Bracken SP, Ramsey EW. N,N-diethyl-2-[4-(phenylmethyl)phenoxy]ethanamine in combination with cyclophosphamide: an active, low-toxicity regimen for metastatic hormonally unresponsive prostate cancer. J Clin Oncol 1995;13:1398–1403.

37. Raghavan D, Brandes KK, Snyder T, et al. Mitoxantrone plus DPPE in hormone-refractory prostate cancer (HR-CAP) with symptomatic metastases—response in 70% of cases: abstract # 786. American Society of Clinical Oncology, Annual Meeting. 2002.

38. Beer TM, Javle M, Henner W, et al. Pharmcokinetics (PK) and tolerability of DN-101, a new formulation of calcitriol, in patients with cancer [abstract]. American Association for Cancer Research Annual Meeting, Orlando, FL . 3-27-2004.

39. Beer TM. Development of weekly high-dose calcitriol based therapy for prostate cancer. Urol Oncol 2003;21:399–405.

40. Beer TM, Myrthue A. Calcitriol in cancer treatment: from the lab to the clinic. Mol Cancer Ther 2004;3:373–381.

41. Beer TM, Eilers KM, Garzotto M, et al. Quality of life and pain relief during treatment with calcitriol and docetaxel in symptomatic metastatic androgen-independent prostate carcinoma. Cancer 2004;100:758–763.

42. Beer TM, Garzotto M, Eilers KM, et al. Targeting FSH in androgen-independent prostate cancer: abarelix for prostate cancer progressing after orchiectomy. Urology 2004;63:342–347.

43. Beer TM, Garzotto M, Eilers KM, et al. Phase II study of abarelix depot for androgen independent prostate cancer progression during gonadotropin-releasing hormone agonist therapy. J Urol 2003;169:1738–1741.

44. Ben Josef E, Yang SY, Ji TH, et al. Hormone-refractory prostate cancer cells express functional follicle-stimulating hormone receptor (FSHR). J Urol 1999;161:970–976.

45. Garnick MB, Campion M. Abarelix Depot, a GnRH antagonist, v LHRH superagonists in prostate cancer: differential effects on follicle-stimulating hormone. Abarelix Depot study group. Mol Urol 2000;4:275–277.

46. Carducci MA, Padley RJ, Breul J, et al. Effect of endothelin-A receptor blockade with atrasentan on tumor progression in men with hormone-refractory prostate cancer: a randomized, phase II, placebo-controlled trial. J Clin Oncol 2003;21:679–689.

47. Carducci MA, Nelson JB, et al. Effects of altrasentan on disease progression and biological markers in men with metastatic hormone-refractory prostate cancer: phase 3 study;[abstract]. American Society of Clinical Oncology, 40th Annual Meeting, June 2004;4508.

48. Immediate versus deferred treatment for advanced prostatic cancer: initial results of the Medical Research Council Trial. The Medical Research Council Prostate Cancer Working Party Investigators Group. Br J Urol 1997;79:235–246.

49. Soloway MS, Pareek K, Sharifi R, et al. Neoadjuvant androgen ablation before radical prostatectomy in cT2bNxMo prostate cancer: 5-year results. J Urol 2002;167:112–116.

50. Schulman CC, Debruyne FM, Forster G, et al. 4-Year follow-up results of a European prospective randomized study on neoadjuvant hormonal therapy prior to radical prostatectomy in T2-3N0M0 prostate cancer. European Study Group on Neoadjuvant Treatment of Prostate Cancer. Eur Urol 2000;38:706–713.

51. Gleave ME, La Bianca SE, Goldenberg SL, et al. Long-term neoadjuvant hormone therapy prior to radical prostatectomy: evaluation of risk for biochemical recurrence at 5-year follow-up. Urology 2000;56:289–294.

52. Wirth M, Frohmuller H, Marz F, et al. Randomized multicenter trial on adjuvant flutamide therapy in locally advanced prostate cancer after radical surgery: Interim analysis of treatment effect and prognostic factors. Br J Urol 1997;80:263 [abstract].

53. See WA, McLeod D, Iversen P, et al. The bicalutamide Early Prostate Cancer Program. Demography. 2001;6:43–47.

54. Ditonno P, Battaglia M, Selvaggi FP. Adjuvant hormone therapy after radical prostatectomy: indications and results. Tumori 1997;83:567–575.

55. Roach M, III. Hormonal therapy and radiotherapy for localized prostate cancer: who, where and how long? J Urol 2003;170:S35–S40.

56. Pilepich MV, Winter K, John MJ, et al. Phase III radiation therapy oncology group (RTOG) trial 86-10 of androgen deprivation adjuvant to definitive radiotherapy in locally advanced carcinoma of the prostate. Int J Radiat Oncol Biol Phys 2001;50:1243–1252.

57. Sato N, Akakura K, Isaka S, et al. Intermittent androgen suppression for locally advanced and metastatic prostate cancer: preliminary report of a prospective multicenter study. Urology 2004;64:341–345.

58. Klotz LH, Herr HW, Morse MJ, et al. Intermittent endocrine therapy for advanced prostate cancer. Cancer 1986;58:2546–2550.

59. Sato N, Gleave ME, Bruchovsky N, et al. Intermittent androgen suppression delays progression to androgen-independent regulation of prostate-specific antigen gene in the LNCaP prostate tumour model. J Steroid Biochem Mol Biol 1996;58:139–146.

60. Wolf J, Tunn U. Intermittent androgen blockade in prostate cancer: rationale and clinical experience. Eur Urol 2000;38:365–371.

61. Bruchovsky N, Klotz LH, Sadar M, et al. Intermittent androgen suppression for prostate cancer: Canadian Prospective Trial and related observations. Mol Urol 2000;4:191–199.

62. Grossfeld GD, Small EJ, Carroll PR. Intermittent androgen deprivation for clinically localized prostate cancer: initial experience. Urology 1998;51:137–144.

63. Bales GT, Sinner MD, Kim.J.H., et al. Impact of intermittent androgen deprivation on quality of life. J Urol 2004;155:1069.

64. Lawton CA, Winter K, Murray K, et al. Updated results of the phase III Radiation Therapy Oncology Group (RTOG) trial 85-31 evaluating the potential benefit of androgen suppression following standard radiation therapy for unfavorable prognosis carcinoma of the prostate. Int J Radiat Oncol Biol Phys 2001;49:937–946.

65. Chao D, Harland SJ. The importance of continued endocrine treatment during chemotherapy of hormone-refractory prostate cancer. Eur Urol 1997;31:7–10.

66. D'Amico AV, Schultz D, Loffredo M, et al. Biochemical outcome following external beam radiation therapy with or without androgen suppression therapy for clinically localized prostate cancer. JAMA 2000;284:1280–1283.

67. Boccon-Gibod L, Bertaccini A, Bono AV, et al. Management of locally advanced prostate cancer: a European consensus. Int J Clin Pract 2003;57:187–194.

68. Merrick GS, Butler WM, Galbreath RW, et al. Five-year biochemical outcome following permanent interstitial brachytherapy for clinical T1-T3 prostate cancer. Int J Radiat Oncol Biol Phys 2001;51:41–48.

69. Stone NN, Stock RG, Unger P. Effects of neoadjuvant hormonal therapy on prostate biopsy results after (125)I and (103)Pd seed implantation. Mol Urol 2000;4:163–168.

70. Potters L, Torre T, Ashley R, et al. Examining the role of neoadjuvant androgen deprivation in patients undergoing prostate brachytherapy. J Clin Oncol 2000;18:1187–1192.

71. Fleshner NE, Trachtenberg J. Combination finasteride and flutamide in advanced carcinoma of the prostate: effective therapy with minimal side effects. J Urol 1995;154:1642–1645.

72. Ornstein DK, Rao GS, Johnson B, et al. Combined finasteride and flutamide therapy in men with advanced prostate cancer. Urology 1996;48:901–905.

73. Kirby R, Robertson C, Turkes A, et al. Finasteride in association with either flutamide or goserelin as combination hormonal therapy in patients with stage M1 carcinoma of the prostate gland. International Prostate Health Council (IPHC) Trial Study Group. Prostate 1999;40:105–114.

74. Brufsky A, Fontaine-Rothe P, Berlane K, et al. Finasteride and flutamide as potency-sparing androgen-ablative therapy for advanced adenocarcinoma of the prostate. Urology 1997;49:913–920.

75. Ornstein DK, Smith DS, Andriole GL. Biochemical response to testicular androgen ablation among patients with prostate cancer for whom flutamide and/or finasteride therapy failed. Urology 1998;52:1094–1097.

76. Dupont A, Labrie F, Giguere M, et al. Combination therapy with flutamide and [D-Trp6]LHRH ethylamide for stage C prostatic carcinoma. Eur J Cancer Clin Oncol 1988;24:659–666.

77. Labrie F. Androgen blockade in prostate cancer in 2002: major benefits on survival in localized disease. Mol Cell Endocrinol 2002;198:77–87.

78. Adis International Inc. Adis Clinical Trials Insight: DIALOG File 173; Database search. Langhorne, PA: Adis International Inc, 2004.

79. PJP Publications. Pharmaprojects: DIALOG file 128; Database search. Richmond, Surrey, UK: PJP Publications, 2004.

80. Chen J, Hwang DJ, Bohl CE, et al. A Selective Androgen Receptor Modulator (SARM) for hormonal male contraception. J Pharmacol Exp Ther 2004.

81. Gao W, Kearbey JD, Nair VA, et al. Comparison of the pharmacological effects of a novel selective androgen receptor modulator (SARM), the 5{alpha}-Reductase inhibitor finasteride, and the antiandrogen hydroxyflutamide in intact rats: New approach for benign prostate hyperplasia (BPH). Endocrinology 2004.

82. Inhale Therapeutic Systems Inc. Inhale announces positive phase I clinical results of inhaleable peptide, leuprolide. Media Release. Available from: URL: http://www.inhale.com 2001.

83. Laufer M, Thortone D, et al. Phase I study of escalating doses of the dual-action 5-alpha reductase inhibitor LY320236 in patients with advanced prostate cancer: preliminary clinical and hormonal results. Proceedings of 36th Annual Meeting of the American Society of Clinical Oncology 2000;19:369.

84. Periti P, Mazzei T, Mini E. Clinical pharmacokinetics of depot leuprorelin. Clin Pharmacokinet 2002;41:485–504.

85. Balchen T, Agerso H, et al. Single subcutaneous administration of a novel, fast-acting gonadotropin-releasing hormone antagonist degarelix (FE200486) with depot characteristics in healthy men. Clinical and Experimental Pharmacology and Physiology 2004;31 (Suppl.1):126.

86. Weston P, Hammonds J, Vaughton K, et al. Degarelix: a novel GnRH antagonist tested in a multicenter, randomized, dose-finding study in prostate cancer patients: [podium presentation, no. PD-4.03]. Congress of the Societe Internationale d'Urologie, 27th, Hawaii, October 5 2004.

87. Lorenzo A. Spectrum deals for rights to clinical-stage LHRH antagonist. Bioworld Today 2004;15:156.

88. Erb K, Pechstein B, Schueler A, et al. Pituitary and gonadal endocrine effects and pharmacokinetics of the novel luteinizing hormone-releasing hormone antagonist teverelix in healthy men—a first-dose-in-humans study. Clin Pharmacol Ther 2000;67:660–669.

89. Jungwirth A, Pinski J, Galvan G, et al. Inhibition of growth of androgen-independent DU-145 prostate cancer in vivo by luteinising hormone-releasing hormone antagonist Cetrorelix and bombesin antagonists RC-3940-II and RC-3950-II. Eur J Cancer 1997;33:1141–1148.

90. Kaisary AV, Bowsher WG, Gillatt DA, et al. Pharmacodynamics of a long acting depot preparation of avorelin in patients with prostate cancer. Avorelin Study Group. J Urol 1999;162:2019–2023.

91. Mieda M, Ohta Y, Saito T, et al. Antiandrogenic activity and endocrinological profile of a novel antiandrogen, TZP-4238, in the rat. Endocr J 1994;41:445–452.

92. Shukeir N, Arakelian A, Chen G, et al. A synthetic 15-mer peptide (PCK3145) derived from prostate secretory protein can reduce tumor growth, experimental skeletal metastases, and malignancy-associated hypercalcemia. Cancer Res 2004;64:5370–5377.

93. Shukeir N, Arakelian A, et al. Prostate secretory protein PSP-94 decreases tumor growth and hypercalcemia of malignancy in a syngenic in vivo model of prostate cancer. Cancer Res 2003;63:2072–2078.

94. Brandes LJ, Hogg GR. Study of the in-vivo antioestrogenic action of N,N-diethyl-2-[4-(phenylmethyl)phenoxy]ethanamine HCl (DPPE), a novel intracellular histamine antagonist and antioestrogen binding site ligand. J Reprod Fertil 1990;89:59–67.

95. Stein S, Zoltick B, Peacock T, et al. Phase II trial of toremifene in androgen-independent prostate cancer: a Penn cancer clinical trials group trial. Am J Clin Oncol 2001;24:283–285.

96. Steiner MS, Pound CR. Phase IIA clinical trial to test the efficacy and safety of Toremifene in men with high-grade prostatic intraepithelial neoplasia. Clin Prostate Cancer 2003;2:24–31.

97. Gonzalez-Barcena D, Schally AV, Vadillo-Buenfil M, et al. Response of patients with advanced prostatic cancer to administration of somatostatin analog RC-160 (vapreotide) at the time of relapse. Prostate 2003;56:183–191.

98. Pinski J, Schally AV, Halmos G, et al. Effect of somatostatin analog RC-160 and bombesin/gastrin releasing peptide antagonist RC-3095 on growth of PC-3 human prostate-cancer xenografts in nude mice. Int J Cancer 1993;55:963–967.

99. Pollak MN, Schally AV. Mechanisms of antineoplastic action of somatostatin analogs. Proc Soc Exp Biol Med 1998;217:143–152.

100. Chertin B, Spitz IM, Lindenberg T, et al. An implant releasing the gonadotropin hormone-releasing hormone agonist histrelin maintains medical castration for up to 30 months in metastatic prostate cancer. J Urol 2000;163:838–844.

101. Schlegel PN, Kuzma P, Frick J, et al. Effective long-term androgen suppression in men with prostate cancer using a hydrogel implant with the GnRH agonist histrelin. Urology 2001;58:578–582.

102. McLeod D, Zinner N, Tomera K, et al. A phase 3, multicenter, open-label, randomized study of abarelix versus leuprolide acetate in men with prostate cancer. Urology 2001;58:756–761.

103. Tomera K, Gleason D, Gittelman M, et al. The gonadotropin-releasing hormone antagonist abarelix depot versus luteinizing hormone releasing hormone agonists leuprolide or goserelin: initial results of endocrinological and biochemical efficacies in patients with prostate cancer. J Urol 2001;165:1585–1589.

104. Trachtenberg J, Gittleman M, Steidle C, et al. A phase 3, multicenter, open label, randomized study of abarelix versus leuprolide plus daily antiandrogen in men with prostate cancer. J Urol 2002;167:1670–1674.

105. Holzbeierlein JM, Castle E, Thrasher JB. Complications of androgen deprivation therapy: prevention and treatment. Oncology (Huntingt) 2004;18:303–309.

106. Hellerstedt BA, Pienta KJ. The current state of hormonal therapy for prostate cancer. CA Cancer J Clin 2002;52:154–179.

107. DIALOG. Diogenes Adverse Reaction Database. 2002.

108. Peters JL, Fairney A, Kyd P, et al. Bone loss associated with the use of LHRH agonists in prostate cancer. Prostate Cancer Prostatic Dis 2001;4:161–166.

109. Stepan JJ, Lachman M, Zverina J, et al. Castrated men exhibit bone loss: effect of calcitonin treatment on biochemical indices of bone remodeling. J Clin Endocrinol Metab 1989;69:523–527.

110. Kiratli BJ, Srinivas S, Perkash I, et al. Progressive decrease in bone density over 10 years of androgen deprivation therapy in patients with prostate cancer. Urology 2001;57:127–132.

111. Smith MR. The role of bisphosphonates in men with prostate cancer receiving androgen deprivation therapy. Oncology (Huntingt) 2004;18:21–25.

112. Lasser KE, Allen PD, Woolhandler SJ, et al. Timing of new black box warnings and withdrawals for prescription medications. JAMA 2002;287:2215–2220.

113. Roden DM. Drug-induced prolongation of the QT interval. N Engl J Med 2004;350:1013–1022.

114. Garnick MB, Pratt C, Campion M, et al. The effect of hormonal therapy for prostate cancer on the electrocardiographic QT interval: Phase 3 results following treatment with leuprolide and goserelin, alone or with bicalutamide, and the GnRH antagonist abarelix. J Clin Oncol 2004;22:4578 [abstract].

115. Debruyne FM. ABACAS 1: a comparison of the efficacy and safety of abarelix versus goserelin plus bicalutamide in patients with advanced or metastatic prostate cancer: a one year randomized open-label multicenter, Phase III trial [abstract]. Presented by P. Teillac at a workshop entitled "Advances in the Biology of Hormonal Therapy in the Treatment of Prostate Cancer". European Association of Urology 18th Congress, Madrid, Spain, 2003.

116. Strum SB, McDermed JE, Scholz MC, et al. Anaemia associated with androgen deprivation in patients with prostate cancer receiving combined hormone blockade. Br J Urol 1997;79:933–941.

117. Berman KF, Schmidt PJ, Rubinow DR, et al. Modulation of cognition-specific cortical activity by gonadal steroids: a positron-emission tomography study in women. Proc Natl Acad Sci USA 1997;94:8836–8841.

118. Warnock JK, Bundren JC, Morris DW. Depressive symptoms associated with gonadotropin-releasing hormone agonists. Depress Anxiety 1998;7:171–177.

119. Warnock JK, Bundren JC. Anxiety and mood disorders associated with gonadotropin-releasing hormone agonist therapy. Psychopharmacol Bull 1997;33:311–316.

120. Green HJ, Pakenham KI, Headley BC, et al. Quality of life compared during pharmacological treatments and clinical monitoring for non-localized prostate cancer: a randomized controlled trial. BJU Int 2004;93:975–979.

121. Green HJ, Pakenham KI, Headley BC, et al. Altered cognitive function in men treated for prostate cancer with luteinizing hormone-releasing hormone analogues and cyproterone acetate: a randomized controlled trial. BJU Int 2002;90:427–432.

122. Aventis Pharmaceuticals. Nilandron (Aventis) Nilutamide Tablets, Prescribing information as of July 2001 in Physician's Desk Reference Electronic Library. Thomson, Micromedex, 2004.

123. Bennett CL, Raisch DW, Sartor O. Pneumonitis associated with nonsteroidal antiandrogens: presumptive evidence of a class effect. Ann Intern Med 2002;137:625.

124. Ahmad SR, Graham DJ. Pneumonitis with antiandrogens. Ann Intern Med 2003;139:528–v529.

125. Praecis Pharmaceuticals Incorporated. Plenaxis [package insert]. Waltham, MA: PRAECIS PHARMACEUTICALS INCORPORATED, 2003.

126. Melton LJ, III, Alothman KI, Khosla S, et al. Fracture risk following bilateral orchiectomy. J Urol 2003;169:1747–1750.

127. Bogdanos J, Karamanolakis D, Milathianakis C, et al. Combined androgen blockade-induced anemia in prostate cancer patients without bone involvement. Anticancer Res 2003;23:1757–1762.

128. Almeida OP, Waterreus A, Spry N, et al. One year follow-up study of the association between chemical castration, sex hormones, beta-amyloid, memory and depression in men. Psychoneuroendocrinology 2004;29:1071–1081.

129. Shioi K, Yoshida M, Sakai N. Interstitial pneumonitis induced by bicalutamide and leuprorelin acetate for prostate cancer. Int J Urol 03;10:625–626.

39

Intermittent androgen suppression for prostate cancer: rationale and clinical experience

Martin Gleave, S Larry Goldenberg

Abstract

Since the mid-1980s, research on hormonal treatments for prostate cancer have focused on maximizing androgen ablation through combination therapy. Unfortunately, maximal androgen ablation increases treatment-related side effects and expense and has not significantly prolonged time to androgen-independent (AI) progression. The rationale behind intermittent androgen suppression (IAS) is based on: 1) observations that androgen ablation delays tumor progression but is rarely curative in most patients, and hence quality of life must be considered; 2) the assumption that immediate androgen ablation is superior to delayed therapy in improving survival of patients with prostate cancer; and 3) the hypothesis that if tumor cells surviving androgen withdrawal can be forced along a normal pathway of differentiation by androgen replacement, then apoptotic potential might be restored, androgen dependence may be prolonged, and progression to androgen independence may be delayed. Observations from animal model studies suggest that progression to androgen independence involves adaptive responses to androgen deprivation, which are, in turn, modulated by intermittent androgen replacement.

Supported by these animal model observations, several centers have now tested the feasibility of IAS therapy in nonrandomized groups of patients with prostate cancer using serum prostate-specific antigen (PSA) as trigger points. Experimental and clinical data suggest that prostate cancer is amenable to control by IAS, and so IAS may offer clinicians an opportunity to improve quality of life in patients with prostate cancer by balancing the benefits of immediate androgen ablation (delayed progression and prolonged survival) while reducing treatment-related side effects and expense. Whether time to progression and survival is affected in a beneficial or adverse way is being studied in randomized, prospective protocols. This chapter will review the rationale behind IAS, compare observations from published series, and discuss potential indications and treatment strategies using IAS.

Introduction

More than 80% of men with advanced prostate cancer have symptomatic and objective responses following androgen suppression, and serum PSA levels decrease in almost all patients. Surgical or medical castration results in a median progression-free survival of 12 to 33 months and a median overall survival of 23 to 37 months in patients with stage D2 disease.[1,2] However, for reasons that are only partly defined, the apoptotic process induced by androgen ablation fails to eliminate the entire malignant cell population. Another limitation of conventional androgen ablation is that it accelerates the rate of progression of prostate cancer to an androgen-independent state,[3] and after a variable period of time averaging 24 months, progression inevitably occurs with rising serum PSA levels and androgen-independent growth. Since the mid-1980s, many efforts have focused on maximizing the degree of androgen suppression therapy by combining agents that inhibit or block both testicular and adrenal androgens. Unfortunately, maximal androgen ablation (i.e., the addition of an antiandrogen to medical or surgical castration) increases treatment-related side effects and expense and has not significantly prolonged time to androgen-independent progression in most patients.[2,4,5]

The idea of intermittent cycling of endocrine therapies arose through a realization that treatment resistance emerges from a Darwinian interplay of genetic and epigenetic factors and selective pressures of treatment. Early observations that prostatic involution after castration is an active process involving rapid elimination of most epithelial cells led to the postulate that replacement of androgens, even in small amounts, would have a conditioning effect on surviving cells and allow them to conserve or regain desirable traits of differentiation.[6,7] In the case of tumors, several lines of evidence obtained by Foulds[7] and Noble[8] implied that long periods of hormone deprivation simply accelerated progression towards autonomous growth and thus were better avoided. Although, no practical method of countering progression by hormonal means emerged from this work, the subsequent demonstration that consecutive episodes of testosterone-induced regeneration of involuted prostate completely restored the susceptibility of the epithelium to further androgen withdrawal,[9] was an incentive to try similar experiments on tumors. The potential benefits of intermittent, rather than continuous, therapy include improved quality of life through reduced therapy-induced side effects, decreased costs, and possibly improved control over progression to androgen-independence. However, IAS is a feasible treatment option only if immediate hormone therapy is superior to delayed, and if adaptive mechanisms help mediate androgen-independent progression. The following section will review evidence that supports this rationale.

Rationale for intermittent androgen suppression

Balancing the benefits of "early" androgen ablation

While early diagnosis and treatment is a long-held paradigm in oncology, the controversy surrounding optimal time to initiate hormone therapy in prostate cancer remains relevant considering how wide the spectrum of advanced prostate cancer has become. Although androgen ablation has been the standard therapy for advanced prostate cancer for over 60 years, the optimal time to begin this treatment in asymptomatic patients remains controversial: whether to start treatment early after diagnosis or wait until the disease burden is larger and causes symptoms. This issue is especially relevant in the PSA era, with its expanding proportion of PSA-relapses after failed local therapy, many of whom may be candidates for androgen ablation therapy.

The rationale for IAS would be weak if time to disease progression and overall survival were similar between early (i.e., at the time of diagnosis of metastatic or recurrent disease) and delayed (i.e., waiting for the development of symptoms) androgen ablation. Measuring serum PSA after radical prostatectomy or radiotherapy would be a waste of time and resources, and only patients with clinical symptomatic recurrences would require hormonal therapy. Accumulating theoretical, preclinical, and clinical evidence support treatment at the time of diagnosis of locally advanced or metastatic disease. The Goldie–Coldman[10] hypothesis of increasing somatic genomic alterations and tumor heterogeneity over time provides a theoretical basis to support initiation of therapy as early as possible. Also, data from several xenograft models support initiation of androgen ablation when tumor burden is small.[11,12] For example, using the androgen-dependent Shionogi mouse model, So et al[12] reported that large tumor volume and corresponding delay of castration reduced the time to androgen-independent recurrence and death. Earlier androgen ablation, at time of subclinical (nonpalpable) disease, significantly delayed the rate and time to androgen-independent recurrence compared with delayed therapy when tumor burden was high.

Many clinical studies also report prolonged time to androgen-independence and improved survival with early therapy in men with advanced prostate cancer. While the first Veterans Administration Cooperative Urological Research Group (VACURG) study[13] reported that delayed endocrine therapy was equivalent to immediate treatment, reanalysis by Byar[14] indicated that earlier therapy, when corrected for the cardiovascular mortality associated with diethylstilbestrol (DES), was more effective. The Medical Research Council (MRC) study from the UK randomized over 800 men with advanced M0 or M1 disease to immediate or deferred therapy and showed that palliative surgery for bladder outlet or ureteral obstruction was reduced by almost 50% and disease-specific survival improved with immediate therapy.[15] Another, more recent study from the European Organisation for Research and Treatment of Cancer (EORTC) also demonstrated significant improvement in time to disease progression, and 5-year survival (58% versus 78%) in patients with locally advanced disease treated with radiotherapy and either immediate androgen ablation for 3 years or delayed therapy until symptomatic progression.[16] In an Eastern Collaborative Oncology Group (ECOG) trial, Messing et al[17] reported dramatically improved overall and recurrence-free survival in patients with node-positive disease that underwent radical prostatectomy treated

with immediate androgen ablation compared with deferred therapy. Finally, recent data from the Early Prostate Cancer (EPC) trials demonstrates that those patients treated immediately with the antiandrogen bicalutamide had a lower risk of progression of disease.[18] Importantly, however, data from Trial 25 (Scandinavia) also reported that time to death is accelerated in men with T1/T2 prostate cancer treated with bicalutamide compared with watchful waiting alone (hazard ratio [HR] 1.47; $P = 0.0195$). This decrease in overall survival in T1/T2 watchful waiting patients treated with bicalutamide is significant, appears to be drug related, and is biologically plausible. While the effects may be due to bicalutamide itself and not be related to androgen receptor blockade, the effects are most plausibly due to androgen blockade. In contrast, in Trial 25 in T3/T4 prostate cancer patients, time to death was significantly longer (HR 0.67; $P = 0.0125$) in bicalutamide- compared with placebo-treated men. Accelerated rate of death in watchful waiting T1/T2 tumors with a reverse trend in watchful waiting T3/T4 patients is consistent with the hypothesis that bicalutamide treatment improved survival in men at high risk of progression, but worsened survival in men at low risk of progression.

Coincident with accumulating evidence supporting immediate therapy is a shift in the target population eligible to receive androgen ablation from metastatic disease to PSA failures after radical prostatectomy or radiotherapy. Use of PSA for early detection has produced a stage migration and 50% decrease in the incidence of stage D2 disease over the last 2 years.[19] Because the median survival in hormone-naive M+ disease is only 2 to 3 years, the long-term side-effects of androgen ablation do not become apparent and are, therefore, not clinically relevant. However, use of PSA and stage migration has resulted in earlier diagnosis at younger ages and earlier stages of disease, with the prospect of much longer therapy and risk of chronic complications. Furthermore, the use of PSA to detect biochemical recurrences following radical prostatectomy or radiotherapy identifies men at risk to recur and who may benefit from early adjuvant therapy but who have life expectancies exceeding 10 years. Hence, combinations of stage migration, earlier diagnosis of PSA recurrences, longer life expectancies, and trend towards immediate therapy will force clinicians to balance the potential benefits of early adjuvant therapy with risks of development of metabolic complications, as well as the increased expense, associated with long-term continuous androgen withdrawal therapy. These metabolic complications include loss of bone mass (osteoporosis) and fractures, loss of muscle mass, anemia with easy fatigue and decreased energy levels, changes in lipid profile with increased risk of cardiovascular complications, glucose intolerance, and depressive and/or irritable personality changes.[20] Decreased overall survival in low risk watchful waiting patients treated with bicalutamide in the EPC trials further emphasize the need to carefully select patients at high risk of disease progression who are most likely to benefit from early hormone therapy. In this regard, IAS may offer clinicians an opportunity to improve quality of life in patients with prostate cancer by balancing the benefits of immediate androgen ablation (delayed progression and prolonged survival) while reducing treatment-related side effects and expense.

Modulating adaptive responses mediating androgen independence

The development of therapeutic resistance, after hormone- or chemotherapy, for example, is the underlying basis for most cancer deaths. Therapeutic resistance and tumor progression result from multiple, stepwise changes in DNA structure and gene expression—a Darwinian interplay of genetic and epigenetic factors, many arising from selective pressures of treatment. This highly dynamic process cannot be attributed to singular genetic events, involving instead cumulative changes in gene expression that facilitate escape from normal regulatory control of cell growth and survival. Prostate cancer initially progresses as an androgen-dependent tumor, manifested by apoptosis, cell cycle arrest, and changes in androgen-regulated gene expression after androgen ablation.[21] Unfortunately, progression to androgen-independence nearly always occurs in prostate cancer after androgen ablation. It is somewhat ironic that the very same agents used to kill or control cancer cells also trigger cascades of events that lead to a hormone-resistant phenotype.

Progression to androgen independence is a multifactorial process by which cells acquire the ability to both survive in the absence of androgens and proliferate using non-androgenic stimuli for mitogenesis, and involves variable combinations of clonal selection, adaptive upregulation of antiapoptotic cytoprotective genes (e.g., *BCL2*, clusterin *HSP27*), androgen receptor transactivation in the absence of androgen from mutations or increased levels of coactivators and alternative growth factor pathways, including HER2/NEU, epidermal growth factor receptor (EGFR), transforming growth factor-β (TGFβ), and insulin-like growth factor 1 (IGF1).[3,23–31] A complete review of these mechanisms is beyond the scope of this review, but likely all variably operate in heterogenous tumors like prostate cancer.

Bruchovsky et al[3] described a model whereby prostate cancer cells surviving androgen withdrawal are derived from adaptive cell survival mechanisms in a small number of initially androgen-dependent stem cells. High-throughput bioprofiling using gene and tissue microarrays is used by many research groups to characterize genetic and signaling networks that enable tumors to progress and adapt to treatments. In general, there is a reproducible, programmatic drift in gene expression in prostate tissues after androgen ablation. Of interest, while clusterin, BCL2, BCLXL, HSP27, insulin-like growth factor binding proteins 2 and 5 (IGFBP2, IGFBP5) are expressed at very low levels in androgen-dependent tumors, they are all upregulated after castration and remain constitutively overexpressed in recurrent androgen-independent tumors. Increased expression of BCL2,[25,27] androgen receptor,[26] clusterin,[28,32] IGFBP5,[29] IGFBP2,[30] and HSP27[31] after castration help confer androgen resistance and represent adaptive responses by malignant cells to activate survival and mitogenic pathways to compensate for androgen withdrawal.

Based on the above observations, it is reasonable to postulate that the adaptive changes in gene expression precipitated by androgen ablation may be modulated by re-exposure to the differentiating effects of androgen. The ability of benign or malignant prostate cells to undergo apoptosis, and to express PSA, is acquired as a feature of differentiation of prostatic cells under the influence of androgens. Even in malignancy, the ability to undergo apoptosis is acquired as a feature of differentiation under the influence of androgens. Therefore, in the absence of androgens, dividing cells cannot differentiate and become pre-apoptotic (to androgen withdrawal) again, which explains why recurrent tumor growth after castration is characterized by androgen independence.[3] The rationale behind IAS is based on the hypothesis that if tumor cells surviving androgen withdrawal are forced along a pathway of differentiation by androgen replacement, then apoptotic potential might be restored and progression to androgen independence delayed. It follows that, if androgens are replaced soon after regression of tumor, it should be possible to bring about repeated cycles of androgen-stimulated growth, differentiation, and androgen-withdrawal regression of tumor.

Preclinical studies of intermittent androgen suppression

Dunning R3327 rat prostatic adenocarcinoma

Using the Dunning rat carcinoma as a model of progression to androgen-independence, Isaacs et al[11,22] emphasized the importance of genetic instability, which increases tumor heterogeneity by increasing the number of distinctly different clones of cells, analogous to the Goldie–Coldman hypothesis of tumor progression.[10] Androgen-independent progression results from selective outgrowth of one or more androgen resistant clones after androgen ablation. Trachtenberg et al[33] reported no significant growth reduction in Dunning R3327 tumors treated with IAS, and concluded that IAS was inferior to early castration in inhibiting tumor growth. Similarly, Russo et al[34] reported that Dunning R3327 tumors treated with continuous or intermittent DES had tumor volumes at death smaller than control or castrate rats, but a survival advantage was achieved only in the castrate or continuous DES groups. Although the intermittent regimen was successful in delaying tumor growth, it did not yield a survival advantage and in this respect was inferior to castration. The foregoing experiments using the Dunning R3327 model draw attention to the importance of using cyclic androgen deprivation only for the treatment of androgen-dependent cancer. Dunning tumors are androgen-sensitive, not androgen-dependent, and apoptotic regression does not occur following castration. Hence, the failure to improve outcome with IAS in Dunning tumors is not an unexpected result. Indeed, IAS may be detrimental because of stimulation of androgen-sensitive cells when testosterone levels increase. Androgen ablation with the addition of cytotoxic agents appears to be the most effective therapy in this model.[22]

Shionogi mouse carcinoma

Intermittent androgen suppression of the androgen-dependent Shionogi carcinoma has been carried out experimentally by transplanting tumors into a succession of male mice. The cycle of transplantation and castration-induced apoptosis was successfully repeated four times before growth became androgen-independent during the fifth cycle.[3,35] The mean time to androgen independence increased three-fold compared with one-time castration, consistent with a retarding effect of cyclic therapy on tumor progression. Some caution is required in the interpretation of these results since the procedure of transplanting a regressing tumor from a castrated to a noncastrated animal temporarily may reduce the rate of cell division and give rise to an apparent delay in progression. However, in addition to tumor growth, other markers of androgen dependence such as castration-induced apoptosis and *TRPM2* (clusterin) gene expression were maintained three times longer with IAS compared with continuous therapy, paralleling and supporting the changes in tumor volume.

LNCaP xenograft model

As in human prostate cancer, serum PSA levels in LNCaP xenografts are androgen-regulated and proportional to tumor volume.[36,37]

After castration, serum and tumor-cell PSA levels decrease by 80% and remain suppressed for 3 to 4 weeks before increasing again. With intermittent testosterone withdrawal and replacement in castrated mice bearing LNCaP tumors, androgen-independent regulation of the PSA gene was delayed three-fold.[38] Taking an alternative approach, Thalmann et al[39] reported evidence suggesting that contin-uous androgen suppression may facilitate develop-ment of androgen-independent osseous metastasis. Characterization of androgen-independent-LNCaP cell lines produced a subline (C4-2) that metastasized to bone, and, interestingly, the incidence of osseous metastases appeared higher in castrated than in intact male hosts. Additional indirect evidence supporting the concept of IAS come from two independent reports that isolated androgen-repressed LNCaP cell lines that grew faster in castrated than in intact hosts, and exhibited growth rates that were actually suppressed by androgens.[40,41] Taken together, these data emphasize the potentially diverse biologic effects that androgens have on a heterogeneous and adapting tumor population and supports the concept that progression to androgen-independence involves loss of androgen-induced differentiation and/or upregulation of androgen-repressed growth regulatory pathways.

Clinical studies of intermittent androgen suppression

The intermittent regulation of serum testosterone levels for therapeutic purposes in prostate cancer was first attempted with cyclic administration of estrogenic hormone.[42] Nineteen patients with advanced prostate cancer received DES until a clinical response was clearly demonstrated, and then it was withheld until symptoms recurred. One additional patient was treated with flutamide using a similar schedule. The mean duration of initial therapy was 30 months (range 2–70 months). Subjective improvement was noted in all patients during the first 3 months of treatment. When therapy was stopped, 12 of 20 patients relapsed after a mean interval of 8 months (range 1–24 months) and all subsequently responded to re-administration of drug. Therapy-induced impotency was reversed in 9 of 10 men within 3 months of the break in treatment. An improved quality of life was achieved owing to the reduced intake of DES, and no adverse effects on survival were apparent.

The first nonsteroidal antiandrogens became available around the same time as this study, and subsequently most clinical research focused on the combined use of luteinizing hormone releasing hormone (LHRH) agonists and antiandrogens. Little attention has been given to the reversibility of action of LHRH agonists, the significance of which is far-reaching. The potential for a full recovery from therapy makes it possible to alternate a patient between periods of treatment and no treatment. Furthermore, serial serum PSA measurements, which were not available at the time of the study by Klotz et al,[42] permit accurate monitoring of disease activity and serve as trigger points for stopping and restarting therapy. In response to this androgenic stimulus, atrophic cells are recruited into a normal pathway of differentiation where the risk of progression to androgen-independence is reduced. With the associated movement through the division cycle, the cells become pre-apoptotic again making it possible to repeat therapy.

Preliminary results of IAS in 47 patients using reversible medical castration and serum PSA as trigger points were reported by Goldenberg et al[43] in 1995, and updated to include 80 patients in 1999[44] and 2002.[45] Patients with a minimum follow-up of 12 months and

either recurrent or metastatic disease were followed for a mean of 46 months. Mean initial serum PSA was 110 ng/mL. Treatment was initiated with combined androgen blockade and continued for an average of 9 months. Because prognosis is poor in patients who do not achieve normal PSA levels after androgen ablation, only patients with PSA nadir levels below 4 ng/mL were candidates for this IAS protocol. Medication was withheld after 9 months of therapy until serum PSA increased to mean values between 10 and 20 ng/mL. This cycle of treatment and no treatment was repeated until the regulation of PSA became androgen independent (Figure 39.1).

Thirty-two men are currently in their second cycle and 24 are in their third or higher cycle. The mean time to PSA nadir during the first three cycles was 5 months. The first two cycles averaged 18 months in length with 45% of the time off therapy, while the third cycle averaged 15.5 months. Serum testosterone returned to the normal range within a mean of 8 weeks of stopping treatment. The off-treatment period in all cycles was associated with an improvement in sense of well-being, and the recovery of libido and potency in the men who reported normal or near-normal sexual function before the start of therapy. Androgen-independent progression occurred in 10 of 29 stage D patients and 7 of 41 with localized disease after a mean follow-up of 43 months (Table 39.1). Of 21 stage D2 patients, 12 remained on study with stable disease. Nine patients died, three from noncancer-related illness, with median time to progression and overall survival of 26 and 42 months, respectively.

Since these initial reports, other investigators have confirmed the feasibility of IAS in patients with advanced or recurrent prostate cancer. Higano et al[46] reported their experience in Seattle using IAS with a cohort of 22 patients (7 stage D2, 3 stage D1, 2 stage T2/T3, and 10 biochemical failures after definitive local therapy). The median follow-up was 26 months, and all patients remained alive, with two patients (1 biochemical relapse and 1 D1) progressing to androgen-independence at 33 and 22 months, respectively. Time off therapy for stage D2 patients was 35%, slightly less than the percentage of time off for biochemical failures (44%). All patients cycled off therapy for three or more months noted some improvement in overall quality of life.

Oliver et al[47] in London reviewed 20 patients with localized or metastatic prostate cancer who elected to stop androgen ablation therapy after median of 12 months (range 3–48 months). After a median of 9 months off therapy, 13 patients progressed and were restarted on androgen ablation, and 10 of these remain progression-free after 2 years. Of particular interest were 7 patients who were on therapy for 3, 3, 3, 16, 12, 5, and 12 months and subsequently off hormone therapy for 33, 43, 36, 36, 36, 40, and 42 months, respectively. These authors commented on trends in their small series for better duration off therapy in older patients and in those with non-metastatic disease.

Carrol et al[48] in San Francisco reported on their initial experience with 47 patients with clinically localized prostate cancer treated with an IAS protocol. Patients were followed for a mean of 24 months and completed on average two treatment cycles. Only one patient failed to respond to reinstitution of treatment, and no other patients demonstrated progression during the follow-up period, illustrating the ability of reversible medical castration to induce repeated cycles of therapeutic response. Average cycle length was 16 months for the first cycle and 11 months for the second, and patients averaged 50% of their time off therapy.

A prospective phase II study in post-radiotherapy recurrences accrued over 100 men at 4 centers across Canada.[49] Patients were treated for 9 months and cycled off therapy until serum PSA rose back to levels between 8 and 15 ng/mL (Figure 39.2). Study endpoints included monitoring length of time off therapy,

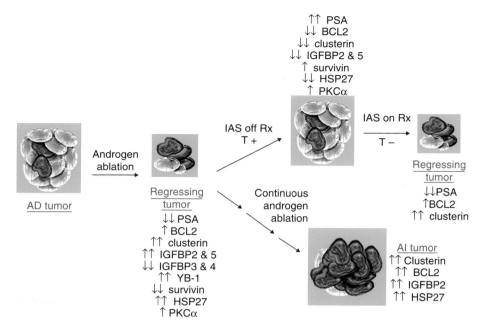

Figure 39.1
Androgen ablation results in apoptosis and upregulation of previously androgen-repressed genes (e.g., Bcl-2, clusterin). However, not all cells are eliminated and, in the absence of androgens, proliferating cells do not differentiate to become pre-apoptotic again, which results in development of the androgen-independent phenotype and constitutive overexpression of resistance-associated genes like *BCL2*, clusterin, and HSP27. With intermittent re-exposure to testosterone (T+), proliferating cells differentiate, expression of resistance associated genes decrease, and cells become pre-apoptotic again, permitting another round of androgen ablation-induced apoptosis and tumor regression (T–). (IAS, intermittent androgen suppression; IGFBP, insulin-like growth factor binding protein; PKC, protein kinase C; PSA, prostate-specific antigen;

Table 39.1 Clinical studies of intermittent androgen suppression (IAS)

Investigator	Sample size	Clinical stage	Mean follow-up (months)	Cycle 1 start PSA (mg/L)	Cycle 2 start PSA, mg/L	Cycle 3 start PSA, mg/L	Mean cycle length (months),* cycle 1, 2, 3	Mean time off therapy (%)	Mean time to PSA nadir (months)
Goldenberg[43]	47	local + metastatic	30	128	15 (n = 30)	18 (n = 15)	18, 18, 16	47	5
Oliver[46]	20	local + metastatic	n/a	n/a	n/a	n/a	n/a	n/a	n/a
Grossfeld[48]	47	local	24	21	7.0 (n = 17)	20.5 (n = 3)	16, 11, n/a[†]	50	4
Higano[47]	22	local + metastatic	26	25	7.7 (n = 12)	n/a (n = 0)	15, 18	38	3.5
Crook[55]	54	Local	33	43	n/a	n/a	18	46	5
Hurtado-Coll[45]	70	local + metastatic	46	110	16 (n = 56)	12 (n = 24)	18, 18, 16	47	5

PSA, prostate-specific antigen.
*Length of time spent on drug therapy and off therapy during each cycle of IAS; [†]Treatment was continued for 1–2 months after nadir PSA reached.

quality-of-life measurements, and time to androgen-independent progression. First cycle analysis demonstrated improved quality-of-life measurements when men were cycled off therapy.

Observations from these series, as well as those from recently published studies[50–52] add to and are consistent with the initial reports from Vancouver[42–44] in terms of response rates and time off therapy. Each of these small series collectively illustrate that relatively short on-therapy periods may result in off-therapy intervals of several years in some men, which suggests that continuous androgen ablation may represent over-treatment in a proportion of men. These IAS series use serum PSA as the marker of response to therapy and tumor progression, as well as a guide for when to restart therapy. Serum PSA increases before evidence of tumor progression becomes apparent in more than 90% of patients with progressive disease treated with continuous therapy.[53] As a result, bone scans for monitoring disease progression are used in patients with new symptoms or biochemical progression. Dissociation between biochemical and clinical progression occasionally occurs, however, and

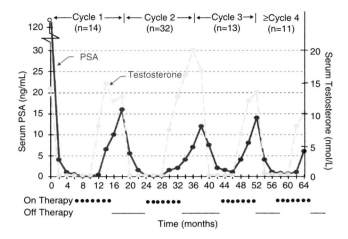

Figure 39.2
Composite results on 70 patients with prostate cancer treated with intermittent androgen suppression, of whom 14 are in their first cycle of treatment, 32 in their second cycle, 13 in their third, 5 in their fourth cycle, and 6 in their fifth cycle. Mean serum prostate-specific antigen (PSA) at the start of the first, second, third and fourth cycles was 110, 16, 12, and 14 ng/mL, respectively. The first three cycles averaged 18, 18, and 15.5 months in length, respectively.

stopping therapy with IAS in this scenario would likely accelerate progression. Although unusual, dissociation between biochemical and clinical progression emphasizes the need for phase III controlled data to better characterize the risks and benefits of IAS.

Candidates for intermittent androgen suppression

Failure of serum PSA to nadir below 4 ng/mL after 6 months of therapy is associated with a short duration of response to androgen ablation and poor prognosis,[54] and IAS is not offered to these patients. Men with TxN1–3M0 who are sexually active, compliant to close follow-up, or who do not tolerate the side effects of androgen ablation can be considered for IAS as long as they realize it is investigational. Biochemical failures after radiotherapy or surgery are groups most likely to benefit from IAS, which permits flexibility in applying and achieving survival benefits of immediate therapy[48,49,55] while balancing potential long-term side effects and costs of continuous therapy. The authors believe that most men with TxNxM1 should be treated with continuous therapy and not be offered IAS except when enrolled in a clinical trial.

Length of treatment cycle

Conceptually, a cycle of androgen ablation should continue until maximal castration-induced apoptosis and tumor regression is induced, but stopped before constitutive development of an androgen-independent phenotype. Premature termination of therapy may permit some cancer cells destined to undergo apoptosis to survive upon re-exposure to testosterone. Some investigators treated

for 1 to 2 months past PSA nadir, which results in shorter "on" cycles and shorter "off" cycles, but similar percentages of time spent off therapy. The definition of nadir must be consistent, however, and should be the lowest, plateau serum PSA level attained following initiation of androgen ablation. Standardization of treatment regimens is necessary for comparison of future series.

A 9 month treatment on cycle is used in most series for the following reasons. First, PSA nadir and maximal soft tissue regression is not reached until 8 or 9 months in many patients on IAS.[44,45] Similarly, the duration of time necessary for PSA to reach its nadir in clinically confined disease after institution of neoadjuvant hormone therapy is often longer than 6 months.[56,57] Using a lower limit of sensitivity of 0.2 ng/mL, PSA nadir was reached in only 34% after 3 months, 60% after 5 months, 70% after 6 months, and 84% at 8 months.[56] The initial rapid decrease in PSA results from cessation of androgen-regulated PSA synthesis and apoptosis, while the ongoing slower decline reflects decreasing tumor volume. Second, immunostaining for proliferation markers (Ki67 and proliferating cell nuclear antigen [PCNA]) showed minimal or reduced activity in radical prostatectomy specimens after 8 months of neoadjuvant therapy compared to pretreatment biopsy specimens.[58,59] Third, levels of the antiapoptotic cytoprotective proteins like BCL2 and clusterin, increase beginning during the first 3 months of neoadjuvant hormone therapy (NHT), and remain elevated after 8 months of therapy, consistent with their role in prevention of castration-induced apoptosis.[25,32,59] These observations indicate that stress-induced increases in BCL2 and clusterin occur early after castration and that concerns regarding constitutively elevated levels that are indicative of developing androgen independence are less likely. Interestingly, androgen can downregulate BCL2 expression in LNCaP cells in vitro[27] and clusterin levels in Shionogi tumors in vivo,[60] observations that may be significant when considering mechanisms by which IAS delays time to androgen-independent progression. Based on time to PSA nadir, reduced proliferation marker staining, and early upregulation of cytoprotective proteins, treatment duration of 9 months is recommended prior to stopping therapy, as illustrated in Figure 39.3.

When to restart

Trigger points for reinstitution of androgen withdrawal therapy are similar among investigators reporting on their IAS experience.[43–49] Although the optimal time remains undefined and empirical, time off therapy should be long enough to permit normalization of improved quality of life and testosterone-induced tumor cell differentiation. Re-exposure of tumor cells to testosterone during the off-treatment cycles of IAS is critical to the underlying hypothesis and rationale behind IAS. Furthermore, recovery of testosterone between treatment cycles is necessary for recovery of sexual function, reduced side effects, and normal sense of well-being. Until more information is obtained, PSA trigger points are regarded as tentative settings only. Trigger points are individualized and factors that are considered include pretreatment PSA levels, stage, PSA velocity, presence of symptoms, and tolerance of androgen ablation therapy. In general, in patients with metastatic disease and high pretreatment PSA levels, therapy is restarted when PSA increases to 20 ng/mL; in patients with locally recurrent disease and moderately elevated pretreatment PSA levels, therapy is restarted when PSA reaches 6 to 15 ng/mL, and earlier for post-radical prostatectomy recurrences.

Phase III trials

Several trials are underway comparing continuous versus intermittent therapy. Both quality of life and cancer outcome events are being measured. These studies include:

- NCIC CTG (PR.7)—for patients with *biochemical failure* following radiotherapy and without radiographic evidence of metastatic disease. Target sample size is 1360 patients, with over 800 accrued by the end of 2004.

- SWOG 9346 (NCIC PR.8)—for newly diagnosed *metastatic* prostate cancer. This group recently reported some early data on PSA normalization rates. 84% of 527 patients had their PSA fall to within the normal range during the induction (first) cycle. This was more likely to occur in men who had: a younger age, a lower initial PSA, no weight change, no bone pain, no visceral metastases or distant nodal metastases. 96% of men whose PSA normalized, did so within 180 days. Target enrollment of 1360 patients should be met by 2006.

The mature results of these trials will be keenly awaited and hopefully will determine the role of IAS in the treatment of prostate cancer.

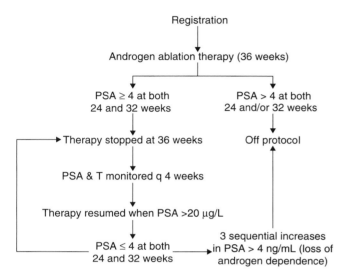

Figure 39.3

Schema of intermittent androgen suppression therapy for patients with biochemical recurrences following radiation therapy for clinically localized prostate cancer. (PSA, prostate-specific antigen; T, testosterone.)

Future directions

Observations from phase II studies suggest that IAS does not have a negative impact on time to progression or survival, both of which appear similar to continuous combined therapy. However, the available information about IAS remains limited and leaves several questions unanswered. The issue of survival is the most important and phase III randomized studies are required to accurately assess the effects of IAS on this critical parameter. Intermittent androgen suppression appears to improve quality of life by permitting recovery of libido and potency, increasing energy levels, and enhancing sense of well-being during off-treatment periods. Preclinical and preliminary clinical studies have identified groups of patients who are most likely to benefit from IAS, trigger points on when to restart therapy, and determined optimal duration of treatment. It is important to look for other signs of progressive disease when serum PSA is used to monitor disease activity, in case of the unusual scenario of PSA-negative disease progression.

The possibility of expanding the use of IAS to earlier stage disease should be examined in greater detail. Conceivably, IAS may become

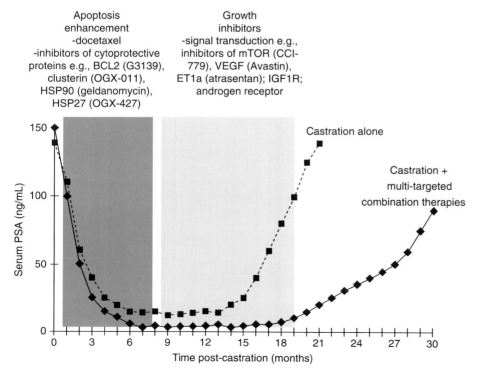

Figure 39.4

Illustrative example of how integration of targeted biologic agents with active cytotoxic agents like docetaxel into cycles of intermittent androgen suppression (IAS) may prolong the length of each IAS cycle by enhancing castration-induced apoptosis and/or inhibiting activation of alternative growth factor signaling pathways. (ET, endothelin; IGF1R, insulin-like growth factor 1 receptor; VEGF, vascular endothelial growth factor.)

an alternative to radical prostatectomy or irradiation for the primary treatment of localized prostate cancer in some men with life expectancies of less than 15 years. The prospect of improving the results of IAS by increasing the length and number of cycles is attractive. Prolongation of the length of each off treatment cycle may be possible with 5α-reductase inhibitors like finasteride. As illustrated in Figure 39.4, augmentation of intermittent therapy might be accomplished by the administration of apoptotic-enhancing agents, like cytotoxic agents (docetaxel) or targeted biologic agents (e.g., antisense clusterin, angiogenesis inhibitors, atrasentan), administered at specific times during a cycle of treatment when the modality-of-choice would have its maximum effect.

References

1. Miyamoto H, Messing EM, Chang C. Androgen deprivation therapy for prostate cancer: current status and future prospects. Prostate 2004;61:332–53.
2. Denis L, Murphy GP. Overview of phase III trials on combined androgen treatment in patients with metastatic prostate cancer. Cancer 1993;72:3888–3895.
3. Bruchovsky N, Rennie PS, Coldman AJ, et al. Effects of androgen withdrawal on the stem cell composition of the Shionogi carcinoma. Cancer Res 1990;50:2275–2282.
4. Crawford ED, Eisenberger M, McLeod DG, et al. Comparison of bilateral orchiectomy with or without flutamide for the treatment of patients with stage D2 adenocarcinoma of the prostate: Results of NCI intergroup study 0105 (SWOG and ECOG). Br J Urol 1997;80:278 [Abstract].
5. Prostate Cancer Trialists' Collaborative Group. Maximum androgen blockade in advanced prostate cancer: an overview of 22 randomised trials with 3283 deaths in 5710 patients. Lancet 1995;346:265–269.
6. Bruchovsky N, Lesser B, Van Doorn E, et al. Hormonal effects on cell proliferation in rat prostate. Vitamin Horm 1975;33:61–102.
7. Foulds L. Neoplastic Development 1. New York, Academic Press, 1969.
8. Noble RL. Hormonal control of growth and progression in tumors of Nb rats and a theory of action. Cancer Res 1977;37:82–94.
9. Sanford NL, Searle JW, Kerr JFR. Successive waves of apoptosis in the rat prostate after repeated withdrawal of testosterone stimulation. Pathology 1984;16:406–410.
10. Goldie JH, Coldman AJ. A mathematical model for relating the drug sensitivity of tumours to their spontaneous mutation rate. Cancer Treat Rep 1979;63:1727–1733.
11. Isaacs JT. The timing of androgen ablation therapy and / or chemotherapy in the treatment of prostatic cancer. Prostate 1984;5: 1–17.
12. So AI, Bowden M, Gleave M. Effect of time of castration and tumour volume on time to androgen-independent recurrence in Shionogi tumours. BJU Int 2004;93:845–850.
13. Mellinger GT. Veterans Administration Cooperative Urological Research Group. Carcinoma of the prostate: a continuing co-operative study. J Urol 1964;91:590–594.
14. Byar DP. Proceedings: The Veterans Administration Cooperative Urological Research Group's studies of cancer of the prostate. Cancer 1973;32:1126–1130
15. Immediate vs deferred treatment for advanced prostate cancer: Initial results of the MRC trial. The Medical Research Council Prostate Cancer Working Party Investigators Group. Br J Urol 1997;79: 235–246.
16. Bolla M, Gonzalez MD, Warde P, et al. Improved survival in patients with locally advanced prostate cancer treated with radiotherapy and goserilin. N Engl J Med 1997;337:295–300.
17. Messing EM, Manola J, Sarosdy M, et al. Immediate hormonal therapy compared with observation after radical prostatectomy and pelvic lymphadenectomy in men with node-positive prostate cancer. N Engl J Med 1999;341:1781–1788

18. Iversen P, Johansson JE, Lodding P, et al. Scandinavian Prostatic Cancer Group. Bicalutamide (150 mg) versus placebo as immediate therapy alone or as adjuvant to therapy with curative intent for early nonmetastatic prostate cancer: 5.3-year median followup from the Scandinavian Prostate Cancer Group Study Number 6. J Urol 2004;172:1871–1876.
19. Stanford JL, Blumenstein BA, Brawer MK. Temporal trends in prostate cancer rates in the Pacific Northwest. J Urol 1996;155:604A.
20. Townsend MF, Sanders WH, Northway RO, et al. Bone fractures associated with luteinizing hormone-releasing hormone agonists used in the treatment of prostatic carcinoma. Cancer 1997;79:545–550.
21. Tenniswood M. Apoptosis, tumour invasion and prostate cancer. Br J Urol 1997;79:27–34.
22. Isaacs JT, Wake N, Coffey DS, et al. Genetic instability coupled to clonal selection as a mechanism for progression in prostatic cancer. Cancer Res 1982;42:2353–2361.
23. Craft N, Shostak Y, Carey M, et al. A mechanism for hormone-independent prostate cancer through modulation of androgen receptor signaling by the HER-2/neu tyrosine kinase. Nat Med 1999;5: 280–285.
24. Feldman BJ, Feldman D. The development of androgen-independent prostate cancer. Nature Rev 2001;1:34–45.
25. Raffo AJ, Periman H, Chen MW, et al. Overexpression of bcl-2 protects prostate cancer cells from apoptosis in vitro and confers resistance to androgen depletion in vivo. Cancer Res 1995;55:4438–4445.
26. Chen CD, Welsbie DS, Tran C, et al. Molecular determinants of resistance to antiandrogen therapy. Nat Med 2004;10:33–39.
27. Gleave ME, Tolcher A, Miyake H, et al. Progression to androgen-independence is delayed by antisense Bcl-2 oligodeoxynucleotides after castration in the LNCaP prostate tumor model. Clinical Cancer Res 1999;5:2891–2898.
28. Miyake H, Rennie P, Nelson C, et al. Testosterone-repressed prostate message-2 (TRPM-2) is an antiapoptotic gene that confers resistance to androgen ablation in prostate cancer xenograft models. Cancer Res 2000;60:170–176.
29. Miyake H, Nelson C, Rennie P, et al. Overexpression of Insulin-Like Growth Factor Binding Protein-5 helps accelerate Progression to Androgen-Independence in the human prostate LNCaP tumor model through activation of phosphatidylinositol 3′-kinase pathway. Endocrinology 2000;141:2257–2265.
30. Kiyama S, Morrison K, Zellweger T, et al. Castration-induced increases in insulin-like growth factor-binding protein-2 promotes proliferation of androgen-independent human prostate LNCaP tumors. Cancer Res 2003;63:3575–3584.
31. Rocchi P, So A, Kojima S, et al. Heat shock protein 27 increases after androgen ablation and plays a cytoprotective role in hormone refractory prostate cancer. Cancer Research, 2004;64:6595–6602
32. July LV, Akbari M, Zellweger T, et al. Clusterin expression is significantly enhanced in prostate cancer cells following androgen withdrawal therapy. Prostate 2002;50:179–188.
33. Trachtenberg J. Experimental treatment of prostatic cancer by intermittent hormonal therapy. J Urol 1987;137:785–788.
34. Russo P, Liguori G, Heston WDW, et al. Effects of intermittent diethyl-stilbestrol diphosphate administration on the R3327 rat prostatic carcinoma. Cancer Res 1987;47:5967–5970.
35. Akakura K, Bruchovsky N, Goldenberg SL, et al. Effects of intermittent androgen suppression on androgen-dependent tumours: apoptosis and serum prostate specific antigen. Cancer 1993;71:2782–2790.
36. Gleave ME, Hsieh JT, Wu H-C, et al. Serum PSA levels in mice bearing human prostate LNCaP tumors are determined by tumor volume and endocrine and growth factors. Cancer Res 1992;52:1598–1605.
37. Sato N, Gleave M, Bruchovsky N, et al. A metastatic and androgen-sensitive human prostate cancer model using intraprostatic inoculation of LNCaP cells in SCID mice. Cancer Res 1997;57: 1584–1589.
38. Sato N, Gleave ME, Bruchovsky N, et al. Intermittent androgen suppression delays time to non-androgen regulated prostate specific

antigen gene expression in the human prostate LNCaP tumour model. J Steroid Biochem Molec Biol 1996;58:139–146.

39. Thalmann, GN, Anezinis, PE, Chang SH, et al. Androgen-independent cancer progression and bone metastasis in the LNCaP model of human prostate cancer. Cancer Res 1994;54:2577–2581.

40. Umekita Y, Hiipakka RA, Kokontis JM, et al. Human prostate tumor growth in athymic mice: inhibition by androgens and stimulation by finasteride. Proc Natl Acad Sci USA 1996;93:11802–11807.

41. Zhou HYE, Chang S-H, Chen B-Q, et al. Androgen-repressed phenotype in human prostate cancer. Proc Natl Acad Sci USA 1996;93:15152–15157.

42. Klotz LH, Herr HW, Morse MJ, et al. Intermittent endocrine therapy for advanced prostate cancer. Cancer 1986;58:2546–2250.

43. Goldenberg SL, Bruchovsky N, Gleave ME, et al. Intermittent androgen suppression in the treatment of prostate cancer: a preliminary report. Urology 1995;45:839–845.

44. Goldenberg SL, Gleave ME, Taylor D. Clinical experience with intermittent androgen suppression for prostate cancer: Minimum 3 years of follow-up. Molecular Urology 1999;3:287–292.

45. Hurtado-Coll A, Goldenberg SL, Gleave ME, et al. Intermittent androgen suppression in prostate cancer: the Canadian experience. Urology 2002;60:52–56.

46. Oliver RT, Williams G, Paris AM, et al. Intermittent androgen deprivation after PSA-complete response as a strategy to reduce induction of hormone-resistant prostate cancer. Urology 1997;49:79–82.

47. Higano CS, Ellis W, Russell K, et al. Intermittent androgen suppression with leuprolide and flutamide for prostate cancer. A pilot study. Urology 1996;48:800–804.

48. Grossfeld GD, Small EJ, Lubeck DP, et al. Androgen deprivation therapy for patients with clinically localized (stages T1 to T3) prostate cancer and for patients with biochemical recurrence after radical prostatectomy. Urology 2001;58:56–64.

49. Bruchovsky N, Klotz LH, Sadar M, et al. Intermittent androgen suppression for prostate cancer: Canadian prospective trial related observations. Mol Urol 2002;4:191–199.

50. Sato N, Akakura K, Isaka S, et al. Chiba Prostate Study Group. Intermittent androgen suppression for locally advanced and metastatic prostate cancer: preliminary report of a prospective multicenter study. Urology 2004;64:341–345.

51. Albrecht W, Collette L, Fava C, et al. Intermittent maximal androgen blockade in patients with metastatic prostate cancer: an EORTC feasibility study. Eur Urol 2003;44:505–511.

52. Lane TM, Ansell W, Farrugia D, et al. Long-term outcomes in patients with prostate cancer managed with intermittent androgen suppression. Urol Int 2004;73:117–122.

53. Stamey TA, Kabalin JN, Ferrari M, et al. Prostate specific antigen in the diagnosis and treatment of adenocarcinoma of the prostate. IV. Anti-androgen treated patients. J Urol 1989;141:1088–1090.

54. Miller JI, Ahmann FR, Drach GW, et al. The clinical usefulness of serum prostate specific antigen after hormonal therapy of metastatic prostate cancer. J Urol 1992;147:956–961.

55. Crook JM, Szumacher E, Malone S, et al. Intermittent androgen suppression in the management of prostate cancer. Urology 1999;53:530–534.

56. Gleave ME, Goldenberg SL, Jones EC, et al. Maximal biochemical and pathological downstaging requires 8 months of neoadjuvant hormonal therapy prior to radical prostatectomy. J Urol 1996;155:213–219.

57. Gleave ME, Goldenberg SL, Chin J, et al. Phase III randomized comparative study of 3 vs 8 months of neoadjuvant hormone therapy prior to radical prostatectomy: Biochemical and pathologic endpoints. J Urol 2001;166:500–506.

58. Patterson R, Gleave M, Jone E, et al. Immunohistochemical analysis of radical prostatectomy specimens after 8 months of neoadjuvant hormone therapy. Mol Urol 1999;3:277–286.

59. Tsuji M, Murakami Y, Kanayama H, et al. Immunohistochemical analysis of Ki-67 antigen and Bcl-2 protein expression in prostate cancer: effect of neoadjuvant hormonal therapy. Br J Urol 1998;81:116–121.

60. Rennie PS, Bruchovsky N, Akakura K, et al. Effect of tumour progression on the androgenic regulation of the androgen receptor, TRPM-2 and YPT1 genes in the Shionogi carcinoma. J Steroid Biochem Mol Biol 1994;50:31–40.

40

Antiandrogen withdrawal syndromes: pathophysiology and clinical implications

Kathleen W Beekman, Grant Buchanan, Wayne D Tilley, Howard I Scher

Introduction

The "antiandrogen withdrawal syndrome" describes the anti-prostate cancer effects following the selective discontinuation of an antiandrogen such as flutamide, bicalutamide, or nilutamide in a patient with progressive prostate cancer treated with a combination of an antiandrogen and testicular androgen ablation. The effects, when they occur, do so in castrate patients with rising prostate-specific antigen (PSA) and/or clinical metastatic disease-points in the illness where the tumor is considered by many to be "hormone-refractory" (Figure 40.1)[1]. While the withdrawal syndrome was originally described with flutamide by three groups including our own in 1993,[2-4] it was soon recognized that withdrawal responses could occur following the selective discontinuation of other hormones including estrogens, progestational agents, and glucocorticoids (reviewed by Kelly et al[5]). The responses were similar to what had been observed previously in breast cancer patients following discontinuation of tamoxifen.[6,7] It would thus appear that designating these prostate tumors as "hormone-refractory" is a misnomer.

Since the original description of the antiandrogen withdrawal syndrome, much has been learned about the mechanisms associated with prostate cancer progression. Indeed, in retrospect, a "bedside to bench" observation helped to focus researchers on the clinical significance of continued signaling through the androgen receptor (AR) in tumors that progress following castration. The antiandrogen withdrawal syndromes provides an in-vivo demonstration of how a specific treatment influences both the biology and clinical behavior of the disease. This phenomenon, now termed "therapy-mediated selection pressure,"[8] illustrates why localised prostate cancers at the time of diagnosis may have different molecular profiles than tumors than metastatic tumors that progress following castration. As such, when considering a targeted therapy, it is essential to understand the targets that are present within the context of the specific clinical state[1] in which the therapy will be utilized or studied.[9]

Historical perspective

The original descriptions of the palliative effects of diethylstilbestrol or surgical orchiectomy on progressive prostate cancer, made over 6 decades ago,[10,11] highlighted an important management principle that is still valid today: blocking the production or action of testicular androgens by medical or surgical means does not eliminate all of the malignant cells within a tumor mass, and as such is not curative. Reports of the palliative benefits of surgical[12] or medical[13] adrenalectomy to eliminate androgens from non-testicular sources followed, which, coupled with studies showing incomplete suppression of intratumoral dihydrotestosterone with medical castration alone,[14] suggested that strategies to eliminate both testicular and adrenal androgens as the initial therapeutic approach might be more beneficial than the elimination of testicular androgens alone. Estimates were that androgens from adrenal sources might represent 5% to 45% of the residual androgens present in tumors after surgical castration alone.[15]

The anti-prostate cancer effects of androgen ablative therapies include an apoptotic response in a proportion of cells within a mass, producing a decrease in size but not the complete elimination of the tumor; followed by a period of apparent stability in which PSA levels do not change and the tumor is viable but not proliferating; followed by a period of regrowth as a castration resistant lesion. Because ablation of testicular androgens alone was not curative, an important clinical question in the 1980s was whether an approach designed to ablate both testicular and adrenal androgens as initial hormone therapy would prove to be superior to those directed solely at testicular sources. It was postulated that superiority would be demonstrated in several ways: 1) an increase in the proportion of patients who are cured; 2) a delay in time to progression as assessed by post-therapy PSA changes (after 1990 when the test became available), new metastases on an imaging study, or the development of prostate cancer related symptoms; 3) prolongation of life; and 4) an improved safety profile.

It was also during this era that a range of medical approaches became available that obviated the need for both a surgical orchiectomy and surgical adrenalectomy to ablate androgens from these sources. Among the medications introduced and subsequently approved for use were the gonadotropin-releasing hormone (GnRH) agonists and antagonists, steroidal and nonsteroidal antiandrogens, 5α-reductase inhibitors, and inhibitors of adrenal androgen synthesis. With surgical orchiectomy the least preferred method by patients to ablate testicular androgens,[16] and the recognized morbidity of surgical adrenalectomy, medical therapies soon replaced surgery (both adrenalectomy and orchiectomy) as the so-called "treatment of choice." It was at this point that prospective, randomized trials comparing GnRH agonists/antagonists (leuprolide acetate and goserelin) and antiandrogens (flutamide and later bicalutamide and nilutamide) to gonadrotropin-releasing hormone

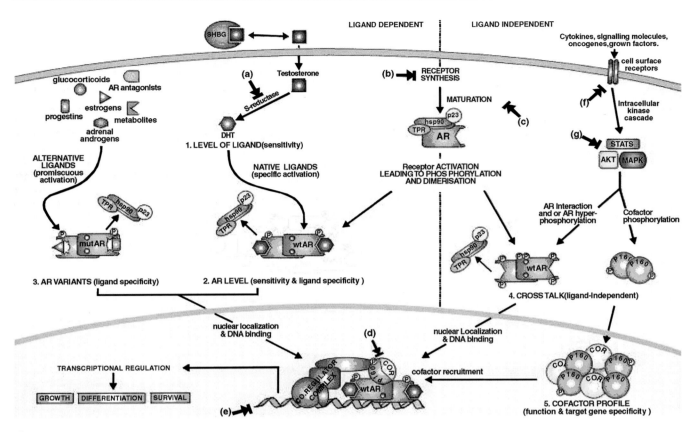

Figure 40.1

Mechanisms by which signaling through the androgen receptor (AR) continues following castration. Following synthesis, the AR exists in dynamic equilibrium between an immature state and an active form capable of binding high affinity androgenic ligands via association/dissociation with a complex that includes heat-shock proteins. (*a*) Receptor-dependent, ligand-mediated signaling. Ligand binding results in the dissociation of this complex, receptor dimerization and phosphorylation, nuclear transport, DNA binding, the recruitment of components of the transcription machinery and other cofactor molecules, such as the p160 coactivators, and ultimately, the activation of particular gene pathways. (*b*) Receptor-dependent, ligand-independent. The AR can also be activated in the absence of ligand by membrane bound tyrosine kinase receptors such as HER2/neu, as well as by signaling molecules, growth factors and cytokines. Intracellular kinase cascades result in receptor activation, transport, binding to androgen response elements and the transactivation of target genes. *1 to 5*, Mechanisms of continued androgen signaling implicated in maintaining prostate cancer growth in a castrate environment following androgen ablation therapy. *1*, Tumor cells may acquire mechanisms to accumulate androgens, such as sequestration by steroid hormone binding globulin or altered regulation of enzymes involved in the synthesis and metabolism of androgens. *2*, Castrate-resistant clinical prostate cancer samples often exhibit increased AR levels compared with early stage tumors or normal prostate cells. This may result from amplification or overexpression of the AR gene. *3*, AR gene mutations can allow promiscuous activation of the AR by alternative ligands, such as glucocorticoids, estrogens, adrenal androgens, progestins and traditional receptor antagonists such as hydroxyflutamide. Other mutations may alter the recruitment of cofactors. *4*, Cross-talk with other signaling pathways may activate the AR in the absence of native ligands. *5*, An altered profile of AR coregulators (coactivators and corepressors) may facilitate ligand-independent AR signaling, or enhance AR activation by low levels of ligand. (i) to (vii), Represent potential new points of therapeutic intervention.

Reproduced with permission from Scher et al[53]

agonists/antagonists alone were begun. Similar trials were designed and initiated with surgical orchiectomy as the method of testicular androgen ablation. Using a variety of combinations of medical and surgical approaches, over 27 prospective randomized comparisons were initiated and completed. Two in particular were perhaps the most influential on clinical practice: SWOG Intergroup 1, which compared the combination of leuprolide acetate plus flutamide to leuprolide acetate plus placebo[17]; and EORTC 30893, which compared goserelin plus flutamide to surgical orchiectomy.[18] Both trials showed a survival benefit for the combined or maximal androgen blockade approach relative to a monotherapy approach that reduced testicular androgens alone. However, despite the survival benefit, the combined androgen blockade was not curative for the

majority of men. Consequently, a large number of men with progressive disease who had either undergone an orchiectomy or who received GnRH hormone agonists/antagonists in combination with flutamide presented for further therapy.

Clinical observation of antiandrogen withdrawal response

The antiandrogen withdrawal syndrome was first described when clinical responses were observed following selective discontinuation of flutamide in combination with a GnRH analog or surgical orchiectomy. No additional therapy was added at the point that flutamide was stopped, and those patients who had not undergone surgical castration were continued on medical therapies to maintain testosterone levels in the castrate range.[2–4] At the University of Michigan and Memorial Sloan-Kettering Cancer Center (MSKCC), the observation was the result in part of our focus on how to reduce the methodologic difficulties associated with drug development in this disease, and in particular how to base eligibility and outcomes on pre- and post-therapy changes in PSA.[19] In the first patient, a withdrawal response was observed, and flutamide was discontinued to avoid the potential hepatic toxicities associated with an investigational agent prior to enrollment on an experimental protocol we were conducting for the palliation of pain secondary to osseous metastases. Following flutamide discontinuation, and prior to protocol enrollment, the PSA level was observed to decline and bone pain decreased. A repeat PSA performed 2 weeks later showed a further PSA reduction, and protocol therapy was not administered.[4] Suspecting this might be an effect similar to what had been reported with tamoxifen,[6,7] flutamide was selectively discontinued in additional patients and additional responses were observed.[20] A most important finding was that effects were not limited to declines in PSA, as objective tumor regressions were documented. Tumor sites in which objective regressions were observed included the epidural space, nodal disease, and in the viscera visceral sites such as the liver. The responses to flutamide withdrawal, when they occurred, did so rapidly, consistent with the short half-life of the drug. As shown in Table 40.1, a range of response rates were reported, with estimates that up to 40% of patients would experience subjective and objective benefits.[2,3,20–23]

Predictive factors for a response to flutamide discontinuation included high baseline alkaline phosphatase and prolonged drug exposure.[24,25] Factors associated with prolonged drug exposure, included the disease extent at the start of therapy, clinical characteristics associated with minimal disease burdens (such as a good performance status), and low PSA levels. For example, in study INT-0105, in which men with non-castrate metastatic tumor with or without prior local therapy were randomized to receive an orchiectomy plus flutamide versus orchiectomy alone, progression-free survival times were 20.4 months in the flutamide arm versus 18.6 months in the placebo arm ($P = 0.2$).[26] These results contrasted with those of another study, in which 309 men in the rising PSA

state following prostatectomy had a median response duration of 10.8 years.[27] This contrast in response reflects differences between the two studies in the extent of disease.

It is important to note that at the time withdrawal responses to flutamide were first described, flutamide was the only antiandrogen in general use. Currently, there are two general classes of antiandrogens in clinical use: steroidal and nonsteroidal. Steroidal antiandrogens, which have progestational as well as antiandrogenic effects, include cyproterone acetate (available primarily in Europe) and megestrol acetate. In addition to differences in clearance and side effect profiles, the agents have variable affinity for the androgen receptor and the exact site of binding to the receptor, as evidenced by the effectiveness of these agents in second and third-line settings. It was hypothesized that patients that progressed while receiving bicalutamide or nilutamide in combination with a GnRH analog or orchiectomy would exhibit a withdrawal response as well, and reports soon followed of withdrawal responses to the selective discontinuation of bicalutamide[28–32] and nilutamide,[33] thus establishing the "antiandrogen withdrawal syndrome" as a clinical entity.[29,34] In addition, similar withdrawal responses were observed with the progestational agents megestrol acetate,[35–37] diethyl-stilbestrol,[38] and chlormadinone acetate.[39]

The paradox of the antiandrogen withdrawal response is that both the steroidal and nonsteroidal agents used initially to inhibit tumor growth could, in certain situations, stimulate tumor growth to the point where discontinuation of the agent became a "therapeutic intervention" for the individual patient. The range of agents associated with this phenomenon, and the fact that most of them acted through the AR, suggested promiscuity in ligand binding and receptor activation. Additional evidence of the agonist effect of these agents is the clinical flare of disease associated with the use of progestational agents administered to treat cachexia, consistent with aberrant receptor activation.[40]

An obvious consideration is that a withdrawal response cannot be observed in a patient who is not receiving the drug, which implies that under the "selection pressure" of prolonged exposure a drug initially used to antagonize androgen action transforms into an agonist that promotes tumor growth. The withdrawal response occurs only in patients who are otherwise medically or surgically castrated and serum testosterone levels are low (<50 ng/mL). It is not observed in patients who are receiving nonsteroidal antiandrogens as monotherapy—when testosterone levels are elevated due to

Table 40.1 Responses to antiandrogen withdrawal

Reference	Antiandrogen	Median exposure (months)	>50% PSA decline, n (%)	Time to progression (months)
Scher HI 1993[20]	Flutamide	NA	10/25 (40)	5+
Dupont 1993[2]	Flutamide	57	32/40 (80)	14.5
Sartor 1994[22]	Flutamide	27	14/29 (48)	8
Figg 1995[36]	Flutamide	28	7/21 (33)	3.7
Scher 1995[101]	Flutamide	16	16/57 (28)	4
Small 1995[29]	Flutamide	21.5	12/82 (15)	3.5
Herrada 1996[23]	Flutamide	19	11/39 (28)	3.3
Sella 1988[102]	Cyproterone acetate	10.5	4/12 (33)	7.2
Small 1997[103]	Flutamide	NA	4/8 (50)	NA
Nieh J Urol 1997[31]	Bicalutamide	26	1/3 (33)	6
Schelhammer 1997[32]	Flutamide	NA	4/8 (50)	NA
Schelhammer 1997[32]	Bicalutamide	NA	4/14 (29)	NA
Small 2004[43]	Bicalutamide 59%	NA	15/132 (11)	5.9

increased hypothalamic release of GnRH and consequent increased luteinizing hormone release from the anterior pituitary gland. The response is rarely seen when the antiandrogen is added at the time of progression following an initial response to orchiectomy or GnRH analog. Overall, the frequencies of response to bicalutamide or nilutamide discontinuation are less than observed with flutamide.[29,41] In addition, withdrawal responses to bicalutamide and nilutamide may not occur for as long as 10 to 12 weeks following discontinuation of the drug, reflecting the long half-life (greater than 7 days) of the two agents.[29,34] This presents a dilemma for the clinician as to whether there is sufficient time to wait for a withdrawal response that occurs infrequently, or whether to simply start a new therapy immediately. There is no straightforward answer.

Combined antiandrogen withdrawal and adrenal androgen ablation

Several studies reported even more "dramatic" responses to flutamide discontinuation when combined with a direct inhibitor of adrenal androgen synthesis such as aminoglutethimide[22] or ketoconazole.[42] This ultimately led to a prospective, randomized comparison of the combination of antiandrogen discontinuation and ketoconazole to antiandrogen discontinuation alone.[43] In this trial, patients who received the combination of antiandrogen withdrawal and ketoconazole had a higher PSA response (27%; 95% confidence interval [CI] 20–35%) and longer median time to progression (8.6 months) than patients who received antiandrogen alone (11%; 95% CI 7–17% and 6 months) ($P = 0.0002$). There was no survival difference. The lower overall PSA decline rate may reflect the fact that over two-thirds of the patients in the population received bicalutamide and one-third flutamide. Whether a survival difference would have been observed if only flutamide was used is unknown.

Second-line antiandrogens therapy

The role of second- and third-line hormonal therapy for patients who progress despite castration and antiandrogen withdrawal is largely undefined. As many trials of second- and third-line therapy were conducted prior to PSA based standards of reporting,[44] interpreting the literature is difficult. Flutamide has been the most widely studied in the second-line setting, primarily following castration alone, with response rates ranging from 35% to 45%.[45,46] Similar results have been demonstrated with other nonsteroidal antiandrogens. Retrospective analyses of patients treated with nilutamide after progression on another antiandrogen resulted in PSA declines in up to 50% of patients.[47,48] In addition, several studies have suggested that the response rate to an antiandrogen increases following exposure to another antiandrogen,[25,49] and that different antiandrogens can be non-cross-resistant even though they are all directed toward the AR and represent the same class of drug. Large studies testing the utility of flutamide after antiandrogen withdrawal have not been conducted. However, one small study reported a response rate of 50% (5 of 10) in patients treated with flutamide following progression with a GnRH and bicalutamide.[50]

Currently, it is not known whether the survival advantage observed with taxotere-based chemotherapy is affected by the number of prior hormonal manipulations a patient has experienced. A phase III trial which sought to clarify this issue by testing whether docetaxel is superior to ketoconazole (ECOG 1899),[51] was closed secondary to poor accrual, most likely because many physicians feel that maximizing hormonal therapy, especially for asymptomatic patients, is preferable to initiating chemotherapy. Although we agree with this approach, there has been no prospectively designed trial that has shown a survival benefit for second-line hormonal therapy.

Biology of antiandrogen withdrawal response

Studies to understand the mechanisms contributing to withdrawal responses have been limited in part by the lack of appropriate tumor tissue for study. It is compounded by the nature of progressive prostate cancers which are often manifest by a rising PSA or bony metastases, neither of which are conducive to tissue acquisition. As noted previously, the change in the clinical behavior of the disease under the selection pressure of a drug mandates characterization of the tumor both at the time of relapse and at the time therapy is first initiated. The results of these studies, along with the characterization of prostate cancer cell lines and xenografts, show that androgen receptor signaling is maintained or enhanced in the majority of tumors that are progressing despite castrate levels of testosterone. The result is an altered androgen signaling pathway that has enhanced sensitivity to castrate levels of dihydrotestosterone, is promiscuous for activation by alternative ligands, or is activated by cross talk with cytokine and/or growth factor pathways.

Androgen receptor structure

The cellular mediator of androgen action is the AR, a transcription factor that modulates expression of genes involved in differentiation, homeostasis, and angiogenesis. The AR has a modular structure, consisting primarily of a large amino-terminal transactivation domain (NTD), a centrally located DNA-binding domain (DBD), and a carboxy-terminal ligand binding domain (LBD) that confers high affinity and specificity for androgen binding.

Mutations of the AR gene have been reported in prostate cancer at frequencies of 5% to 50%, depending upon disease stage and prior treatment. The majority involve a small number of discrete regions of the LBD.[52] Most of these mutations confer promiscuity or sensitivity for receptor activation by other steroid hormones and/or by the specific antiandrogen used in clinical management of the disease.[52,53] The concept of "therapy-mediated selection pressure" is exemplified by the detection of AR variants in tumors from patients treated with hydroxyflutamide, as part of a combined androgen blockade strategy, which confers enhanced receptor activity in response to flutamide, but which retains sensitivity to other antiandrogens.[54,55] This has been observed clinically, as patients who have progressed on flutamide do respond to bicalutamide. This has also been described for several other antiandrogens, and can be recapitulated in vitro. Culture of LNCaP cells with bicalutamide resulted in outgrowth of a subline containing a mutation at codon 741, which conferred increased cell growth and PSA secretion in response to bicalutamide but not flutamide.[56] These data suggest that each antiandrogen may elicit a specific mechanism that can lead to a withdrawal response, consistent with clinical observations that second-line therapy with antiandrogens often results in tumor regression. Studies of the autochthonous TRAMP model of prostate cancer[57,58] demonstrate that therapy mediated selection of AR mutations is not limited to antiandrogen treatment. Whereas noncastrate mice develop mutations in the AR LBD, mice castrated at 12 weeks of age developed mutations in the NTD.[59] Importantly, mutations in the NTD can affect the AR function in a manner distinct from those in the LBD. Enforced expression in the mouse prostate of the AR-NTD variant, Gln231Glu, conferred rapid development of prostatic intraepithelial neoplasia that progressed to invasive and metastatic disease in 100% of mice.[60] In contrast, enforced expression of the wild-type AR or a common LBD AR variant responsive to other steroid hormones had no discernible effect.[60] This study highlights the potential functional significance of mutations in the AR-NTD, and demonstrates that specific mutations can turn the AR into a potent oncogene sufficient to promote metastatic prostate cancer.

While AR gene mutations likely are an important part of antiandrogen agonist activity and subsequent withdrawal responses, they cannot be detected in all patients.[61] Although this may be due to technical issues, differences in patient populations, stage of disease, tumor burden, and/or time on antiandrogen therapy,[61] it is likely that multiple mechanisms will play a role in antiandrogen agonist activity and subsequent withdrawal response, with AR mutations being only one contributing mechanism.

Androgen receptor expression

Xenograft models of human prostate cancer are useful models in which to study the AR, as most grow initially in an androgen-dependent state, undergo regression upon castration, and subsequently regrow in the castrate environment. In support of the hypothesis that AR continues to play an important role in growth of progressive castrate prostate cancer, several studies have demonstrated an increase in the level of AR and/or AR-regulated genes in xenograft tumors with castrate levels of testosterone in comparison to untreated tumors.[62–66] In particular, comprehensive gene expression profiling determined that the AR was the only gene upregulated in the progression from androgen-sensitive to castration-resistant growth in all 7 human prostate cancer xenograft models analyzed.[67] In clinical disease, recent studies have show an analogous increase in both AR mRNA and protein levels in metastatic castrate-resistant prostate cancer compared with localized disease.[53] Moreover, increased AR levels in the prostate of clinically localized disease has been shown to predict relapse following radical prostatectomy, suggesting that increased AR may predispose to castrate resistance and/or metastatic spread.[68] Importantly, increased levels of AR may be all that is required to switch antagonists such as bicalutamide to receptor agonists,[67] providing a mechanism distinct from AR mutations to explain disease progression and antiandrogen withdrawal.

There are likely to be several mechanisms that contribute to increased AR levels, including AR gene amplification (as demonstrated in up to 29% of tumors)[69–71] and increased stability or reduced degradation of the AR protein in progressive disease.[72] However, not all progressive tumors demonstrate an increase in AR, and some may have actually shown a decrease.[73] These differences highlight that the AR alone is probably not sufficient to ensure continued signaling, but is probably dependent upon multiple factors that impact on its pathway.

Increased levels of androgenic steroids, combined with an increase in the amount of receptor protein (see below), could contribute to maintenance of AR signaling despite castrate levels of testosterone in the blood.[71] A recent study using laser capture mass spectrometry documented levels of androgenic steroids in tumors from men with progressive disease after hormonal therapy that were sufficient to induce signaling.[63]

Role of coregulatory molecules

Transcriptional activity of the AR is mediated, in part, by the recruitment of coregulator proteins that enhance (coactivators) or repress (corepressors) receptor function. An increase in coactivator proteins has been shown to develop in the setting of castrate disease,[62,74,75] coinciding with an increase in AR expression during the growth phase of prostate cancer cells following androgen deprivation.[72] The clinical consequence of an increase in coactivator proteins may be manifested as an increased sensitivity of the AR to lower concentrations of androgen or an alteration in AR specificity. In support of this hypothesis, several studies have shown that AR coactivators, such as ARA70 and ARA55, selectively enhance the ability of 17-β-estradiol and hydroxyflutamide to activate the AR.[60,76,77] Important coactivators include transcriptional intermediary factor (TIF2) and steroid receptor co-activator-1 (SRC1), which have been shown to be increased in prostate tumors following castration. TIF2 broadens the ligand-binding specificity of certain AR mutants to include activation of the receptor by adrenal androgens.[72] Nuclear corepressors mediate transcriptional repression and may play an important role in prostate cancer growth as well. Nuclear hormone receptor corepressor (NCoR) is recruited to the ligand-bound AR and can mediate the antagonist action of bicalutamide, flutamide, and mifepristone on the AR; the lack of NCoR may allow for an increase in the agonist activity of these agents on the AR.[78,79]

Although a large array of nuclear coregulators has been described thus far, the exact mechanism of how coregulators affect transcription is still being elucidated. Aberrant regulation of coregulators may result in androgen independent growth and provide a mechanism for agonist activity of antiandrogens resulting in therapy-mediated alterations of progressive prostate cancers. Disruption of coregulator-mediated growth may prove to be an important therapeutic target.

Crosstalk with other signaling pathways

Activation of the AR by tyrosine kinase receptors, growth factors, or cytokines is thought to provide a mechanism by which prostate cancer growth can bypass the requirement for native ligand.[77,80–86] Activation of the AR by these factors results in the proliferation of prostate cancer cells, and increased tumor cell survival during androgen deprivation.[87,88] Indeed, several studies have reported increased HER2/NEU expression in prostate cancer at all stages of disease.[89–91] In a recent study analyzing radical prostatectomy specimens obtained at surgery for clinically organ-confined prostate cancer, 90% of patients who subsequently developed extensive metastatic disease requiring androgen ablation therapy already expressed high levels of both HER2/NEU and AR (Dr Camela Ricciardelli,

University of Adelaide; personal communication). It is currently thought that HER2/NEU can promote DNA binding and stability of the AR through activation of MAPK and AKT, which can bind to and activate the AR.[88,92] Other mechanisms that directly activate MAPK and AKT elicit a similar effect.[88] Hydroxyflutamide has been shown to potentiate this pathway by allowing rapid phosphorylation of MAPK, possibly via RAS/RAF association.[87]

Clinical significance of antiandrogen withdrawal response

While the antiandrogen withdrawal response has been critical in propelling an improved understanding of the biology of prostate cancer, it is important not to overstate the clinical significance of withdrawal response for patients with castration resistant disease. As noted earlier in the chapter, an obvious consideration is that a withdrawal response cannot be observed in a patient who is not receiving the drug. One potential reason that the antiandrogen withdrawal response is less prominent in clinical practice than would be predicted is the use of bicalutamide over flutamide. The approval of bicalutamide on the basis of a prospective, randomized trial demonstrating similar anti-prostate cancer effects, similar survival times, and an improved safety profile relative to flutamide, when each was combined with a GnRH agonist,[93] led to a dramatic decrease in flutamide use. Although never studied on a comparative basis, cumulative reports suggest that withdrawal responses occur more frequently following flutamide discontinuation relative to bicalutamide. It can, therefore, be anticipated that, on a cumulative basis, the frequency of responses to antiandrogen withdrawal will decrease.

Nevertheless, it is still reasonable to consider a trial of antiandrogen withdrawal alone at the time of progression in the appropriate setting because the degree and duration of response when it occurs in the individual patient can be significant. In this context, subsequent therapy is withheld until progression is documented after the steroidal or nonsteroidal antiandrogen is discontinued, allowing a sufficient observation period for a response to occur as a function of the half-life of agent that was discontinued.[94]

The clinical significance of the antiandrogen withdrawal response is also affected by a decrease in the duration of antiandrogen treatment when combined with a GnRH analog. A number of randomized trials have been conducted comparing different hormonal approaches as monotherapy and/or as a part of so-called combined androgen blockade strategies. A meta-analysis of trials evaluating LHRH agonists/antagonists, orchiectomy, DES, or choice of DES or orchiectomy as monotherapy showed that, in general, hormonal interventions that lower serum testosterone levels to castrate levels result in similar survival times.[95] Other meta-analyses have repeatedly shown a modest survival benefit at 5 years with combined androgen blockade.[96–99] One report included 21 trials with 6871 patients and showed a modest but significant survival advantage at 5 years for combined therapy (hazard ratio 0.87; 95% CI 0.80–0.94), favoring combined therapy. The analysis was most influenced by three trials in which a 3.7- to 7-month median survival difference was observed.[100] These findings are in direct contrast, however, to the results of the INT-0105 comparing orchiectomy alone with orchiectomy and flutamide, which did not show any benefit with combined therapy. Based on the knowledge that GnRH

analogs produce a rise in testosterone for the first few weeks of administration, and that no difference is observed when the antiandrogen is combined with a surgical orchiectomy, the authors suggested that the likely benefit of the approach is elimination of the negative effects of the testosterone surge on prostate cancer growth observed in the first 2 to 3 weeks of treatment with GnRH agonist/antagonist, rather than the superiority of the combination approach itself. The result has led many physicians to change their practice to limit the total duration of antiandrogen treatment (e.g., 1–3 months), as opposed to long-term continuous therapy. Given that one of the predictive factors for response to antiandrogen withdrawal is the duration of antiandrogen treatment, this likely will result in fewer patients progressing on antiandrogen based combination therapy, further reducing the frequency of withdrawal responses that are observed.

Conclusions

Until recently, patients with progressive prostate cancer in the setting of castrate levels of testosterone were considered to have "hormone-refractory" disease. However, this notion is not supported by recent evidence that the AR continues to play an important role in the growth of castration resistant prostate cancers. Moreover, the observations that the AR has increased sensitivity for activation and may be activated by non-classical ligands in the castrate state, makes a compelling case for the development of AR targeted strategies that are effective, even in the progressive castrate state. Such new therapies are necessary for significant therapeutic advances for the majority of patients with advanced prostate cancer who will ultimately fail androgen ablation. Elucidation of the mechanisms contributing to the antiandrogen withdrawal response provides a window into this process.

References

1. Scher HI, Heller G. Clinical states in prostate cancer: towards a dynamic model of disease progression. Urology 2000;55:323–327.
2. Dupont A, Gomez J, Cusan L, et al. Response to flutamide withdrawal in advanced prostate cancer in progression under combination therapy. J Urol 1993;150:908–913.
3. Collinson MP, Daniel F, Tyrell CJ, et al. Response of carcinoma of the prostate to withdrawal of flutamide. Br J Urol 1993;72:662–663.
4. Kelly WK, Scher HI. Prostate specific antigen decline after antiandrogen withdrawal: the flutamide withdrawal syndrome. J Urol 1993;149:607–609.
5. Kelly WK, Slovin S, Scher HI. Steroid hormone withdrawal syndromes: pathophysiology and clinical significance. Urol Clin North Am 1997;24:421–433.
6. Belani CP, Pearl P, Whitley ND, et al. Tamoxifen withdrawal response. Arch Intern Med 1989;149:449–450.
7. Howell A, Dodwell DJ, Anderson H, et al. Response after withdrawal of tamoxifen and progestins in advanced breast cancer. Ann Oncol 1992;3:611–617.
8. Buchanan G, Greenberg NM, Scher HI, et al. Collocation of androgen receptor gene mutations in prostate cancer. Clin Cancer Res 2001;7:1273–1281.
9. Scher H, Shaffer D. Prostate cancer: a dynamic disease with shifting targets. Lancet Oncology 2003;4:407–414.
10. Huggins C, Hodges CV. Studies on prostatic cancer. I. The effect of castration, of estrogen and of androgen injection on serum

phosphatases in metastatic carcinoma of the prostate. Cancer Res 1941;1:193–197.

11. Huggins C, Stevens RE Jr, Hodges CV. Studies on prostatic cancer. II. The effect of castration on advanced carcinoma of the prostate gland. Arch Surg 1941;43:209–223.

12. Huggins C, Bergenstal DM. Effect of bilateral adrenalectomy on certain human tumors. Proc Natl Acad Sci USA 1952;38:73–76.

13. Robinson MR, Shearer RJ, Fergusson JD. Adrenal suppression in the treatment of carcinoma of the prostate. Br J Urol 1974;46: 555–559.

14. Geller J, Albert JD, Nochstein DA, et al. Comparison of prostatic cancer tissue dehydrotestosterone levels at the time of relapse following orchiectomy or estrogen therapy. J Urol 1984;132:693–696.

15. Labrie F, Dupont A, Belanger A, et al. New approach in the treatment of prostate cancer: complete instead of partial withdrawal of androgens. Prostate 1983;4:579–594.

16. Cassileth BR, Soloway MS, Vogelzang NJ, et al. Patients' choice of treatment in stage D prostate cancer. Urology 1989;33:57–62.

17. Crawford ED, Eisenberger MA, McLeod DG, et al. A controlled trial of leuprolide with and without flutamide in prostatic carcinoma. N Engl J Med 1989;321:419–424.

18. Denis LJ, Keuppens F, Smith PH, et al. Maximal androgen blockade: final analysis of EORTC phase III trial 30853. EORTC Genito-Urinary Tract Cancer Cooperative Group and the EORTC Data Center. Eur Urol 1998;33:144–151.

19. Scher HI, Mazumdar M, Kelly WK. Clinical trials in relapsed prostate cancer: defining the target. J Natl Cancer Inst 1996;88:1623–1634.

20. Scher HI, Kelly WK. The flutamide withdrawal syndrome: its impact on clinical trials in hormone-refractory prostatic cancer. J Clin Oncol 1993;11:1566–1572.

21. Scher H, Kelly WK, Cohen L, et al. Flutamide withdrawal response in patients with metastatic prostate cancer (PC) progressing on hormonal therapy. Proc Am Soc Clin Oncol 1993;12:723.

22. Sartor O, Cooper M, Weinberger M, et al. Surprising activity of flutamide withdrawal, when combined with aminoglutethimide, in treatment of "hormone-refractory" prostate cancer. J Natl Cancer Inst 1994;86:222–227.

23. Herrada J, Dieringer P, Logothetis CJ. Characterization of patients with androgen-independent prostatic carcinoma whose serum prostate specific antigen decreased following flutamide withdrawal. J Urol 1996;155:620–623.

24. Scher HI, Zhang ZF, Kelly WK. Hormone and anti-hormone withdrawal therapy: implications for management of androgen independent prostate cancer. Urology 1996;47:61–69.

25. Scher HI, Kolvenbag GJ. The antiandrogen withdrawal syndrome in relapsed prostate cancer. Eur Urol 1997;31:3–7; discussion 24–27.

26. Eisenberger MA, Blumenstein BA, Crawford ED, et al. Bilateral orchiectomy with or without flutamide for metastatic prostate cancer. N Engl J Med 1998;339:1036–1042.

27. Bianco FJ, Dotan ZA, Kattan MW, et al. Duration of response to androgen deprivation therapy and survival after subsequent biochemical relapse in men initially treated with radical prostatectomy. Proc Am Soc Clin Onc 2004;23:393 [Abstract #4552].

28. Small EJ, Carroll PR. Prostate-specific antigen decline after casodex withdrawal: evidence for an antiandrogen withdrawal syndrome. Urology 1994;43:408–410.

29. Small EJ, Srinivas S. The antiandrogen withdrawal syndrome: experience in a large cohort of unselected patients with advanced prostate cancer. Cancer 1995;76:1428–1434.

30. Schellhammer P, Kolvenbag GJCM. Serum PSA decline after casodex withdrawal. Urology 1994;44:790–791.

31. Nieh PT. Withdrawal phenomenon with the antiandrogen casodex. J Urol 1995;153:1070–1072.

32. Schellhammer PF, Venner P, Haas GP, et al. Prostate specific antigen decreases after withdrawal of antiandrogen therapy with bicalutamide or flutamide in patients receiving combined androgen blockade. J Urol 1997;157:1731–1735.

33. Haun SD, Gerridzen RG, Yau JC, et al. Antiandrogen withdrawal syndrome with nilutamide. Urology 1997;49:632–634.

34. Wirth MP, Froschermaier SE. The antiandrogen withdrawal syndrome. Urol Res 1997;25:S67–71.

35. Dawson NA, McLeod DG. Dramatic prostate specific antigen decrease in response to discontinuation of megestrol acetate in advanced prostate cancer: expansion of the antiandrogen withdrawal syndrome. J Urol 1995;153:1946–1947.

36. Figg WD, Sartor O, Cooper MR, et al. Prostate specific antigen decline following the discontinuation of flutamide in patients with stage D2 prostate cancer. Am J Med 1995;98:412–414.

37. Burch PA, Loprinzi CL. Prostate-specific antigen decline after withdrawal of low-dose megestrol acetate. J Clin Oncol 1999;17:1087–1088.

38. Bissada NK, Kaczmarek AT. Complete remission of hormone refractory adenocarcinoma of the prostate in response to withdrawal of diethylstilbesterol. J Urol 1995;153:1944–1945.

39. Akakura K, Akimoto S, Furuya Y, et al. Incidence and characteristics of antiandrogen withdrawal syndrome in prostate cancer after treatment with chlormadinone acetate. Eur Urol 1998;33:567–571.

40. Tassinari D, Fochessati F, Panzini I, et al. Rapid progression of advanced "hormone-resistant" prostate cancer during palliative treatment with progestins for cancer cachexia. J Pain Symptom Manage 2003;25:481–484.

41. Small E, Schellhammer P, Venner P, et al. A double-blind assessment of antiandrogen withdrawal from casodex (C) or eulexin (E) therapy while continuing luteinizing hormone releasing hormone analogue (LHRH-A) therapy for patients (pts) with stage D2 prostate cancer (PCA). Proc Am Soc Clin Oncol 1996;15.

42. Small EJ, Baron A, Apodaca D. Simultaneous anti-androgen withdrawal (AAWD) and treatment with ketoconazole (KETO)/hydrocortisone (HD) in patients with advanced "hormone-refractory" prostate cancer (HRPC). Proc Am Soc Clin Oncol 1997;16:313a.

43. Small EJ, Halabi S, Dawson NA, et al. Antiandrogen withdrawal alone or in combination with ketoconazole in androgen-independent prostate cancer patients: a phase III trial (CALGB 9583). J Clin Oncol 2004;22:1025–1033.

44. Bubley GJ, Carducci M, Dahut W, et al. Eligibility and response guidelines for phase II clinical trials in androgen-independent prostate cancer: recommendations from the PSA Working Group. J Clin Oncol 1999;3461–3467.

45. Labrie F, Dupont A, Giguere M, et al. Benefits of combination therapy with flutamide in patients relapsing after castration. Br J Urol 1988;61: 341–346.

46. Fossa SD, Slee PH, Brausi M, et al. Flutamide versus prednisone in patients with prostate cancer symptomatically progressing after androgen-ablative therapy: a phase III study of the European organization for research and treatment of cancer genitourinary group. J Clin Oncol 2001;19:62–71.

47. Kassouf W, Tanguay S, Aprikian AG. Nilutamide as second line hormone therapy for prostate cancer after androgen ablation fails. J Urol 2003;169:1742–1744.

48. Desai A, Stadler WM, Vogelzang NJ. Nilutamide: possible utility as a second-line hormonal agent. Urology 2001;58:1016–1020.

49. Joyce R, Fenton MA, Rode P, et al. High dose bicalutamide for androgen independent prostate cancer: effect of prior hormonal therapy. J Urol 1998;159:149–153.

50. Kojima S, Suzuki H, Akakura K, et al. Alternative antiandrogens to treat prostate cancer relapse after initial hormone therapy. J Urol 2004;171:679–683.

51. Walczak JR, Carducci MA. Phase 3 randomized trial evaluating second-line hormonal therapy versus docetaxel-estramustine combination chemotherapy on progression-free survival in asymptomatic patients with a rising prostate-specific antigen level after hormonal therapy for prostate cancer: an Eastern Cooperative Oncology Group (E1899), Intergroup/Clinical Trials Support Unit study. Urology 2003;62:141–146.

52. Buchanan G, Yang M, Nahm SJ, et al. Mutations at the boundary of the hinge and ligand binding domain of the androgen receptor confer increased transactivation function. Mol Endocrinol 2000;15: 46–56.

53. Scher HI, Buchanan G, Gerald W, et al. Targeting the androgen receptor: improving outcomes for castration-resistant prostate cancer. Endocrine Rel Cancer 2004;11:459–476.

54. Taplin ME, Bubley GJ, Ko YJ, et al. Selection for androgen receptor mutations in prostate cancers treated with androgen antagonist. Cancer Res 1999;59:2511–2515.

55. Fenton MA, Shuster TD, Fertig AM, et al. Functional characterization of mutant androgen receptors from androgen-independent prostate cancer. Clin Cancer Res 1997;8:1383–1388.

56. Hara T, Miyazaki J, Araki H, et al. Novel mutations of androgen receptor: a possible mechanism of bicalutamide withdrawal syndrome. Cancer Res 2003;63:149–153.

57. Greenberg NM, DeMayo F, Finegold MJ, et al. Prostate cancer in a transgenic mouse. Proc Natl Acad Sci USA 1995;92:3439–3443.

58. Gingrich JR, Barrios RJ, Kattan MW, et al. Androgen-independent prostate cancer progression in the TRAMP model. Cancer Res 1997;57:4687–4691.

59. Han G, Foster BA, Mistry S, et al. Hormone status selects for spontaneous somatic androgen receptor variants that demonstrate specific ligand and cofactor dependent activities in autochthonous prostate cancer. J Biol Chem 2001;276:11204–11213.

60. Han G, Buchanan G, Ittmann M, et al. Mutation of the androgen receptor causes oncogenic transformation of the prostate. Proc Natl Acad Sci USA 2005;102:1151–1156.

61. Taplin ME, Rajeshkumar B, Halabi S, et al. Androgen receptor mutations in androgen-independent prostate cancer: Cancer and Leukemia Group B Study 9663. J Clin Oncol 2003;21:2673–2678.

62. Gregory CW, Hamil KG, Kim D, et al. Androgen receptor expression in androgen-independent prostate cancer is associated with increased expression of androgen-regulated genes. Cancer Res 1998;58:5718–5724.

63. Mohler JL, Gregory CW, Ford 3rd OH, et al. The androgen axis in recurrent prostate cancer. Clinical Cancer Res 2004;10:440–448.

64. Culig Z, Hobisch A, Hittmair A, et al. Expression, structure, and function of androgen receptor in advanced prostatic carcinoma. Prostate 1998;35:63–70.

65. Takeda H, Akakura K, Masai M, et al. Androgen receptor content of prostate carcinoma cells estimated by immunohistochemistry is related to prognosis of patients with stage D2 prostate carcinoma. Cancer 1996;77:934–940.

66. Sadi MV, Barrack ER. Image analysis of androgen receptor immunostaining in metastatic prostate cancer. Cancer 1993;71:2574–2580.

67. Chen CD, Welsbie DS, Tran C, et al. Molecular determinants of resistance to antiandrogen therapy. Nat Med 2004;10:33–39.

68. Ricciardelli C, Choong CS, Buchanan G, et al. Androgen receptor levels in prostate cancer epithelial and peritumoral stromal cells identify non-organ confined disease. Prostate 2005;63:19–28.

69. Bubendorf L, Kolmer M, Konenen J, et al. Hormone therapy failure in human prostate cancer: analysis by complementary DNA and tissue microarrays. J Natl Cancer Inst 1999;91:1758–1764.

70. Koivisto P, Visakorpi T, Kallioniemi OP. Androgen receptor gene amplification: a novel molecular mechanism for endocrine therapy resistance in human prostate cancer. Scand J Clin Lab Invest Suppl 1996;226:57–63.

71. Holzbeierlein J, Lal P, LaTulippe E, et al. Gene expression analysis of human prostate carcinoma during hormonal therapy identifies androgen-responsive genes and mechanisms of therapy resistance. Am J Pathol 2004;164:217–227.

72. Gregory CW, He B, Johnson RT, et al. A mechanism for androgen receptor-mediated prostate cancer recurrence after androgen deprivation therapy. Cancer Res 2001;61:4315–4319.

73. Kinoshita H, Shi Y, Sandefur C, et al. Methylation of the androgen receptor minimal promoter silences transcription in human prostate cancer. Cancer Res 2000;60:3623–3630.

74. Debes JD, Schmidt LJ, Huang H, et al. P300 mediates androgen-independent transactivation of the androgen receptor by interleukin 6. Cancer Res 2002;62:5632–5636.

75. Fujimoto N, Yeh S, Kang HY, et al. Cloning and characterization of androgen receptor coactivator, ARA55, in human prostate. J Biol Chem 1999;274:8316–8321.

76. Yeh S, Miyamoto H, Shima H, et al. From estrogen to androgen receptor: A new pathway for sex hormones in prostate. Proc Natl Acad Sci USA 1998;95:5527–5532.

77. Yeh S, Chang HC, Miyamoto H, et al. Differential induction of the androgen receptor transcriptional activity by selective androgen receptor coactivators. Keio J Med 1999;48:87–92.

78. Berrevoets CA, Umar A, Trapman J, et al. Differential modulation of androgen receptor transcriptional activity by the nuclear receptor corepressor (N-CoR). Biochem J 2004;379:731–738.

79. Hodgson MC, Astapova I, Cheng S, et al. The androgen receptor recruits nuclear receptor CoRepressor (N-CoR) in the presence of mifepristone via its N and C termini revealing a novel molecular mechanism for androgen receptor antagonists. J Biol Chem 2005;280:6511–6519.

80. Kim D, Gregory CW, French FS, et al. Androgen receptor expression and cellular proliferation during transition from androgen-dependent to recurrent growth after castration in the CWR22 prostate cancer xenograft. Am J Pathol 2002;160:219–226.

81. Culig Z, Hobisch A, Cronauer MV, et al. Androgen receptor activation in prostatic tumor cell lines by insulin-like growth factor-I, keratinocyte growth factor, and epidermal growth factor. Cancer Res 1994;54:5474–5478.

82. Nazareth LV, Weigel NL. Activation of the human androgen receptor through a protein kinase: A signaling pathway. J Biol Chem 1996;271:19900–19907.

83. Craft N, Chhor C, Tran C, et al. Evidence for clonal outgrowth of androgen-independent prostate cancer cells from androgen-dependent tumors through a two-step process. Cancer Res 1999;59:5030–5036.

84. Grossmann ME, Huang H, Tindall DJ. Androgen receptor signaling in androgen-refractory prostate cancer. J Natl Cancer Inst 2001;93:1687–1697.

85. Ueda T, Mawji NR, Bruchovsky N, et al. Ligand-independent activation of the androgen receptor by interleukin-6 and the role of steroid receptor coactivator-1 in prostate cancer cells. J Biol Chem 2002;277:38087–38094.

86. Ueda T, Bruchovsky N, Sadar MD. Activation of the androgen receptor N-terminal domain by interleukin-6 via MAPK and STAT3 signal transduction pathways. J Biol Chem 2002;277:7076–7085.

87. Lee SO, Lou W, Hou M, et al. Interleukin-6 promotes androgen-independent growth in LNCaP human prostate cancer cells. Clin Cancer Res 2003;9:370–376.

88. Wen Y, Hu MC, Makino K, et al. HER-2/neu promotes androgen-independent survival and growth of prostate cancer cells through the AKT pathway. Cancer Res 2000;60:6841–6845.

89. Shi Y, Brands FH, Chatterjee S, et al. Her-2/neu expression in prostate cancer: high level of expression associated with exposure to hormone therapy and androgen independent disease. J Urol 2001;166: 1514–1519.

90. Reese DM, Small EJ, Magrane G, et al. HER2 protein expression and gene amplification in androgen-independent prostate cancer. Am J Clin Pathol 2001;116:234–239.

91. Lara PN Jr, Meyers FJ, Gray CR, et al. HER-2/neu is overexpressed infrequently in patients with prostate carcinoma. Results from the California Cancer Consortium Screening Trial. Cancer 2002;94:2584–2589.

92. Mellinghoff IK, Vivanco I, Kwon A, et al. HER2/neu kinase-dependent modulation of androgen receptor function through effects on DNA binding and stability. Cancer Cell 2004;6:517–527.

93. Schellhammer P, Sharifi R, Block N, et al. A controlled trial of bicalutamide versus flutamide, each in combination with luteinizing hormone-relapsing hormone analogue therapy, in patients with advanced prostate cancer. Urology 1995;45:745–752.

94. Carducci M, Nelson BJ, Saad F, et al. Effects of atrasentan on disease progression and biological markers in men with metastatic hormone-refractory prostate cancer: Phase 3 study. Proc Am Soc Clin Onc 2004;23:383 [Abstract # 4058].

95. Seidenfeld J, Samson DJ, Hasselblad V, et al. Single-therapy androgen suppression in men with advanced prostate cancer: a systematic review and meta-analysis. Ann Intern Med 2000;132:566–577.

96. Bennett CL, Tosteson TD, Schmitt B, et al. Maximum androgen-blockade with medical or surgical castration in advanced prostate cancer: A meta-analysis of nine published randomized controlled trials and 4128 patients using flutamide. Prostate Cancer Prostatic Dis 1999;2:4–8.

97. Caubet J, Tosteson TD, Dong EW, et al. Maximum androgen blockade in advanced prostate cancer: a meta-analysis of published randomized controlled trials using nonsteroidal antiandrogens. Urology 1997;49:71–78.

98. Schmitt B, Bennett C, Seidenfeld J, et al. Maximal androgen blockade for advanced prostate cancer. Cochrane Database Sys Rev; 2000 CD001526.

99. Group PCTC. Maximum androgen blockade in advanced prostate cancer: an overview of 22 randomized trials with 3283 deaths in 5711 patients. Lancet 1995;346:265–269.

100. Samson DJ, Seidenfeld J, Schmitt B, et al. Systematic review and meta-analysis of monotherapy compared with combined androgen blockade for patients with advanced prostate carcinoma. Cancer 2002;95: 361–376.

101. Scher HI, Zhang Z-F, Cohen L, et al. Hormonally relapsed prostatic cancer: lessons from the flutamide withdrawal syndrome. Adv Urol 1995;8:61–95.

102. Sella A, Flex D, Sulkes A, et al. Antiandrogen withdrawal syndrome with cyproterone acetate. Urology 1998;52:1091–1093.

103. Small EJ, Baron A, Bok R. Simultaneous and antiandrogen withdrawal and treatment with ketoconazol and hydrocortisone in patients with advanced prostate carcinoma. Cancer 1997;80:1755–1759.

41

Chemotherapy for advanced prostate cancer

Andrew J Armstrong, Michael A Carducci

Introduction

Prostate cancer will result in approximately 30,000 annual deaths in men in the United States in 2005 and is the second leading cause of cancer deaths in men after lung cancer.[1,2] While the death rate from prostate cancer has been declining due to a number of factors such as earlier diagnosis and effective, less morbid local treatment options, approximately 6% of men will present with distant metastases and approximately 40% to 60% will relapse following local treatments.[2–4] In general, androgen suppression leads to the response and stabilization of metastatic hormone-sensitive disease for approximately 18 to 24 months with a historic median survival from the time of diagnosis of metastases ranging from 24 to 30 months.[5,6] A recent update of select patients from the Pound database from Johns Hopkins has demonstrated a median survival from development of metastases to death of 6.5 years.[7] Prostate-specific antigen (PSA) doubling time at relapse following radical prostatectomy, time to recurrence, and original Gleason score were predictive of metastasis-free survival, illustrating the heterogeneity of this disease.[7] However, eventually these patients will develop progressive hormone-refractory metastatic prostate cancer and these patients have a median survival of approximately 12 to 18 months.[8–11]

The concept that hormone-refractory metastatic prostate cancer is a chemo-resistant disease has been challenged by recent clinical trials. The use of surrogate outcomes such as PSA response has led to the more rapid identification of novel agents with activity in hormone-refractory metastatic prostate cancer (HRPC). Docetaxel (Taxotere), a taxoid with a more manageable benefit-to-toxicity ratio than historic cytotoxic agents used in prostate cancer, has demonstrated a clinical benefit and overall survival advantage in recent multi-institutional trials. Further refinements of the definitions of hormone independence, quality-of-life outcomes, and surrogate markers of response have led to improved standardization across clinical trials that allow for head to head comparisons of active agents.[12,13] The earlier detection of biochemical recurrence and asymptomatic metastatic disease with the use of serum PSA measurements and improved imaging techniques may also translate into the earlier initiation of therapy before disease burden and pain become overwhelming factors. While hormone-refractory metastatic prostate cancer remains an incurable disease, chemotherapy has come to play a role in prolonging patient survival with meaningful quality-of-life endpoints and has generated optimism about progress among both clinicians and patients.

Currently, approved chemotherapy regimens in hormone refractory metastatic prostate cancer include docetaxel, mitoxantrone, and estramustine but these agents have not yet demonstrated consistent clinical benefits in earlier stages of disease. The use of chemotherapy in high-risk patients either as neoadjuvant treatment or adjuvant to local therapy, as well as in nonmetastatic high-risk patients with PSA-only recurrence, is an active area of clinical investigation and these patients should be encouraged to enroll in clinical trials to answer these questions.

Definition of hormone-refractory prostate cancer

The most widely accepted criteria for the hormone-refractory state has been the demonstration of progressive, measurable, or evaluable disease in the face of castrate levels of serum testosterone (<50 ng/dL).[12] Biochemical progression after antiandrogen (bicalutamide, flutamide, nilutamide) withdrawal, as measured consecutively over a 4 to 6 week period, has been proposed for eligibility into clinical trials for HRPC. Patients are usually continued on luteinizing hormone releasing hormone (LHRH) agonists during this time if tolerable. There is at this time no universally accepted definition of progression of hormone-refractory disease, however, and patients may have no measurable or evaluable disease with PSA-only progression and be termed hormone refractory. These PSA-only hormone refractory patients represent a heterogeneous group depending on when hormonal therapy was initiated, and, therefore, time to progression is highly variable. Survival in this group that is increasingly encountered in the clinic is generally better when compared with patients with metastatic hormone-refractory disease, and chemotherapy trials such as ECOG 1899 attempted to define this population prospectively (see below).

The demonstration of progressive disease in the face of continuous androgen suppression with gonadotropin releasing hormone (GnRH) agonists often leads to the introduction of combined androgen blockade with antiandrogens, followed shortly by antiandrogen withdrawal and trials of third-line hormonal therapy, often with the combination of ketoconazole and hydrocortisone. The response time to each of these manipulations is brief, on the order of several months, with likely survival benefits for responders.[14] Eventually, prostate cancer growth becomes refractory to these manipulations. Consequently, until recently, the indication for chemotherapy in practical terms has generally been progression despite the utilization of all hormonal options, manifested generally by clinically measurable disease. This paradigm is likely to shift as new chemotherapeutic and biologic agents are shown to be more active.

Chemotherapy for early advanced prostate cancer

The use of chemotherapy for high-risk patients following local therapy, or in high-risk patients with a rising PSA following local therapy, is an active area of clinical investigation. Modeling therapy after adjuvant or neoadjuvant therapy for localized breast cancer, several groups are using combination chemotherapy before and after radical prostatectomy or external-beam radiation therapy. CALGB trial 90203 is examining pre-radical prostatectomy estramustine and docetaxel in high-risk men with a predicted 5-year survival of less than 60%.[15] SWOG 9921 will look at adjuvant androgen deprivation with or without mitoxantrone in high-risk men following radical prostatectomy.[16] RTOG P-0014 is a multicenter trial examining the role of chemotherapy in the adjuvant setting for high-risk men who have failed local therapy or are at high risk for recurrence (Gleason >7, or >6 with positive lymph nodes or capsular penetration). Four cycles of chemotherapy in this trial will be selected from one of a number of trial approved regimens, including docetaxel and combination regimens, and will be given either upfront with androgen ablation or at progression after androgen ablation.[17] In addition ECOG 1899 randomized men with biochemical progression after androgen suppression to either second line hormonal manipulation with ketoconazole and hydrocortisone or to chemotherapy with docetaxel and estramustine (closed in 2005 due to poor accrual).[18] Until these studies are complete and confirmed, it is difficult to recommend the use of chemotherapy in these settings outside of a clinical trial.

Historical perspective of chemotherapy for metastatic prostate cancer

Objective, measurable response rates of metastatic prostate cancer to single agent chemotherapy has ranged from 10% to 30%, while multi-agent chemotherapy response rates have ranged from 20% to 60%.[19,20] Trials reporting PSA declines of greater than 50% for single agents have ranged from 4% to 48%, and for combination therapies from 25% to 82% (see Tables 41.1 and 41.2). These objective response rates are similar in magnitude to the response rates of other advanced, metastatic malignancies such as colon and breast cancer.[21,22] Historically, however, the demonstration of improved survival and time to progression was not demonstrated with chemotherapy for metastatic prostate cancer. Until recently, approval of the major active agents, estramustine and mitoxantrone, were based on response rates and quality of life outcomes, respectively, rather than quantity of life gained. Only in the last several years have newer docetaxel-based approaches demonstrated both improved response rates and prolonged survival.[8,9]

Biology of chemoresistance in prostate cancer

During the progression of human prostate cancer, multiple steps leading to drug resistance, resistance to apoptosis, and increased growth fraction, as well as immune evasion lead to the general concept of treatment resistance. Many of these changes may be related to genomic instability and acquired somatic mutations, possibly as a result of increased susceptibility of prostate cancer cells to environmental toxins and oxidative damage.[23] The methylation and subsequent loss of expression of glutathione S-transferase-π, a phase II detoxification enzyme likely involved in genome protection from carcinogens, is one of the earliest changes seen during prostate cancer progression.[24] Increased expression of multidrug resistance protein (MRP), BCL2, vascular endothelial growth factor (VEGF), cyclin-D1, and p53 have all been correlated with progression to the androgen-independent state, as have diminished levels of the tumor suppressors phosphatase and tensin homolog deleted on chromosome ten (PTEN), and P27KIP1.[24–28] *BCL2* is a unique protooncogene expressed in the basal regenerating compartment of the prostate that extends cell viability in the absence of cell proliferation, by preventing programmed cell death, or apoptosis.[25] While the cell of origin in prostate cancer is unclear, these basal cells are typically androgen independent and may contain the putative prostate cancer stem cell responsible for relapse following androgen ablation.[23] Destruction of the more differentiated compartment of luminal type cells that are androgen dependent would not be expected to eradicate these stem cells. Whether these regenerating cells are present from the beginning of prostate cancer development or acquired during progression remains to be determined. However, BCL2 was found to be expressed in 6 of 19 androgen-dependent carcinomas compared with 9 of 12 androgen-independent patient samples, with overexpression generally correlating with androgen independence.[25] Currently, therapies are under evaluation that target BCL2 and examine the impact of chemotherapy on global markers of apoptosis.

Resistance to cytotoxic therapy-induced programmed cell death may also be related to the relative inactivation of the *PTEN* tumor suppressor gene during the progression to the hormone refractory state.[29] Loss of heterozygosity of *PTEN* is seen in approximately 60% of prostate metastases, compared with 15% of early malignancies.[30,31] This tumor suppressor gene regulates the activity of the AKT/PI3K survival pathway, which is important in contributing to apoptotic resistance to cytotoxic agents, cell-anchorage independent growth, angiogenesis, and nutrient-driven proliferation.[32,33] Inhibition of this overactive pathway in conjunction with cytotoxic therapy may correct this resistance seen in prostate cell lines exposed to long-term androgen deprivation.[31]

Resistance to cytotoxic therapy may be related to concurrent resistance to androgen deprivation and progression to HRPC. Upregulation of the androgen receptor has been observed during progression to the androgen refractory state.[34] Alterations in coactivators and corepressors of the androgen receptor may function as a biologic signal amplification switch associated with increased androgen receptor expression, and may explain some of the lack of benefit, and even paradoxical growth, seen during treatment with antiandrogens.[34] Androgen receptor mutations, about 45% of which are activating mutations, have been observed in a minority of patients with HRPC and may lead to increased sensitivity to estrogens, progestins, and other non-androgen ligands.[35–37] Increased sensitivity to local autocrine and paracrine stromal growth factors (i.e. epidermal growth factor [EGF], heregulin, insulin-like growth factor 1 [IGF1], interleukin 6 [IL6]) that act either through the androgen receptor or bypass it downstream have been reported.[35,38] Transition to the hormone-refractory state may thus be accompanied by an amplification of androgen signaling, the transition to codependence on growth factor pathways, and a resistance to apoptotic death due to the overactivity of these survival pathways, such as AKT/PI3K. Prostate-specific antigen production may also become driven by non-androgen signals.[31,38] These changes may also lead to chemoresistance, and so represent novel targets for combination therapies.

Early chemotherapy trials

In the pre-PSA era, the first cytotoxic agents tested in metastatic prostate cancer were nitrogen mustard (1947), thio-tepa (1959), diphenylthiocarbazone (1960), and mithramycin (1963), with some objective and subjective responses in small numbers of patients.[39] In the 1960s, cyclophosphamide (1965), fluorouracil (1968), and vinblastine, often in combination with nitrogen mustards, demonstrated anecdotal responses but no large studies were conducted until 1976.[39,40] The first randomized trial was conducted with cyclophosphamide and fluorouracil showing a 41% and 36% objective response respectively (7% and 12% partial responses with stable disease excluded) in 74 patients.[41] In the 1970s, multiple randomized trials compared single and combination agents often in comparison to standard treatment with glucocorticoids and second line hormonal agents.[39,42] Several agents, such as diethylstilbestrol in the 1960s, had initial high response rates, but were later categorized into hormonal therapies.

Before 1976, few agents were systematically studied, due to the difficulties of defining measurable disease and the relative biochemical success of hormonal therapy, which relegated chemotherapy trials to those patients with the poorest prognosis and most advanced stages.[39] The initial National Prostatic Cancer Projects (NPCP) in the 1970s found between a 10-40% response rate among multiple single agents, if stabilized disease was excluded. Highest objective response rates on the order of 30% to 40% were seen in lomustine (CCNU), cisplatin, and cyclophosphamide, while the lowest responses (<10%) were seen with fluorouracil, melphalan, and prednimustine.[39] Combination regimens involving cyclophosphamide and fluorouracil, as well as doxorubicin-based regimens, improved on response rates and subjective pain measures, but did not demonstrate overall cohort survival superiority.[39,43] In all of these early chemotherapy trials, the control groups received what was then standard therapy, including synthetic estrogens and secondary hormonal manipulations, radiation, and steroids. Baseline characteristics of the groups were not uniform in terms of prior treatment, making results difficult to interpret. Response rates in the 1980s were reported most often as measurable disease response, but were not standardized and generally had wide 95% confidence intervals and inter-investigator variability, and, therefore, conclusions about relative efficacy were difficult.[43] In general, no single agent or combination of agents was shown to improve survival, despite response rates that ranged from 10% to 70%. In their review of the current status of chemotherapy for prostate cancer in 1985, Eisenberger et al concluded that no single agent or combination of agents changed the overall downward slope of the survival curve, and that most trials were difficult to interpret due to non-uniformity, the use of stable disease as a response criteria, crossover, and the lack of power in the studies to demonstrate small survival benefits.[43] The overall complete remission (CR) and partial remission (PR) rates of 17 randomized trials combined in this review in 1985, based on variable response criteria, was 4.5%, with no change in survival compared with standard palliative care.[43] It was felt that even a potential small incremental benefit in survival at the expense of

chemotherapy toxicity was not clinically useful, thus contributing to the therapeutic nihilism of the era.

A 1992 review by Yagoda et al found a similarly disappointing 8.7% overall CR/PR rate among different chemotherapy agents ranging from 2% to 10% for cyclophosphamide, 10% for cisplatin and continuous fluorouracil, and 21% for vinblastine.[44] The notion that prostate cancer was intrinsically chemoresistant has been questioned, however, as less toxic, more active agents became available, notably docetaxel and other microtubule targeted therapies. The development of PSA as a surrogate marker of response has certainly contributed to our ability to select for active agents.

Clinical endpoints in management of androgen-independent prostate cancer

Quality-of-life outcomes

The first chemotherapy agent to be USFDA approved in prostate cancer based on quality-of-life (QoL) outcomes was mitoxantrone in 1996, although many of the above chemotherapy agents studied in the past demonstrated anecdotal and even some randomized data in temporarily improving pain from prostate cancer.[39] Kantoff et al studied 242 men with HRPC randomized to mitoxantrone and hydrocortisone, or hydrocortisone alone, with survival, response, and QoL parameters as primary outcomes.[45] While no survival benefit was observed (12.3 months versus 12.6 months), there was a trend to symptomatic pain improvement in terms of severity and frequency. This was similar to the Canadian trial by Tannock et al that demonstrated a 29% palliative response with mitoxantrone and prednisone compared with 12% in the prednisone only group, with a longer duration of pain control and overall improved cost-effectiveness in the chemotherapy arm (43 weeks versus 18 weeks).[46] Since these publications in the 1990s, newer agents have been examined with QoL outcomes among the secondary measured outcomes, notably docetaxel in the TAX327 trial (vida infra).

Quality-of-life outcomes are subjective and determined by the patient, and are consequently difficult to quantify and standardize across groups and among different instruments for measurement. The QoL outcomes are unlikely to change clinical practice if the survival of two comparison groups are significantly disparate. However, prostate cancer-specific questionnaires and instruments such as the functional assessment of cancer therapy for prostate cancer (FACT-P), the EORTC quality-of-life questionnaire (QLQ), the functional living index in cancer (FLIC) and other validated measures of prostate cancer-specific QoL scales may be useful in helping clinicians and patients determine the appropriate individualized therapies, especially when two comparison agents have similar survival endpoints.[46–49] Importantly, QoL outcomes should ideally be considered as a primary endpoint in phase III trials, in addition to survival, and measured at baseline and serially throughout treatment and follow-up as for other standard measured variables. Emphasis by physicians to patients on the importance of these QoL questionnaires may lead to more compliance and the development of less toxic, effective therapies based on outcomes that are important to the patient.

Prostate-specific antigen declines as surrogate marker

Prostate-specific antigen levels are a sensitive indicator of response to multiple modalities of treatment, including radical prostatectomy, external-beam radiation, brachytherapy, and hormonal manipulation. After hormonal treatment of metastatic prostate cancer, a greater than 90% decline in the serum PSA has correlated with progression-free survival.[50] A greater than 90% decline corresponded to a probability of progression at 1 year of 25%, compared with a probability of 80% to 90% progression for smaller percent declines.[50] The use of this surrogate endpoint for disease activity in the setting of chemotherapy for HRPC has also been validated as a predictor of objective disease progression and survival. A greater than 50% decline in serum PSA in the absence of clinical or radiographic evidence of disease progression, and confirmed 4 weeks later, was established in 1999 by the Prostate Specific Antigen Working Group (NCI) as clinical guidelines for HRPC trials.[12,51,52] In general, these recommendations were made as a guide to the design of larger, randomized, survival-based trials, rather than as a true surrogate for survival. Expression of PSA is generally regulated by autocrine, paracrine, and hormonal activity, and levels may be altered independent of disease activity if this activity is affected by the investigational agent.[53,54] Generally, cytotoxic agents have not been shown to alter PSA levels independently of their clinical responses, but it has been recommended that new agents examine the effect on PSA expression independently before entering into large-scale trials. Multiple analyses have demonstrated a correlation between a greater than 50% serum PSA decline at 8 weeks and overall survival, with some demonstrating a three-fold increase in survival compared with smaller responses.[51,52] Thus for most cytotoxic agents, serum PSA declines of greater than 50% may be a useful surrogate outcome in early clinical trials until larger, randomized trials are able to be conducted to examine progression-free and overall survival. For biologic agents, PSA changes are generally considered in the context of the independent effects of these agents on secretion of PSA.

Survival and disease progression

The natural history of untreated metastatic hormone-refractory prostate cancer is heterogeneous but generally that of progressive disease, skeletal metastases, and impairment in quality of life related to bony pain, fractures, and deterioration in functional status. Prior to the recent USFDA approval of docetaxel, no agents had been shown to alter the natural history of this progression and thus extend life. Median survival of untreated symptomatic disease has generally been less than 12 months, with 6 to 10 months median survival.[43,45,55] Recently, a CALGB prognostic model for predicting survival in HRPC has been developed and validated.[55] Four risk groups were identified using the following factors: lactate dehydrogenase (LDH); Prostate specific antigen (PSA), alkaline phosphatase, Gleason score, ECOG performance status, hemoglobin, and presence of visceral metastases (Box 41.1). Median survival by quartiles for each of these four groups were 8.8, 13.4, 17.4, and 22.8 months, illustrating the heterogeneity of this disease and the need for standardization among potential treatment groups.[55] A similar nomogram has been developed and validated at Memorial

---

> **Box 41.1** Adverse prognostic variables in metastatic hormone refractory prostate cancer[10,53]
>
> - Poor performance status
> - Elevated lactate dehydrogenase
> - Liver metastases
> - Low hemoglobin
> - Elevated alkaline phosphatase
> - Less than 2 year interval from onset of hormonal therapy to chemotherapy initiation
> - PSA kinetics (likely)

Sloan-Kettering Cancer Center.[10] Prostate-specific antigen kinetics have not yet been validated as a surrogate marker for survival in the hormone refractory state, unlike the utility of PSA doubling time in men with rising PSA preceding and following local treatment.[56,57] However, larger scale studies are anticipated to show a correlation of overall survival and the rate of rise of PSA. Thus, men with HRPC are a diverse group whose survival is affected by multiple variables that have confounded the search for therapeutic agents in the past.

Measurable disease has been difficult to quantify in metastatic HRPC, given that many patients have bone-only metastases that may change over time, independently of treatment effect. Initial clinical trials of cytotoxic agents, therefore, included stable disease as a measure of response, clouding the ability to assess the efficacy of these agents.[43] The criteria for evaluating objective responses to therapy have been updated to include the RECIST (response evaluation criteria in solid tumors) criteria, but bony disease remains an unmeasurable quantity.[58] Survival as a primary endpoint has become an indisputable and necessary approach to advancing newer agents toward approval and into the clinic. The plenary sessions of the American Society of Clinical Oncology (ASCO) 2004 demonstrated for the first time that chemotherapy is able to prolong survival in this population, with TAX327 demonstrating a 2.5 month survival advantage of docetaxel over mitoxantrone, and SWOG 9916 demonstrating a similar increment with the combination of docetaxel and estramustine.[8,9] Both studies correlated improved PSA responses and objective response rates with overall survival. Progression-free survival was improved in both trials by similar magnitudes, and tended to correlate with improved QoL scores and pain outcomes. Thus, these two large scale phase III trials demonstrate the feasibility, tolerability, and improved outcomes of doceaxel based chemotherapy, and should serve as a new baseline with which to compare new agents.

Pivotal trials of chemotherapy in metastatic hormone-refractory prostate cancer

Tables 41.1 and 41.2 present a selected comparison of modern PSA-era trials of single agent and combination therapies examined in phase II and III trials. A further historical review is well summarized by Yagoda et al in 1992[44] and by Beer in 2004.[19] The major pivotal trials that have changed clinical practice are discussed below.

Table 41.1 Selected single agent activity in high-risk prostate cancer

Agent	References	Number of patients	Survival (months)	Time to progression (months)	Measurable RR (%)	PSA RR (95% CI)
Docetaxel	8, 56–59	810	9–18.9	4.6–5.1	12–28	38–48
Paclitaxel	60–62	126	9–13.5	NR	17	4–39
Mitoxantrone	43, 44, 63	255	12.3-23	3.7–8.1	13	33–48
Epirubicin	64–67	260	9–13	NR	31	24–32
Vinorelbine	68–71	154	10.2–17	2.9–7	7	4–28
Estramustine	72	113	NR	NR	40	21
Cyclophosphamide	73–74	53	8–12.7	NR	14	4
Doxorubicin	65, 75	135	9–13	NR	22	NR
Gemcitabine	76	50	14.7	2.7	NR	NR
Cisplatin	77	29	NR	NR	10	NR

Table 41.2 Selected combination chemotherapy activity in high-risk prostate cancer

Agents	Refs	No. of patients	Survival (months) (months)	Time to progression	Clinical response (%)	PSA response (%)
Paclitaxel, estramustine, etoposide, and carboplatin (TEEC)	78	19	14.2	5.5	58	58
Docetaxel/estramustine	9, 79–83	619	12–20	6–10	17–42	50–82
Paclitaxel/estramustine	84–87	119	13–17.3	4.6–5.6	49	53–62
Vinorelbine/estramustine	88–90	72	10.5–15.1	3.5–5.8	6	24–71
Vinblastine/estramustine	91	95	11.9	3.7	20	25
Ketoconazole, doxorubicin, vinblastine, estramustine (KAVE)	92–93	80	19–23.4	NR	61	56–67
Estramustine/etoposide	93–97	211	11–14	NR	48	14–58
Docetaxel/vinorelbine	98	21	NR	NR	60	66
Docetaxel/capecitabine	99	23	NR	NR	30	71
Mitoxantrone, Estramustine, vinorelbine	100	70	18.4	NR	20	50
Cyclophosph., Dexamethasone, Vincristine	101	52	10.6	2.5	25	29

Estramustine

The oral microtubule inhibitor estramustine sodium phosphate (EMP) was the first cytotoxic chemotherapy agent to be approved for use in metastatic prostate cancer, receiving FDA approval in 1981. Estramustine was conceived as a novel targeted agent and is a conjugate of estradiol and nitrogen mustard, and its principle mechanism has been felt to be microtubule disassembly.[57,59] In addition to estrogenic effects, it may additionally cause disruption to the nuclear matrix and chromatin structure independently. Its use as monotherapy has generally been disappointing in terms of response rate (see Table 41.1), and limited by systemic toxicity, notably thromboembolic events seen in about 6% to 7% of patients.[9,60] Response rates in combination regimens have been higher but also limited by these toxicities.[61–63] The recent SWOG 9916 trial of estramustine and docetaxel was unable to reduce this risk with an adult aspirin and low dose coumadin given concurrently.[9]

Combination therapy with estramustine and other microtubule inhibitors in phase II trials has demonstrated additive PSA declines (greater than 50%) on the order of 60%–70%, with a median survival of 20 months (see Table 41.1). The recent phase III trial of docetaxel and estramustine given every 3 weeks with low dose prednisone confirmed the efficacy of this regimen. This trial, SWOG 9916, examined

770 men with progressive HRPC, and randomized to two 21-day regimens: estramustine 280 mg orally on days 1 to 5 with docetaxel 60 mg/m^2 i.v. day 2 and dexamethasone given 20 mg t.i.d. on day 1; versus mitoxantrone 12 mg/m^2 i.v. day 1 with prednisone 5 mg b.i.d. continuously.[9] The estramustine/docetaxel combination demonstrated a 20% improvement in overall survival and a 27% improvement in progression-free survival. Overall median survival improved from 16 to 18 months favoring estramustine/docetaxel with an improved time to progression from 3 to 6 months. This modest improvement, however, has been counterbalanced by the similar results obtained in phase III trials of docetaxel alone (vida infra), thus likely limiting the clinical utility of estramustine in combination regimens. Additionally, the 7% risk of thromboembolic complications in a recent meta-analysis, and the cumulative gastrointestinal toxicities of estramustine/docetaxel combinations likely preclude this combination therapy from standard of care.[19,60]

Mitoxantrone/prednisone

Mitoxantrone is an anthracenedione with cytotoxic activity, and was the first drug to be tested in phase III trials for HRPC in which clinically meaningful QoL parameters were used as an assessment of response.[45,46] Monotherapy PSA response rates (RRs) have ranged from 33% to 48%, with measurable RRs of 13%, without demonstrable improvements in overall survival. The USFDA approval of mitoxantrone in 1996 was the result of two large phase III randomized trials that showed a clinically beneficial response measured in pain ratings and palliative response.[45,46] Tannock et al demonstrated a significantly longer duration of palliation with mitoxantrone and prednisone versus prednisone alone (43 versus 18 weeks), but no difference in overall survival.[46] Kantoff et al confirmed this in a large CALGB trial reported in 1999, which showed improved secondary QoL outcomes and delayed disease progression of about 2 months.[45] Toxicity with mitoxantrone has been primarily hematologic including about a 40% to 50% incidence of grade 3 and 4 neutropenia. However, neutropenic fever has been reported in less than 1% of cases, and no toxic deaths have been reported in the large phase III trials. Cardiac toxicity, mostly congested heart failure (CHF) has been observed in less than 5% of patients. Mitoxantrone has additionally been studied in a large phase II trial of men with HRPC and asymptomatic metastatic disease.[64] While no overall difference in survival was seen, men on the chemotherapy arm had a prolonged disease-free period and time to progression as compared with prednisone alone (8.1 months versus 4.1 months). Toxicity in these trials have mostly consisted of hematologic toxicity (grade 3/4 neutropenia in about 60–70%) and cardiac toxicity (5%).

Docetaxel

Docetaxel is a cytotoxic agent and member of the taxoid family. It induces apoptosis in cancer cells through p53-independent mechanisms that are felt to be due to its inhibition of microtubule depolymerization and inhibition of antiapoptotic signaling.[65,66] The induction of microtubule stabilization intracellularly through β-tubulin interactions causes GTP-independent polymerization and cell cycle arrest at G2/M, and some have reported a two-fold greater microtubule affinity compared with paclitaxel.[65,67] Additionally, docetaxel has been found to induce BCL2 phosphorylation in vitro, a process which has been correlated with caspace activation and loss of its normal antiapoptotic activity.[68] Unable to inhibit the proapoptotic molecule BAX, phosphorylated BCL2 may also induce apotosis through this independent mechanism. However, additional mechanisms may be important such as P27KIP1 induction and repression of BCLXL.[67,69]

Weekly docetaxel has been studied in several phase II trials and the phase III TAX327 trial with favorable results and toxicity profiles. Berry et al conducted a multi-institutional phase II study that gave 36 mg/m[2] docetaxel weekly for 6 out of 8 weeks per cycle with dexamethasone premedication, which demonstrated a 9.4 month survival and 46% PSA response (greater than 50% decline) among men with HRPC, 25% of whom were previously treated with mitoxantrone.[70] Likewise, a trial by Beer et al in previously untreated men demonstrated improved pain outcomes in 48% and a 46% PSA "response" using a similar regimen.[71] The every 3-week schedules of docetaxel were developed in two large randomized trials[72,73] that demonstrated a 38% to 46% PSA-response rate and median survival of 9 months using docetaxel at 75 mg/m[2] every 21 days with dexamethasone premedication. Responders had a median survival of 27 months with favorable quality of life outcomes. It has generally been felt that the every 3-week schedule has had more neutropenia (43–71% versus 3–25%) compared with the weekly regimens, but all regimens have been well tolerated without any significant clinical differences.

Docetaxel has become the agent of choice as of 2004 for metastatic HRPC, based on a large phase III randomized trial, TAX 327, which demonstrated its superiority to the past standard, mitoxantrone and prednisone.[8] TAX 327 built on the work of the above four phase II trials,[72,73] which demonstrated the safety and efficacy of weekly and every 3-week schedules of docetaxel. TAX-327 enrolled 1006 patients with progressive HRPC, no prior chemotherapy, and stable pain scores to one of three arms, all with concomitant prednisone at 5 mg p.o. b.i.d.: mitoxantrone 12 mg/m[2] i.v. q21 days; docetaxel 75 mg/m[2] i.v. q21 days; and docetaxel 30 mg/m[2] i.v. weekly. Patents remained on gonadal suppression but had all other hormonal agents discontinued within 4 to 6 weeks. Treatment duration was 30 weeks in all arms, or a maximum of 10 cycles in the every 3-week arms, with more patients completing treatment in the every 3-week docetaxel arm than the mitoxantrone arm due mostly to differences in disease progression (46% versuss 25%).[8] After a median 20.7 month follow-up, overall survival in the every 3-week docetaxel arm was 18.9 months with a pain response rate of 35% and a PSA response of 45%, contrasted with weekly docetaxel at 17.3 months, 31%, and 48% respectively. This translated into a 24% relative risk reduction in death (95% CI 6–48%; p = 0.0005) with every 3-week docetaxel (Figure 41.1).[8] The mitoxantrone arm performed favorably against historic mitoxantrone-treated patients, with a median survival of 16.4 months, a pain response of 22%, and a PSA response of 32%.[8]

Toxicity in the every 3-week versus weekly docetaxel arms was notable for more hematologic toxicity in the every 3-week arm (3% neutropenic fever versus 0%; 32% grade 3/4 neutropenia versus 1.5%), but slightly lower rates of nausea and vomiting, fatigue, nail changes, hyperlacrimation, and diarrhea. Neuropathy was slightly more common in the every 3-week arm (grade 3/4 in 1.8% versus 0.9%).[8] Quality of life as measured by the FACT-P scores did not

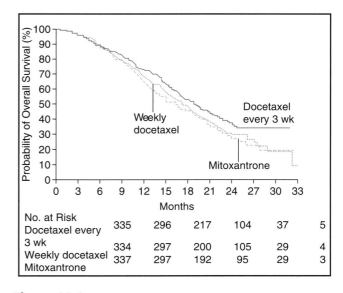

Figure 41.1

Kaplan–Meier estimates of overall survival in the three arms of the TAX 327 trial involving 1006 men with hormone-refractory metastatic prostate cancer randomized to prednisone plus docetaxel (every 3 weeks or weekly) versus mitoxantrone and prednisone.

differ significantly among the docetaxel schedules but were more favorable than the mitoxantrone arm.[8] In extrapolating the use of docetaxel to large populations of men with HRPC, it is also important to be point out significant reports of interstitial pneumonitis, extravasation injuries, colitis, excess tearing, and maculopapular rash that may occur with docetaxel but were not seen in TAX327.[65]

Of note, paclitaxel has been studies in several phase II trials with similar response rates to docetaxel using prolonged 24-hour infusion schedules.[74–76] However, no phase III trials of paclitaxel have been advanced nor any head-to-head comparisons with docetaxel and are unlikely to be performed given the likely minor differences in clinical outcomes expected.

Combination chemotherapy

Docetaxel/estramustine

Based on the success of multiple phase II studies with the combination of docetaxel and estramustine, SWOG conducted the large phase III trial SWOG 99-16, the results of which were reported in 2004.[9,61–63,77,78] The rationale for the addition of two microtubule targeted therapies has been the in-vitro synergism observed in some hormone-sensitive cell lines between estramustine and docetaxel, the clinical experience of improved PSA, and objective response rates historically and when compared with docetaxel alone.[62,79]

SWOG 99-16 randomized 770 patients with progressive HRPC to oral estramustine 280 mg p.o. t.i.d. with docetaxel 60 mg/m² every 21 days or mitoxantrone 12 mg/m² every 21 days with low dose prednisone. The protocol was amended due to a high rate of cardiovascular thromboembolic events to include prophylactic low dose coumadin and aspirin, which unfortunately was unable to demonstrate a reduction in thromboembolism. While the docetaxel/estramustine arms demonstrated improvement over the control group in terms of overall survival by 2 months and progression-free survival by 3 months, the clinical utility of the regimen suffered as a result of the excessive grade 3 and 4 gastrointestinal and cardiovascular toxicities (20% and 15%, respectively).[9] Given the similar magnitude of survival benefit and response rates with single agent docetaxel with substantially less toxicity than estramustine regimens, it is likely that the use of estramustine combinations will drop off considerably. While head-to-head comparisons of separate phase III trials are impossible due to differences in schedule, patient populations, and docetaxel dosing (60 mg/m² in SWOG 9916 and 75 mg/m² in TAX 327), it is unlikely that a large survival benefit with estramustine will be missed despite the combination's improved response rate.

While multiple other chemotherapy agents have been studied in phase II clinical trials, none have advanced into phase III trials or demonstrated improved survival over the currently approved drugs: docetaxel, estramustine, and mitoxantrone. Table 41.1 lists selected active combination regimens with phase II and III activity in HRPC. In general, combination therapies with active single agents, such as paclitaxel, etoposide, estramustine, and carboplatin (TEEC), or ketoconazole, doxorubicin, vinblastine, and estramustine (KAVE), have shown improved response rates and increased toxicity but comparable survival times to single agent docetaxel, precluding their use as standard therapy.[80–82] Doublets of microtubule-based therapies, including vinorelbine and vinblastine with docetaxel or estramustine, have not demonstrated significantly improved response or progression-free survival rates.[61–63,77,78,81–95]

Certain agents, such as oral continuous "metronomic" cyclophosphamide and dexamethasone in combination have shown activity in a retrospective trial of a mixed population of men with HRPC.[96] A decline of more than 50% PSA was seen in 78% of 34 men, 13 of whom had been treated with prior chemotherapy, with a 9-month duration of response. This appealing well-tolerated oral treatment may be a reasonable alternative in select patients who have progressed despite chemotherapy, suffered adverse reactions to standard chemotherapy, or, given the nearly 10% cerebrospinal-fluid bioavailability of cyclophosphamide, have central nervous system or leptomeningeal disease.[96] Dividing doses into more frequent, or metronomic fractions, such as weekly docetaxel, has not been shown to be less toxic and has not demonstrated improved durable responses prospectively; however, continued prospective study of this low toxicity, patient friendly approach with new agents is warranted.[97]

Modifying chemotherapy response

Androgen priming

Given the theoretical sensitivity of rapidly dividing cells to cytotoxic therapy, the rationale for the addition of androgen to chemotherapy as a way of inducing cell cycle turnover was tested in 1988 by Manni et al.[98] They theorized that priming with the androgen fluoxymesterone 3 days prior to and concurrent with chemotherapy administration would synchronize tumor growth and lead to a greater response rate than placebo. Eight-five patients with prostate cancer who had progressed despite orchiectomy were treated initially with aminoglutethamide and hydrocortisone to induce androgen depletion and then with cyclophosphamide, fluorouracil, and doxorubicin every 3 weeks. Randomization was to androgen or no androgen. Median response and duration of response was no different, and median survival was shorter in the androgen arm (10 versus 15 months).[98] There were significant toxicities related to tumor growth during androgen administration, including cord compression, increased bone pain, and worsening liver function. While this does not address androgen priming in the modern era with active cytotoxic M-phase specific agents, it has not currently been shown to be more effective than no treatment or continued hormonal ablation.[99]

Androgen deprivation

While metastatic HRPC may remain androgen responsive, it is unclear if continued androgen suppression in the face of disease progression and trials of cytotoxic therapy has clinical utility. The specific question of whether clinicians should continue GnRH agonists while initiating chemotherapy has not been addressed in modern randomized clinical trials. However, retrospective and anecdotal reports have documented progressive disease and inferior outcomes on discontinuation of androgen suppression during chemotherapy with resumption of response on restarting hormonal therapy.[100,101] In one small series, PSA progression was documented during chemotherapy for HRPC, with resumption of PSA response with reinstitution of hormone ablation.[100] This may indicate that HRPC is not truly androgen independent, but rather maintains features of androgen driven growth. However, androgen ablation alone is insufficient to maintain responses in HRPC, and antiandrogen withdrawal remains a therapeutic measure in a fraction of patients. Currently, the PSA working group has recommended that patients stay on LHRH agonists during chemotherapy and chemotherapy trials and all recently reported studies maintain this level of hormonal therapy.

Role of corticosteroids

The role of glucocorticoids as adjunctive treatment to chemotherapy in HRPC is controversial, based on the fact that most current clinical trials have allowed the use of these agents in both treatment and control arms. Prednisone or hydrocortisone alone have demonstrated more than 50% PSA declines on the order of 20% and relief of QoL parameters such as pain control in 20% to 50% of patients.[102] Time to progression in men with symptomatic metastatic HRPC treated with low dose prednisone alone has been comparable to flutamide, with a time to progression of 3.4 months and 56% subjective response rate.[103] As glucocorticoids suppress pituitary adrenocorticotrophic hormone (ACTH) production and thus adrenal androgen levels, one mechanism may be this third-line antiandrogen effect. However, glucocorticoids also have direct cytopathic effects and immunomodulatory effects that may interfere with intracellular growth and survival pathways. For example, dexamethasone has been shown to reduce IL–6 and nuclear factor κB (NFκB) levels, factors which may be important in hormone refractory prostate cancer cell growth.[104] Alternatively, one potential mechanism wherein glucocorticoids may worsen outcome in men with HRPC has been the demonstration of androgen receptor mutations that lead to steroidal agonism and tumor growth rather than growth inhibition.[105] It may continue to be difficult to separate out these effects due to the approval of recent agents that included low dose prednisone as part of the treatment arm.

Novel biologic agents in combination with chemotherapy

Novel targeted combination therapies of biologic agents to enhance the efficacy chemotherapy are being extensively investigated, and include such agents as EGF receptor tyrosine kinase inhibitors (gefitinib, erlotinib), platelet-derived growth factor (PDGF) receptor tyrosine kinase inhibitors (imatinib), thalidomide and other immunomodulatory agents, differentiating agents such as DN101 (calcitriol), radioimmunotherapies, antiangiogenic agents such as bevacizumab, proapoptotic agents, and others. These will be discussed extensively in subsequent chapters, as primary first-line therapy and for relapsed progressive disease after chemotherapy. However, a brief discussion of the more active agents is warranted here, and these are listed in Box 41.2.

Thalidomide in combination with docetaxel was investigated in a recent phase II study based on the principle that an immunomodulatory and anti-angiogenic molecule would enhance the efficacy of a traditional cytotoxic agent.[106] Thalidomide inhibits IL6 and tumor necrosis factor-α (TNF-α), and has other immunostimulatory

---

Box 41.2 Novel biologic agents in development for advanced prostate cancer in combination with chemotherapy

- Thalidomide
- CC5013 (Revlimid) and CC-4047 (Actimid)
- DN-101 (calcitriol)
- Imatinib (Gleevec)
- Bortezomib (Velcade)
- Bevacizumab (Avastin)
- Proapoptotic agents, i.e., BCL2 antisense oligonucleotides (oblimersen sodium)
- CCI-779 and inhibitors of AKT and mTOR pathways
- Lapatinib and other EGFR, PDGFR, HER2/HER3 inhibitors
- Bisphosphonates (pamidronate, clodronate, zoledronic acid)
- Atrasentan (Xinlay)
- Radiolabeled isotopes and monoclonal antibodies (samarium, strontium, lutetium, yttrium)
- Vaccine strategies

EGFR, epithelial growth factor receptor; PDGFR, platelet-derived growth factor receptor

---

effects, while metabolites of thalidomide have been found to have antiangiogenic activity in rat aortic ring assays.[107,108] This trial randomized patients with chemotherapy naive metastatic HRPC to either weekly docetaxel alone or in combination with 200 mg/day of oral thalidomide. Prostate-specific antigen and objective responses were seen in 53% and 35% of the combined group, respectively, compared with 37% and 27% in the docetaxel alone arm. Progression-free survival was improved from 3.7 months to 5.9 months in the combined group, and at 26 months of follow-up, overall survival was improved from 14.7 months to 28.9 months, the longest seen yet of any combination therapy in HRPC.[106] Adverse effects in the thalidomide group included the expected sedation and dizziness seen in 43%, grade 1 and 2 peripheral neuropathy in 76%, thrombosis in 18%, and slightly more constipation. Although this trial was underpowered, with only 75 patients, it is suggestive of an incremental benefit in disease progression and stabilization. Other novel immunomodulatory and potentially anti-angiogenic agents such as Revlimid and CC-4047 that are structurally based on thalidomide but without the neurotoxicity and sedative properties are currently moving into phase II studies after initial studies demonstrated their activity and safety.[109,110]

DN101 represents a new formulation of calcitriol, a vitamin D analog that has demonstrated preclinical synergy with docetaxel and improved PSA responses and median survival in phase II trials when used in combination with docetaxel.[111] In 37 patients treated on this trial with weekly docetaxel and pretreatment with oral calcitriol 0.5 μg/kg, median time to progression was 11.4 months, and median survival was 19.5 months, comparing favorably with historic controls. The phase II/III ASCENT trial will examine the combination of DN101, a high-dose oral calcitriol formulation, and weekly docetaxel, in a larger population compared with the current docetaxel standard.

Other agents such as imatinib (Gleevec) as a targeted therapy of the PDGF receptor pathway, bortezomib (Velcade) as a novel proteasome inhibitor, and bevacizumab (Avastin) as a VEGF inhibitor have demonstrated preclinical and phase I activity and are moving forward to larger scale trials currently, such as the CALGB trial 90006 of estramustine and docetaxel in combination with Avastin in men with HRPC.[112–114] The antiapoptotic protein BCL2 is a rational target of therapy and is being investigated as a predictor of clinical response. The inhibitory antisense oligonucleotide oblimersen sodium is being tested in phase II/III trials in combination with docetaxel and has shown some promising early results.[115] Correlation of antiapoptotic gene protein levels with response has not yet been clinically correlated, and this theory is being examined by ECOG 1899, discussed earlier in this chapter. Epidermal growth factor receptor (EGFR) and other growth factor receptor inhibitors hold some promise in combination with cytotoxic agents based on responses seen in NSCLC; however only modest PSA responses and no clinical activity has been demonstrated with single agent use of gefitinib in HRPC.[116] Improved responses with multitargeted tyrosine kinase inhibition (i.e., lapatinib) or inhibition of additional cell survival pathways important to prostate cancer such as mTOR (i.e., CCI-779) or AKT/PI3K remain to be demonstrated but are eagerly anticipated.[115] Bone targeted agents such as bisphosphonates and atrasentan, a novel endothelin receptor antagonist, have also shown clinical activity in HRPC and will be discussed in subsequent chapters.[114]

Therapy for progressive disease following chemotherapy

To date, there remains no FDA approved therapies for second- or third-line treatment of metastatic prostate cancer that has progressed after chemotherapy, and this unfilled niche represents an active area of clinical investigation that should encourage enrollment on clinical trials. Overall survival in this group of patients is approximately 12 months based on time to progression and overall survival in large phase III trials.[8,9] As stated above, combination therapies may result in higher response rates but at increased toxicity, especially in heavily pretreated individuals, with lower response rates generally seen in those who have failed first line chemotherapy.

One agent that is currently under evaluation as second line therapy is the oral platinum agent, Satraplatin, which has shown in vivo activity against taxane and cisplatin refractory prostate cell lines. A small phase III trial has shown improved response rates and progression free survival of Satraplatin 100 mg/m^2 × 5 days in combination with prednisone every 28 days, with a trend toward improved overall survival, although the study was not powered to detect a difference.[118] Median progression-free (5.2 versus 2.5 months) and overall survival (14.9 versus 11.9 months) were slightly better compared with prednisone alone, and has led to the initiation of the SPARC trial (Satraplatin and prednisone against refractory cancer) for second line HRPC chemotherapy. It remains to be seen if this agent has improved toxicity and survival data over standard palliative care or currently available well tolerated agents, such as oral cyclophosphamide and dexamethasone or other active agents.

The epothilones are a class of microtubule targeting cytotoxic agents in development for second line HRPC as well, and their activity in this scenario is an area of active investigation. The epothilones are derived from the myxobacterium *Sorangium cellulosum*, and in preclinical models they have demonstrated a wide range of clinical activity, including taxane-resistant models, with a mechanism similar to the taxanes.[119] By suppressing microtubule depolymerization, these agents induce G2/M arrest and apoptosis. However, while taxanes are susceptible to P-glycoprotein-induced drug efflux, the epothilones are not.[119] One such agent, Epothilone-B analog BMS-247550 (Ixabepilone) has been studied in a phase II trial of men with HRPC. Initial results demonstrate a 34% PSA response and 30% objective response, with a progression-free survival of 8 months, comparable to the best results seen with taxane based therapy.[16] The use of BMS 247550 in taxane-resistant HRPC is being investigated currently by Rosenberg et al in NCI protocol 6046 compared with mitoxantrone and prednisone.[120] Additional schedules are being evaluated in other phase II studies that may be less neurotoxic than the initial phase II trials.

It is worth mentioning that studies of chemotherapy in combination with radiolabeled antibodies or radioisotopes for metastatic prostate cancer are also under development for progressive disease following chemotherapy. The most advanced of these approaches involves strontium-89 (^{89}Sr) given with doxorubicin as consolidation following induction chemotherapy on the MD Anderson KAVE regimen. This approach has shown significant palliation of pain (>50%), prolongation of survival (from 17 to 28 months), and improved time to progression with ^{89}Sr as consolidation with doxorubicin compared with doxorubicin alone in a randomized phase II trial.[17] While involving a fairly toxic, nonstandard chemotherapy regimen and a small number[57] of patients that require confirmation testing, this trial demonstrated the potential additive benefits of radioisotopes such as samarium-153 (^{153}Sm)or ^{89}Sr to chemotherapy. Whether these agents can add benefit following or in combination with docetaxel chemotherapy remains unanswered. The use of these agents as salvage therapy for symptomatic metastases has been studied in several randomized trials and will be discussed in a subsequent chapter. While survival benefits have not been demonstrated to date, radioisotopes have been shown to reduce analgesic requirements in symptomatic men with multiple metastatic sites at the expense of myelosuppression.[121] Prostate-specific membrane antigen (PSMA) monoclonal antibody-tagged radioisotopes such as Yttrium-90 (^{90}Y) or Lutetium-177 (^{177}Lu) are also in development and have begun to enter phase II trials.[122]

Current indications for chemotherapy

In conclusion, chemotherapy with docetaxel or mitoxantrone for metastatic HRPC has become the standard of care given the improved survival demonstrated in recent phase III trials. The benefits or the addition of estramustine is likely offset by its toxicity profile and lack of demonstrable survival benefit over docetaxel alone. Treatment with docetaxel seems to favor an every 3-week schedule, given up to 10 cycles, but may be continued as long as objective responses are seen. The use of chemotherapy in earlier phases of advanced disease, such as biochemical only HRPC, asymptomatic metastatic HRPC subgroups, and as adjuvant or neoadjuvant to definitive local therapies remains to be proven but these clinical trials are moving forward quickly to change the treatment paradigms in high-risk men.[123,124] Surrogate markers such as PSA doubling time and changes in PSA velocity are under investigation to facilitate the development of these therapies in a more rapid manner.[125,126] A large number of novel agents with diverse mechanisms of action that target many of the critical checkpoints in prostate cancer growth, invasion, apoptosis, and metastasis are additionally bringing a great deal of excitement to this rapidly changing field. Whether these agents will replace chemotherapy or be used in conjunction with cytotoxic chemotherapy remains to be seen.

Conflict-of-interest statement

Funding for some of the studies described in this article was provided by Aventis Pharmaceuticals and Abbott Laboratories. Dr Carducci is on the Speakers Bureau for Aventis Pharmaceuticals and is a consultant to Abbott Laboratories. The terms of this arrangement are being managed by the Johns Hopkins University in accordance with its conflict of interest policies.

References

1. Weir, HK, Thun MJ, Hankey BF, et al. Annual Report to the Nation on the Status of Cancer 1975-2000, Featuring the Uses of Surveillance Data for Cancer Prevention and Control. J Natl Cancer Inst 2003;95:1276–1299.
2. Jemal A, Murray T, Ward E, et al. Cancer Statistics 2005. CA Cancer J Clin 2005;55:10–30.
3. Han M, Partin AW, Piantadosi S, et al. Era Specific Biochemical Recurrence-Free Survival Following Radical Prostatectomy for Clinically Localized Prostate Cancer. J Urol 2001;166:416–419.
4. Zietman AL, Coen JJ, Dallow KC, et al. The Treatment of Prostate Cancer by Conventional Radiation Therapy:an Analysis of Long-Term Outcome. Int J Radiat Oncol Biol Phys 1995;32:287–292.
5. Goktas S, Crawford ED. Optimal Hormonal Therapy for Advanced Prostatic Carcinoma. Semin Oncol 1999;26:162–173.
6. Eisenberger MA, Partin AW, Pound C, et al. Natural History of Progression of Patients with Biochemical (PSA) Relapse Following Radical Prostatectomy: Update. Proc Am Soc Clin Oncol 2003;22:280 [abstract 1527].
7. Eisenberger MA, Blumenstein BA, Crawford ED, et al. Bilateral Orchiectomy with or without Flutamide for Metastatic Prostate Cancer. N Engl J Med 1998;339:1036–1042.
8. Eisenberger MA, de Wit R, Berry W, et al. A Multicenter Phase III Comparison of Docetaxel (D) + Prednisone (P) and Mitoxantrone (M) + P in Patients with Hormone-Refractory Prostate Cancer. Proc Am Soc Clin Oncol 2004 [abstract 4].
9. Petrylak D, Tangen C, Hussain M, et al. SWOB 99-16:Randomized Phase III Trial of Docetaxel (D)/Estramustine (E) versus Mitoxantrone (M)/Prednisone (P) in Men with Androgen-Independent Prostate Cancer. Proc Am Soc Clin Oncol 2004 [abstract 3].
10. Smaletz O, Scher HI, Small EJ, et al. Nomogram for Overall Survival of Patients with Progressive Metastatic Prostate Cancer After Castration. J Clin Oncol 2002;20:3972–3982.
11. Kantoff PW, Halabi S, Conaway M, et al. Hydrocortisone with or without Mitoxantrone in Men with Hormone-Refractory Prostate Cancer: Results of the Cancer and Leukemia Group B 9182 Study. J Clin Oncol 1999;17:2506–2513.
12. Bubley GJ, Carducci MA, Dahut W, et al. Eligibility and Response Guidelines for Phase II Clinical Trials in Androgen-Independent Prostate Cancer: Recommendations from the Prostate-Specific Antigen Working Group. J Clin Oncol 1999;17:3461–3467.
13. Scher HI, Eisenberger M, D'Amico AV, et al. Eligibility and Outcomes Reporting Guidelines for Clinical Trials for Patients in the State of a Rising Prostate Specific Antigen: Recommendations from the Prostate-Specific Antigen Working Group. J Clin Oncol 2004;22:537–556.
14. Small EJ, Halabi S, Dawson NA, et al. Antiandrogen Withdrawal Alone or in Combination with Ketoconazole in Androgen-Independent Prostate Cancer Patients: A Phase III Trial (CALGB 9583). J Clin Oncol 2004;22:1025–1033.
15. Eastham JA, Kelly WK, Grossfeld GD, et al. Cancer and Leukemia Group B (CALGB) 90203:a Randomized Phase 3 Trial of Radical Prostatectomy Alone versus Estramustine and Docetaxel Before Radical Prostatectomy for Patients with High Risk Localized Disease. Urology 2003;62 Suppl 1:55–62.
16. Hussain M, Faulkner J, Vaishampayan U, et al. Epothilone B Analogue BMS-247550 Administered Every 21 Days in Patients with Hormone Refractory Prostate Cancer. A Southwest Oncology Group Study (S0111). Proc Am Soc Clin Oncol 2004 [abstract 4510].
17. Tu SM, Millikan RE, Mengistu RE, et al. Bone Targeted Therapy for Advanced Androgen-Independent Carcinoma of the Prostate: a Randomized Phase II Trial. Lancet 2001;357:336–341.
18. Walczak JR, Carducci MA. Phase III Randomized Trial Evaluating Second Line Hormonal Therapy versus Docetaxel-Estramustine Combination Chemotherapy on Progression-Free Survival in Asymptomatic Patients with a Rising PSA After Hormonal Therapy for Prostate Cancer:an Eastern Cooperative Oncology Group (E1899), Intergroup/Clinical Trials Support Unit Study. Urology 2003;62 Suppl 1:141–146.
19. Beer TM. Advances in Systemic Therapy for Prostate Cancer: Chemotherapy for Androgen-Independent Prostate Cancer. Proc Am Soc Clin Oncol 2004;225–232.
20. Martel CL, Gumerlock PH, Meyers FJ, et al. Current Strategies in the Management of Hormone Refractory Prostate Cancer. Cancer Treat Rev 2003;29:171–187.
21. Fosati R, Confalonieri C, Torri V, et al. Cytotoxic and Hormonal Treatment for Metastatic Breast Cancer:A Systematic Review of Published Randomized Trials Involving 31, 510 Women. J Clin Oncol 1998;16:3439–3460.
22. Goldberg RM, Sargent DJ, Morton RF, et al. A Randomized Controlled Trial of Fluorouracil Plus Leukovorin, Irinotecan, and Oxaliplatin Combinations in Patients with Previously Untreated Metastatic Colorectal Cancer. J Clin Oncol 2004;22:23–30.
23. Isaacs JT. The Biology of Hormone Refractory Prostate Cancer: Why does it Develop? Urol Clin NA 1999;26:263–273.
24. Lee WH, Morton RA, Epstein JI, et al. Cytidine Methylation of Regulatory Sequences near the P-class Glutathione-S-Transferase Gene Accompanies Human Prostate Cancer Carcinogenesis. Proc Natl Acad Sci USA 1994;91:11733–11737.
25. McDonnell TJ, Troncoso P, Brisbay SM, et al. Expression of the Protooncogene bcl-2 in the Prostate and its Association with Emergence of Androgen-Independent Prostate Cancer. Cancer Res 1992;52:6940–6944.
26. Sullivan GF, Amenta PS, Villanueva JD, et al. The Expression of Drug Resistance Gene Products during the Progression of Human Prostate Cancer. Clin Cancer Res 1998;4:1393–1403.
27. Apakama I, Robinson MC, Walter NM, et al. Bcl-2 Overexpression Combined with p53 Protein Accumulation Correlates with Hormone-Refractory Prostate Cancer. Br J Cancer 1996;74:1258–1262.
28. Graff JR. Emerging Targets in the AKT Pathway for Treatment of Androgen-Independent Prostatic Adenocarcinoma. Expert Opin Ther Targets 2002;6:103–113.
29. Whang YE, Wu X, Suzuki H, et al. Inactivation of the Tumor Suppressor PTEN/MMAC1 in Advanced Human Prostate Cancer Through Loss of Expression. Proc Natl Acad Sci USA 1998;95:5246–5250.
30. McMenamin ME, Soung P, Perera S, et al. Loss of PTEN Expression in Paraffin-Embedded Primary Prostate Cancer Correlates with High Gleason Score and Advanced Stage. Cancer Res 1999;59:4291–4296.
31. Pfeil K, Eder IE, Putz T, et al. Long Term Androgen-Ablation Causes Increased Resistance to PI3K/Akt Pathway Inhibition in Prostate Cancer Cells. Prostate 2004;58:259–168.
32. Cantley LC, Neel BG. New Insights into Tumor Suppression: PTEN Suppresses Tumor Formation by Restraining the Phosphoinositide 3-kinase/AKT Pathway. Proc Natl Acad Sci USA 1999;96:4240–4245.
33. Ramaswamy S, Nakamura N, Vazquez F et al. Regulation of the G1 Progression by the PTEN Tumor Suppressor Protein is Linked to Inhibition of the Phosphatidylinositol 3-kinase/akt Pathway. Proc Natl Acad Sci USA 1999;96:2110–2115.
34. Chen CD, Welsbie DS, Tran C, et al. Molecular Determinants of Resistance to Antiandrogen Therapy. Nature Medicine 2004;10:33–38.
35. Tilley WD, Buchanan G, Hickey TE, et al. Mutations in the Androgen Receptor Gene are Associated with Progression of Human Prostate Cancer to Androgen Independence. Cancer Res 1996;2:277–285.
36. Taplin ME, Bubley GJ, Chuster TD, et al. Mutation of the Androgen-Receptor Gene in Metastatic Androgen-Independent Prostate Cancer. N Engl J Med 1995;332:1393–1398.
37. Marcelli M, Ittman M, Mariani S, et al. Androgen Receptor Mutations in Prostate Cancer. Cancer Res 2000;60:944–949.

38. Culig Z, Hobisch A, Cronauer MV, et al. Androgen Receptor Activation in Prostatic Tumor Cell Lines by Insulin-Like Growth Factor-I, Keratinocyte Growth Factor, and Epidermal Growth Factor. Cancer Res 1994;54:5474–5478.

39. Torti, FM, Carter SK. The Chemotherapy of Prostatic Adenocarcinoma. Ann Int Med 1980;92:681–689.

40. Schmidt, JD. Chemotherapy of Hormone-Resistant Stage D Prostatic Cancer. J Urol 1980;123:797–805.

41. Scott W, Johnson DE, Schmidt JE, et al. Chemotherapy of Advanced Prostatic Carcinoma with Cyclophosphamide or 5-Fluorouracil: Results of First National Randomized Study. J Urol 1976;114:909–911.

42. Klein LA. Prostatic Carcinoma. N Eng J Med 1979;300:824–833.

43. Eisenberger MA, Simon R, O'Dwyer PJ, et al. A Reevaluation of Nonhormonal Cytotoxic Chemotherapy in the Treatment of Prostatic Carcinoma. J Clin Oncol 1985;3:827–841.

44. Yagoda A, Petrylak D. Cytotoxic Chemotherapy for Advanced Hormone-Resistant Prostate Cancer. Cancer 1993;71 Supp 3:1098–1109.

45. Kantoff PW, Halabi S, Conaway M, et al. Hydrocortisone with or without Mitoxantrone in Men with Hormone-Refractory Prostate Cancer: Results of the Cancer and Leukemia Group B 9182 Study. J Clin Oncol 1999;17:2506–2513.

46. Tannock IF, Osoba D, Stocklet MR. Chemotherapy with Mitoxantrone plus Prednisone or Prednisone Alone for Symptomatic Hormone-Resistant Prostate Cancer: a Canadian Randomized Trial with Palliative Endpoints. J Clin Oncol 1996;14:1756–1764.

47. Esper P, Fei M, Chodak G, et al. Measuring Quality of Life in Men with Prostate Cancer using the Functional Assessment of Cancer Therapy-Prostate Instrument. Urology 1997;50:920–928.

48. Schipper CJ, McMurray A, Levitt M. Measuring the Quality of Life of Cancer Patients: The Functional Living Index-Cancer: Development and Validation. J Clin Oncol 1984;2:472–483.

49. Fossa S, Aaronson N, Newling D. Quality of Life and Treatment of Hormone-Resistant Metastatic Prostate Cancer. Eur J Cancer 1990;26:1133–1136.

50. Matzkin, H, Eber P, Todd B, et al. Prognostic Significance of Changes in Prostate-Specific Markers after Endocrine Treatment of Stage D2 Prostatic Cancer. Cancer 1992;70:2302–2309.

51. Scher HI, Kelly WK, Zhang ZF, et al. Post-Therapy Serum Prostate-Specific Antigen Level and Survival in Patients with Androgen-Independent Prostate Cancer. J Natl Cancer Inst 1999;91:244–251.

52. Smith DC, Dunn RL, Strawderman MS, et al. Change in Serum Prostate-Specfic Antigen as a Marker of Response to Cytotoxic Therapy for Hormone-Refractory Prostate Cancer. J Clin Oncol 1998;16:1835–1843.

53. Horti J, Dixon SC, Logothetis C, et al. Increased Transcriptional Activity of PSA in the Presences of TNP-470, an Angiogenesis Inhibitor. Br J Cancer 1999;79:1588–1593.

54. Wasilenkko WJ, Palad AJ, Somers KD, et al. Effect of the Calcium Influx Inhibitor Carboxyamido-triazole on the Proliferation and Invasiveness of Human Prostate Tumor Cell Lines. Int J Cancer 1996;68:259–264.

55. Halabi S, Small EJ, Katoff PW, et al. Prognostic Model for Predicting Survival in Men with Hormone-Refractory Metastatic Prostate Cancer. J Clin Oncol 2003;21:1232–1237.

56. Loberg, RD, Fielhauer JR, Peinta BA, et al. Prostate-Specific Antigen Doubling Time and Survival in Patients with Advanced Metastatic Prostate Cancer. Urology 2003;62 Suppl 6B:128–133.

57. Eklov S, Nilsson S, Larson A. Evidence for a Non-Estrogenic Cytostatic Effect of Estramustine on Human Prostatic Carcinoma Cells In Vivo. Prostate 1992;20:43–50.

58. Therasse P, Arbuck SG, Eisenhauer EA, et al. New Guidelines to Evaluate the Response to Treatment in Solid Tumors. J Natl Cancer Inst 2000;92:205–216.

59. Hartley-Asp B. Estramustine-Induced Mitotic Arrest in Two Human Prostatic Carcinoma Cell Lines DU 145 and PC-3. Prostate 1984;5:93.

60. Lubinieki GM, Berlin JA, Weinstein RB, et al. Risk of Thromboembolic Events (TE) with Estramustine-Based Chemotherapy in Hormone-Refractory Prostate Cancer: Results of a Meta-analysis. Proc Am Soc Clin Oncol 2003 [abstract 1581].

61. Savarese DM, Halabi S, Hars V, et al. Phase II Study of Docetaxel, Estramustine, and Low-Dose Hydrocortisone in Men with Hormone-Refractory Prostate Cancer: A Final Report of CALGB 9780. J Clin Oncol 2001;19:2509–2515.

62. Eymard JC, Joly F, Priou F, et al. Phase II Randomized Trial of Docetaxel plus Estramustine (DE) versus Docetaxel (D) in Patients with Hormone Refractory Prostate Cancer: A Final Report. Proc Am Soc Clin Oncol 2004 [abstract 4603].

63. Petrylak D, Shelton G, England-Owen C, et al. Response and Preliminary Survival Results of a Phase II Study of Docetaxel and Estramustine in Patients with Androgen-Independent Prostate Cancer. Proc Am Soc Clin Oncol 2000 [abstract 1312].

64. Berry W, Dakhil S, Modiano M, et al. Phase III Study of Mitoxantrone plus Low Dose Prednisone versus Low Dose Prednisone Alone in Patients with Asymptomatic Hormone Refractory Prostate Cancer. J Urol 2002;168:2539–2443.

65. Khan MA, Carducci MA, Partin AW. The Evolving Role of Docetaxel in the Management of Androgen Independent Prostate Cancer. J Urol 2003;170:1709–1716.

66. Ringel I, Horwitz SB. Studies with RP 56976 (Taxotere): A Semisynthetic Analogue of Taxol. J Natl Cancer Inst 1991;83:288–291.

67. Stein CA. Mechanisms of Action of Taxanes in Prostate Cancer. Semin Oncol 1999;26:3–7.

68. Haldar S, Chintapalli J, Croce CM. Taxol Induces Bcl-2 Phosphorylation and Death of Prostate Cancer Cells. Cancer Res 1996;56:1253–1255.

69. Lara PN Jr, Kung HJ, Gumerlock PH, et al. Molecular biology of prostate carcinogenesis. Crit Rev Oncol Hematol 1999;32:197–208

70. Berry W, Rohrbaugh T. Phase II Trial of Single Agent, Weekly Taxotere in Symptomatic, Hormone-Refractory Prostate Cancer. Proc Am Soc Clin Oncol 1999 [abstract 1290].

71. Beer T, Pierce W, Lowe B, et al. Phase II Study of Weekly Docetaxel (Taxotere) in Hormone Refractory Metastatic Prostate Cancer. Proc Am Soc Clin Oncol 2000 [abstract 1368].

72. Picus J, Schultz M. Docetaxel (Taxotere) as Monotherapy in the Treatment of Hormone-Refractory Prostate Cancer: Preliminary Results. Semin Oncol 1999;26:14–18.

73. Friedland D, Cohen J, Miller R, et al. A Phase II Trial of Docetaxel (Taxotere) in Hormone Refractory Prostate Cancer: Correlation of Antitumor Effect to Phosphorylation of Bcl-2. Semin Oncol 1999;26:19–23.

74. Roth BJ, Yeap BY, Wilding G, et al. Taxol in Advanced Hormone-Refractory Carcinoma of the Prostate: A Phase II Trial of the Eastern Cooperative Oncology Group. Cancer 1993;72:2457–2460.

75. Trivedi C, Redman B, Flaherty LE, et al. Weekly 1-hour Infusion of Paclitaxel: Clinical Feasibility and Efficacy in Patients with Hormone Refractory Prostate Carcinoma. Cancer 2000;89:431–436.

76. Berry W, Gregurich M, Dakhil S, et al. Phase II Randomized Trial of Weekly Paclitaxel with or without Estramustine Phosphate in Patients with Symptomatic Hormone Refractory, Metastatic Carcinoma of the Prostate. Proc Am Soc Clin Oncol 2001 [abstract 696].

77. Sinibaldi VJ, Carducci MA, Moore-Cooper S, et al. Phase II Evaluation of Docetaxel plus One-Day Oral Estramustine Phosphate in the Treatment of Patients with Androgen Independent Prostate Carcinoma. Cancer 2002;94:1457–1465.

78. Birch R, Kalman L, Holt L, et al. Randomized Phase IIb Trial Comparing Two Schedules of Docetaxel (D) plus Estramustine (E) for Metastatic Hormone Refractory Prostate Cancer. Proc Am Soc Clin Oncol 2004 [abstract 4622].

79. Kreis W, Budman DR, Calabro A. Unique Synergism or Antagonism of Combinations of Chemotherapeutic and Hormonal Agents in Human Prostate Cancer. Br J Urol 1997;79:196–202.

80. Smith DC, Chay CH, Dunn RL. Phase II Trial of Paclitaxel, Estramustine, Etoposide, and Carboplatin in the Treatment of Patients with Hormone-Refractory Prostate Carcinoma. Cancer 2003;98:269–276.

81. Ellerhorst JA, Tu SM, Amato RJ, et al. Phase II Trial of Alternating Weekly Chemohormonal Therapy for Patients with Androgen-Independent Prostate Cancer. Clin Cancer Res 1997;3:2371–2376.

82. Millikan R, Thall PF, Lee SJ, et al. Randomized Multicenter Phase II Trial of Two Multicomponent Regimens in Androgen-Independent Prostate Cancer. J Clin Oncol 2003;21:878–883.

83. Hudes GR, Nathan F, Khater C, et al. Phase II Trial of 96-Hour Paclitaxel plus Oral Estramustine Phosphate in Metastatic Hormone-Refractory Prostate Cancer. J Clin Oncol 1997;15:3156–163.

84. Vaishampayan U, Fontana J, Du W, et al. An Active Regimen of Weekly Paclitaxel and Estramustine in Metastatic Androgen-Independent Prostate Cancer. Urology 2002;60:1050–1054.

85. Athanasiadis A, Tsavdaridis D, Rigatos SK, et al. Hormone Refractory Prostate Cancer Treated with Estramustine and Paclitaxel Combination. Anticancer Res 2003;23:3085–3088.

86. Ferrari AC, Chachoua A, Singh H, et al. A Phase I/II Study of Weekly Paclitaxel and 3 Days of High Dose Oral Estramustine Phosphate in Metastatic Androgen-Independent Prostate Cancer. Cancer 2001;91:2039–2045.

87. Smith MR, Kaufman D, Oh W, et al. Vinorelbine and Estramustine in Androgen-Independent Metastatic Prostate Cancer: a Phase II Study. Cancer 2000;89:1824–1828.

88. Sweeney CJ, Monaco FJ, Jung SH, et al. A Phase II Hoosier Oncology Group Study of Vinorelbine and Estramustine Phosphate in Hormone-Refractory Prostate Cancer. Ann Oncol 2002;13:435–440.

89. Carles J, Domenech M, Gelabert-Mas A, et al. Phase II Study of Estramustine and Vinorelbine in Hormone-Refractory Prostate Carcinoma Patients. Acta Oncol 1998;37:187–191.

90. Hudes G, Einhorn L, Ross E, et al. Vinblastine versus Vinblastine plus Oral Estramsutine Phosphate for Patients with Hormone-Refractory Prostate Cancer: A Hoosier Oncology Group and Fox Chase Phase III Trial. J Clin Oncol 1999;17:3160–3166.

91. Pienta KJ, Redman B, Hussain M, et al. Phase II Study of Oral Estramustine and oral Etoposide in Hormone-Refractory Adenocarcinoma of the Prostate. J Clin Oncol 1994;12:2005–2012.

92. Pienta KJ, Redman B, Bandekar R, et al. A Phase II Study of Oral Estramustine and Oral Etoposide in Hormone-Refractory Prostate Cancer. Urology 1997;50:401–406.

93. Pienta KJ, Fisher EI, Eisenberger MA, et al. A Phase II Trial of Estramustine and Etoposide in Hormone Refractory Prostate Cancer:A Southwest Oncology Group Trial (SWOG 9407). Prostate 2001;46:257–261.

94. Dimopoulos MA, Panopoulos C, Bamia C, et al. Oral Estramustine and Oral Etoposide for Hormone-Refractory Prostate Cancer. Urology 1997;50:754–758.

95. Koletsky AJ, Guerra ML, Kronish L. Phase II Study of Vinorelbine and Low Dose Docetaxel in Chemotherapy-Naïve Patients with Hormone-Refractory Prostate Cancer. Cancer J 2003;9:286–292.

96. Glode LM, Barqawi A, Crighton F. Metronomic Therapy with Cyclophosphamide and Dexamethasone for Prostate Carcinoma. Cancer 2003;98:1643–1648.

97. DiPaola RS, Durvage HJ, Kamen BA. High Time for Low-Dose Prospective Clinical Trials. Cancer 2003;98:1559–1561.

98. Manni A, Bartholomew M, Caplan R, et al. Androgen Priming and Chemotherapy in Advanced Prostate Cancer: Evaluation of Determinants of Clinical Outcome. J Clin Oncol 1988;6:1456–1466.

99. Morris MJ, Kelly WK, Slovin S, et al. Phase I Trial of Exogenous Testosterone for the Treatment of Castrate Metastatic Prostate Cancer. Proc Am Soc Clin Oncol 2004 [abstract 4560].

100. Chao D, Harland SJ. The Importance of Continued Endocrine Treatment during Chemotherapy of Hormone-Refractory Prostate Cancer. Eur Urol 1997;31:7–10.

101. Taylor CD, Elson P, Trump DL. Importance of Continued Testicular Suppression in Hormone-Refractory Prostate Cancer. J Clin Oncol 1993;11:2167–2172.

102. Tannock I, Gospodarowicz M, Meakin W, et al. Treatment of Metastatic Prostate Cancer with Low Dose Prednisone:Evaluation of Pain and Quality of Life as Pragmatic Indices of Response. J Clin Oncol 1989;7:590–597.

103. Fossa SD, Slee PH, Brausi M, et al. Flutamide versus Prednisone in Patients with Prostate Cancer Symptomatically Progressing After Androgen-Ablative Therapy: a Phase III Study of the European Organization for Research and Treatment of Cancer Genitourinary Group. J Clin Oncol 2001;19:62–71.

104. Nishimura K, Nonomura N, Satoh E, et al. Potential Mechanism for the Effects of Dexamethasone on Growth of Androgen-Independent Prostate Cancer. J Natl Cancer Inst 2001;93:1739–1746.

105. Matias PM, Carrondo MA, Coelho R, et al. Structural Basis for the Glucocorticoid Response in a Mutant Human Androgen Receptor Derived from an Androgen-Independent Prostate Cancer. J Med Chem 2002;45:1439–1446.

106. Dahut WL, Gulley JL, Arlen PM, et al. Randomized Phase II Trial of Docetaxel Plus Thalidomide in Androgen-Independent Prostate Cancer. J Clin Oncol 2004;22:2532–2539.

107. Bauer KS, Dixon SC, Figg WD. Inhibition of Angiogenesis by Thalidomide Requires Metabolic Activation, which is Species-Dependent. Biochem Pharmacol 1998;55:1827–1834.

108. Bartlett JB, Dredge K, Dalgleish AG. The Evolution of Thalidomide and its IMiD Derivatives as Anticancer Agents. Nat Rev Cancer 2004;4:314–322.

109. Liu Y, Tohnya TM, Figg WD, et al. Phase I Study of CC-5013 (Revlimid), a Thalidomide Derivative in Patients with Refractory Metastatic Cancer. Proc Am Soc Clin Oncol 2003;22 [abstract 927].

110. Sison B, Bond T, Amato RJ, et al. Phase II Study of CC-4047 in Patients with Metastatic Hormone-Refractory Prostate Cancer. Proc Am Soc Clin Oncol 2004 [abstract 4701].

111. Beer TM, Eilers KM, Garzotto M, et al. Weekly High Dose Calcitriol and Docetaxel in Metastatic Androgen-Independent Prostate Cancer. J Clin Oncol 2003;21:123–128.

112. Chatta GS, Fakih M, Ramalingam S, et al. Phase I Pharmacokinetic Study of Daily Imatinib in Combination with Docetaxel for Patients with Advanced Solid Tumors. Proc Am Soc Clin Oncol 2004 [abstract 2047].

113. Papandreou CN, Daliani DD, Nix D, et al. Phase I Trial of the Proteasome Inhibitor Bortezomib in Patients with Advanced Solid Tumors with Observations in Androgen-Independent Prostate Cancer. J Clin Oncol 2004;22:2108–2121.

114. Picus J, Halabi S, Rini B, et al. The Use of Bevacizumab with Docetaxel and Estramustine in Hormone Refractory Prostate Cancer:Initial Results of CALGB 90006. Proc Am Soc Clin Oncol 2003;22:393 [abstract 1578].

115. Schroder FH, Wldhagen MF. ZD1839 (Gefitinib) and Hormone Resistant Prostate Cancer-Final Results of a Double Blind Randomized Placebo-Controlled Phase II Study. J Clin Oncol 2004;22 [abstract 4698].

116. Tolcher AW, Chi K, Juhn K, et al. A phase II, pharmacokinetic, and biological correlative study of oblimersen sodium and docetaxel in patients with hormone-refractory prostate cancer. Clin Cancer Res 2005;11:3854–3861.

117. Carducci M, Nelson JB, Saad F. Effects of atrasentan on disease progression and biological markers in men with metastatic hormone-refractory prostate cancer: Phase 3 study. Proc Am Soc Clin Oncol 2004 [abstract 4508].

118. Sternberg CN, Hetherington J, Paluchowska PHTJ, et al. Randomized Phase III Trial of a New Oral Platinum, Satraplatin (JM-216) plus Prednisone or Prednisone Alone in Patients with Hormone Refractory Prostate Cancer. Proc Am Soc Clin Oncol 2003;22:395 [abstract 1586].

119. Goodin S, Kane MP, Rubin EH. Epothilones: Mechanism of Action and Biologic Activity. J Clin Oncol 2004;22:2105–2125.

120. Rosenberg JE, Galsky MD, Weinberg V, et al. Response to second-line taxane based therapy after first-line epothdone B analogue BMS 247550(BMS) therapy in hormone refractory prostate cancer (HRPC). Proc Am Soc Clin Oncol 2004 [abstract 4564].

121. Porter AT, McEwan AJ, Powe JE, et al. Results of a Randomized Phase III Trial to Evaluate the Efficacy of Strontium-89 Adjuvant to Local Field External Beam Irradiation in the Management of Endocrine Resistant Metastatic Prostate Cancer. Int J Radiat Oncol Biol Phys 1993;25:805–813.

122. Glode LM. Phase III Randomized Study of Adjuvant Androgen Deprivation Therapy with or without Mitoxantrone and Prednisone after Prostatecomy in Patients with High Risk Adenocarcinoma of the Prostate. Retrieved Aug 17, 2004 from NCI Clinical Trials website:http://cancer.gov/search/viewclinicaltrials.aspx?version=healthprofessional&cdrid=67352.

123. Bander N, Milowsky MI, Nanus DM, et al. Phase I trail . 177 Lutetium-labeled J591, a monoclonal antibody to prostate-specific membrane antigen, in patients with androgen-independent prostate cancer. J Clin Oncol 2005;23:4591–4601.

124. Pienta KJ. Radiation Therapy Oncology Group P-0014:A Phase 3 Randomized Study of Patients with High Risk Hormone-Naïve Prostate Cancer: Androgen Blockade with 4 Cycles of Immediate Chemotherapy versus Androgen Blockade with Delayed Chemotherapy. Urology 2003;62:95–101.

125. D'Amico AV, Halabi S, Vogelzang NJ, et al. A Reduction in the Rate of PSA Rise Following Chemotherapy in Patients with Metastatic Hormone Refractory Prostate Cancer Predicts Survival:Results of a Pooled Analysis or CALGB HRPC Trials. Proc Am Soc Clin Oncol 2004 [abstract 4506].

126. Crawford ED, Pauler DK, Tangen CM, et al. Three-month Change in PSA as a Surrogate Endpoint for Mortality in Advanced Hormone-Refractory Prostate Cancer: Data from SWOG 9916. Proc Am Soc Clin Oncol 2004 [abstract 4505].

42

Radiotherapy for the treatment of locally advanced and metastatic prostate cancer

Danny Y Song, Salma K Jabbour, Theodore L DeWeese

Radiotherapy in the management of locally advanced prostate cancer

Introduction

The value of radiotherapy in the treatment of prostate cancer has been recognized for nearly a century. The use of transurethral radium was first described in 1911 by Pasteau and Degrais.[1] In 1930, Smith and Pierson described the utility of high voltage X-ray therapy in the treatment of prostate cancer, and, in 1930, Widmann subsequently noted an improvement in survival for patients with advanced prostate cancer treated with kilovoltage X-rays.[2,3] Prior to the advent of prostate-specific antigen (PSA), the majority of patients were diagnosed based on clinically evident disease, which was often more advanced than the presentations commonly seen today. The activity of radiation in prostate cancer was evident by its effect on large palpable tumors that resolved following treatment. Widespread screening for prostate cancer has led to an increasing frequency of the disease being detected in its early stages, but there remains a significant proportion of patients who are diagnosed with locally advanced or even metastatic disease.

The historical definition of locally advanced prostate cancer refers to patients with advanced clinical stage based on direct extension of disease beyond the prostatic capsule either felt on digital rectal examination or seen on imaging—i.e., stage T3 or T4. Such patients are at high risk for disease recurrence following surgical or nonsurgical treatment. In addition to tumor stage, a number of studies have correlated histologic tumor grade and pretreatment PSA with not only extracapsular extension of disease found at radical prostatectomy, but also risk of disease recurrence following any therapy.[4–7] Therefore, a more contemporary and commonly used method of defining locally advanced disease also includes patients who have biologically more aggressive and, therefore, higher risk disease as predicted by prognostic factors such as PSA level and tumor grade. High-risk patients are generally considered to be those who have advanced clinical stage disease, high presenting PSA, and/or poorly differentiated histology (Gleason 8–10).[8] In addition, patients with involvement of regional pelvic lymph nodes are also frequently included in the category of locally advanced disease. As a result, patients seen in modern clinical practice who are classified as having locally advanced disease differ significantly from those termed to have locally advanced disease in prior eras, and

this should be kept in mind when reviewing older data. Although the optimal treatment of this group of patients remains undefined, radiation is a commonly utilized primary modality. Historical results with either radical prostatectomy or radiation therapy alone are suboptimal, with biochemical control rates of less than 40% at 5 years.[9–12] We describe the innovations in radiation oncology that have been developed in an attempt to improve on these results via the use of dose escalation (using either external-beam radiation therapy [EBRT] or brachytherapy as a boost), whole pelvic radiation therapy (WPRT), and androgen suppression (AS).

Dose-escalated radiotherapy

Rationale

Although many patients with locally advanced prostate cancer develop metastatic disease as the first sign of failure, local control with standard radiotherapy is poor and intraprostatic tumor may serve as a reservoir for metastatic dissemination.[11,13] Coen et al analyzed 1469 patients treated with radiation therapy who had more than 2 years of follow-up data. Gleason score of 7 or more, PSA greater than 15 ng/mL, and T3/T4 stage predicted a higher incidence of distant failure. On multivariate analysis, local failure was the strongest predictor for distant metastasis, with 77% versus 61% distant metastasis-free survival at 10 years for patients with locally controlled versus uncontrolled disease.[14] Several retrospective studies of long-term data in patients treated with conventional techniques in the 1970s and 1980s describe a direct relationship between radiation dose and local control in men with locally advanced prostate cancer. Valicenti et al reviewed the data from Radiation Therapy Oncology Group (RTOG) phase III trials of EBRT, and on multivariate analysis found that a dose of more than 66 Gy significantly reduced the relative risk of prostate cancer-related death in men with Gleason scores of 8 to 10.[15] Data from the American College of Radiology Patterns of Care study on 624 patients with stage T3 disease revealed the actuarial 7-year local recurrence rate was 36% with doses of 60 to 64.9 Gy, 32% for 65 to 69.9 Gy, and 24% for 70 Gy and over.[16] Multivariate analysis of the MD Anderson experience in 1127 patients with stage T1 to T4 disease treated with radiotherapy from 1987 to 1997 found radiation dose to be an independent predictor of biochemical control in addition to pretreatment PSA, Gleason score, and palpable stage. The patients who benefited most from higher doses were those with pretreatment PSA greater than 10 ng/mL.[17]

The radiotherapy technique utilized in the majority of patients in these studies relied on estimations of prostate boundaries based on surrogate landmarks such as the pubic bones and rectal and bladder contrast media. The ability to escalate radiation dose to greater than 70 Gy with such conventional radiotherapy techniques was limited by rectal and bladder complications. In the Patterns of Care study, the rate of grade 3 or 4 complications increased from 3.5% to 6.9% when doses exceeding 70 Gy were delivered.[18] Smit et al reported up to 30% incidence of late proctitis after conventional prostate radiation therapy to 70 Gy, with the incidence of proctitis correlating with the maximum rectal dose.[19] Schultheiss et al attempted to identify factors predictive of late genitourinary (GU) and gastrointestinal (GI) morbidity in patients treated with doses above 65 Gy. Central axis dose was the only independent variable significantly related to the incidence of late GI morbidity.[20]

The past two decades have witnessed the development of innovative radiotherapy techniques including three-dimensional conformal radiation therapy (3DCRT), which utilizes computed tomography (CT)-based targeting as well as more sophisticated beam delivery and treatment plan assessment techniques. In conjunction with the development of 3DCRT, improvements in the accuracy of patient positioning and the quantitation of prostate motion have created the ability to more accurately as well as conformally target the shape and location of the prostate while minimizing treatment of surrounding tissues.[21] These benefits have resulted in the ability to decrease toxicity of treatment at iso-effective dose levels. A randomized trial of 64 Gy conventional radiotherapy versus similar doses delivered with 3DCRT demonstrated grade 1 or higher proctitis occurring in 37% of the 3DCRT group versus 56% of the conventional group ($P = 0.004$). Grade 2 proctitis was also significantly lower at 5% in the 3DCRT group versus 15% in the conventional group. There were no significant differences in bladder function after treatment between the groups.[22] A similar study by Koper et al utilizing doses of 66 Gy found a significant reduction in grade 2 GI toxicity with the use of 3DCRT compared to conventional techniques (19 versus 32%; $P = 0.02$). Again, there was similar grade 2 or higher GU toxicity between the arms, despite a significant reduction in bladder volumes treated in patients receiving 3DCRT.[23]

Trials

The combination of the enhanced therapeutic ratio of 3DCRT and evidence of a dose response effect in prostate cancer have led to clinical trials of dose escalated radiotherapy in an attempt to improve on the results seen with conventional treatment.

Long-term, 12-year follow-up of the initial Fox Chase dose escalation study cohort of 232 patients has been reported by Hanks. Doses ranged from 67 to 81 Gy, with median total dose (at the center of the prostate) being 74 Gy. The American Society for Therapeutic Radiology and Oncology (ASTRO) consensus definition of three consecutive rises in PSA was used to determine biologic no evidence of disease (bNED) status.[24] For purposes of analysis, patients were divided into six prognostic subgroups by pretreatment PSA, clinical stage, Gleason score, and presence of perineural invasion. Patients with pretreatment PSA levels of 10 to 20 ng/mL had statistically significant differences in bNED control when stratified by dose on univariate analysis. On multivariate analysis, radiation dose was a statistically significant predictor of bNED control for all patients and for unfavorable patients with a pretreatment PSA less than 10 ng/mL. No radiation dose response was seen for patients with pretreatment PSA greater than 20 ng/mL, but only 44 patients were in this group.

No difference was noted in the frequency of Grade 2 and 3 GU and Grade 3 GI morbidity when patients were stratified by radiation dose, although a significant increase in Grade 2 GI complications occurred as the dose increased.[25]

Pollack recently updated the Fox Chase experience, reporting on 839 patients treated to doses from 63 to 84 Gy (median 74 Gy) with a median follow-up of 63 months. Multivariate analysis found radiotherapy dose and pretreatment PSA to be the most significant factors prognostic for bNED survival, followed by Gleason score and T stage. Perineural invasion was no longer a significant predictor of PSA outcome. Within six prognostic groups, higher radiotherapy dose was significantly associated with outcome in all but the most favorable (PSA < 10 ng/mL and Gleason 2–6) and least favorable (PSA > 20 ng/mL and T3/T4) groups. However, there were only 22 patients available for analysis within the latter group. For patients with PSA over 20 ng/mL and T1/T2 clinical stage, dose was significant for bNED survival when analyzed by the Wilcoxon test.[26]

Preliminary results of a multi-institutional, prospective dose escalation study performed by a collaboration of French centers has been reported by Bey et al. Eligible patients had T1b-T3 disease: Gleason score and PSA were not criteria for study entry. Thirty-one percent of patients had stage T3 disease, and 9% had pretreatment PSA greater than 20 ng/ml. The inital cohort received 66 Gy prescribed to the center of the prostate, with subsequent cohorts receiving escalating doses to a maximum of 80 Gy. With mean follow-up time of 32 months, no statistical differences were observed in Grade 2 or higher GI or GU late toxicity between the 66–70 Gy vs. 74–80 Gy groups. The probabilty of achieving a post-treatment PSA nadir of 1 ng/ml or more was significantly greater in the 74–80 Gy group, and directly related to the dose of radiation given.

Investigators at Memorial Sloan-Kettering have also performed a dose-escalation trial using 3DCRT in patients with clinical stage T1–T3 disease. Doses were 64.8 to 75.6 Gy prescribed at the prostate periphery, with isocenter doses approximately 5% to 7% higher than the stated dose. Patients were stratified into three risk groups based on PSA level, Gleason score, and clinical stage. At 10 years, bNED survival (ASTRO definition) was significantly better with higher doses in all three risk groups. For intermediate risk patients, 10-year bNED survival was 50% in patients receiving 75.6 Gy, versus 42% in patients receiving 70.2 Gy ($P = 0.05$); for unfavorable risk patients, the corresponding rates were 42% versus 24% ($P = 0.04$). Grade 2 and grade 3 or higher rectal toxicity was 17% and 1.5%, respectively, while grade 2 and grade 3 or higher urinary toxicity were 15% and 2.5%.[28]

Cooperative group trial

Preliminary toxicity results of a prospective phase I/II 3DCRT dose-escalation study performed by the RTOG have been reported. RTOG 94-06 enrolled patients with T1–T3 tumors to sequentially escalated dose levels beginning at 68.4 Gy at 1.8 Gy per fraction, to 78 Gy at 2 Gy per fraction daily. Patients were grouped into three categories based on risk of seminal vesicle invasion greater than or less than 15% and presence of T3 disease. Patients with more than 15% risk of seminal vesicle involvement were treated to both prostate and seminal vesicles to 55.8 Gy, followed by a reduction in target volume to the prostate alone. Patients with T3 disease received the full dose to both prostate and seminal vesicles. Doses were prescribed as a minimum dose to a target volume. Michalski et al evaluated late effects in 424 patients treated on the first two dose levels of 68.4 Gy (level I) and 73.8 Gy (level II). Average months at risk after completion of therapy ranged from 21.4 to 40.1 months for patients on dose level I, and 10.0 to 34.2 months for patients on dose level II. The incidence of RTOG grade 2 or higher GU toxicity was 10% to 13%, and RTOG grade 2 or higher GI toxicity was 7% to 8%, with most toxicity occurring within the first 2 years after therapy. When compared with historical RTOG data derived from prior studies using pre-3DCRT techniques, the incidence of grade 3 or higher toxicity was reduced for all groups (despite the administration of higher doses), but this was associated with an increase in the rate of grade 1 complications. This resulted in an overall statistically significant increase in the number of patients with any late effects when compared with expected complications derived from the historical data. These data implied a reduction of higher grade toxicity occurred with the toxicity being shifted to lower grades, as well as an overall increase in low-grade toxicity presumably due to dose escalation.[29] Results in 173 patients with stage T1 and T2 disease treated on dose level III (79.2 Gy) have also been reported (T3 patients were excluded due to poor accrual). No patients experienced grade 3 or higher acute toxicity. The incidences of late grade 1 and 2 GU toxicity were 31% and 11%, respectively, while the rates of grade 1 and 2 GI toxicity were 24% and 7%. The overall rate of toxicity was comparable to previous dose levels. With a median follow-up of 3.3 years, 4 patients (2.4%) experienced grade 3 late toxicity, with 3 GU events and one related to the rectum. There were no grade 4 or 5 late complications. Again, comparison with historical controls revealed that the observed rate of grade 3 or higher late effects was significantly lower than expected.[30]

Randomized trials

In order to validate the hypothesis that dose escalation results in improved outcomes in prostate cancer, Shipley et al at the Massachusetts General Hospital carried out a phase III randomized study of dose escalation using proton beam irradiation as method of delivering higher doses to the prostate. Unlike the more commonly utilized photon beams, proton beams penetrate surrounding tissues depositing only a small amount of energy until they reach a specified distance, at which point the dose is delivered. This gives the ability to minimize doses to the tissues around the target. Currently, proton beam for routine clinical use is available at only two centers within the United States, although construction is underway at additional facilities. The study enrolled only patients with locally advanced (stages T3/T4) disease, randomizing them to either 67.2 Gy with conventional radiotherapy, or 75.6 Gy equivalent with the last 25.2 Gy delivered by proton beam. The trial was performed from 1982 to 1992, and, therefore, used older definitions of treatment effectiveness, namely disease-specific survival was defined as PSA less than 4 ng/mL, negative digital rectal exam, and negative rebiopsy (if performed). With a median follow-up of 61 months, there were no significantly differences in disease-specific survival, overall survival, or local control between the two arms. The only statistically significant benefit seen was in the planned subgroup analysis of patients with poorly differentiated tumors (Gleason 4 or 5 of 5), where the rates of local control were 19% versus 84% at 8 years (P = 0.0014). For the entire group, the incidence of grades 1 and 2 rectal bleeding was greater in the high dose arm (32 versus 12%; P = 0.002).[31] It must be noted that, due to stage migration from the widespread adoption of PSA screening, the patients treated in the era when this study was performed are significantly different from the majority of patients seen today, even within the same category of T3/T4 disease, and, therefore, the applicability of this study to current practice is uncertain.

A more contemporary dose-escalation study utilizing proton beam irradiation was recently reported by researchers at Massachusetts General Hospital and Loma Linda University. This study randomized 393 patients with stages T1b–T2b prostate cancer and PSA less than 15 ng/mL to either 19.8 GyE (photon Gy equivalents) or 28.8 GyE, followed by a 3DCRT dose of 50.4 Gy (total doses 70.2 GyE versus 79.2 GyE, respectively). Only 2% of patients receiving 70.2 GyE and 1.5% receiving 79.2 GyE had acute RTOG morbidity greater than grade 2. At a median follow-up of 4 years, the 5-year biochemical failure rate was significantly lower in the patients receiving higher dose radiation (19.1% versus 37.3%; P = 0.00001); this difference also held true when patients with intermediate risk disease were analyzed. The majority of the patients treated on this study had low- to intermediate-risk disease (only 8.4% had Gleason grade 8), but this study deserves mention because it strongly supports the concept of dose escalation in prostate cancer.[32]

Pollack et al have also performed a phase III randomized trial at the MD Anderson Cancer Center comparing 70 Gy versus 78 Gy radiotherapy using 3DCRT. A total of 305 patients with stage T1 to T3 tumors were treated using 2 Gy daily fractions prescribed to the isocenter; androgen ablation was not given as part of initial therapy. Treatment failure was defined by the ASTRO consensus definition or the initiation of salvage treatment. For the entire cohort, the freedom-from-failure (FFF) rates at 5 years were 64% and 70% for the 70 Gy and 78 Gy arms, respectively (P = 0.03). The patients who benefited most from the dose escalation were the subgroup with PSA greater than 10 ng/mL, where the FFF rates were 43% and 62% (P = 0.01). Within this subgroup there was also a significant difference in the rates of metastasis-free survival (98% versus 88%; P = 0.056), although no differences in overall survival were seen during the follow-up period to date. Among patients with stage T3 disease, there were also statistically significant differences in FFF (36% versus 61%; P = 0.047). The data did not indicate a difference in FFF for the patients with Gleason scores of 7 through 10, where FFF rates were 64% and 68%, respectively (P = 0.39). Although bladder toxicity was not increased in the high-dose group, there was an increase in the rate of grade 2 or higher late rectal toxicity with a significant, direct correlation between the extent of treated rectal volume and grade 2 or higher rectal toxicity. Among patients with detailed dose–volume histogram information available, 8 of 9 patients with grade 3 or higher rectal toxicity had more than 25% of rectum receiving at least 70 Gy, and the majority of grade 2 or higher rectal toxicity was also in patients with more than 25% of rectum receiving at least 70 Gy.[33,34]

Nonrandomized data for high-grade tumors

A retrospective analysis of a larger number of patients with high grade (Gleason 8–10) tumors is available from Roach et al at the University of California-San Francisco. Fifty patients with T1 to T4 clinical stage and median PSA of 22.7 ng/mL were treated with a variety of doses of external-beam radiation. Biochemical failure was defined as increase in PSA of 0.5 ng/mL per year, PSA level more than 1.0 ng/mL, or positive post-treatment biopsy. The overall actuarial probability of freedom from biochemical failure at 4 years was 23%. Multivariate analysis of all patients revealed pretreatment PSA to be the only predictor of PSA failure. In a multivariate analysis restricted to patients with PSA less than 20 ng/mL, 83% of those treated to more than 71 Gy were free of progression compared with none of those treated to lower doses (P = 0.03).[35] Fiveash et al reported on the combined results of a group of 180 patients treated at the University of Michigan, University of California-San Francisco, and Fox Chase Cancer Center. Patients had T1 to T4 N0 to Nx adenocarcinoma with a pretreatment PSA; 27% received adjuvant or neoadjuvant hormonal therapy. The total dose received was less than 70 Gy in 30%, 70 to 75 Gy in 37%, and more than 75 Gy in 33%. At a median follow-up of 3.0 years, the 5-year freedom from PSA failure was 62.5% for all patients and 79.3% in T1/T2 patients. Univariate analysis revealed T-stage, pretreatment PSA, and radiotherapy (RT) dose predictive of freedom from PSA failure. Univariate analysis of likelihood of 5-year overall survival revealed RT dose to be the only significant predictive factor. When Cox proportional hazards model was performed separate for T1/2 and T3/4 tumors, none of the prognostic factors achieved statistical significance for overall survival or freedom from biochemical progression in the T3/4 group, but lower RT dose and higher pretreatment PSA did predict for PSA failure within the T1/2 patients.[36]

In summary, the available randomized evidence suggests that dose escalation with 3DCRT results in significant improvements in PSA-defined disease control in patients with "intermediate-risk" prostate cancer. The impact on disease control in patients with higher risk features such as stage T3/T4, Gleason 8 to 10, and PSA greater than 20 ng/mL in these studies is unclear, although most suffer from low accrual within this subgroup. However, retrospective data suggest that patients with high-grade, low-stage tumors benefit from dose escalation. It remains to be seen whether these improvements will result in differences in overall survival. Only with very long-term follow-up will these differences become evident. While the use of 3DCRT results in improvements in toxicity profile compared to conventional radiotherapy, escalated doses with these techniques do seem to result in increased rectal toxicity, although mostly limited to grade 2 or less. Further study will allow for development of better estimates of late toxicity associated with higher doses, as well as agreement on what constitutes an acceptable level of toxicity.

The "next" technologic advancement beyond 3DCRT is intensity-modulated radiotherapy (IMRT). Compared with 3DCRT, IMRT gives the ability to create steeper dose gradients around the target, thereby reducing the volume of surrounding tissues receiving high doses of radiation. It also allows for even greater conformality of the treatment volume to the target. Since IMRT is a more recently developed technique than 3DCRT, there is less available data regarding clinical experience with dose escalation. However, it offers the possibility of reduced toxicity and thus dose escalation to even higher levels without concomitant increase in risk.[37] Investigators at Memorial Sloan-Kettering have reported 6-year results in a cohort of 171 patients with T1c to T3 prostate cancer treated with 81 Gy using IMRT. Doses were prescribed to the isodose line encompassing the target volume. Fifty-four percent of patients received neoadjuvant androgen deprivation therapy prior to radiation. The 6-year PSA relapse-free survival rates for favorable, intermediate, and unfavorable risk disease were 91%, 73%, and 64% using the ASTRO consensus definition. Notably, the 6-year likelihood of grade 2 rectal bleeding was 4%, and 1.1% of patients developed grade 3 rectal toxicity. The 6-year risk of grade 2 GU toxicity was 10%. There were no grade 4 toxicities. These results appear favorable when compared with the toxicity profiles described previously for 3DCRT treatment.[38]

Dose escalation via high-dose rate brachytherapy

The use of brachytherapy is another means by which it is possible to increase local dose to the prostate. Conformal high dose rate

brachytherapy (HDR) is an alternative means of dose escalation, which offers a potential advantage over EBRT in that a steep dose gradient between the prostate and adjacent normal tissues can be generated. Other theoretical advantages are the elimination of inter-and intrafraction motion of the prostate gland, random and systemic treatment setup errors, gland edema, and imprecise target localization.[39,40] Briefly, the technique utilizes catheters placed into the prostate under intraoperative transrectal ultrasound guidance. The catheters are subsequently attached to an afterloading unit that sequentially feeds a high-activity (iridum-192) source into predetermined positions within the catheters. The dwell times within each position can be adjusted, thus allowing for development of a treatment plan which optimally conforms to the target volume. Typically, the patient receives HDR in one to three fractions (separated by 4–6 hours) after each intraoperative catheter placement session, with the catheters remaining in place between fractions. Between one and three sessions may take place during a treatment course, either following or interdigitated with conformal EBRT.

There may be radiobiologic advantages to the use of large doses per HDR fraction. Traditionally, tumors have been considered to be less sensitive to large doses per fraction than normal tissues, and, therefore, delivering an increased number of fractions to the same total dose was associated with decreased normal tissue late effects. More recent analyses of clinical and laboratory data suggest that prostate cancer is more sensitive to large doses per fraction relative to normal tissues.[41,42] If true, this would also mean that iso-effective doses of hypofractionated HDR could be delivered with less acute toxicity than possible with smaller fractions.

One of the largest published experiences to date comes from Deger et al, who analyzed 230 patients with T2 (35%) and T3 (58%) tumors. The median PSA was 12.8 ng/mL; 60% and 16% of patients had Grade 2 and Grade 3 histologic grade, respectively. The mean time to PSA nadir was 15 months, and 47% of patients reached a nadir less than 0.5 ng/mL. The 5-year biochemical progression-free survival rate was 75% for T2 and 60% for T3 tumors. Following modifications to technique and a decrease in the HDR fractional dose to 9 Gy, complications were reported to decrease from 16.4% to a rate of 6.9%.[43]

Investigators at William Beaumont Hospital have described their experience in a dose escalation trial of HDR with EBRT in 207 patients with poor prognostic factors of PSA 10 ng/mL or higher, Gleason 7 or above, or clinical stage T2b or higher. No patient received hormonal therapy, and the ASTRO consensus definition was used for determining biochemical failure. Treatment consisted of EBRT 46 Gy to the prostate, with a total of two HDR treatments given during the first and third weeks of treatment. The majority of patients (57%) had T2b/T2c disease; 19.8% had Gleason 8 to 10 tumors, and most patients had pretreatment PSA between 4 and 10 ng/mL. At a mean follow-up of 4.7 years, the 5-year actuarial biochemical control rate was 74%. The 5-year biochemical control rate was 85% for one poor prognostic factor, 75% for two and 50% for all three. On Cox regression analysis, lower HDR dose and higher Gleason score were associated with biochemical failure.[44] Table 42.1 summarizes several institutional reports on HDR.

Due to the heterogeneity of patient groups treated in many of the reported experiences, it is difficult to draw conclusions about the efficacy of HDR relative to other treatments. However, the biochemical control rates appear favorable compared to historic results.[9–12] Given the comparably short median follow-up times, longer observation will be needed to better determine the incidence of late complications.

Table 42.1 Reports from several institutions on high dose rate brachytherapy (HDR)

Group	# Patients	T-Stage	Mean (median) PSA, ng/mL	Median FU, months	Biochem. control, %	HDR fractional dose, Gy	# Fractions	GU toxicity	GI Toxicity
William Beaumont	207	T1c–T3c	11.5	52.8	74 @ 5 yrs	5.5–11.5	2–3	8% late grade 3	1% late Grade 3-4
Seattle	104	T1b–T3c	(8.1)	45	84 @ 5 yrs	3–4	4	6.7% stricture	2% spotty bleeding
Kiel	144	T1b–T3	25.6	96	69 @ 8 yrs	9.0	2	2.1% late grade 3	4.1% late Grade 3
Goteburg	50	T1b–T3b	Not stated	45	78 @ 5 yrs	10	2	8% acute; 4% chronic dysuria	26% mild diarrhea, 8% moderate diarrhea
Berlin	230	T2–T3	(12.8)	40	T2: 75	9–10	2	10% frequency/dysuria @ 3 months	1.7% recto-urehtral fistula
Munich	40	T2–T3	40.7	74	79.5	9	2	5% prostate necrosis	2.5% recto-vesical fistula
Lahey Clinic	52	T1–T2	10.4	11.8	92.2	6	3	11% Grade 2	18% Grade 2
Long Beach	200	T1c–T3b	10	30	93 @ 25 months	5–6.5	3–4	10% acute grade 3–4	20% acute grade 3–4
Offenbach	102	T1–T3	(15.3)	31	82 @ 3 yrs	5–7	4	27% acute grade 2–3	8% Acute Grade 2
Gothenburg	214	T1–T3	(9.6)	48	Low risk 92 @ 5 yrs	10	2	6% urethral stricture	
Kawasaki, Japan	98	T1c–T3b	(11.7)	43	T1–T2 95.9 @ 5 yrs	6	4	29.6% cystourethritis or proctitis	29.6% cystourethritis or proctitis
California Endocurietherapy	491	T1c–T3b	Not stated	Not stated	Not stated	6	4	0.6% incontinence	0.2% rectal bleeding

FU, follow-up; PSA, prostate-specific antigen.

Dose escalation via permanent interstitial seed implantation

A similar means of performing dose escalation is by performing permanent interstitial seed implantation (low dose rate brachytherapy) in addition to EBRT. The vast majority of the low dose rate brachytherapy experiences reported have not included patients with high-risk disease due to concerns about extraprostatic involvement or microscopic systemic disease minimizing the impact of increased local dose. D'Amico et al retrospectively analyzed outcomes with radical prostatectomy, permanent interstitial seed implantation, or EBRT in 1872 men treated at two institutions. High-risk patients were defined as those with stage T2c or PSA greater than 20 ng/mL or Gleason score of 8 or above. Within the 590 patients in this category, those treated with seed implantation or seed implantation combined with AS had significantly inferior PSA outcomes compared with patients receiving radical prostatectomy or EBRT (relative risk of failure 3.0 and 3.1, respectively).[45] Potential criticisms of this study include the relatively small cohort of patients in the implant group and the fact that no EBRT was utilized as is more commonly practiced today. However, if improved disease control in locally advanced disease via dose escalation is a valid concept, then permanent interstitial implantation may offer a method of achieving safe dose escalation when used in addition to EBRT. Stock et al treated 139 patients with high-risk features (defined as Gleason score 8–10, PSA 20 ng/mL, stage T2b, or positive seminal vesicle biopsy) with 9 months of AS, seed implantation, and 45 Gy EBRT. Negative laparoscopic pelvic lymph node dissections were performed in 44% of patients. At 5 years, the actuarial overall freedom from PSA failure rate was 86%. Post treatment prostate biopsies performed in 47 patients were negative in 100% at last biopsy.[46] Sylvester et al reported results of combined EBRT and seed implantation in 232 patients and evaluated the subset of high-risk patients as defined by the D'Amico risk criteria (Gleason 8–10, PSA > 20 ng/mL, or stage T2c).[8] The 10-year biochemical relapse-free survival in these patients was 48%.[47] Dattoli et al reported results using 41 Gy EBRT followed by palladium-101 (^{101}Pd) seed implantation in a more favorable group of patients (Gleason 7 and/or PSA > 10 ng/mL). The 10-year freedom from biochemical progression rate was 79% using a strict PSA failure criteria of a nadir greater than 0.2 ng/mL.[48] These results may come at a cost of increased morbidity compared with brachytherapy alone. Brandeis et al prospectively evaluated quality of life following combined modality therapy or seed implantation alone, and found urinary, bowel, and sexual function as well as American Urological Association symptom score to be all statistically worse in patients receiving combined treatment.[49] Others have not found combined modality treatment to be more toxic than seed implantation alone.[50]

Androgen deprivation therapy

In conjunction with radiation in locally advanced prostate cancer

Human prostate cancer cells vary in their in-vitro sensitivity to both acute radiation (like that delivered as EBRT) and low dose rate radiation (like that used in prostate brachytherapy). The radiosensitivity does not appear to be dependent on p53 status or the ability of the cell to initiate G1 cell cycle arrest—both previously thought to be important to radiation response. These studies also do not reveal dependence on androgen responsiveness.[51] Androgen-responsive prostate cells undergo programmed cell death (apoptosis) when deprived of androgens.[52,53] Like radiation, this death does not seem to be p53-dependent.[52] Several authors have performed in-vivo analyses of radiation combined with androgen deprivation on androgen-responsive tumors of both prostate and nonprostate origin.[54,55] None of these studies have conclusively demonstrated synergy between radiation and androgen deprivation but do suggest that timing of the androgen deprivation may be critical. In one study of androgen withdrawal in the Shionogi breast tumor model, Zietman et al found that a lower dose of radiation was required to control 50% of the tumors if androgens were used in combination with radiation. Specifically, animals treated with radiation following maximal androgen withdrawal-mediated tumor regression required 42.1 Gy of radiation to control 50% of the tumors compared with 89.0 Gy in animals treated with radiation only. The most direct interpretation of these data is that following androgen withdrawal, there is a smaller number of tumor clonogens for the radiation to eradicate.

As early as 1967, hormonal therapy was being added to radiation therapy in an attempt to modify the outcome of patients with stage C (T3) prostate cancer.[56] Historically, the rationale for the treatment of these patients was based on the knowledge that these patients had an inferior outcome compared with patients with earlier stage prostate cancer treated with radiation therapy. In addition, these T3 tumors were quite large, and it was thought that a course of cytoreductive therapy might provide a more favorable geometry for external irradiation, as well as reduce tumor burden.[57]

In the early 1980s, two institutional series reported encouraging results with the use of AS and EBRT in this group of patients.[57,58] Pilepich et al also found that patients with histologically unfavorable lesions who had been treated on the Radiation Therapy Oncology Group (RTOG) 75-06 trial receiving AS and EBRT had a similar disease-free survival and overall survival as patients with more favorable tumors who did not receive the AS.[59] In part, these studies provided the basis for the next series of RTOG phase II studies designed to test the efficacy of combined EBRT and AS, with the hypothesis that preradiation cytoreduction as well as concomitant radiation- and AS-induced cell death would improve local control in patients with locally advanced prostate tumors.[60,61] Based on this experience, RTOG study 86-10 was initiated.[62] This was a randomized, phase III trial of EBRT alone (standard treatment arm) versus neoadjuvant and concomitant total androgen suppression (TAS) and EBRT (experimental treatment arm). Eligible patients were those with bulky, locally advanced tumors (>25 cm²), stage T2b to T4, N0 to N1, M0. Those patients randomized to receive TAS were treated with goserelin acetate 3.6 mg every 28 days and flutamide 250 mg t.i.d. for 2 months prior to the start of radiation and during radiation therapy. A total of 471 patients were enrolled and randomized to one of the two treatment arms. Analysis of this series revealed that those patients treated with TAS and radiation had a statistically significant improvement in local control at 5 years compared with those patients treated with radiation only ($P < 0.001$). An update of this study at a median follow-up of 6.7 years for all patients and 8.6 years for patients who were still alive continued to show statistically significant differences in local control (42% versus 30%), biochemical disease-free survival (24% versus 10%), and cause-specific mortality (23% versus 31%). Subset analysis indicated a preferential effect in patients with Gleason score 2 to 6, where there was a significant difference in overall survival between the arms (70% versus 52%).[63] To date, there is no difference in the overall survival of the two groups of patients. This may have several possible explanations. It is possible that there may not be an overall survival benefit to patients when TAS is added to EBRT in this fashion and/or this patient population. However, it is important to note that this study was limited in that it did not routinely collect serum PSA on all patients prior to entry, a parameter that is now recognized to be an extremely important prognostic factor and indicator of disease extension. Therefore, there likely were a large number of patients with elevated serum PSA in the range frequently associated with a high risk of micrometastatic disease. The study also included patients with node-positive disease, also recognized as a poor risk factor, and one in which the value of any treatment modality to overall survival can be debated. Nonetheless, this is an important study, performed in a rigorous fashion, revealing important and measurable benefit with the addition of AS to radiation therapy for this high-risk group of patients.

A concurrent study, the RTOG 85-31, trial compared EBRT alone with EBRT followed by adjuvant goserelin indefinitely for patients with clinical or pathologic stage T3 or node-positive prostate cancer. At a median follow-up of 6 years, investigators reported statistically significant differences in rates of local failure (23% versus 37%), distant metastasis (27% versus 37%), and disease-free survival (36% versus 25%). However, these differences did not translate into improvements in cause-specific or overall survival for the cohort as a whole. In contrast to RTOG 86-10, subset analysis did reveal that patients with Gleason 8 to 10 tumors who had not undergone prostatectomy received a significant improvement in absolute survival with the addition of immediate and long-term goserelin ($P = 0.036$).[64]

Bolla et al have published a long-term analysis of the EORTC 22863 trial.[65] This phase III trial enrolled 415 patients with stage T3/T4 any grade, or stage T1/T2 WHO grade 3, prostate cancer with no evidence of nodal or metastatic disease. Patients were randomized to receive either EBRT alone (control arm) or AS plus EBRT (experimental arm). Androgen suppression consisted of oral cyproterone acetate (50 mg t.i.d.) for 4 weeks prior to radiation and an luteinizing hormone releasing hormone (LHRH) agonist started on the first day of radiation and continued every month for 3 years. A total of 401 patients were analyzed with a median follow-up of 66 months. The 5-year locoregional recurrence-free survival was 98% in the experimental arm versus 84% in the control arm ($P < 0.001$), and clinical relapse-free survival 74% in the experimental arm versus 40% in the control arm ($P < 0.001$). There was also a difference in favor of AS in the 5-year incidence of distant metastases (29% versus 9.8%; $P < 0.0001$). Most significantly, this study was the first to report that there was an overall survival advantage with the addition of AS to radiation with an estimated 5-year survival of 78% in the experimental arm versus 62% in the control arm ($P = 0.001$). It still remains to be determined whether the intriguing results generated in the EORTC 22863 trial regarding improved overall survival using 3 years of adjuvant AS are reproducible and broadly applicable.

A more recent study from Harvard is the only other trial to demonstrate an overall survival advantage with the addition of AS to EBRT. This was a phase III randomized study comparing 70 Gy of 3DCRT alone versus 3DCRT and 6 months of LHRH agonist and flutamide. Eligible patients had PSA of at least 10 ng/mL, Gleason score of 7 or higher, or radiographic evidence of extraprostatic disease. Patients also underwent cardiac stress testing prior to enrollment to rule out competing causes of mortality. Although the majority of these patients had "intermediate-risk" disease, 13% had PSA values of 20 to 40 ng/mL, and 64% had Gleason score of 7 or higher. Patients who developed biochemical failure (PSA > 1.0 ng/mL with two consecutive PSA) received salvage AS when PSA reached approximately 10 ng/mL. The trial was stopped after interim analysis at median follow-up of 4.5 years revealed an overall survival benefit in favor of the AS arm (5-year survival 88% versus 78%, $P = 0.04$).[66]

Duration of treatment

The EORTC series and others raise several significant issues. One in particular concerns the optimum duration of androgen deprivation administration. Although results of the EORTC study and RTOG 85-31 suggest that long-term AS may be beneficial for disease control, prolonged AS has been associated with other causes of patient morbidity including osteopenia, anemia, muscle wasting, and impotence.[67] These toxicities are especially worthy of consideration given that patients treated for prostate cancer tend to be older.

The study by Laverdiere et al provided important information in this regard. In this study, patients with stage T2a to T4 disease were randomized to receive either EBRT alone, 3 months of neoadjuvant AS (LHRH-agonist plus flutamide) followed by EBRT, or 3 months of TAS then AS plus EBRT followed by another 6 months of adjuvant AS. Interestingly, the addition of 3 months of TAS prior to radiation reduced the two year positive prostate biopsy rate from 65% (radiation only) to 28%. Those patients receiving neoadjuvant, concomitant and adjuvant TAS and radiation had only a 5% positive prostate biopsy rate. These data would seem to confirm the idea that a more protracted course of AS is important, at least in terms of local control. While impressive, the length of follow-up is too short to determine if the addition of AS to radiation has made any significant impact on other meaningful endpoints such as disease-free survival (DFS) or overall survival.[68] In contrast to the above results, Laverdiere et al. have also reported an analysis based on patients with T2-T3 disease enrolled in 2 studies of AS with EBRT, including the study described above. The second study randomized patients to neoadjuvant and concomitant AS (total 5 months) versus neoadjuvant, concomitant and short-course adjuvant (total 10 months) AS; both groups received EBRT. At a median follow-up of 5 years, there was a significant advantage in bNED survival rate with the addition of neoadjuvant and concomitant AS, but no advantage with the addition of short-course adjuvant AS after EBRT.[69]

The RTOG has also performed a phase III randomized study (RTOG 92-02) to ascertain the benefit of prolonged AS following neoadjuvant and concomitant AS with EBRT. Patients with locally advanced (T2c–T4) prostate cancers with PSA of less than 150 ng/mL received 4 months of goserelin and flutamide, 2 months before and 2 months during RT. A dose of 65 to 70 Gy was given to the prostate, and 44 to 50 Gy to the pelvic lymph nodes. Randomization was between no additional AS therapy following completion of RT, versus 24 months of additional goserelin; 1554 patients entered the study. The 5-year rate of biochemical DFS was 46.4% versus 28.1% in the long-term and short-term AS arms, respectively ($P < 0.0001$). The long-term AS arm showed significant improvement in all end points except overall survival (80% versus 78.5% at 5 years, $P = 0.73$), although an unplanned subset analysis revealed a significant survival benefit for patients with Gleason 8 to 10 tumors as determined by the institution (but not on central pathology review). Despite a statistically significant reduction in the rate of prostate cancer-related deaths in the long-term arm (38% versus 24%, $P = 0.001$), there was an absolute increase in the number of deaths as a result of other causes, resulting in a similar rate of overall survival. Cardiovascular disease at the time of enrollment was more prevalent in the patients treated on the long-term arm (55% versus 44%, respectively), but a detrimental effect of long-term AS therapy on other causes of death cannot be excluded.[70]

Other data also suggest that the benefit of long-term AS may be greater in patients with high Gleason scores. Roach et al analyzed patients enrolled on five randomized RTOG studies that treated patients with radiotherapy and AS. Patients with stage T3 disease, nodal involvement, or Gleason 7 grade had a disease-specific survival benefit with the addition of 4 months of goserelin and flutamide, whereas patients with Gleason 8 to 10 disease or multiple high-risk factors had an approximately 20% higher survival at 8 years with the use of up-front, long-term hormonal therapy.[71] However, it is unclear how much of this conclusion overlaps with that from RTOG 85-31, since it was included in the analysis. Another re-analysis of RTOG data comes from Horwitz et al, who assessed the benefit of long-term versus short-term androgen deprivation in studies 85-31 and 86-10. The benefit in bNED control, distant metastasis-free survival, and cause-specific survival from long-term AS was limited to those patients with centrally reviewed Gleason score of 7 to 10; multivariate analysis demonstrated Gleason score and the use of long-term AS to be independent predictors for all three outcome measures.[72]

Related data comes from a number of surgical series investigating the use of AS therapy prior to radical prostatectomy. Several of these series have shown reduction in the positive margin rate, inferring AS-induced cell death. Relevant to this discussion is that a longer course of AS (i.e., 8 months) resulted in the greatest reduction in serum PSA, and only a 12% incidence of positive surgical margins compared with 23% in the 3-month AS arm.[73]

While these data are not conclusive and the studies assess differing endpoints, they provide some useful information. Taken together, they would seem to support the theory that a longer course of AS may very well lead to improved locoregional control of large tumors or high-risk tumors that possess an elevated risk of extraprostatic extension. However, although differences have been shown in biochemical and clinical disease control, so far there is no demonstrated overall survival advantage of prolonged versus short-course AS.

Sequencing of androgen deprivation and radiation therapy

The question of optimal sequencing of AS and radiation is similarly unanswered. As will be discussed later, it is not clear whether the effects of AS on tumor control are merely additive to the tumoricidal effects of radiation or whether they are synergistic, providing an enhancement of tumor killing that cannot be simply explained by the killing of each modality individually.

In order to assess the importance of AS timing in relation to EBRT, the RTOG performed a phase III trial (RTOG 94-13) where patients were randomized to either 2 months of neoadjuvant AS followed by AS and EBRT (control arm) or EBRT followed by 4 months of adjuvant AS.[74] Patients were also randomized in a 2×2 factorial design to receive WPRT versus prostate-only radiation. Eligibility included localized prostate cancer with risk of lymph node involvement of 15% or more (based on an equation using pretreatment PSA, Gleason score, and stage).[75] At a median follow-up of 59 months, patients treated with neoadjuvant and concomitant AS experienced a similar 4-year progression-free survival compared with those receiving adjuvant AS (52% versus 49%; $P = 0.56$). However, the group that received WPRT and neoadjuvant and concomitant AS had a significantly improved progression-free survival rate compared with the other three arms (60% versus 44–50%; $P = 0.008$). Further information regarding the most effective duration of neoadjuvant treatment will be provided by RTOG 99-10, which randomized patients to either 6 months or 2 months of neoadjuvant AS followed by concurrent AS and radiation.

Alteration of toxicity

In addition to improved tumor control, androgen deprivation therapy adds its own side-effect profile but may also alter possible radiation-induced side effects. In the randomized study by D'Amico et al, patients receiving AS with 3DCRT had statistically significant increases in grade 3 impotence (26% versus 21%) as well as gynecomastia, but no other significant differences in late toxicity were noted in this trial.[66] In contrast, Chen et al found no significant differences in 1-year potency rates between men receiving 3DCRT with AS versus 3DCRT alone, and patients treated in RTOG 86-10 had no differences in frequency or time to return of sexual potency.[63,76]

Reductions in prostatic volume after neoadjuvant AS can result in smaller treatment fields and consequent reductions in the amount of surrounding normal tissue that is secondarily irradiated. Reduction in the volume of irradiated rectum, for example, is associated with a significant decrease in long-term rectal injury.[77] Comparisons of dose–volume histograms from 3DCRT plans generated on patients pre- and post-neoadjuvant AS reveal a median reduction in prostate volume of 27% to 42%. This was also correlated with a decrease in the amount of irradiated rectum, bladder, and bowel.[78–80] Despite this expected benefit of AS, most studies do not support such a hypothesis. Late grade 1 to 3 incontinence was increased within the combined therapy group in the Bolla study (29% versus 16%; $P = 0.002$).[81] In a retrospective analysis by Sanguineti et al, rectal dose and the use of adjuvant AS were both significantly associated with higher risk of late rectal toxicity. The 2-year estimates of grade 2 to 4 late rectal toxicity were 30.3% versus 14.1% in patients receiving or not receiving AS, respectively.[82] The RTOG 94-13 study found the acute and 2-year rates of late grade 3 or higher GU/GI toxicity to be higher on the arm receiving whole pelvic EBRT with neoadjuvant and concomitant AS, but these differences did not reach statistical significance.[74] Valicenti et al compared toxicity rates in patients enrolled in RTOG 94-06, where approximately half of men received neoadjuvant AS (with variable dose levels of radiation). On univariate analysis, AS significantly increased the incidence of grade 2 acute GU complications, but was not significant in the multivariate analysis when volume of bladder treated was taken into account. The use of AS did increase risk of acute GU effects in men with preexisting obstructive symptoms.[83] Long-term AS may increase toxicity in and of itself. In RTOG 92-02, there was a small but statistically significant increase in the frequency of late grade 3 to 5 GI toxicity in the long-term compared with the short-term AS arm (2.6% versus 1.2% at 5 years; $P = 0.037$), although there is no clear explanation for this difference.[70]

The combination of AS and EBRT for the treatment of locally advanced prostate cancer results in an apparent increase in local control and disease-free survival as supported by several prospective, randomized trials. There are conflicting data from such trials as to the benefit in overall survival, and the most favorable duration as well as timing of AS in relation to radiation is not yet known. These are important questions to answer because of the potential added toxicity of AS, especially when administered long-term. Besides the well-recognized side effects of AS such as hot flashes and decreased libido, there are other important physiologic changes that occur with long-term use, including anemia, loss of muscle mass, decreased bone density, and depression.[67] Consideration of these potentially limiting side effects is required before instituting therapy.

Whole pelvic radiation therapy for occult nodal metastasis

A significant proportion of patients with locally advanced prostate cancer will have clinically occult pelvic lymph node spread. The primary nodes at risk for involvement include the external iliac, hypogastric, presacral, and obturator nodes.[84] Theoretically, treatment of these nodal areas in patients with meaningful risk of nodal involvement might be of therapeutic benefit if sufficient doses of radiation are given to eradicate microscopic tumor.

Partin et al developed predictive nomograms for lymph node involvement as well as other surgical findings based on multi-institutional data from radical prostatectomy specimens. Using these tables, it is possible to estimate the risk of lymph node involvement based on a patient's preoperative Gleason score, clinical stage, and PSA.[85] Roach et al developed an equation that estimates the risk of lymph node involvement based on the Partin tables[86]:

$$\text{Lymph node risk} = \{2/3\}\ \text{PSA} + ([\text{Gleason score} - 6] \times 10) \qquad [42.1]$$

The true incidence of nodal involvement is most likely underestimated in data based on surgical series, due to the inherent false-negative rate of lymph node dissections as typically performed in modern surgical practice. Heidenreich et al compared results in patients with similar risk characteristics undergoing extended pelvic lymphadenectomy versus standard pelvic lymphadenectomy. The incidence of lymph node detection was significantly higher in the extended lymphadenectomy group (26% versus 12%), and 42% of nodal metastases in the extended lymphadenectomy group were outside of areas dissected in a standard pelvic lymphadenectomy, including external iliac and obturator nodes. All except one patient with lymph node involvement had PSA greater than 10.5 ng/mL and Gleason score of 7 or higher.[87] Therefore, a larger proportion of patients may benefit from pelvic nodal irradiation than might be estimated by using the Partin nomograms.

Several retrospective, single institutional analyses have shown conflicting results as to the benefit of WPRT. Some of these studies are flawed by the fact that they are from the pre-PSA era, making the determination of patients at risk of nodal involvement as well as evaluation of treatment efficacy more difficult. They also suffer from low patient numbers and use of dated radiotherapy techniques.[88–90] However, some studies did find a benefit to the use of larger treatment fields that encompassed pelvic nodal areas.[91] Ploysongsang et al reported statistically significant improvements in 5-year survival rates amongst stage B and stage C patients receiving WPRT in comparison with stage-matched controls treated to prostate only.[92] Seaward et al analyzed a group of 506 patients treated at the University of California San Francisco who had a 15% or greater risk of nodal involvement (based on the Roach equation: Eq. 101.1). The median biochemical progression-free survival was significantly higher (34 months versus 21 months; $P = 0.0001$) in patients who received initial WPRT followed by prostate boost as opposed to prostate only radiation.[93]

Three randomized trials have been performed to evaluate the benefit of WPRT. Bagshaw reported a series of 57 patients with surgically staged, node-negative prostate cancer who were randomized to either WPRT and prostate boost versus prostate-only radiotherapy. Although the disease-free survival was improved with the use of WPRT, the results were not statistically significant, possibly due to the small sample size.[94] The RTOG has reported results of two randomized studies performed to date on the value of WPRT in

prostate cancer. RTOG 77-06 evaluated WPRT in patients with stage A2 and stage B prostate cancer with no evidence of lymph node involvement on lymphangiogram or biopsy. Randomization was to either 65 Gy to the prostate alone or to 45 Gy WPRT with 20 Gy prostatic boost. At a median follow-up of 7 years, there was no beneficial effect of WPRT on local control, distant metastases, disease-free or overall survival.[95] Given that the patients on this study were at low risk of lymph node involvement, it is inconclusive in determining whether patients at moderate to high risk of nodal metastasis benefit from WPRT.

As discussed above in the section on AS, RTOG 94-13 also looked at the role of WPRT in patients with either risk of nodal involvement of 15% or greater (based on the Roach equation: Eq. 42.1) or with T2c to T4 disease; the maximum allowable pre-treatment PSA was 100 ng/mL. Whole pelvic radiation therapy was associated with a 4-year progression-free survival of 54%, compared with 47% in the arms treated with prostate-only radiation. Interestingly, when comparing all four treatment arms there was a progression-free survival advantage for WPRT plus neoadjuvant/concurrent AS compared with the other arms (60% versus 44–50%; $P = 0.008$). No overall survival differences were seen.[74]

The positive results in this study for WPRT may be attributed to the use of AS in addition to WPRT, which has been shown to be synergistic with radiation.[54] The optimal dose of WPRT associated with durable control of microscopic nodal disease has not been determined, but doses beyond 50 to 55 Gy have not been utilized due to the limited radiation tolerance of small bowel which is often in whole pelvic radiotherapy fields. In a retrospective analysis on 963 patients performed by Perez et al, patients receiving whole pelvic doses of 50 to 55 Gy had fewer pelvic failures compared with those receiving 40 to 45 Gy ($P = 0.07$). A statistically significant reduction in pelvic failures was noted in stage C poorly differentiated tumors when the pelvic nodes received doses greater than 50 Gy compared with lower doses (23% versus 46%; $P = 0.01$).[96] In RTOG 94-13, the addition of AS to an otherwise modest dose of radiation may have allowed the WPRT to cross a threshold of efficacy.

Another factor that may enhance the benefit of WPRT is the use of CT-based treatment planning, which allows for better targeting of lymphatic regions at risk. The "standard" 4-field pelvic radiation portal as practiced in the conventional radiotherapy era (including RTOG 94-13) often underdosed or missed portions of at-risk nodal chains entirely. With CT, the location of the pelvic vasculature can be used as approximations of the lymph node locations, with margin added to cover the associated lymph nodes.[97,98]

Conclusions

Radiation therapy is the current standard of care for patients with locally advanced prostate cancer. The addition of AS to EBRT results in increased local control and disease-free survival, and data are emerging to show an improvement in overall survival as well. The optimal sequencing and duration of AS when combined with radiotherapy remains to be determined, and considerations must be made for the impact of prolonged AS on overall health and quality of life. The use of dose-escalated radiotherapy using modern treatment planning and delivery techniques results in increased biochemical control rates in patients with "intermediate-risk" disease, but further study is needed regarding its impact on patients with "high-risk" prognostic features. The use of WPRT combined with

AS in patients at meaningful risk of lymph node involvement is now supported by prospective randomized data. Finally, radiotherapy delivered either by external beam or radioisotope remains an important adjunct in the management of patients with metastatic prostate cancer, especially in the palliation of bony metastases.

Radiation therapy in the treatment of metastatic prostate cancer

Background

Fortunately, relatively few men now present with metastatic disease. According to Jemal et al, currently, only 6% of men present at the time of diagnosis with distant metastases, whereas between 1984 and 1990, up to 25% of men presented with distant metastases.[99,100] Unfortunately, a number of men who are diagnosed with prostate cancer and receive definitive therapy for their disease still ultimately progress to and die of metastatic cancer. A recent study from a large Midwestern hospital found that 8.9% of a cohort of 2056 patients had metastatic progression at a mean follow-up of 3.6 years.[101] Another study found that after 21 years of follow-up for patients who underwent an observational approach for T0 to T2 disease, 17% of patients experienced metastatic disease.[102] Pound et al reported that up to one quarter of men who demonstrated biochemical recurrence after prostatectomy had a recurrence after 5 years.[103]

Prostate cancer has a proclivity to spread to bone, causing predominantly osteoblastic metastases with frequent components of osteosclerosis. Hematogenous dissemination of prostate cancer cells tends to favor the axial skeleton, where red marrow is abundant, likely because blood flow to these areas is high.[104] In a meta-analysis of autopsies of 1589 patients who died of prostate cancer from 1967 to 1995, it was found that hematogenous metastases were present in one third of patients. The site of most frequent involvement was bone (90%), followed by lung (46%), liver (25%), pleura (21%), and adrenals (13%).[105] The previously held concept that Batson's venous plexus acts as a direct conduit of spread of prostate cancer[106] was disproved in a study that analyzed the distribution of bone metastases using technicium-99 whole-body scans. The distribution of metastases in patients with prostate cancer were largely identical to those of patients with other cancers, and one quarter of prostate cancer patients had lesions exclusively outside of the pelvis, sacrum or lumbar spine.[107] A more contemporary theory is that tumors with propensity to metastasize to bone possess the ability to not only survive but also proliferate and colonize in bone and bone marrow.[108] It has been shown that tumor cells produce cell adhesion molecules that allow them to bind to and penetrate bone marrow sinusoids.[109] Bone also harbors inactive but multiple important growth factors, which are thought to support metastatic cell deposit growth.[110] In turn, the presence of tumor cells causes reactions of bone destruction and new bone formation, and the resulting products from bone resorption may act as chemoattractants for more tumor cells.[111–114] Prostate-specific antigen, a serine protease with trypsin-like activity, has also been implicated in the development of prostate cancer bone metastases. It has been shown to be a protease for insulin-like growth factor binding protein, a molecule that can inhibit the osteoblastic activity of insulin-like growth factors.[115,116]

Patients who experience bone metastases may suffer from pain, fractures, and spinal cord compression (Figure 42.1), all of which may require hospitalization, affect patient functionality and independence, and contribute to increased healthcare costs.[117] Many patients with bone metastases will develop other medical complications or become bed-ridden. Not surprisingly, the presence of skeletal metastases is associated with a significant reduction in quality of life.[118]

Clinical assessment of bone metastases

Any patient with a diagnosis of prostate cancer who presents with new complaints of bone pain must have a full history and physical exam performed. Important components of the history of review include the patient's disease status (last PSA, androgen sensitivity, and prior treatments) and pain characteristics such as onset, location, duration, radiation, and alleviating or exacerbating factors. Metastatic bone pain may have an insidious and nonspecific onset and typically increases in severity at a focal or referred location over weeks to months. However, a pathologic fracture may cause acute pain, and spinal cord compression may present with acute onset of pain with paresthesias, weakness, or bladder or bowel incontinence. The pain is most typically somatic in nature. The differential diagnosis of bone pain should include nonmalignant causes such as arthritis, muscle strain or spasm, hyperparathyroidism, or osteopenic vertebral body collapse.

A general physical examination should be performed, including palpation and percussion of the painful sites and full neurologic exam. Laboratory data should be obtained including serum PSA (although poorly differentiated prostate cancer may not produce PSA) and

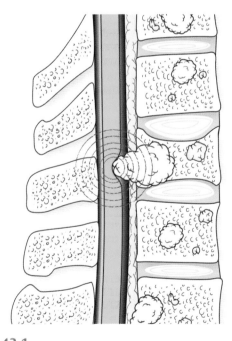

Figure 42.1
Spinal cord compression resulting from metastatic involvement of the spine by prostate cancer may require treatment by radiotherapy.

alkaline phosphatase. Occasionally urinary hydroxyproline, a collagen metabolite, can also be useful.

Radiographic assessment of a patient with presumed bone metastases should include a radionuclide bone scan to evaluate the presence and distribution of metastases. Plain X-rays are useful in evaluating a specific, symptomatic area or as part of further evaluation of a lesion seen by bone scan, but are generally less sensitive than bone scans for detecting new, metastatic foci of disease. X-rays do, however, remain particularly helpful in evaluating a bone risk for the risk of pathologic fracture and whether prophylactic fixation is required.

Radiation therapy for palliation of bone metastases

For patients with hormone-naive metastatic disease, initial management with AS will often provide substantial symptom relief.[119] However, patients may present with pain not completely alleviated by AS, or may develop painful metastases in the setting of androgen-unresponsive disease. Focal EBRT is a well-established modality for palliation of bone pain occurring in one or several sites. Studies have shown that up to 90% of patients receiving EBRT for painful bony metastases obtain some degree of pain relief, and more than half of patients experience complete pain relief.[120,121]

The mechanism of the pain-modulating effects of EBRT are not well elucidated and not completely explained by reduction in tumor size, as pain relief may be rapid and precede the onset of tumor response.[122] The goals of palliative radiotherapy are to alleviate pain, prevent pathologic fracture, and improve quality of life by increasing mobility and functional status. Also, patients experiencing side effects from large doses of opioids may be treated with EBRT in order to minimize pain medication requirements. Acute morbidities related to skeletal radiation are usually modest and can include local erythema, lowered blood counts, and tiredness. Nausea and vomiting can occur if the abdomen is in the treatment portal, but effective prophylaxis is achievable with antiemetic agents.[123] No significant differences have been noted in the toxicities associated with single fraction or multifraction regimens. Pathologic fractures occur in approximately 5% of patients, probably due to unresponsive or recurrent disease.[129,131]

External-beam radiation therapy fractionation schedules for bone metastases

Controversy surrounds the optimal dose and fractionation schedule for palliating bone metastases with radiation. RTOG 74-02 was an early, randomized clinical trial that assessed the difference in pain relief among various fractionation schemes in 1000 patients. The fractionation schemes were 40.5 Gy in 15 fractions versus 20 Gy in 5 fractions for solitary metastases, and 30 Gy in 10 fractions versus 25 Gy in 5 fractions for multiple metastases. All of the schedules appeared equally effective in initially alleviating pain, but patients receiving higher doses of radiation appeared to have better outcome with less need for re-treatment and less narcotic use.[120,124] Twice daily treatment done three times per week (2 Gy per fraction) was

found to have no advantage over conventional schedules of 30 Gy in 15 fractions and 22.5 Gy in 5 fractions.[125] Therefore, most palliative fractionation schemes appear reasonable and have a high probability of achieving adequate pain relief.[126–129]

Single fraction versus multiple fraction regimens

In a trial from the UK, 765 patients with painful skeletal metastases were randomly assigned to receive either 8 Gy in a single fraction, 20 Gy in 5 fractions, or 30 Gy in 10 fractions and were followed for 1 year after treatment. Overall survival at 12 months was 44%, and no survival differences were seen among the three groups. There were no differences in time to first improvement in pain, with more than 50% of patients achieving pain relief by 1 month after the start of treatment, time to complete pain relief with a two-thirds chance of having no pain by one year, or time to first increase in pain up to 12 months from EBRT. Re-treatment was twice as common after 8 Gy than after multifraction radiotherapy, but may have been due to a greater readiness to prescribe additional radiotherapy after a single fraction.[130]

In the Dutch Bone Metastases Study, 1171 patients were randomized to receive either 8 Gy in one fraction or 24 Gy in six fractions. A median survival of 7 months was observed. Seventy one percent of patients experienced a response at some time during the first year. No difference between the two groups were found with regard to pain medication, quality of life, and side effects. Re-treatment was needed in 25% of the 8 Gy group and 7% of the 24 Gy group. More pathologic fractures also were observed in the single fraction group.[131] Both the Dutch and British multicenter trials reaffirmed the palliative benefit both of single and fractionated schedules but suggested that re-treatment was required more frequently with single dose EBRT.

A large North American trial, RTOG 97-14, has also investigated the question of single (8 Gy in one fraction) versus multiple (30 Gy in 10 fractions) fractions in the palliative management of painful prostate and breast cancer bone metastases and enrolled 949 patients. Preliminary results at 3 months follow-up has demonstrated no difference in partial or complete pain relief between the two groups (65% versus 66%), and one-third no longer required narcotic medications.[132] Quality-of-life analyses showed little differences between the two treatment arms. The increased utility in changes of emotion in the 30 Gy arm was hypothesized to be due to a benefit from increased social support gained with longer treatment time.[133]

Two meta-analyses, each evaluating over 3000 patients, showed that re-irradiation rates were consistently different between low-dose and high-dose arms, with more frequent re-irradiation required in the lower dose arms. No dose response relationships could be detected.[134] Re-treatment rates and pathologic fracture rates were higher with single fraction EBRT compared with multifraction EBRT (21%, 3% versus 7.4%, 1.6%). Both single and multifraction EBRT were effective in achieving pain relief.[135] Single-fraction EBRT was found to be most cost-effective palliative treatment when compared with pain medication, chemotherapy, and multifraction RT.[136] Nevertheless, further studies prospectively evaluating quality of life and cost are warranted.

There is variation among patterns of care among physicians. When American radiation oncologists were questioned about four hypothetical clinical scenarios concerning painful osseous metastases, the most commonly used schedule was 30 Gy in 10 fractions.[137] Canadian radiation oncologists were more likely to recommend treatment with 20 Gy in 5 fractions.[138] In deciding on the optimal palliative EBRT dosing for any single patient, the physician must consider multiple factors for each individual patient including the patient's life expectancy, extent of disease, volume of the treatment field, rate of disease progression, performance status, and cost of therapy. For those cases in which the patient is estimated to have a one- to two-year survival or more, doses of 40 to 50 Gy over 4 to 5 weeks should be considered to maximize duration and response to treatment. In patients whose life expectancies are less than 1 year, 30 Gy in 10 fractions are typically given and in instances where survival is estimated to be 3 months or less, 8 Gy in one fraction may be appropriate.[119]

Systemic radionuclides

The reactive bone formation that frequently occurs in the presence of metastatic bone involvement from prostate cancer results in new bone, which has increased avidity for bone-seeking molecules such as bisphosphonates.[139] This is the basis by which radionuclides such as samarium-153 and rhenium-186, when complexed to bone-avid molecules, may be selectively delivered to sites of metastatic bone involvement. Other radionuclides (including strontium-89) have a natural affinity for metabolically active bone.[140] The advantage of radionuclide treatment is the ability to simultaneously target multiple sites of involvement with a single intravenous administration. After administration with [153]Sm chelated to ethylenediaminetetramethylene phosphonic acid (EDTMP) , 65% to 80% of patients report pain relief, and symptom response usually occurs within 1 week of treatment. The average duration of response is 2 to 3 months. An initial pain flare may occur in approximately 10% of patients, and the major toxicity of treatment is myelosuppression.[141–143] A detailed discussion of radionuclide therapy is presented elsewhere in this text.

Wide-field radiation therapy/ hemibody radiation therapy

Hemibody radiation therapy (HBRT) was first developed in the 1960s for patients with multiple sites of painful bone metastases. Although blood counts are lowered with wide-field radiation therapy (WFRT), the body can regenerate the marrow supply when at least 10% of the bone marrow is spared from radiation. Ordinarily, sequential treatments to the upper and lower halves were possible provided that the treatments were separated by 4 to 6 weeks. These treatments could be used alone or as an adjunct to local-field irradiation. The optimal single doses were found to be 6 Gy to the upper hemibody and 8 Gy for the middle or lower segment, with increasing doses showing no benefit in pain response.[149] The maximum tolerated dose of fractionated (2.5 Gy) HBRT was found to be 17.5 Gy; however it was found that pain from prostate cancer osseous metastases is sufficiently treated with 3 Gy on 2 consecutive days and was as effective as 3 Gy for 5 days.[144,145] Fractionated schedules allow for a higher total dose without increased toxicity. Fractionated schemes may also give longer duration of relief and more complete relief, as well as improved overall and progression free survival with less toxicity.[146] RTOG 82-06 sought to explore the possibility that HBRT (8 Gy in one fraction) added to local-field radiotherapy (30 Gy in 10 fractions) might delay the onset of metastases in the affected hemibody

and decrease the frequency of further treatment. The addition of HBRT to local-field EBRT was found to delay the progression of existing disease and prolong the median time to new disease (12.6 versus 6.3 months). Time to new treatment within the hemibody segment was delayed and 16% fewer patients were retreated. There was also a trend to improved survival in prostate cancer patients treated with HBRT. These findings suggest that hemibody irradiation may eradicate micrometastases.[147]

Despite these potential advantages, the morbidity of HBRT is greater than localized radiotherapy. Patients may experience thromboleukopenia, emesis, rigors and fevers, pneumonitis, xerostomia, and cataracts. Nowadays, WFRT/HBRT is used in 1% to 2% of cases since patients with widespread painful bone metastases can usually be palliated with radioisotopes.[137] However, unlike radioisotopes, HBRT can palliate both osseous and extraosseous metastases. Moreover, in those cases in which systemic radioisotopes cannot be given, HBRT may be a reasonable alternative. Hemibody radiation therapy is thought to provide more rapid relief of pain compared with radioisotope therapy.[148,149] Pain relief with HBRT is rapid in onset, and 50% of patients were found to have pain relief within 48 hours, 80% had pain relief within 1 week, and all had pain relief within 2 weeks. One fifth of all patients had a complete response in their pain.

Irradiation of previously treated areas

Although most patients have a good initial response to radiotherapy, approximately 10% to 25% of patients will have pain relapse necessitating retreatment.[32,33] Local-field radiation may need to be repeated at the same site and can generally be recommended with a similar probability of response. Overall response rates with re-treatment are reported to be 84% to 87%.[150] The patients who benefit most from re-irradiation are those who relapse 4 months or more beyond initial treatment, have good performance status, and have a solitary metastasis.[151] In patients with vertebral metastases, the risk of re-irradiation must be carefully considered against the risk of radiation-induced myelopathy if the re-irradiation dose would exceed the normal tolerance of the spinal cord.[152] Nevertheless, because of the short life expectancy of most patients considered for this therapy, the immediate benefits of re-irradiation may outweigh the potential for long-term toxicities.

In an attempt to increase the safety and efficiency of vertebral body re-irradiation by limiting dose to the spinal cord, intensity-modulated radiotherapy and stereotactic body radiation therapy have been utilized. Stereotactic body radiation therapy refers to a variety of techniques that have in common the ability to increase the precision of radiation delivery.[153] One series evaluated 19 patients retreated for recurrent spinal cord metastases with IMRT or fractionated conformal RT with a maximal re-treatment dose of less than 20 Gy. Most patients achieved an improvement in pain. Although there were no significant late toxicities after a median follow-up of 1 year, 12 patients had died within this timeframe.[154] Another series of 125 patients treated with stereotactic body radiation therapy included 78 who had received prior spinal radiation. Patients received a mean dose of 17.5 Gy in a single fraction to the 80% isodose line. No acute radiation toxicity or new neurological deficits occurred during a median follow-up of 18 months. Axial and radicular pain improved in 74 of 79 patients who were symptomatic before treatment.[155]

Postoperative radiation therapy

Pathologic fractures occur in approximately 10% to 20% of cancer patients with bony metastatic disease, and orthopedic stabilization is frequently performed either prophylactically or after the occurrence of fracture.[156] Postoperative radiotherapy has been shown to help patients attain an improved functional status and use of the extremity following orthopedic stabilization. For patients who do not initially receive postoperative radiation therapy, 15% require a second orthopedic procedure after an average of 1 year, compared with 3% in patients receiving radiotherapy. Postoperative radiation therapy may also contribute to an increase in overall survival.[157]

For patients with spinal cord compression due to metastatic disease, a combined surgical and radiotherapeutic approach is warranted. Regine et al randomized patients with spinal cord compression to either radical decompressive surgical resection followed by radiation therapy or radiation therapy alone. Surgery was performed within 24 hours of study entry with the intent in all cases to remove as much tumor as possible, provide immediate decompression, and stabilize the spine. Radiation therapy in both groups was given to a total dose of 30 Gy in fractions of 3 Gy. The combined modality group required fewer steroids and narcotics, and was able to maintain ambulatory ability and functional status longer than the patients receiving radiotherapy alone.[158]

Conclusions

Radiotherapy is an important therapeutic modality in the management of metastatic prostate cancer, and should be used to alleviate symptoms from bone pain or in the postoperative setting. It has been shown that the use of EBRT for metastatic bone lesions provides pain relief regardless of the fractionation scheme chosen, although the data also suggest that a more prolonged course of radiotherapy may be associated with reduced risk of fracture and less relapse of pain. Radiation therapy should be considered as a first line treatment for the palliation of a few symptomatic bone metastases. For diffuse bony metastases causing widespread pain, for areas that have been treated with previous EBRT to maximal normal tissue tolerances, or for painful areas that have recurred, patients should be considered for treatment with radionuclides or wide-field radiation.[27] Patients undergoing surgical treatment of bone metastases should receive postoperative radiation to maximize functional recovery and limit risk of recurrence.

References

1. Pasteau O, Degrais J. The radium treatment of cancer of the prostate. Rev Malad Nutr 1911;363–367.
2. Smith GS, Pierson EL. The value of high voltage x-ray therapy in carcinoma of the prostate. J Urol 1930;23:331.
3. Widmann BP. Cancer of the prostate. The result of radium and roentgen ray treatment. Radiology 1934;22:153.
4. Kupelian P, Katcher J, Levin H, et al. Stage T1-2 prostate cancer. Int J Radiat Oncol Biol Phys 1997;37:1043–1052.
5. Partin A, Mangold L, Lamm D, et al. Contemporary update of prostate cancer staging nomograms (Partin tables) for the new millennium. Urology 2001;58:843–848.
6. Roach M, Lu J, Pilepich M, et al. Four prognostic groups predict long-term survival from prostate cancer following radiotherapy alone on Radiation Therapy Oncology Group clinical trials. Int J Radiat Oncol Biol Phys 2000;47:609–615.
7. D'Amico AV, Whittington R, Malkowicz SB, et al. Biochemical outcome after radical prostatectomy, EBRT, or interstitial radiation therapy for clinically localized prostate cancer. JAMA 1998;280:969–974.
8. D'Amico AV. Combined-modality staging for localized adenocarcinoma of the prostate. Oncology (Huntington) 2001;15:49–59.
9. Zietman AL, Coen JJ, Shipley WU, et al. Radical radiation therapy in the management of prostatic adenocarcinoma: the initial prostate specific antigen value as a predictor of treatment outcome. J Urol 1994;151:640–645.
10. Kuban DA, el-Mahdi AM, Schellhammer PF. Prostate-specific antigen for pretreatment prediction and posttreatment evaluation of outcome after definitive irradiation for prostate cancer. Int J Radiat Oncol Biol Phys 1995;32:307–316.
11. Hanks GE, Hanlon AL, Hudes G, et al. Patterns-of-failure analysis of patients with high pretreatment prostate-specific antigen levels treated by radiation therapy: the need for improved systemic and locoregional treatment. J Clin Oncol 1996;1093–1097.
12. Shipley WU, Thames HD, Sandler HM, et al. Radiation therapy for clinically localized prostate cancer. JAMA 1999;281:1598–1604.
13. Coen JJ, Zietman AL, Thakral H, et al. Radical radiation for localized prostate cancer: local persistence of disease results in a late wave of metastases. J Clin Oncol 2002;20:3199–3205.
14. Kuban DA, el-Mahdi AM, Schellhammer PF. Potential benefit of improved local tumor control in patients with prostate carcinoma. Cancer 1995;75:2373–2382.
15. Valicenti R, Lu J, Pilepich M. Survival advantage from higher-dose radiation therapy for clinically localized prostate cancer treated on the radiation therapy oncology group trials. J Clin Oncol 2000;18:2740–2746.
16. Hanks GE, Martz KL, Diamond JJ. The effect of dose on local control of prostate cancer. Int J Radiat Oncol Biol Phys 1988;15:1299–305.
17. Pollack A, Smith LG, von Eschenbach AG. External beam radiotherapy dose response characteristics of 1127 men with prostate cancer treated in the PSA era. Int J Radiat Oncol Biol Phys 2000;48:57–512.
18. Leibel SA, Hanks GE, Kramer S. Patterns of care outcome studies: results of the national practice in adenocarcinoma of the prostate. Int J Radiat Oncol Biol Phys 1984;10:401–409.
19. Smit WG, Helle PA, Van Putten WL. Late radiation damage in prostate cancer patients treated by high dose external radiotherapy in relation to rectal dose. Int J Radiat Oncol Biol Phys 1990;18:23–29.
20. Schultheiss TE, Lee WR, Hunt MA, et al. Late GI and GU complications in the treatment of prostate cancer. Int J Radiat Oncol Biol Phys 1997;37:3–11.
21. Roach M. Reducing the toxicity associated with the use of radiotherapy in men with localized prostate cancer. Urol Clin N Am 2004;31:353–366.
22. Dearnaley DP, Khoo VS, Norman AR, et al. Comparison of radiation side-effects of conformal and conventional radiotherapy in prostate cancer: a randomised trial. Lancet 1999;23:267–272.
23. Koper PC, Stroom JC, van Putten WL, et al. Acute morbidity reduction using 3DCRT for prostate carcinoma: a randomized study. Int J Radiat Oncol Biol Phys 1999;43:727–734.
24. American Society for Therapeutic Radiology and Oncology Consensus Panel. Consensus statement: Guidelines for PSA following radiation therapy. Int J Radiat Oncol Biol Phys 1997;37:1035–1041.
25. Hanks GE, Hanlon AL, Epstein B, et al. Dose response in prostate cancer with 8-12 years' follow-up. Int J Radiat Oncol Biol Phys 2002;54:427–435.
26. Pollack A, Hanlon AL, Horwitz EM, et al. Prostate cancer radiotherapy dose response: an update of the Fox Chase experience. J Urol 2004;171:1132–1136.
27. Bey P, Carrie C, Beckendorf V, et al. Dose escalation with 3D-CRT in prostate cancer: French study of dose escalation with conformal 3D radiotherapy in prostate cancer-preliminary results. Int J Radiat Oncol Biol Phys 2000;48:513–517.
28. Zelefsky M, Fuks Z, Chan H, et al. Ten-year results of dose escalation with 3-dimensional conformal radiotherapy for patients with clinically localized prostate cancer. Int J Radiat Oncol Biol Phys 2003;57S:149–150.

29. Michalski JM, Winter K, Purdy JA, et al. Preliminary evaluation of low-grade toxicity with conformal radiation therapy for prostate cancer on RTOG 9406 dose levels I and II. Int J Radiat Oncol Biol Phys 2003;56:192–198.

30. Ryu JK, Winter K, Michalski JM, et al. Interim report of toxicity from 3D conformal radiation therapy for prostate cancer on 3DOG/RTOG 9406, level III (79.2 Gy). Int J Radiat Oncol Biol Phys 2002;54:1036–1046.

31. Shipley WU, Verhey LJ, Munzenrider JE, et al. Advanced prostate cancer: the results of a randomized comparative trial of high dose irradiation boosting with conformal protons compared with conventional dose irradiation using photons alone. Int J Radiat Oncol Biol Phys 1995;32:3–12.

32. Zietman AL, DeSilvio M, Slater JD, et al. A randomized trial comparing conventional dose (70.2GyE) and high-dose (79.2GyE) conformal radiation in early stage adenocarcinoma of the prostate: results of an interim analysis of PROG 95-09. Int J Radiat Oncol Biol Phys 2004;60:S131.

33. Pollack A, Zagars GK, Smith LG, et al. Preliminary results of a randomized radiotherapy dose-escalation study comparing 70 Gy with 78 Gy for prostate cancer. J Clin Oncol 2000;18:3904–3911.

34. Pollack A, Zagars GK, Starkschall G, et al. Prostate cancer radiation dose response: results of the M.D. Anderson phase III randomized trial. Int J Radiat Oncol Biol Phys 2002;53:1097–1105.

35. Roach M 3rd, Meehan S, Kroll S, et al. Radiotherapy for high grade clinically localized adenocarcinoma of the prostate. J Urol 1996;156:1719–1723.

36. Fiveash JB, Hanks G, Roach M 3rd, et al. 3D conformal radiation therapy (3DCRT) for high grade prostate cancer: a multi-institutional review. Int J Radiat Oncol Biol Phys 2000;47:335–342.

37. Luxton G, Hancock SL, Boyer AL. Dosimetry and radiobiologic model comparison of IMRT and 3D conformal radiotherapy in treatment of carcinoma of the prostate. Int J Radiat Oncol Biol Phys 2004;59:267–284.

38. Chan HM, Zelefsky MJ, Fuks Z, et al. Long-term outcome of high dose intensity modulated radiotherapy for clinically localized prostate cancer. Int J Radiat Oncol Biol Phys 2004;60:S169–S170.

39. Ghilezan M, Yan D, Liang J, et al. Online image-guided intensity-modulated radiotherapy for prostate cancer: how much improvement can we expect? A theoretical assessment of clinical benefits and potential dose escalation by improving precision and accuracy of radiation delivery. Int J Radiat Oncol Biol Phys 2004;60:1602–1610.

40. Yan D, Xu B, Lockman D. The influence of interpatient and intrapatient rectum variation on external beam treatment of prostate cancer. Int J Radiat Oncol Biol Phys 2001;51:1111.

41. Fowler J, Chappell R, Ritter M. Is alpha/beta for prostate tumors really low? Int J Radiat Oncol Biol Phys 2001;50:1021–1031.

42. Duchesne GM, Peters LJ. What is the alpha/beta ratio for prostate cancer? Rationale for hypofractionated high-dose-rate brachytherapy. Int J Radiat Oncol Biol Phys 1999;44:747–748.

43. Deger S, Boehmer D, Turk I, et al. High dose rate brachytherapy of localized prostate cancer. Eur Urol 2002;41:420–426.

44. Martinez A, Gonzalez J, Spencer W, et al. Conformal high dose rate brachytherapy improves biochemical control and cause specific survival in patients with prostate cancer and poor prognostic factors. J Urol 2003;169:974–980.

45. D'Amico AV, Whittington R, Malkowicz B, et al. Biochemical outcome after radical prostatectomy, external beam radiation therapy, or interstitial radiation therapy for clinically localized prostate cancer. JAMA 1998;280:969–974.

46. Stock RG, Cahlon O, Cesaretti JA, et al. Combined modality treatment in the management of high-risk prostate cancer. Int J Radiat Oncol Biol Phys 2004;1352–1359.

47. Sylvester JE, Blasko JC, Grimm PD, et al. Ten-year biochemical relapse-free survival after external beam radiation and brachytherapy for localized prostate cancer: the Seattle experience. Int J Radiat Oncol Biol Phys 2003;57:944–952.

48. Dattoli M, Wallner K, True L, et al. Long-term outcomes after treatment with external beam radiation therapy and palladium 103 for patients with higher risk prostate carcinoma. Cancer 2003;97:979–983.

49. Brandeis JM, Litwin MS, Burnison CM, et al. Quality of life outcomes after brachytherapy for early stage prostate cancer. J Urol 2000;163:851–857.

50. Gelblum DY, Potters L. Rectal complications associated with transperineal interstitial brachytherapy for prostate cancer. Int J Radiat Oncol Biol Phys 2000;48:119–124.

51. DeWeese TL, Shipman JM, Dillehay LE, et al. Sensitivity of human prostatic carcinoma cell lines to low dose rate radiation exposure. J Urol 1998;159:591–598.

52. Furuya Y, Lin XS, Walsh JC, et al. Androgen ablation-induced programmed death of prostatic glandular cells does not involve recruitment into a defective cell cycle or p53 induction. Endocrinology 1995;136:1898–1906.

53. Denmeade SR, Lin XS, Isaacs JT. Role of programmed (apoptotic) cell death during the progression and therapy for prostate cancer. Prostate 1996;28:251–265.

54. Zietman AL, Nakfoor BM, Prince EA, et al. The effect of androgen deprivation and radiation therapy on an androgen-sensitive murine tumor: an in vitro and in vivo study. Cancer J Sci Am 1997;3:31–36.

55. Joon DL, Hasegawa M, Sikes C, et al. Supraadditive apoptotic response of R3327-G rat prostate tumors to androgen ablation and radiation. Int J Radiat Oncol Biol Phys 1997;38:1071–1077.

56. Del Regato J. Radiotherapy for carcinoma of the prostate. A report from the Committee for the Cooperative Study of Radiotherapy for Carcinoma of the Prostate. Colorado Springs, Colo: Penrose Cancer Hospital, 1968.

57. Green N, Bodner H, Broth E, et al. Improved control of bulky prostate carcinoma with sequential estrogen and radiation therapy. Int J Radiat Oncol Biol Phys 1984;10:971–976.

58. Mukamel E, Servadio C, Lurie H. Combined external radiotherapy and hormonal therapy for localized carcinoma of the prostate. Prostate 1983;4:283–287.

59. Pilepich MV, Krall JM, Johnson RJ, et al. Prognostic factors in carcinoma of the prostate-analysis of the RTOG 75-06. Int J Radiat Oncol Biol Phys 1987;13:339–349.

60. Pilepich MV, Krall JM, John MJ, et al. Hormonal cytoreduction in locally advanced carcinoma of the prostate treated with definitive radiotherapy: Preliminary results of RTOG 83-07. Int J Radiat Oncol Biol Phys 1989;16:813–817.

61. Pilepich MV, John MJ, Krall JM, et al. Phase II Radiation Therapy Oncology Group study of hormonal cytoreduction with flutamide and zoladex in locally advanced carcinoma of the prostate treated with definitive radiotherapy. Am J Clin Oncol 1990;13:461–464.

62. Pilepich MV, Krall JM, al-Sarraf M, et al. Androgen deprivation with radiation therapy alone for locally advanced prostatic carcinoma: a randomized comparative trial of the Radiation Therapy Oncology Group. Urology 1995;45:616–623.

63. Pilepich MV, Winter K, John MJ, et al, Phase III radiation therapy oncology group (RTOG) trial 86-10 of androgen deprivation adjuvant to definitive radiotherapy in locally advanced carcinoma of the prostate. Int J Radiat Oncol Biol Phys 2001;50:1243–1252.

64. Lawton CA, Winter K, Murray K, et al. Updated results of the phase III radiation therapy oncology group (RTOG) trial 85-31 evaluating the potential benefit of androgen suppression following standard radiation therapy for unfavorable prognosis carcinoma of the prostate. Int J Radiat Oncol Biol Phys 2001;49:937–946.

65. Bolla M, Collette L, Blank L, et al. Long-term results with immediate androgen suppression and external irradiation in patients with locally advanced prostate cancer (an EORTC study): a phase III randomized trial. Lancet 2002;360:103–108.

66. D'Amico AV, Manola J, Loffredo M, et al. 6-month androgen suppression plus radiation therapy vs radiation therapy alone for patients with clinically localized prostate cancer. JAMA 2004;292:821–827.

67. Holzbeierlein JM, Castle E, Thrasher JB. Complications of androgen deprivation therapy: prevention and treatment. Oncology 2004;18:303–309.

68. Laverdiere J, Gomez JL, Cusan L, et al. Beneficial effect of combination hormonal therapy administered prior and following external beam radiation therapy in localized prostate cancer. Int J Radiat Oncol Biol Phys 1997;37:247–252.

69. Laverdiere J, Nabid A, de Bedoya LD, et al. The efficacy and sequencing of a short course of androgen suppression on freedom from biochemical failure when administered with radiation therapy for T2-T3 prostate cancer. J Urol 2004;171:1137–1140.

70. Hanks GE, Pajak TF, Porter A, et al. Phase III trial of long-term adjuvant androgen deprivation after neoadjuvant hormonal cytoreduction and radiotherapy in locally advanced carcinoma of the prostate: the Radiation Therapy Oncology Group protocol 92-02, J Clin Oncol 2003;21:3972–3978.

71. Roach M, Lu J, Pilepich MV, et al. Predicting long-term survival and the need for hormonal therapy: a meta-analysis of RTOG prostate cancer trials. Int J Radiat Oncol Biol Phys 2000;47:617–627.

72. Horwitz EM, Winter K, Hanks GE, et al. Subset analysis of RTOG 85-31 and 86-10 indicates an advantage for long-term vs. short-term adjuvant hormones for patients with locally advanced nonmetastatic prostate cancer treated with radiation therapy. Int J Radiat Oncol Biol Phys 2001;49:947–956.

73. Gleave ME, Goldenberg SL, Chin JL, et al. Randomized comparative study of 3 versus 8-month neoadjuvant hormonal therapy before radical prostatectomy: biochemical and pathological effects. J Urol 2001;166:500–507.

74. Roach M 3rd, DeSilvio M, Lawton C, et al. Phase III trial comparing whole-pelvic versus prostate-only radiotherapy and neoadjuvant versus adjuvant combined androgen suppression: radiation therapy oncology group 9413. J Clin Oncol 2003;21:1904–1911.

75. Roach M 3rd, Marquez C, Yuo HS, et al. Predicting the risk of lymph node involvement using the pre-treatment prostate specific antigen and Gleason score in men with clinically localized prostate cancer. Int J Radiat Oncol Biol Phys 1994;28:33–37.

76. Chen CT, Valicenti RK, Lu J, et al. Does hormonal therapy influence sexual function in men receiving 3D conformal radiation therapy for prostate cancer? Int J Radiat Oncol Biol Phys 2001;50:591–595.

77. Dearnaley DP, Khoo VS, Norman AR, et al. Comparison of radiation side-effects of conformal and conventional radiotherapy in prostate cancer: a randomised trial. Lancet 1999;353:267–272.

78. Zelefsky MJ, Harrison A. Neoadjuvant androgen ablation prior to radiotherapy for prostate cancer: Reducing the potential morbidity of therapy. Urology 1997;49:38–45.

79. Forman JD, Kumar R, Haas G, et al. Neoadjuvant hormonal downsizing of localized carcinoma of the prostate: Effects on the volume of normal tissue irradiation. Cancer Invest 1995;13:8–15.

80. Yang FE, Chen GTY, Ray P, et al. The potential for normal tissue dose reduction with neoadjuvant hormonal therapy in conformal treatment planning for stage C prostate cancer. Int J Radiat Oncol Biol Phys 1995;33:1009–1017.

81. Bolla M, Gonzalez D, Warde P, et al. Improved survival in patients with locally advanced prostate cancer treated with radiotherapy and goserelin. N Eng J Med 1997;337:295–300.

82. Sanguineti G, Agostinelli S, Foppiano F, et al. Adjuvant androgen deprivation impacts late rectal toxicity after conformal radiotherapy of prostate carcinoma. Br J Cancer 2002;86:1843–1847.

83. Valicenti RK, Winter K, Cox JD, et al. RTOG 94-06: is the addition of neoadjuvant hormonal therapy to dose-escalated 3D conformal radiation therapy for prostate cancer associated with treatment toxicity? Int J Radiat Oncol Biol Phys 2003;57:614–620.

84. Gray H. Anatomy of the Human Body. Philadelphia: Lea & Febiger, 1985.

85. Partin AW, Mangold LA, Lamm DM, et al. Contemporary update of prostate cancer staging nomograms (Partin Tables) for the new millennium. Urology 2001;58:843–848.

86. Roach M 3rd, Marquez C, Yho HS, et al. Predicting the risk of lymph node involvement using the pre-treatment prostate specific antigen and Gleason score in men with clinically localized prostate cancer. Int J Radiat Oncol Biol Phys 1994;28:33–37.

87. Heidenreich A, Varga Z, Von Knobloch R. Extended pelvic lymphadenectomy in patients undergoing radical prostatectomy: high incidence of lymph node metastasis. J Urol 202;167:1681–1686.

88. Rosen E, Cassady JR, Connolly J, et al. Radiotherapy for prostate carcinoma: the JCRT experience (1968–1978). II. Factors related to tumor control and complications. Int J Radiat Oncol Biol Phys 1985;11:723–730.

89. Aristizabal SA, Steinbronn D, Heusinkveld RS. External beam radiotherapy in cancer of the prostate. The University of Arizona experience. Radiother Oncol 1984;1:309–315.

90. Zagars GK, von Eschenbach AC, Johnson DE, et al. Stage C adenocarcinoma of the prostate. An analysis of 551 patients treated with external beam radiation. Cancer 1987;60:1489–1499.

91. McGowan DG. The value of extended field radiation therapy in carcinoma of the prostate. Int J Radiat Oncol Biol Phys 1981;7:1333–1339.

92. Ploysongsang SS, Aron BS, Shehata WM. Radiation therapy in prostate cancer: whole pelvis with prostate boost or small field to prostate? Urology 2002;40:18–26.

93. Seaward SA, Weinberg V, Lewis P, et al. Improved freedom from PSA failure with whole pelvic irradiation for high-risk prostate cancer. Int J Radiat Oncol Biol Phys 1998;42:1055–1062.

94. Bagshaw M. Radiotherapeutic treatment of prostatic carcinoma with pelvic node involvement. Urol Clin N Am 1984;11:297–304.

95. Asbell SO, Krall JM, Pilepich MV, et al. Elective pelvic irradiation in Stage A2, B carcinoma of the prostate: analysis of RTOG 77-06. Int J Radiat Oncol Biol Phys 1988;15:1307–1316.

96. Perez CA, Michalski J, Brown KC, et al. Nonrandomized evaluation of pelvic lymph node irradiation in localized carcinoma of the prostate. Int J Radiat Oncol Biol Phys 1996;36:573–584.

97. Forman JD, Lee Y, Robertson P, Montie JE, et al. Advantages of CT and beam's eye view display to confirm the accuracy of pelvic lymph node irradiation in carcinoma of the prostate. Radiology 1993;186:889–892.

98. Taylor A, Rockall AG, Usher C, et al. Delineation of a reference target volume for pelvic lymph node irradiation using MR imaging with ultrasmall superparamagnetic iron oxide particles. Int J Radiat Oncol Biol Phys 2004;60:S225.

99. Jemal A, Tiwari RC, Murray T, et al. Cancer statistics 2004. CA Cancer J Clin 2004;54:8–29.

100. Guinan P, Stewart AK, Fremgen AM, et al. Patterns of care for metastatic carcinoma of the prostate gland: results of the American College of Surgeons' patient care evaluation study. Prostate Cancer Prostatic Dis 1998;1:315–320.

101. Penson DF, Moul JW, Evans CP, et al. The economic burden of metastatic and prostate specific antigen progression in patients with prostate cancer: findings from a retrospective analysis of health plan data. J Urol 2004;161:2250–2254.

102. Johansson JE, Andren O, Andersson SO, et al. Natural history of early, localized prostate cancer. JAMA 2004;291:2713–2719.

103. Pound CR, Partin AW, Eisenberger MA, et al. Natural history of progression after PSA elevation following radical prostatectomy. JAMA 1999;281:1591–1597.

104. Kahn D, Weiner GJ, Ben-Haim S, et al. Positron emission tomographic measurement of bone marrow blood flow to the pelvis and lumbar vertebrae in young normal adults. Blood 1994;83:958–963. Erratum in Blood 1994;84:3602.

105. Bubendorf L, Schopfer A, Wagner U, et al. Metastatic patterns of prostate cancer: an autopsy study of 1,589 patients. Hum Pathol 2000;31:578–583.

106. Batson OV. The role of the vertebral veins in metastatic processes. Ann Intern Med 1942;16:38–45.

107. Dodds PR, Caride VJ, Lytton B. The role of the vertebral veins in the dissemination of prostatic carcinoma. J Urol 1981;126:753–755.

108. Roodman GD. Mechanisms of bone metastasis. N Engl J Med 2004;350:1655–1664.

109. Cooper CR, Pienta KJ. Cell adhesion and chemotaxis in prostate cancer metastasis to bone: a minireview. Prostate Cancer Prostatic Dis 2000;3:6–12.

110. Hauschka PV, Mavrakos AE, Iafrati MD, et al. Growth factors in bone matrix: isolation of multiple types by affinity chromatography on heparin-sepharose. J Biol Chem 1986;261:12665–12674.

111. Galasko CSB. Mechanisms of lytic and blastic metastatic disease of bone. Clin Orthop 1982;169:20–27.

112. Jacob K, Webber M, Benayahu D, et al. Osteonectin promotes prostate cancer cell migration and invasion: a possible mechanism for metastasis to bone. Cancer Res 1999;59:4453–4457.

113. Dodwell DJ. Malignant bone resorption: cellular and biochemical mechanisms. Ann Oncol 1992;3:257–267.

114. Schneider A, Kalikin LM, Mattos AC, et al. Bone turnover mediates preferential localization of prostate cancer in the skeleton. Endocrinology 2005;146:1727–1736.

115. Watt KW, Lee PJ, M'Timkulu T, et al. Human prostate-specific antigen: structural and functional similarity with serine proteases. Proc Natl Acad Sci USA 1986;83:3166–3170.

116. Fielder PJ, Rosenfeld RG, Graves HC, et al. Biochemical analysis of prostate specific antigen-protelyzed insulin-like growth factor finding protein-3. Growth Regul 1994;4:164–172.

117. Coleman RF. Skeletal complications of malignancy. Cancer 1997;80:1588–1594.

118. Jonler M, Nielsen OS, Groenvold M, et al. Quality of life in patients with skeletal metastases of prostate cancer and status prior to start of endocrine therapy: results from the Scandinavian Prostate Cancer Group study 5. Scan J Urol Nephrol 2005;39:42–48.

119. Sartor OA, DiBiase SJ. Management of bone metastases in advanced prostate cancer. UpToDate Online 12.3, http://www.uptodate.com.

120. Tong D, Gillick L, Hendrickson FR. The palliation of symptomatic osseous metastases: final results of the Study by the Radiation Therapy Oncology Group. Cancer 1982;50:893–899.

121. Arcangeli G, Giovinazzo G, Saracino B, et al. Radiation therapy in the management of symptomatic bone metastases: the effect of total dose and histology on pain relief and response duration. Int J Radiat Oncol Biol Phys 1998;42:1119–1126.

122. Zelefsky MJ, Scher HI, Forman JD, et al. Palliative hemiskeletal irradiation for widespread metastatic prostate cancer: a comparison of single dose and fractionated regimens. Int J Radiat Oncol Biol Phys 1989;17:1281–1285.

123. Franzen L, Nyman J, Hagberg H, et al. A randomised placebo controlled study with ondansetron in patients undergoing fractionated radiotherapy. Ann Oncol 1996;7:587–592.

124. Blitzer PH. Reanalysis of the RTOG study of the palliation of symptomatic osseous metastasis. Cancer 1985;55:1468–1472.

125. Okawa T, Kita M, Goto M, et al. Randomized prospective clinical study of small, large and twice-a-day fraction radiotherapy for painful bone metastases. Radiother Oncol 1988;13:99–104.

126. Madsen EL. Painful bone metastasis: efficacy of radiotherapy assessed by the patients: a randomized trial comparing 4 Gy × 6 versus 10 Gy × 2. Int J Radiat Oncol Biol Phys 1983;9:1775–1779.

127. Martin WM. Multiple daily fractions of radiation in the palliation of pain from bone metastases. Clin Radiol 1983;34:245–249.

128. Cole DJ. A randomized trial of a single treatment versus conventional fractionation in the palliative radiotherapy of painful bone metastases. Clin Oncol 1989;1:59–62.

129. Nielsen OS, Bentzen SM, Sandberg E, et al. Randomized trial of single dose versus fractionated palliative radiotherapy of bone metastases. Radiother Oncol 1998;47:233–240.

130. Yarnold JR. 8 Gy single fraction radiotherapy for the treatment of metastatic skeletal pain: randomised comparison with a multifraction schedule over 12 months of patient follow-up. Bone Pain Trial Working Party. Radiother Oncol 1999;52:111–121.

131. Steenland E, Leer JW, van Houwelingen H, et al. The effect of a single fraction compared to multiple fractions on painful bone metastases: a global analysis of the Dutch Bone Metastasis Study. Radiother Oncol 1999;52:101–109.

132. Hartsell WF, Scott C, Bruner CW, et al. Phase III randomized trial of 8 Gy in 1 fraction vs 30 Gy in 10 fractions for palliation of painful bone metastases: preliminary results of RTOG 97-14. Int J Radiat Oncol Biol Phys 2003;57:S124.

133. Bruner DW, Winter K, Hartsell A. Prospective Health-Related Quality of Life Valuations (Utilities) of 8 Gy in 1 fraction vs 30 Gy in 10 fractions for palliation of painful bone metastases: preliminary results of RTOG 97-14. Int J Radiat Oncol Biol Phys 2004;60:S142.

134. Wu JS, Wong R, Johnston M, et al. Meta-analysis of dose-fractionation radiotherapy trials for the palliation of painful bone metastases. Int J Radiat Oncol Biol Phys 2003;55:594–605.

135. Wai MS, Mike S, Ines H, et al. Palliation of metastatic bone pain: single fraction versus multifraction radiotherapy – a systematic review of the randomised trials. Cochrane Database Syst Rev 2004;2:CD004721.

136. Konski A. Radiotherapy is a cost-effective palliative treatment for patients with bone metastasis from prostate cancer. Int J Radiat Oncol Biol Phys 2004;60:1373–1378.

137. Ben-Josef E, Shamsa F, Williams AO, et al. Radiotherapeutic management of osseous metastases: a survey of current patterns of care, Int J Radiat Oncol Biol Phys 1998;40:915–921.

138. Chow E, Danjoux C, Wong R. Palliation of bone metastases: a survey of patterns of practice among Canadian radiation oncologists. Radiother Oncol 2000;56:305–314.

139. Fleisch H. Bisphosphonates: pharmacology and use in the treatment of tumor-induced hypercalcaemic and metastatic bone disease. Drugs 1991;42:919–944.

140. Lewington VJ. Bone-seeking radionuclides for therapy. J Nucl Med 2005;46:38S–47S.

141. Collins C, Eary JF, Donaldson G, et al. Samarium-153 -EDTMP in bone metastases of hormone refractory prostate carcinoma: a phase I/II trial. J Nucl Med 1993;34:1839–1844.

142. Farhanghi M, Holmes RA, Volkert WA, et al. Samarium-153-EDTMP: pharmacokinetic, toxicity and pain response using an escalating dose schedule in treatment of metastatic bone cancer. J Nucl Med 1992;33:1451–1458.

143. Dickie GJ, Macfarlane D. Strontium and samarium therapy for bone metastases from prostate carcinoma. Australas Radiol 1999;43:476–479.

144. Scarantino CW, Caplan R, Rotman M, et al. A phase I/II study to evaluate the effect of fractionated hemibody irradiation in the treatment of osseous metastases—RTOG 88-22. Int J Radiat Oncol Biol Phys 1996;36:37–48.

145. Salazar OM, Sandhu T, da Motta NW, et al. Fractionated half-body irradiation (HBI) for the rapid palliation of widespread, symptomatic, metastatic bone disease:a randomized Phase III trial of the International Atomic Energy Agency. Int J Radiat Oncol Biol Phys. 2001;50:765–775.

146. Salazar OM, DaMotta NW, Bridgman SM, et al. Fractionated half-body irradiation for pain palliation in widely metastatic cancers: comparison with single dose. Int J Radiat Oncol Biol Phys 1996;36:49–60.

147. Poulter CA, Cosmatos D, Rubin P. A report of RTOG 8206: a phase III study of whether the addition of single dose hemibody irradiation to standard fractionated local field irradiation is more effective than local field irradiation alone in the treatment of symptomatic osseous metastases. Int J Radiat Oncol Biol Phys 1992;23:207–214.

148. Dearnaley DP, Bayly RJ, A'Hern RP, et al. Palliation of bone metastases in prostate cancer. Hemibody irradiation or strontium-89? Clin Oncol 1992;4:101–107.

149. Salazar OM, Rubin P, Hendrickson FR. Single-dose half-body irradiation for palliation of multiple bone metastases from solid tumors. Final Radiation Therapy Oncology Group report. Cancer. 1986;58:29–36.

150. Mithal NP, Needham PR, Hoskin PJ. Retreatment with radiotherapy for painful bone metastases. Int J Radiat Oncol Biol Phys 1994;29:1011–1014.

151. Hayashi S, Hoshi H, Iida T. Reirradiation with local-field radiotherapy for painful bone metastases. Radiat Med 2002;20:231–236.

152. Grosu AL, Andratschke N, Nieder C, et al. Retreatment of the spinal cord with palliative radiotherapy. Int J Radiat Oncol Biol Phys 2002;52:1288–1292.

153. Song DY, Kavanagh BD, Benedict SH, Schefter TA. Stereotactic Body Radiation Therapy: rationale, techniques, application, and optimization. Oncology (Huntington), 2004;18:1419–1430.

154. Milker-Zabel S, Zabel A, Thilmann C, et al. Clinical results of retreatment of vertebral bone metastases by stereotactic conformal radiotherapy and intensity-modulated radiotherapy. Int J Radiat Oncol Biol Phys 2003;55:162–167.

155. Gerszten PC, Ozhasoglu C, Burton SA. CyberKnife frameless stereotactic radiosurgery for spinal lesions: clinical experience in 125 cases. Neurosurgery 2004;55:89–98.

156. Harrington KD. Orthopaedic management of pelvic and extremity lesions. Clin Orthop Relat Res 1995;312:136–147.

157. Townsend PW, Smalley SR, Cozad SC, et al. Role of postoperative radiation therapy after stabilization of fractures caused by metastatic disease. Int J Radiat Oncol Biol Phys 1995;31:43–49.

158. Regine WF, Tibbs PA, Young A, et al. Metastatic spinal cord compression: a randomized trial of direct decompressive surgical resection plus radiotherapy vs. radiotherapy alone. Int J Radiat Oncol Biol Phys 2003;57S:S125.

43

Use of bisphosphonates in the management of osseous metastases

Roger S Kirby, Jonathan P Coxon

Introduction

Bone is by far the most common site for metastases in prostate cancer, accounting for considerable morbidity (Figure 43.1). Until recently, there have been few viable options for the treatment of the patient with hormone-refractory metastatic disease. This chapter examines the pathophysiology underlying the development of bone metastases. It also summarizes some of the clinical approaches for the management of this common condition, focusing on recent evidence supporting the use of one of the most promising groups of pharmacological agents, the third-generation bisphosphonates.

Etiology and impact of prostate cancer-related bone metastases

Prostate cancer is the most commonly diagnosed malignancy in males in the UK, with nearly 25,000 cases being reported in 1999.[1] Prostate cancer-related morbidity and mortality are closely associated with the formation of metastases. Bone is the preferred site for these metastases, and estimates indicate that bone metastases are present in more than 80% of men with advanced prostate cancer.[2,3] A UK study has shown that bone metastases are present in up to 50% of men at the time of first presentation.[4]

Considerable morbidity arises from the various complications from bone metastases, and it is estimated that the average frequency of a "skeletal related event" in patients with bone metastases is 3 to 4 months, with these events invariably leading to a reduced quality of life.[5] Common presentations include pain, spinal cord compression, pathologic fracture, and abnormalities in serum calcium levels.[6] Patients with hormone-refractory metastatic prostate cancer are particularly prone to incapacitating progressive bone disease.[7]

The normal resculpturing of bone is governed by the coupled processes of bone resorption and formation. Modeling occurs in localized areas of cortical and trabecular bone known as bone metabolic units. Osteoclast-mediated resorption usually takes approximately 7 to 10 days, while the subsequent formation phase, governed by osteoblasts, lasts approximately 3 months (Figure 43.2). Local "coupling" factors produced in the bone marrow regulate the remodeled bone.[8]

The rich milieu of growth factors in the bone environment provide an attractive "soil" for the seeding of certain tumor cells. In the presence of such cells, factors from tumor-induced breakdown of bone stimulate growth of further cancer cells, which in turn leads to further increases in bone resorption (Figure 43.3). This has been described as the vicious cycle.[8] As an example, tumor cells have been shown to release parathyroid hormone-related peptide (PTHrP), which stimulates osteoclastic resorption, via messaging from the osteoblast.[9] Resultant osteolysis releases several bone-derived growth factors, such as transforming growth factor-β (TGFβ). Normally, TGFβ serves to limit bone resorption via a negative feedback mechanism, but in the bone metastasis TGFβ stimulates invading tumor cells, partly accounting for this vicious cycle.[10]

Prostate cancer bone metastases usually appear on radiographs as areas of increased bone density, being principally sclerotic in nature. This suggests the occurrence of osteoblast-mediated excessive bone formation, in response to the presence of tumor cells. However, biochemical and histomorphometric studies indicate that osteolysis (excessive bone destruction) is also concurrently increased, and probably represents a vital initial step in the establishment of the metastases.[6,7,11,12] For example, recent studies using biochemical indices of bone turnover in patients with prostate cancer have found that, although the disease is characterized by osteoblastic metastases, there is also a direct correlation between skeletal metastases and bone resorption markers.[13,14] Indeed, the excretion of these indices was better correlated than plasma alkaline phosphatase, which is an accepted index of bone formation. The classic sclerotic bone lesions seen in prostate cancer represent an uncoupling of normal bone resorption and deposition shifting the balance towards new matrix formation and mineralization. It is now largely accepted that osteolysis is an important component of the influence of malignancy on bone, even when profound increases in new bone formation are also observed.[15] Therefore, it follows that interfering with the process of osteolysis could have an important influence on the development of prostate cancer metastases.

Current treatment options for bone metastases

Given the nature of the vicious cycle described above, options that can be considered for the treatment of metastatic bone disease are: 1) directly reducing tumor cell proliferation, for example, by direct inhibition of growth factors and cytokines; 2) antagonizing the effect of tumor cells on the host; or 3) a combination of these. Direct antitumor treatment options include chemotherapy, surgery, endocrine therapy, or radiotherapy. In practice, chemotherapy has

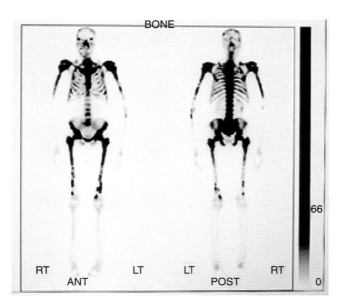

Figure 43.1
Bone metastases from prostate cancer shown on radionuclide bone scan.

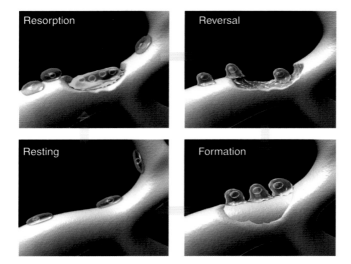

Figure 43.2
Normal bone remodeling. Resorption—stimulated osteoblast precursors release factors that induce osteoclast differentiation and activity. Osteoclasts remove bone mineral and matrix, creating an erosion cavity. Reversal—mononuclear cells prepare bone surface for new osteoblasts to begin forming bone. Formation—successive waves of osteoblasts synthesize an organic matrix to replace resorbed bone and fill the cavity with new bone. Resting—bone surface is covered with flattened lining cells. A prolonged resting period follows with little cellular activity until a new remodeling cycle begins.

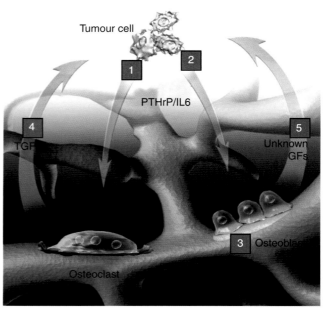

Figure 43.3
Pathogenesis of bone metastases. Factors are released by tumor cells that stimulate both osteoclast *(1)* and osteoblast *(2)* activity. Excessive new bone formation *(3)* occurs around tumor cell deposits, resulting in low bone strength and potential vertebral collapse. Osteoclastic *(4)* and osteoblastic *(5)* activity releases growth factors that stimulate tumor cell growth, perpetuating the cycle of bone resorption and abnormal bone growth. (GFs, growth factors; IL6, interleukin 6; PTHrP, parathyroid hormone-related peptide; TGFβ, transforming growth factor-β.)

refractory state has been reached though, a palliative approach is often sought. Radiotherapy and radiopharmaceuticals can provide local control of symptoms. Calcitonin or gallium nitrate, as indirect antitumor treatments, are occasionally used in a palliative setting for medical control of hypercalcemia, though this condition is rare in prostate cancer.[5] Otherwise, there have been very few options that have proved beneficial in this setting. There is, therefore, a great deal of interest in seeking out alternative therapies for the large number of men suffering with metastatic prostate cancer.

Bisphosphonates: evolution of a therapeutic theory

Bisphosphonates are a well-established class of drugs that have been known for many years to inhibit bone turnover, and have become established therapeutic options in the treatment of diseases such as Paget's disease, osteoporosis, and general tumor-associated bone disease (such as hypercalcemia).

The structure of these drugs is characterized by a central P-C-P bond, which promotes their binding to the mineralized bone matrix, and two variable R chains that determine the relative potency, side effects, and the precise mechanism of action (Figure 43.4). Following administration, bisphosphonates bind strongly to exposed bone mineral around resorbing osteoclasts, leading to very high local concentrations (possibly up to 1000 μM) in the resorption lacunae.[26]

for many years had no established role in prostate cancer, but encouraging results are now indicating some benefit in the most advanced cases, with agents such as mitoxantrone,[16,17] estramustine,[18,19] and in particular, docetaxel,[20–24] thalidomide.[25] Surgical tumor removal is not appropriate in the metastatic setting. For many years, endocrine therapy has represented the mainstay of treatment for the patient with advanced prostate cancer. When the hormone-

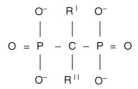

Figure 43.4
Schematic molecular structure of bisphosphonates.

Bisphosphonates have been shown to reduce bone turnover by primarily inhibiting osteoclast function. It has been proposed that these drugs can be thought of as working at three levels.[27] At the tissue level, they decrease bone turnover via initial inhibition of bone resorption, with suppressed bone formation following as a consequence of this. At the cellular level, bisphosphonates exert their activity principally via actions on osteoclasts, inhibiting their formation, migration, and osteolytic activity, as well as directly inducing apoptosis. It has been shown that bisphosphonates also act partly via modulation of signaling from osteoblasts to osteoclasts (Figure 43.5).[28] At the molecular level, the mode of action of bisphosphonates depends on their structure. Non-nitrogen-containing bisphosphonates (in which the R chains contains no N atoms) are metabolized to non-hydrolysable ATP analogs, which become toxic as they accumulate.[29] The more recently developed and more potent nitrogen-containing bisphosphonates act via inhibition of the mevalonate pathway.[30,31] This pathway usually provides the cell with lipids that are required for the normal post-translational modification of GTP-binding proteins, the functions of which are essential for many normal cellular processes.

The action of bisphosphonates on osteoclasts alone represented an initial rationale for investigating their potential use in prostate cancer-associated bone disease, as a reduction in osteoclast activity would reduce the release of growth factors in the bone environment and make it a less fertile soil for the seeding of tumor cells, as indicated above.[32]

Early animal work in the 1980s demonstrated that the bisphosphonates clodronate and etidronate inhibited tumor-mediated osteolysis induced by implanted prostate cancer cells.[33–35] A later exciting development came when in-vitro work established that bisphosphonates also act directly on tumor cells themselves. They have been shown to inhibit cell proliferation and viability, and induce apoptosis in a number of cancer cell lines, including prostate cancer.[36–40] Work in our center with breast cancer cells provided early evidence that inhibition of the mevalonate pathway was again central to the observed apoptotic effects.[41] We recently published similar results for various prostate cancer cell lines,[38] and provided evidence that the resultant apoptosis was dependent on the activation of caspases. Work in our laboratory has confirmed an apoptotic effect on prostate cancer cells at concentrations that are likely to be physiologically relevant.[42] Other work has shown bisphosphonates to inhibit the adhesion of cancer cells to bone slices,[43,44] and to inhibit their invasion through extracellular matrices.[45,46]

In addition to the work outlined above, a number of clinical studies have investigated the usefulness of bisphosphonates in various settings. The results of several small pilot studies encouraged breast cancer investigators to evaluate early-generation bisphosphonates, using either regular intravenous infusions of pamidronate, enteric-coated oral pamidronate, or either oral or parenteral clodronate. A reduction in skeletal morbidity was usually reported. There were initially rather fewer studies in the prostate cancer setting, though some early work showed reductions in bone pain with clodronate,[47,48]

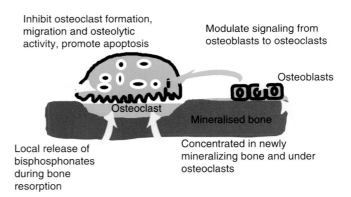

Figure 43.5
Mechanisms of action of bisphosphonates.

though was not later borne out in randomized studies with this drug.[49,50] Early small-scale studies with pamidronate provided encouraging signs of its potential benefit,[51,52] but it was several years before a well-designed randomized study was published on the use of later-generation bisphosphonates in prostate cancer.

Development of more modern bisphosphonates

Pharmacologic advances have led to several newer bisphosphonates being developed in recent years. The question of whether bisphosphonate potency is directly associated with therapeutic efficacy was investigated in work by van der Pluijm et al.[44] They demonstrated that the relative order of potency of six bisphosphonates (etidronate, clodronate, pamidronate, olpadronate, alendronate, and ibandronate) in inhibiting the adhesion of cancer cells to cortical and trabecular bone corresponded to their relative antiresorptive potencies in vivo as well as their ranking in in-vitro bone resorption assays, with predictive value for their clinical efficacy.

It is, therefore, reasonable to suggest that using more potent bisphosphonates could simplify treatment and possibly improve the therapeutic effectiveness of bisphosphonate therapy. Potencies of various bisphosphonates discovered to date are shown in Table 43.1.[53]

The most recent group of bisphosphonates to be developed is the so-called third-generation, the most potent of which is zoledronic acid. Recent large targeted studies indicate that this agent could help clinicians to effectively manage bone metastases in prostate cancer patients.

The most noteworthy trial, whose first results were published by Saad et al in 2002, investigated 643 patients with hormone-refractory prostate cancer and a history of bone metastases. These subjects were randomized to receive a double-blind treatment regimen of intravenous zoledronic acid at either 8 mg (n = 221) or 4 mg (n = 214), or placebo (n = 208), every 3 weeks for 15 months. Infusions were given over 15 minutes. During the trial, renal safety concerns merited the reduction of the 8 mg dose to doses of 4 mg.[54] Primary efficacy measures included proportion of patients with skeletal-related events, time to first event, skeletal morbidity rate, pain and analgesic scores, and disease progression. Safety analyses were also performed.

Results have recently been presented with follow-up extended to 24 months.[55] The study showed that patients receiving 4 mg

Table 43.1 Relative potencies of bisphosphonates. Measured on a molar basis in an in-vivo assay, namely the inhibitory activity on bone resorption induced by 1,25-dihydroxyvitamin D3 in the thyroparathyroidectomized rat[50]

Bisphosphonate	Relative potency
Clodronate	0.05
Pamidronate	1
Olpadronate	2.8
Alendronate	7.4
Risedronate	35.9
Ibandronate	43.6
Zoledronate	847

zoledronic acid experienced 11% fewer skeletal-related events than the placebo cohort (38% versus 49%; p = 0.028). Median time to first skeletal event was 488 days with placebo, and 321 days for patients receiving zoledronic acid 4 mg (p = 0.009). This represents a difference of more than 5 months. The placebo group also witnessed higher increases in pain and analgesic scores. Median survival was extended by 77 days in patients treated with 4 mg zoledronic acid compared with placebo, a non-significant difference. Zoledronic acid was well tolerated, and, although renal function deterioration was seen in approximately 20% of patients in the 8 mg cohort compared with placebo, the 4 mg group showed a relative risk ratio of only 1.07 (p = 0.882).

The authors concluded that in patients with metastatic prostate cancer, treatment with 4 mg zoledronic acid every 3 weeks reduces skeletal-related events, compared with placebo. Further, they confirmed that at this recommended dose and regimen, the benefit-to-risk ratio is acceptable for patients with hormone-refractory prostate cancer metastatic to bone. They proposed that further work is warranted to investigate earlier intervention with zoledronic acid, such as in patients with advanced prostate cancer and rising PSA on endocrine therapy, who have not yet developed metastases. It should be noted though that one such study (Novartis Protocol 704) had to be prematurely closed when an unexpected low frequency of events was observed. Other trials are proposed or underway, under the auspices of the European Organisation for Research and Treatment of Cancer (EORTC), European Association of Urology (EAU) and the Medical Research Council (MRC). These look at the potential benefit of zoledronic acid in hormone-naïve patients who have not developed metastases but who are at high risk of doing so. The MRC trial ("STAMPEDE," looking in addition at celecoxib and docetaxel) is also recruiting those who have had adjuvant or neo-adjuvant hormonal therapy, and those with metastases.

That reducing skeletal-related events (SREs) in prostate cancer patients with bone metastases may well also be economically beneficial is suggested by work that has shown, in the Netherlands at least, around 50% of the total cost of care for such patients is directly attributable to the treatment of SREs.[56]

The results of the study by Saad et al compare favorably to those recently published from the MRC Pr05 trial.[57] This looked at the use of oral clodronate, a first-generation bisphosphonate, in patients with bone metastases who had just started or were responding to first-line therapy. While a tendency towards increased bone progression-free survival was seen with 2080 mg/day clodronate, this difference was not statistically significant. The clodronate group reported significantly more gastrointestinal problems and increased lactate dehydrogenase levels, prompting a significant number of dose adjustments in this group.

A further potential benefit of bisphosphonate treatment is related to the bone loss that is known to occur in prostate cancer patients. It has been shown that many patients with advanced prostate cancer have a low bone mineral density at diagnosis, even before commencing androgen deprivation therapy.[58,59] This is of course compounded by the known osteoporotic effects of luteinizing hormone releasing hormone (LHRH) analogs, to which many patients are now being exposed for longer durations. Recently published results showed that, in patients without bone metastases receiving androgen deprivation therapy, 4 mg zoledronic acid significantly increased the bone mineral density, while a decrease was seen in the placebo group (p < 0.001).[60] A previous study using the second-generation bisphosphonate pamidronate failed to show an increase in bone mineral density,[61] though it did reduce bone loss when compared to placebo.

Zoledronic acid is the only bisphosphonate with the clinically proven indication for use in patients with bone metastases to prevent skeletal related events. Its ease of administration, as a short 15-minute intravenous infusion, is especially important considering that previous-generation bisphosphonates, such as pamidronate, have a standard infusion time of 2 to 4 hours. Such longer infusion times would clearly incur costs in terms of clinical staff time and healthcare resources. The simpler mode of administration with zoledronic acid means that clinicians may shortly be able to offer community-based bisphosphonate treatment, which should benefit healthcare budgets and patients alike. However, further research is required until this can become the standard of care.

Conclusions

- Bone is the most important metastatic site in prostate cancer.
- Skeletal complications, including fractures, are relatively common in prostate cancer.
- Accelerated bone resorption is an important component of the pathophysiology of bone metastases.
- Bisphosphonates are potent, safe, and well-tolerated inhibitors of bone resorption.
- Skeletal morbidity is significantly reduced by administration of bisphosphonates.
- Studies suggest that potent, third-generation bisphosphonates could play a vital role in the management of bone metastases from prostate cancer.

References

1. www.cancerresearchuk.org/statistics/.
2. Carlin BI, Andriole GL. The natural history, skeletal complications, and management of bone metastases in patients with prostate carcinoma. Cancer 2000;88:2989–2994.
3. Pentyala SN, Lee J, Hsieh K, et al. Prostate cancer: a comprehensive review. Med Oncol 2000;17:85–105.
4. George NJ. Natural history of localised prostatic cancer managed by conservative therapy alone. Lancet 1988;1:494–497.
5. Coleman RE. Uses and abuses of bisphosphonates. Ann Oncol 2000;11 Suppl 3:179–184.
6. Scher HI, Chung LW. Bone metastases: improving the therapeutic index. Semin Oncol 1994;21:630–656.
7. Berruti A, Dogliotti L, Bitossi R, et al. Incidence of skeletal complications in patients with bone metastatic prostate cancer and hormone

refractory disease: predictive role of bone resorption and formation markers evaluated at baseline. J Urol 2000;164:1248–1253.

8. Mundy GR. Bone resorption and turnover in health and disease. Bone 1987;8 Suppl 1:S9–16.

9. Thomas RJ, Guise TA, Yin JJ, et al. Breast cancer cells interact with osteoblasts to support osteoclast formation. Endocrinology 1999;140:4451–4458.

10. Guise TA, Mundy GR. Cancer and bone. Endocr Rev 1998;19:18–54.

11. Clarke NW, McClure J, George NJ. Morphometric evidence for bone resorption and replacement in prostate cancer. Br J Urol 1991;68:74–80.

12. Garnero P, Buchs N, Zekri J, et al. Markers of bone turnover for the management of patients with bone metastases from prostate cancer. Br J Cancer 2000;82:858–864.

13. Ikeda I, Miura T, Kondo I. Pyridinium cross-links as urinary markers of bone metastases in patients with prostate cancer. Br J Urol 1996;77:102–106.

14. Takeuchi S, Arai K, Saitoh H, et al. Urinary pyridinoline and deoxypyridinoline as potential markers of bone metastasis in patients with prostate cancer. J Urol 1996;156:1691–1695.

15. Goltzman D. Mechanisms of the development of osteoblastic metastases. Cancer 1997;80:1581–1587.

16. Kantoff PW, Halabi S, Conaway M, et al. Hydrocortisone with or without mitoxantrone in men with hormone-refractory prostate cancer: results of the cancer and leukemia group B 9182 study. J Clin Oncol 1999;17:2506–2513.

17. Tannock IF, Osoba D, Stockler MR, et al. Chemotherapy with mitoxantrone plus prednisone or prednisone alone for symptomatic hormone-resistant prostate cancer: a Canadian randomized trial with palliative end points. J Clin Oncol 1996;14:1756–1764.

18. Savarese DM, Halabi S, Hars V, et al. Phase II study of docetaxel, estramustine, and low-dose hydrocortisone in men with hormone-refractory prostate cancer: a final report of CALGB 9780. Cancer and Leukemia Group B. J Clin Oncol 2001;19:2509–2516.

19. Smith PH, Suciu S, Robinson MR, et al. A comparison of the effect of diethylstilbestrol with low dose estramustine phosphate in the treatment of advanced prostatic cancer: final analysis of a phase III trial of the European Organization for Research on Treatment of Cancer. J Urol 1986;136:619–623.

20. Beer TM, Pierce WC, Lowe BA, et al. Phase II study of weekly docetaxel in symptomatic androgen-independent prostate cancer. Ann Oncol 2001;12:1273–1279.

21. Berry W, Dakhil S, Gregurich MA, et al. Phase II trial of single-agent weekly docetaxel in hormone-refractory, symptomatic, metastatic carcinoma of the prostate. Semin Oncol 2001;28:8–15.

22. Picus J, Schultz M. Docetaxel (Taxotere) as monotherapy in the treatment of hormone-refractory prostate cancer: preliminary results. Semin Oncol 1999;26:14–18.

23. Eisenberger MA, De Wit R, Berry W, et al. A multicenter phase III comparison of docetaxel (D) + prednisone (P) and mitoxantrone (MTZ) + P in patients with hormone-refractory prostate cancer (HRPC). ASCO 2004;Abstract 4.

24. Petrylak DP, Tangen C, Hussain M, et al. SWOG 99–16: Randomized phase III trial of docetaxel (D)/estramustine (E) versus mitoxantrone (M)/prednisone(P) in men with androgen-independent prostate cancer (AIPCA). ASCO 2004;Abstract 3.

25. Figg WD, Arlen P, Gulley J, et al. A randomized phase II trial of docetaxel (taxotere) plus thalidomide in androgen-independent prostate cancer. Semin Oncol 2001;28:62–66.

26. Sato M, Grasser W, Endo N, et al. Bisphosphonate action. Alendronate localization in rat bone and effects on osteoclast ultrastructure. J Clin Invest 1991;88:2095–2105.

27. Fleisch H. Bisphosphonates: mechanisms of action. Endocr Rev 1998;19:80–100.

28. Vitte C, Fleisch H, Guenther HL. Bisphosphonates induce osteoblasts to secrete an inhibitor of osteoclast-mediated resorption. Endocrinology 1996;137:2324–2333.

29. Frith JC, Monkkonen J, Blackburn GM, et al. Clodronate and liposome-encapsulated clodronate are metabolized to a toxic ATP

analog, adenosine 5′-(beta, gamma-dichloromethylene) triphosphate, by mammalian cells in vitro. J Bone Miner Res 1997;12:1358–1367.

30. Amin D, Cornell SA, Gustatson SK, et al. Bisphosphonates used for the treatment of bone disorders inhibit squalene synthase and cholesterol biosynthesis. J Lipid Res 1992;33:1657–1663.

31. Luckman SP, Hughes DE, Coxon FP, et al. Nitrogen-containing bisphosphonates inhibit the mevalonate pathway and prevent post-translational prenylation of GTP-binding proteins, including Ras. J Bone Min Res 1998;13:581–589.

32. Green JR, Clezardin P. Mechanisms of bisphosphonate effects on osteoclasts, tumor cell growth, and metastasis. Am J Clin Oncol 2002;25:S3–S9.

33. Nemoto R, Kanoh S, Koiso K, et al. Establishment of a model to evaluate inhibition of bone resorption induced by human prostate cancer cells in nude mice. J Urol 1988;140:875–879.

34. Pollard M, Luckert PH. Effects of dichloromethylene diphosphonate on the osteolytic and osteoblastic effects of rat prostate adenocarcinoma cells. J Natl Cancer Inst 1985;75:949–954.

35. Pollard M, Luckert PH. The beneficial effects of diphosphonate and piroxicam on the osteolytic and metastatic spread of rat prostate carcinoma cells. Prostate 1986;8:81–86.

36. Aparicio A, Gardner A, Tu Y, et al. In vitro cytoreductive effects on multiple myeloma cells induced by bisphosphonates. Leukemia 1998;12:220–229.

37. Lee MV, Fong EM, Singer FR, et al. Bisphosphonate treatment inhibits the growth of prostate cancer cells. Cancer Res 2001;61:2602–2608.

38. Oades GM, Senaratne SG, Clarke JA, et al. Nitrogen containing bisphosphonates induce apoptosis and inhibit the mevalonate pathway, impairing Ras membrane localization in prostate cancer cells. J Urol 2003;170:246–252.

39. Senaratne SG, Pirianov G, Mansi JL, et al. Bisphosphonates induce apoptosis in human breast cancer cell lines. Br J Cancer 2000;82:1459–1468.

40. Shipman CM, Rogers MJ, Apperley JF, et al. Bisphosphonates induce apoptosis in human myeloma cell lines: a novel anti-tumour activity. Br J Haematol 1997;98:665–672.

41. Senaratne SG, Mansi JL, Colston KW. The bisphosphonate zoledronic acid impairs Ras membrane (correction of impairs membrane) localisation and induces cytochrome c release in breast cancer cells. Br J Cancer 2002;86:1479–1486.

42. Coxon JP, Oades GM, Kirby RS, et al. Zoledronic acid induces apoptosis and inhibits adhesion to mineralized matrix in prostate cancer cells via inhibition of protein prenylation. BJU Int 2004;94:164–170.

43. Boissier S, Magnetto S, Frappart L, et al. Bisphosphonates inhibit prostate and breast carcinoma cell adhesion to unmineralized and mineralized bone extracellular matrices. Cancer Res 1997;57:3890–3894.

44. van der Pluijm G, Vloedgraven H, van Beek E, et al. Bisphosphonates inhibit the adhesion of breast cancer cells to bone matrices in vitro. J Clin Invest 1996;98:698–705.

45. Boissier S, Ferreras M, Peyruchaud O, et al. Bisphosphonates inhibit breast and prostate carcinoma cell invasion, an early event in the formation of bone metastases. Cancer Res 2000;60:2949–2954.

46. Denoyelle C, Hong L, Vannier JP, et al. New insights into the actions of bisphosphonate zoledronic acid in breast cancer cells by dual Rhoα-dependent and -independent effects. Br J Cancer 2003;88:1631–1640.

47. Adami S, Salvagno G, Guarrera G, et al. Dichloromethylene-diphosphonate in patients with prostatic carcinoma metastatic to the skeleton. J Urol 1985;134:1152–1154.

48. Cresswell SM, English PJ, Hall RR, et al. Pain relief and quality-of-life assessment following intravenous and oral clodronate in hormone-escaped metastatic prostate cancer. Br J Urol 1995;76:360–365.

49. Elomaa I, Kylmala T, Tammela T, et al. Effect of oral clodronate on bone pain. A controlled study in patients with metastatic prostatic cancer. Int Urol Nephrol 1992;24:159–166.

50. Kylmala T, Taube T, Tammela TL, et al. Concomitant i.v. and oral clodronate in the relief of bone pain—a double-blind placebo-controlled study in patients with prostate cancer. Br J Cancer 1997;76:939–942.

51. Clarke NW, Holbrook IB, McClure J, et al. Osteoclast inhibition by pamidronate in metastatic prostate cancer: a preliminary study. Br J Cancer 1991;63:420–423.

52. Pelger RC, Nijeholt AA, Papapoulos SE. Short-term metabolic effects of pamidronate in patients with prostatic carcinoma and bone metastases. Lancet 1989;2:865.

53. Green JR, Muller K, Jaeggi KA. Preclinical pharmacology of CGP 42'446, a new, potent, heterocyclic bisphosphonate compound. J Bone Miner Res 1994;9:745–751.

54. Saad F, Gleason DM, Murray R, et al. A randomized, placebo-controlled trial of zoledronic acid in patients with hormone-refractory metastatic prostate carcinoma. J Natl Cancer Inst 2002;94:1458–1468.

55. Saad F, et al. Zoledronic acid is well tolerated for up to 24 months and significantly reduces skeletal complications in patients with advanced prostate cancer metastatic to the bone. Presented at: American Urological Association Annual Meeting 2003 [abstract 1472].

56. Groot MT, Boeken Kruger CG, Pelger RC, et al. Costs of prostate cancer, metastatic to the bone, in the Netherlands. Eur Urol 2003;43:226–232.

57. Dearnaley DP, Sydes MR, Mason MD, et al. A double-blind, placebo-controlled, randomized trial of oral sodium clodronate for metastatic prostate cancer (MRC PR05 Trial). J Natl Cancer Inst 2003;95:1300–1311.

58. Smith MR, McGovern FJ, Fallon MA, et al. Low bone mineral density in hormone-naive men with prostate carcinoma. Cancer 2001;91:2238-2245.

59. Hussain SA, Weston R, Stephenson RN, et al. Immediate dual energy X-ray absorptiometry reveals a high incidence of osteoporosis in patients with advanced prostate cancer before hormonal manipulation. BJU Int 2003;92:690–694.

60. Smith MR, Eastham J, Gleason DM, et al. Randomized controlled trial of zoledronic acid to prevent bone loss in men receiving androgen deprivation therapy for nonmetastatic prostate cancer. J Urol 2003;169:2008–2012.

61. Smith MR, McGovern FJ, Zietman AL, et al. Pamidronate to prevent bone loss during androgen-deprivation therapy for prostate cancer. N Engl J Med 2001;345:948–955.

44

Managing the complications of advanced prostate cancer

Roger S Kirby

Introduction

The most commonly encountered complications of prostate cancer result from either obstructive uropathy or the effects of metastatic spread. Since the favored site of secondary spread is the skeleton, the majority of problems stem from that source. Pathologic fractures may affect the long bones, spine, or pelvis. If the spinal cord is compressed urgent action may be required to prevent permanent paralysis. The first step in management is to accurately establish the diagnosis, treatment selection will depend on whether the cancer is hormone naive or whether one is dealing with a hormone-resistant prostate cancer (HRPC). In the latter situation the prognosis is significantly worse. Recent data suggests that some skeletal-related events may be prevented or delayed by the judicious use of the bisphosphonate zoledronic acid (See Chapter 102).

Lower urinary tract symptoms and obstructive uropathy

Lower urinary tract symptoms

Lower urinary tract symptoms (LUTS) are common among men suffering from locally advanced prostate cancer.[1] Patients often present with symptoms of frequency and poor flow, as well as a sensation of incomplete emptying. Other problems include hematuria, anorexia, and weight loss; these may indicate incipient renal failure and/or widespread metastases. Urinary retention is signified by a palpable bladder.

Diagnosis

A digital rectal examination is mandatory and a palpable nodule, hardening, or irregular asymmetry requires further evaluation. Normally the lateral and upper borders and the median sulcus are identifiable, and the seminal vesicles impalpable. Loss of the median sulcus and irregularity of the seminal vesicle suggests malignant infiltration, which may be confirmed by transrectal ultrasound-guided biopsy. The upper and lower urinary tract is best evaluated by ultrasound and flow studies. A computed tomography (CT) or magnetic resonance imaging (MRI) scan may be required to determine the location and extent of lymphatic metastases, or other soft tissue metastases. A bone scan is the most frequently utilized way of determining the presence of bone metastases (see Figure 102.1). Local MRI can be used to confirm these and to evaluate whether or not spinal cord compression is present.

Management and treatment options

In many patients with metastatic prostate cancer who present with severe LUTS, hormone treatment (usually with an luteinizing hormone releasing hormone [LHRH] analog) will improve voiding function. In patients with acute or chronic retention who fail to void, androgen ablation therapy will generally facilitate voiding and also make a transurethral resection of the prostate (TURP) easier by reducing tumor bulk and vascularity. If voiding does not occur after 8 weeks or so of hormone therapy, a TURP should be considered, although it is associated with a higher incidence of stress incontinence when performed for malignant rather than benign bladder outflow obstruction, and the patient should be informed of this before surgery. Alpha blockers, such as doxazosin, alfuzosin, or tamsulosin, are less effective in malignant prostatic obstruction than in benign prostatic hyperplasia (BPH). However, external-beam radiotherapy to the prostate should be considered even in the presence of bone metastases, as it may arrest local progression and can also control bleeding.

Obstruction of the upper urinary tracts

Obstructive uropathy, caused either by direct compression of the ureterovesical junction, or through invasion of the ureteric orifice and/or the intramural ureter by tumor tissue, can lead to deterioration in renal function, and ultimately, kidney failure if left untreated. In patients with prostate cancer, urinary tract obstruction secondary to the local extension and lymphatic spread of disease is a common finding at both diagnosis, and at later stages of disease,[2] with an incidence varying between 2% and 51%.[3]

Upper and lower urinary tract obstruction may lead to troublesome complications causing significant morbidity, and often indicates a poor prognosis in patients with prostate cancer.[2,4] Recently, the prognosis for patients with advanced-stage disease has been significantly improved through a number of endoscopic interventions,[2] with survival ranging from 4 to 24 months, depending on whether hormone-naive or hormone-resistant prostate cancer is present.[5–9]

Presentation

Patients may sometimes present acutely with ureteric colic.[3] However, patients typically present insidiously either with deranged blood chemistry or the incidental finding of renal cortical atrophy or ureteric dilatation on an upper abdominal imaging study.[4] Both acute and chronic bilateral ureteric obstruction are associated with a decreased urine output, as well as symptoms of uremia, and may lead to renal failure.[4] In cases where upper urinary tract obstruction leads to infection, fever, and urosepsis, this necessitates emergency decompression or percutaneous drainage.[4] Chronic or acute urinary retention should be excluded clinically/sonographically in a patient presenting with bilateral hydronephrosis, and may be treated by the simple measure of urethral or suprapubic catheterization of the bladder.

Investigation of renal failure

When an alteration in serum creatinine is present and obstructive uropathy is suspected, immediate further investigation is indicated. In patients with previously confirmed prostate cancer, possible urologic complications should be anticipated and the patient monitored accordingly.[2] In the majority of cases, initial workup includes serum chemistry and urinary tract ultrasound to check for both lower and upper urinary tract obstruction.[2] Further investigation may include CT to determine the extent of local/nodal disease. Assessment of peak urinary flow rate, symptom scores, or ultrasound of the prostate may be appropriate in some patients.[2] Other imaging modalities available for the diagnosis of obstructive uropathy include intravenous urography, MRI, and radionuclide renography (Figure 44.1).

Ultrasound

Ultrasound is the most commonly employed of investigation in suspected cases of urinary tract obstruction, whether the renal function is normal or abnormal.[2] Ultrasound of the abdomen may show hydronephrosis or hydroureter, suggesting the probable level of an obstruction.

Intravenous urography

While ultrasound has to a large extent replaced the intravenous urogram (IVU), an IVU can provide useful additional information,[10] provided there is adequate renal function (generally a serum creatinine <200 mmol/L). In acute obstruction, a hydronephrosis may not be visible on an early ultrasound and the IVU might then be more informative. A retrograde ureterogram is often technically difficult in locally advanced prostate cancer, and seldom yields information of therapeutic value unless performed as a prelude to attempted ureteric stent insertion.

Computed tomography

Computed tomography plays an important role in determining the etiology of obstructive uropathy when ultrasound and other modalities are not conclusive, and may help to inform subsequent management strategies.[10] A prospective study by Bosniak et al[10] investigated 36 patients with hydronephrosis secondary to obstructive uropathy of uncertain etiology. Abdominal CT was performed following intravenous contrast to establish the cause of ureteric obstruction, and proved to be of value in 92% of cases. In addition, extrinsic masses were demonstrated in 20 patients with metastatic disease.[10]

Ideally, CT is performed with intravenous contrast, but non-contrast-enhanced CT, in particular spiral CT, may still be useful in patients who have an indeterminate ultrasound, or have an allergy to the contrast medium or uremia.[10]

Radionuclide renography

Radionuclide renography is a nuclear imaging technology for the evaluation of renal function. Radionuclides are injected to provide

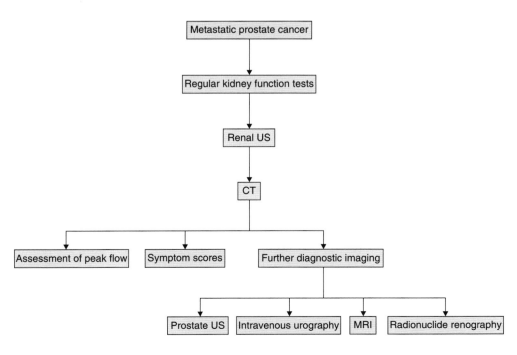

Figure 44.1
Investigation of obstructive uropathy. (CT, computed tomography; MRI, magnetic resonance imaging; US, ultrasound.)

a noninvasive measure of renal split-function.[11] In general, radionuclides establish renal function at the time of examination and not the potential for renal recovery.

Management and treatment

The management of obstructive uropathy is directed by two principles: first, treatment of the causative lesion; second, diagnosis and treatment of the underlying obstructive uropathy. The approach to treatment of obstructive uropathy is dependent on the site of obstruction.[12] In the emergency setting, patients with acute urinary retention resulting from lower tract obstruction can be managed simply by passing a urethral or suprapubic catheter into the bladder.[4] In patients with upper tract obstruction, the placement of a nephrostomy tube, or, more rarely, the retrograde introduction of a ureteric stent, may be necessary.[12] Following drainage, the diagnosis and treatment of the underlying obstructive uropathy can commence. In patients with low-grade acute obstruction or partial chronic obstruction, intervention may be delayed.[12] However, bilateral obstruction and unilateral obstruction accompanied by symptoms of pyonephrosis require prompt management and drainage[12] to prevent irreversible renal damage.

In patients with previously confirmed locally advanced prostate cancer, the choice of treatment for upper tract obstruction is additionally influenced by whether the patient is hormone-naive or has HRPC. Ureteric obstruction in the hormone-naive individual can be treated with androgen blockade or orchidectomy,[7] while in patients with HRPC decompression of ureteric obstruction provides temporary urinary diversion.[2] Lower urinary tract obstruction in patients with significant residual urine and recurrent bouts of urosepsis can be alleviated through the establishment of clean intermittent catheterization.[12] This approach to managing urinary retention requires patient acceptance and training,[4] but can preserve kidney function.[12]

The diagnosis of obstructive uropathy in patients with advanced prostate cancer sometimes raises difficult ethical questions for the treating urologist/oncologist. Although palliative treatment may improve renal function in the short-term, the patient's suffering may be prolonged.[4] Palliative urinary diversion or decompression is usually justified where improvement in renal function facilitates effective treatment options for the primary disease, for example, taxane-based chemotherapy, or for the alleviation of pain.[4] However, the decision to proceed with urinary diversion may not always be in the patient's best interests in end-stage HRPC, particularly if there is advanced symptomatic pelvic disease. Therefore, an individual approach to treatment is required, based on patient age, history, evolution of cancer, as well as ethical and social considerations.[13]

Intervention

Decompression of the urinary tract can help to prolong survival and significantly decrease morbidity in patients with ureteric obstruction.[7,14] Minimally invasive interventions including percutaneous needle nephrostomy (PCNN), long-term ureteric stenting, and endoscopic ureteroneocystostomy have largely replaced traditional open surgical procedures.[7,15] The placement of a stent can provide immediate relief in cases of urinary tract obstruction, but in malignant obstruction urinary flow is via the stent lumen and any blockage of the lumen will cause further obstruction. Percutaneous needle nephrostomy provides direct drainage from the kidneys. If ureteric stenting via the antegrade or retrograde routes is not

achievable, extra-ureteric stenting may be indicated. The role of TURP is only to achieve voiding after retention, or to improve lower urinary tract symptoms. It does not have a principal role in the management of prostate cancer or the management of upper urinary tract obstruction.

Percutaneous needle nephrostomy

Percutaneous needle nephrostomy offers both immediate relief and long-term improvement, with minimum inconvenience if followed by antegrade stenting. In a study[16] of 22 patients with advanced pelvic cancer, 24 nephrostomies were performed (bilateral in 2 patients) for malignant ureteric obstructions. Indications for nephrostomy in this group included renal failure, urosepsis, or pre-treatment before chemotherapy. Sixty-eight percent of patients were able to achieve a useful lifestyle after the procedure, with a survival time ranging from 3 months to 2 years. Similarly, in a study[17] of 77 patients with obstructive uropathy secondary to pelvic malignant disease, a successful nephrostomy insertion rate resulted in an overall median patient survival of over 6 months.

However, although percutaneous drainage via an antegrade or retrograde approach provides a reliable method of renal recovery, the impact of treatment on patient quality of life remains controversial. The studies referred to previously[12,16] included various primary tumor types and the situation in advanced prostate cancer is less clear cut unless the patient is hormonally-naive. A study[5] of 22 HRPC patients with both unilateral (n = 5) and bilateral (n = 17) obstructions, reported that 18 of the patients died with a median survival time of just under 4 months following percutaneous urinary diversion; less than that expected for similar patients without ureteric obstruction. On average, patients spent 41% of their remaining lifetime after PCNN in hospital. The authors concluded that PCNN did not improve the quality of life of these patients.[5]

Conversely, in a later study[7] of 36 patients with bilateral ureteric obstruction and renal failure, the mean survival period for patients in whom androgen depletion had been undertaken after ureteric obstruction was around 21.5 months. In these patients, for whom hormonal therapy remained an option, urinary tract decompression offered a worthwhile improvement in terms of increased survival and reduced in-patient time.[7] However, in patients where androgen depletion had been carried out prior to the diagnosis of ureteric obstruction, survival was significantly worse, at only 2.7 months.[7] The authors of this study concluded that in patients with bilateral ureteric obstruction secondary to prostate cancer who have not undergone hormone manipulation there should be little hesitation in the use of upper tract decompression in either short-term or long-term disease management.[7]

Similar findings were observed by Chiou et al,[6] who reported longer survival rates in 15 prostate cancer patients with both unilateral and bilateral obstructive uropathy following percutaneous nephrostomy, prior to hormone therapy. The 1- and 2-year survival rates of these patients were 73% and 47%, respectively, while those of patients who had previously undergone hormone therapy were lower at 48% and 19%, respectively.[6] However, the authors of this study did not advocate withholding PCNN from patients who had previously undergone hormone manipulation, due to the significant number of patients in this group who survived for longer than a year following treatment.[6]

Ureteric stenting

In patients with prostate cancer, stents provide a palliative and attractive alternative to PCNN in acute relief from ureteric obstruction.[15] Inserted percutaneously or endoscopically into the ureter, longer-term stents may be placed for up to 6 months in patients with obstruction and end-stage disease. However, planned replacement is essential to prevent fractures within the stent wall, or build-up of encrustation.

Endoscopic ureteroneocystostomy

Endoscopic ureteroneocystostomy can restore ureterovesical continuity through the resection of the ureteric meatus following either PCNN or ureteric stent placement. Chefchaouni et al[13] performed endoscopic ureteroneocystostomy in 31 patients with renal failure resulting from advanced unilateral (n = 12) or bilateral (n = 18) obstructive uropathy secondary to prostate cancer, in an attempt to restore continuity of the ureteric orifice. Eleven patients were hormone-naive, whilst 18 had HRPC. All patients underwent PCNN prior to ureteroneocystostomy. Under fluoroscopic guidance the position of the obstruction was then determined, and deep resection of the lateral part of the trigone was performed, enabling the reopening of the ureteric lumen. The nephrostomy tube was removed after normalization or stabilization of renal function. Continuity of the ureteric orifice was achieved in 76% of patients, and a median survival after surgery of 8 months was achieved. Additionally, the average time in hospital was reduced from 27.5 days to

6.8 days following ureteroneocystostomy. The hormonal status of patients had no effect on survival. The authors concluded that ureteroneocystostomy provided an attractive option for patients with obstructive uropathy, due to the short hospital stay and high success rate of this treatment.

Conclusions

Obstructive uropathy is not an uncommon complication among prostate cancer patients.[2] An algorithm for the diagnosis and management of this condition is set out in Figure 44.2. All patients with progressive disease should have their serum creatinine monitored regularly and undergo renal ultrasound if their creatinine becomes deranged. If obstructive uropathy is suspected, an ultrasound or CT scan will assist the diagnosis. The management of obstructive uropathy by urgent upper urinary tract decompression through PCNN or ureteric stenting can significantly reduce patient morbidity and prolong patient survival,[7,14] and is almost always indicated in patients who are hormonally-naive. In patients with HRPC, a palliative approach may sometimes be more appropriate, although the recent publication of data suggesting that taxane-based chemotherapy with docetaxol can prolong survival by several months provides a rationale for a more interventional approach.

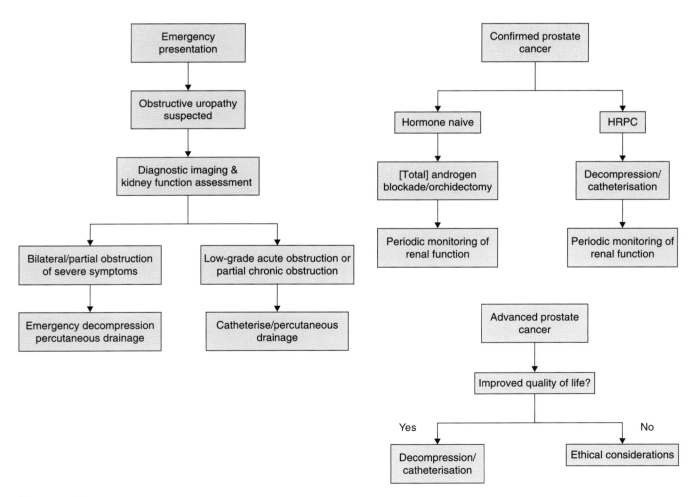

Figure 44.2
Management of obstructive uropathy resulting from prostate cancer. (HRPC, hormone-resistant prostate cancer.)

Management of spinal cord compression due to prostate cancer

As previously mentioned symptomatic spinal cord metastases occur in around 5% to 10% of prostate cancer patients; however, asymptomatic lesions are probably much more common.[18,19] The most common site for spinal metastasis to occur is the vertebral bodies of the thoracic and lumbar regions (See Figure 44.1).[20,21] The most frequent site of symptomatic neural compression is the thoracic region (67%), with 27% in the lumbar spine and 6% in the cervical spine, in part reflecting the narrower volume of the spinal canal in this region.[22,23]

Ninety per cent of prostatic spinal metastases are osteoblastic.[24] Spinal deformity is, therefore, unusual although epidural compression is not uncommon, being the initial sign of malignancy in 36% of patients with epidural metastasis.[25] By contrast, only 7% of breast metastases are osteoblastic, 30% are mixed and 63% are osteolytic.[26] The majority of spinal metastases from other sites are also osteolytic. Osteolytic metastases weaken bone resulting in pathologic fracture with the potential for neurologic compromise as a result of bony compression rather than tumor compression. Recognition of this difference is axiomatic to understanding the difference in clinical presentation and management strategies for prostatic epidural spinal cord compression (ESCC) compared with metastasis from other primary sites. This applies particularly to surgical management, except, in the unusual circumstance (<10%) of osteolytic prostatic metastasis resulting in pathologic fracture with the potential for neurologic compromise.

Several reviews[27–29] emphasize the clinical impact of ESCC, which is defined as a compression at any level of the spinal canal (including cauda equina). Epidural spinal cord compression is, in itself, not fatal; nevertheless, incapacitating pain and subsequent neurologic compromise, such as paraplegia and loss of sphincter control, have major social and clinical implications (Figure 44.3). Complete loss of neurologic function is irretrievable, and, therefore, prevention of ESCC is desirable whenever possible. Several clinically relevant algorithms have been developed to aid the clinician in their early diagnosis and management strategies.[30,31]

Clinical features of presentation

Patients may present via a variety of different routes: as an acute admission, as a referral from a clinic with unexplained musculoskeletal pain or as an existing patient referred by an oncologist or member of the prostate care team.[32] Osborn et al[33] investigated symptoms at presentation in a retrospective study of four large series of spinal metastases from prostate cancer. It was concluded that patients at risk or with actual ESCC, present with four main initial symptoms: back pain, weakness, and autonomic and sensory loss.

Back pain

The most frequent symptom reported in up to 100% of adult ESCC patients is back pain resulting mainly from the involvement of bone with the metastatic tumour[34–38] (Table 44.1).

A recent retrospective analysis by Cereceda et al[35] analyzed 119 patients who had 212 significant episodes of prostatic osseous spinal metastases and confirmed that pain was almost universal (93%). The type of pain and the relieving and aggravating factors reflect the underlying local pathologic process. At first, pain may be local in origin due to periosteal stretching as the metastasis enlarges, sometimes accompanied by somatic referred pain. Radicular pain may also develop with incipient root compression.[33] Prostate cancer patients may suffer this pain for a median duration of 12 months before the onset of ESCC.[39] Localized pain may be relentless and be exacerbated by anything that raises cerebrospinal fluid pressure, such as straining, coughing, or sneezing.[27,33] With increasing occlusion of the spinal canal pain may be aggravated by lying down, in contrast to degenerative spinal disease which is often relieved by recumbency.

Patients often recognize the pain as different to their more long-standing, mechanical, low back pain of degenerative origin, and it is often more proximal given the predilection for the thoracic spine. A retrospective survey of 131 patients with spinal metastases by Stark et al[40] found localized vertebral tenderness in 74% of patients. Care should be taken when attributing pain to degenerative spinal disease in patients with a history of prostate cancer who should be carefully evaluated for spinal metastases.[27,31] Symptomatic neurologic compromise in the form of sensory loss, weakness, and autonomic dysfunction typically develop after pain, commonly but not always in this sequence.

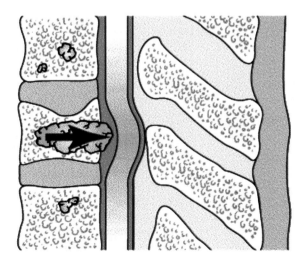

Figure 44.3
Epidural spinal cord compression: neurological complications result from pressure on the spinal cord.

Table 44.1 Pain as a symptom of epidural spinal cord compression in patients with prostate cancer in four retrospective studies

Author	Episodes of spinal metastases	Patients with pain, n (%)
Smith et al[36]	26	25 (96)
Shoskes et al[37]	28	21 (75)
Zelefsky et al[23]	50	48 (96)
Rosenthal et al[38]	31	31 (100)

The neurologic presentation differs with the level of neural compression and its direction. Cord compression above T12 typically results in an upper motor neuron (UMN) picture, while at the conus and below, a lower motor neuron (LMN) picture results. If compression is initially anterior, weakness, loss of pain, and temperature sensitivity may precede compromise of light touch and proprioception (dissociated sensory loss). Conversely, if compression is initially posterior the reverse may apply.

Weakness

Weakness is usually bilateral and frequently involves the muscle groups below the lesion[33] (Table 44.2). The degree of weakness and ambulatory ability at diagnosis are important clinical predictors of outcome.[34,40] Smith et al[36] reported that in patients with prostate cancer and ESCC, 93% of ambulatory patients, 83% of paraparetic patients, and 0% of paraplegic patients were ambulatory after appropriate treatment. Once weakness is present, progression to ESCC in prostate cancer patients is relatively swift.

Autonomic and sensory dysfunction

According to Gilbert et al,[34] autonomic dysfunction in a cancer patient is an unfavorable prognostic sign. Symptoms of bowel and bladder problems, such as incontinence and urinary retention are frequent in these patients at diagnosis (57%) depending on the level of the compression.[27] In addition, Cereceda et al[35] reports that 3% of prostate patients suffered with bladder dysfunction. Over half of patients (51%) report symptoms of numbness and paresthesia, while on examination a sensory loss is found in 78%[27] (Table 44.3). Past medical history may be of importance when considering ESCC; previous radiotherapy, injury, vascular disease, and disk disease may also be indicative of a future risk of ESCC.[27]

Clinical assessment

A complete history and examination with particular attention to neurologic status is necessary in a patient presenting with any combination of these symptoms.[32]

Examination

In addition to a routine general examination with particular attention to excluding visceral metastasis, neurologic examination should assess mental status, cranial nerves, motor and sensory examination, reflexes, and cerebellar function.[31] Posture, stance, and gait in particular, represent an integration of these functions. Assessment in the vertical position, in particular, the ability to tiptoe walk, heel-walk and do single-knee dips will often reveal latent weakness or proprioceptive loss not apparent on bed assessment. If there is a significant history of mechanical spinal pain, plain radiographs of the painful area to exclude incipient spinal collapse should be obtained prior to standing and walking assessment. Precise definition of complete/incomplete neurologic deficit and time after which neurologic recovery cannot be anticipated is not easy to achieve.

Imaging and diagnosis

Magnetic resonance imaging

Magnetic resonance imaging is considered the gold standard diagnostic test for imaging spinal metastases.[33] It is noninvasive, gives excellent anatomical detail of the spinal cord, and is able to image the desired spinal segments irrespective of spinal block. Several studies[41–43] have demonstrated that spinal MRI is as sensitive as other modalities for detecting spinal epidural metastases. However, one potential disadvantage is that it has not been routine to image the whole spinal column, which potentially misses other asymptomatic lesions. In line with other guidelines,[32] it is recommended that all patients should ideally receive an urgent MRI of the entire spine and other affected bones.

Radiography

Prior to the availability of MRI, definitive diagnosis of ESCC required myelography, a highly invasive test for patients who are already in pain. Consequently, routine investigations, such as conventional radiography, were used to determine those patients at low risk of ESCC in whom myelography would not be required. Conventional radiography has the ability to demonstrate vertebral abnormalities in up to 85% of patients with ESCC from both osteoblastic and osteolytic lesions or vertebral collapse.[34,40] Portenoy et al[44] studied the probability of epidural metastatic disease based on the presence of symptoms and radiographic or bone scan changes. It was reported that if there was a localized sign and the radiograph was abnormal the probability of epidural disease was 0.9; however, if the radiograph was normal it was only 0.1 (this was not, however, controlled with MRI). This was increased to 0.95 if both the radiograph and bone scan were abnormal and reduced to 0.02 if the radiograph and bone scan were normal.

For osteolytic metastases, lesions need to be greater than 1 cm and more than 50% of the bone has to be destroyed before these are necessarily evident using conventional radiography. In addition, in HRPC patients, the multiplicity of bony metastases and that the

Table 44.2 Weakness as a symptom of epidural spinal cord compression in patients with prostate cancer in four retrospective studies

Author	Episodes of spinal metastases	Patients with weakness, n (%)
Smith et al[36]	26	14 (54)
Shoskes et al[37]	28	23 (82)
Zelefsky et al[23]	50	25 (50)
Rosenthal et al[38]	31	30 (97)

Table 44.3 Nervous dysfunction as a symptom of epidural spinal cord compression in patients with prostate cancer in four retrospective studies

Author	Episodes of spinal metastases	Patients with autonomic dysfunction, n (%)	Patients with sensory loss, n (%)
Smith et al[36]	26	9 (35)	6 (23)
Shoskes et al[37]	28	14 (50)	19 (68)
Zelefsky et al[23]	50	1 (2)	n/a
Rosenthal et al[38]	31	18 (58)	18 (58)

majority are osteoblastic rather than osteolytic means that a high number of false negatives result. It is, therefore, unlikely that radiographs alone have enough predictive value to warrant their routine use in predicting prostate cancer patients at risk from ESCC.

Myelography

Although MRI has largely replaced myelography, there are still some circumstances in which myelography is useful. Magnetic resonance imaging is contraindicated in those with pacemakers, intracardiac stents and with intraocular metallic foreign bodies. In addition, MR images of the spine are usually grossly distorted by the presence of ferrous implants from previous spinal surgery. If a second episode of ESCC has developed despite prior surgery with implants, myelography combined with CT will usually provide sufficient information on which to base management decisions.

Radionuclide bone scans

Radionuclide bone scans are a useful single test for staging prostate cancer and are more sensitive than radiographs at detecting vertebral metastases.[45,46] A recent study by Soerdjbalie-Maikoe et al,[47] using a new method of evaluating bone scintigraphy concluded that radionuclide bone scans performed at the time of development of hormone refractoriness in HRPC patients is of high predictive value for the inherent risk of ESCC. It does not, however, provide sufficient detail to be of surgical value in discriminating which of the often multiple vertebral site(s) is responsible for neural compression and the direction of that compression. In the context of spinal metastatic disease in practice, isotope bone scans are used only to define extraspinal osseous disease and its extent, and this can usually be delayed until after spinal surgery, if this is necessary. However, if neurology is deteriorating appropriate surgical intervention should not be delayed.

Computed tomography

Computed tomography has for practical purposes been replaced by MRI. This is on the basis of the higher sensitivity of MRI and lack of ionizing radiation. However, there are circumstances in which MRI is contraindicated or the presence of ferrous implants may render it useless.

The usefulness of spinal CT in predicting epidural tumor was investigated by Weissman et al[48] in 30 cancer patients, including four men with prostate cancer. Twenty-one of 23 patients (91%) with cortical disruption at more than one vertebral level on spinal CT had epidural tumor. Spinal CT can, therefore, be a useful test to define a high risk of ESCC if MRI cannot be used. It may also provide additional bony detail to answer particular anatomical questions, for example, bony dimensions for instrumentation or the course of the vertebral artery.

Summary of imaging requirements

Although each case will require a thorough individual assessment the initial assessment of spinal metastases from prostate cancer should include: a neurologic and general assessment, plain radiographs of the spine, an urgent MRI and a chest X-ray. Chest and abdominal CT and radionuclide bone scans are desirable staging investigations, but these should not impede surgical intervention, if neurological status is deteriorating.

Biopsy of spinal lesions

A spinal biopsy is recommended if the lesion is a solitary bony lesion and there is doubt as to the underlying pathology. In these cases imaging with scintigraphy, MRI of the lesion and percutaneous bone biopsy need to be performed before surgery to prevent inappropriate procedures.[32] Experienced surgeons should generally perform percutaneous biopsies, under X-ray control.[32]

Treatment options

Radiotherapy

The response of epidural metastases to radiotherapy is well documented.[49,50] Radiotherapy is the preferred first-line treatment for ESCC in known prostate cancer patients as it is the optimal treatment for what are usually radiosensitive tumors. In 1978 before the advent of modern spinal surgical methods, Gilbert et al[34] reviewed 235 cases of ESCC: 170 patients were treated with radiotherapy alone and 65 patients underwent radiotherapy and decompressive laminectomy. There was no significant difference in functional outcome of the two groups. Zelefsky et al[23] reported similar findings in their analysis of 42 patients with spinal metastases from prostate cancer who had been treated with external-beam radiation. At completion of treatment, it was reported that 92% of patients experienced pain relief, and 67% had significant or complete improvement on neurologic examination. In a further study,[36] which analyzed 35 patients with prostate cancer and suspected spinal cord compression; 26 patients were found to have ESCC. All patients were initially treated with radiation, steroids, and androgen deprivation therapy. In ambulatory or paraparetic patients, radiation, androgen deprivation therapy and steroids can be effective palliative therapy. However, patients who present with paraplegia or in whom paraplegia developed secondary to recurrent compression are often not palliated by this combination of therapies. Surgery is recommended for these patients.[36]

The Radiation Therapy Oncology Group (RTOG) evaluated different dose fractionation irradiation schedules in a randomized, controlled trial[51] to determine their palliative effectiveness in patients with osseous metastases. The frequency, promptness, and duration of pain relief were utilized as measures of response. Ninety percent of patients experienced some relief of pain and 54% achieved eventual complete pain relief. However, the optimal dose fractionation scheme for treating ESCC is still unknown. Most radiation oncologists adhere to standard schedules of 25 to 36 Gy, with an average of 30 Gy over 10 fractions being chosen because it is considered to be a relatively well-tolerated dose for the spinal cord.[27] There may be no optimal plan for every metastatic prostate cancer patient because each plan constructed will represent a compromise between delivery of the highest dose possible to control progression of the tumor and palliate pain effectively, whilst limiting the effect on the spinal cord.

Radiotherapy has minimal side effects in metastatic prostate cancer patients and is efficacious in terms of preventing further tumor growth and ameliorating pain. The neurologic outcome of radiotherapy depends on two factors. Firstly, the degree of functional limitation at initiation of radiotherapy will alter the outcome of therapy. Neurologic status at initiation is important as it has been reported that radiotherapy may preserve the ability to ambulate in 80% to 100% of patients who initiate treatment while still ambulatory.[34,50,52] Secondly, the extent of subarachnoid impingement will also affect the outcome of treatment. Epidural metastases that produce a minor impression on the thecal sac will have a better outcome than a large mass that completely obliterates the subarachnoid space. This has been confirmed in clinical studies, but is the weakest of the two prognostic indicators.[53,54]

In the era of MRI, the response of spinal metastases to radiotherapy has not been thoroughly investigated. Median survival for patients undergoing radiotherapy for ESCC is between 3 and 6 months. Survival rates are higher in patients who were ambulatory when treatment was initiated and in radiosensitive tumors, such as prostate with a single metastasis. The risk of recurrence increases with the length of survival, and 50% of 2-year survivors will develop recurrence.[34] In line with results from other studies, Leviov et al,[55] concluded that a radiotherapeutic success ceiling of 80% existed for metastatic ESCC patients and, in view of this, future investigative studies should focus on educating clinicians in the early detection and diagnosis of this complication. Indications for radiotherapy are given in Box 44.1.

Chemotherapy

Chemotherapy is a reasonable treatment option in patients with ESCC who have undergone previous radiotherapy and are not candidates for surgery when the underlying tumor is likely to be chemosensitive.[27]

Hormone deprivation therapy

Hormonal manipulation has been successfully employed in hormone-naive patients with ESCC from prostate cancer, and there is a definite relationship between neurologic deficit at presentation and response to hormone therapy. Bilateral orchiectomy is the most expeditious method of achieving castrate levels of serum testosterone. If LHRH analogs are utilized, they should be combined with an antiandrogen, as the well-described flare phenomenon may exacerbate the ESCC. However, in patients who have complete paraplegia at the time of presentation, hormone therapy has little benefit.[56] It should not be forgotten that patients with HRPC may respond to second-line therapy, such as estrogens, or taxane-based chemotherapy.

Surgery

A variety of surgical strategies can be employed for neoplastic spinal disease. Appropriate selection is dependent upon the individual case and requires tailoring accordingly. The objectives from a patient perspective are to minimize pain and to maximize or maintain neurologic function with the minimum procedure adequate to the

prognosis. From a spinal perspective, the objectives are to ensure adequate decompression; to ensure the maintenance of, or restoration of, spinal cord or nerve root function, and to eliminate actual or potential spinal instability with preservation of as many normal motion segments as possible.[32]

In the majority of patients with ESCC resulting from prostatic metastases, the clinical problem is local tumor-related pain with accompanying radicular or cord compression syndrome pain rather than spinal instability. In the absence of symptoms or imaging evidence of instability, neural compression symptoms may be adequately managed by decompression alone often in the form of laminectomy with, as necessary, specific root decompression in isolation.

Unusually, if osteolytic metastases are present, or if there is significant instability pain, and/or there is other imaging evidence of potential or actual progressive deformity, techniques of stabilization may be required. They may also be necessary if adequate decompression in itself results in iatrogenic destabilization. For example, distal to T10, if posterior decompression requires removal of one or both facet joints, stabilization would be appropriate. Proximal to this in the thoracic spine, it may be judged that the rib cage may provide adequate stability.

Surgery may also be required if the tumor is found to be radioresistant or is progressing despite adequate radiotherapy.[57] A variety of surgical strategies and techniques are available for treatment of metastatic disease of the spine. Metastatic and HRPC patients may benefit from specific techniques of surgical decompression and stabilization dependent upon the location of their metastases.

Box 44.2 summarizes the indications for and objectives of surgery.

Supportive measures

Analgesics

A systematic approach to regular assessment, review, and treatment needs to be adopted. It is important to elicit the type, nature, and intensity of pain together with the impact on the patient and quality of life. Treatment should be in line with the World Health Organization (WHO) guidance, with medication given regularly (to prevent pain), and by the "ladder": a stepwise progression from non-opioids, to weak opioids, to strong opioids, with appropriate adjuncts.[58]

Steroid treatment

Corticosteroids are an integral part of the therapy of ESCC.[33] Steroids initiated immediately after diagnosis may benefit the prostate cancer patient by relieving pain and improving neurologic

---

Box 44.1 Indications for radiotherapy for spinal metastases[32]

- No spinal instability
- Radiosensitive tumor
- Stable or slow neurological progression
- Multi-level disease
- Surgery precluded by general condition
- Poor prognosis
- Postoperative adjuvant treatment

Box 44.2 Surgery for neoplastic spinal disease

Indications
- Spinal instability
- Clinically significant neurologic compression, in particular by bone
- Unresponsive tumor (to radiotherapy, chemotherapy or androgen ablation)

Objectives
- Maintenance or restoration of spinal cord function
- Correction of spinal instability

function. Corticosteroids such as dexamethasone perform a principle role in supportive treatment and have also been demonstrated to improve outcomes. A randomized trial of dexamethasone in patients undergoing radiotherapy for ESCC from solid tumors found that a significantly higher percentage were ambulatory on dexamethasone at the long-term follow-up.[59] Dexamethasone is the most frequently used agent in the clinical environment; however, no prospective studies have investigated the optimal dose and schedule for patients with ESCC and this remains an area for debate. Supportive evidence of daily doses ranging from 16 to 96 mg is available.[50,60] In the absence of data, an initial dose within this range is justifiable; however, regardless of the dose used, dexamethasone should be tapered as tolerated, since complications can arise rapidly.

Prevention of skeletal related events with bisphosphonates

As well as being a major cause of morbidity, it has now been shown that skeletal fractures correlate negatively with overall survival in men with prostate cancer and are an independent and adverse predictor of survival.[35] It is, therefore, important that skeletal fractures and skeletal morbidity are kept at a minimum. Bisphosphonates seem a promising way ahead in this respect (See Chapter 43).

Biochemical and histomorphometric studies indicate that osteolysis (excessive bone destruction) is present in prostate cancer metastases despite the sclerotic appearance on X-rays. In this respect bisphosphonates, which are pyrophosphate analogs that block osteolysis, may be useful for the treatment of patients with osteoblastic metastases as well as those with osteolytic metastases.

Zoledronic acid is a new nitrogen-containing bisphosphonate that has been evaluated in patients with metastatic HRPC. It has previously been shown to be at least as effective as pamidrinate 90 mg infusion in reducing skeletal complications in patients with myeloma or breast cancer.[36]

In a randomized controlled trial zoledronic acid (4 mg) given intravenously was evaluated against a placebo in patients with metastatic HRPC. A greater proportion of patients who received placebo had skeletal-related events than those who received zoledronic acid at 4 mg (44.2% versus 33.2%; difference, 11.0%; p = 0.021). Median time to first skeletal-related event was 321 days for patients who received placebo, compared with 420 days for patients who received zoledronic acid at 4 mg (p = 0.011 versus placebo) (Figure 44.4). Zoledronic acid 4 mg given as a 15 minute

infusion was well tolerated. The main side effect was influenza-like malaise at the time of and shortly after the infusion.

Conclusions

The treatment of metastatic prostate cancer to the spine differs from that of other spinal metastases, and, in many cases, there is debate as to the optimal management of these patients. Early diagnosis and appropriate imaging are essential. It is imperative to involve spinal surgeons to evaluate neural compromise before deciding on the appropriateness or otherwise of surgical intervention, and the opinion of an experienced radiotherapist should also be sought. Androgen ablation therapy should be urgently instituted in hormone-naive patients; in men with HRPC, second-line therapy should be considered. Early institution of appropriate therapy can make the crucial difference between an independent existence and wheelchair-bound paraplegia.

References

1. Hamilton W, Sharp D. Symptomatic diagnosis of prostate cancer in primary care: a structured review. Br J Gen Prac 2004;54:617–621.
2. Colombel M, Mallame W, Abbou CC. Influence of urological complications on the prognosis of prostate cancer. Eur Urol 1997;31(suppl 3):21–24.
3. Villavicencio H. Quality of life of patients with advanced and metastatic prostatic carcinoma. Eur Urol 1993;24:118–121.
4. Russo P. Urologic emergencies in the cancer patient. Semin Oncol 2000;27:284–298.
5. Dowling RA, Carrasco CH, et al. Percutaneous urinary diversion in patients with hormone-refractory prostate cancer. Urology 1991;37: 89–91.
6. Chiou RK, Chang WY, Horan JJ. Ureteral obstruction associated with prostate cancer: the outcome after percutaneous nephrostomy. J Urol 1990;143:957–959.
7. Paul AB, Love C, Chisholm. The management of bilateral ureteric obstruction and renal failure in advanced prostate cancer. Br J Urol 1994;74:642–645.
8. Sandhu DP, Mayor PE, Sambrook PA, et al. Outcome and prognostic factors in patients with advanced prostate cancer and obstructive uropathy. Br J Urol 1992;70:412–416.
9. Oefelein MG. Prognostic significance of obstructive uropathy in advanced prostate cancer. Urology 2004;63:1117–1121.
10. Bosniak MA, Megibow AJ, Ambos MA, et al. Computed tomography of ureteral obstruction. AJR Am J Roentgenol 1982;138: 1107–1113.
11. Thomsen HS, Hvid-Jacobsen K, Meyhoff HN, et al. Combination of DMSA-scintigraphy and hippuran renography in unilateral obstructive nephropathy. Improved prediction of recovery after intervention. Acta Radiol 1987;28:653–655.
12. Chevalier RL, Klahr S. Therapeutic approaches in obstructive uropathy. Semin Nephrol 1998;18:652–658.
13. Chefchaouni MC, Flam TA, Pacha K, et al. Endoscopic ureteroneocystostomy: palliative urinary diversion in advanced prostate cancer. Tech Urol 1998;4:46–50.
14. Ortlip SA, Fraley EE. Indications for palliative urinary diversion in patients with cancer. Urol Clin North Am 1982;9:79–84.
15. Lang EK. Antegrade ureteral stenting for dehiscence, strictures, and fistulae. AJR Am J Roentgenol 1984;143:795–801.
16. Hoe JW, Tung KH, Tan EC. Re-evaluation of indications for percutaneous nephrostomy and interventional uroradiological procedures in pelvic malignancy. Br J Urol 1993;71:469–472.

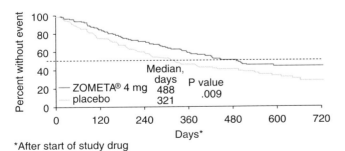

Figure 44.4
Impact of zoledronic acid (Zometa©) on time to first event. The onset of skeletal complications is significantly delayed by more than 5 months.

17. Lau MW, Temperley DE, Mehta S, et al. Urinary tract obstruction and nephrostomy drainage in pelvic malignant disease. Br J Urol 1995;76: 565–569.

18. Sorensen S, Borgesen SE, Rhode K, et al. Metastatic epidural spinal cord compression. Results of treatment and survival. Cancer 1990;65:1502–1508.

19. Rodichok LD, Ruckdeschel JC, Harper GR, et al. Early detection and treatment of spinal epidural metastases: the role of myelography. Ann Neurol 1986;20:696–702.

20. Schiff D. Spinal cord compression. Neuro Clin N Am 2003;21: 67–86.

21. Jacobs SC. Spread of prostatic cancer to bone. Urology 1983;2: 337–344.

22. Flynn DF, Shipley WU. Management of spinal cord compression secondary to metastatic prostatic carcinoma. Urol Clin North Am 1991;18:145.

23. Zelefsky MJ, Scher HI, Krol G, et al. Spinal epidural tumour in patients with prostate cancer: Clinical and radiographic predictors of response to radiation therapy. Cancer 1992 70:2319–2325.

24. Cook GB, Watson FR. Events in the natural history of prostate cancer: using salvage curves, mean age distributions and contingency coefficients. J Urol 1968;99:87.

25. Liskow A, Chang CH, DeSanctis P, et al. Epidural cord compression in association with genitourinary neoplasms. Cancer 1986;59: 949–954.

26. Arseni CN, Simionescu MD, Horwarth L. Tumours of the spine. A follow up study of 350 patients with neurosurgical considerations. Acta Psychiatr Scand 1959;34:398.

27. Grant R, Papadopoulos SM, et al. Metastatic epidural spinal cord compression. Neurol Clin 1991;9:825–841.

28. Byrne TN. Spinal cord compression from epidural metastases. N Engl J Med 1992;327:614–619.

29. Ratanatharathorn V, Powers WE. Epidural spinal cord compression from metastatic tumor: diagnosis and guidelines for management. Cancer Treat Rev 1991;18:55–71.

30. Redmond J, Friedl KE, et al. Clinical usefulness of an algorithm for the early diagnosis of spinal metastatic disease. J Clin Oncol 1988;6: 154–157.

31. Chen TC. Prostate cancer and spinal cord compression. Oncology (Huntington) 15:841–861.

32. British Orthopaedic Association and British Orthopaedic Oncology Society. Metastatic Bone Disease. A guide to good practice. Available at www.boa.ac.uk.

33. Osborn JL, Getzenberg RH, et al. Spinal cord compression in prostate cancer. J Neurooncol 1995;23:135–147.

34. Gilbert RW, Kim JH, et al. Epidural spinal cord compression from metastatic tumor: diagnosis and treatment. Ann Neurol 1978;3:40–51.

35. Cereceda LE, Flechon A, et al. Management of vertebral metastases in prostate cancer: a retrospective analysis in 119 patients. Clin Prostate Cancer 2003;2:34–40.

36. Smith EM, Hampel N, et al. Spinal cord compression secondary to prostate carcinoma: treatment and prognosis. J Urol 1993;149: 330–333.

37. Shoskes DA, Perrin RG. The role of surgical management for symptomatic spinal cord compression in patients with metastatic prostate cancer. J Urol 1989;142:337–339.

38. Rosenthal MA, Rosen D, et al. Spinal cord compression in prostate cancer. A 10-year experience. Br J Urol 1992;69:530–583.

39. Schaberg J, Gainor BJ. A profile of metastatic carcinoma of the spine. Spine 1985 10:19–20.

40. Stark RJ, Henson JA, et al. Spinal metastases. A retrospective survey from a general hospital. Brain1982;105:189–213.

41. Godersky JC, Smoker WR, Knutson R. Use of magnetic resonance imaging in the evaluation of metastatic spinal disease. Neurosurgery 1987;21:676–680.

42. Carmody RF, Yang PJ, et al. Spinal cord compression due to metastatic disease: diagnosis with MR imaging versus myelography. Radiology 1989;173:225–259.

43. Li KC, Poon PY. Sensitivity and specificity of MRI in detecting malignant spinal cord compression and in distinguishing malignant from benign compression fractures of vertebrae. Magn Reson Imaging 1988;6:547–556.

44. Portenoy RK, Galer BS et al. Identification of epidural neoplasm. Radiography and bone scintigraphy in the symptomatic and asymptomatic spine. Cancer 1989;64:2207–2213.

45. Pollen JJ, Gerber K , Ashburn WL, et al. The value of nuclear bone imaging in advanced prostate cancer. J Urol 1981;125:222–223.

46. Merrick MV, Stone AR, Chisolm GD. Prostatic cancer. Nuclear medicine. Recent Res Cancer Res 1981;78:108–118.

47. Soerdjbalie-Maikoe V, Pelger RCM, Lycklama GA, et al. Bone scinigraphy predict the risk of spinal cord compression in hormone refractory prostate cancer. Eur J Nucl Med Mol Imaging 2004;31:958–963.

48. Weissman DE, Gilbert M, Wong H, et al. The use of computed tomography of the spine to identify patients at high risk of epidural metastases. J Clin Oncol 1985;3:1541–1544.

49. Martenson JA, Evans RG, et al. Treatment outcome and complications in patients treated for malignant epidural spinal cord compression (SCC). J Neurooncol 1985;3:77-84.

50. Greenberg HS, Kim JH et al. Epidural spinal cord compression from metastatic tumor: results with a new treatment protocol. Ann Neurol 1980;8:361–366.

51. Tong D, Gillick L, et al. The palliation of symptomatic osseous metastases: final results of the Study by the Radiation Therapy Oncology Group. Cancer 1982;50:893–899.

52. Findlay GF. The role of vertebral body collapse in the management of malignant spinal cord compression. J Neurol Neurosurg Psychiatry 1987;50:151–154.

53. Tomita TJ, Galicich H, et al. Radiation therapy for spinal epidural metastases with complete block. Acta Radiol Oncol 1983;22: 135–143.

54. Helweg-Larsen S Johnsen A, et al. Radiologic features compared to clinical findings in a prospective study of 153 patients with metastatic spinal cord compression treated by radiotherapy. Acta Neurochir (Wien)1997;139:105–111.

55. Leviov M, Dale J, et al. The management of metastatic spinal cord compression: a radiotherapeutic success ceiling. Int J Radiat Oncol Biol Phys 1993;27:231-234.

56. Sasagawa I, Gotoh H, et al. Hormonal treatment of symptomatic spinal cord compression in advanced prostatic cancer. Int Urol Nephrol 1991;23:351–356.

57. McLain RF, Bell GF. Newer management options in patients with spinal metastasis. Cleve Clin J Med 1998;65:359–366.

58. World Health Organization. Cancer pain relief and palliative care. Report of a WHO Expert Committee. World Health Organization Technical Report Series, 804. Geneva, Switzerland, World Health Organization, 1990;1–75.

59. Soresen PS, Helweg-Larsen S, Mouridsen H, et al. Effect of high dose dexamethasone in carcinomatous metastatic spinal cord compression treated with radiotherapy: a randomised trial. Eur J Cancer 1994;30A:22–27.

60. Heimdal K, Hirschberg H, et al. High incidence of serious side effects of high-dose dexamethasone treatment in patients with epidural spinal cord compression. J Neurooncol 1992;12:141–144.

61. Oefelein MG, Ricchiuiti V, Conrad W, et al. Skeletal fractures negatively correlate with overall survival in men with prostate cancer. J Urol 2002;1687:1005–1007.

62. Rosen LS, Gordon D, Antonio BS, et al. Zoledronic acid versus pamidronate in the treatment of skeletal metastases in patients with breast cancer or osteolytic lesions of multiple myeloma: a phase III, double-blind, comparative trial. Cancer J 2001;7:377–387.

45

Principles of palliative care and psychosocial support of the metastatic prostate cancer patient

Donald Newling

Introduction

The principal problem in the management of far advanced prostate cancer is the provision of the best palliative and psychosocial care for those patients who, because of metastatic disease, have a limited longevity and impending reduction of their quality of life.

There are a number of clearly defined problems, which are:

- The management of pain
- The management of urinary obstruction—upper or lower tract
- Skeletal-related events
- Rectal involvement
- Bone marrow failure
- Lymph edema
- Incontinence
- Psychosocial problems

Continuing anticancer therapy

Patients with far advanced metastatic prostate cancer will almost certainly have been medically or surgically castrated and there is evidence to suggest that it is important that the castrate levels of testosterone are maintained even in this advanced state. In addition to hormonal therapy, there is an increasing role for cytotoxic treatment with docetaxel (Taxotere) or mitoxanthrone plus steroids.[1] These treatments, although having minimal effects on survival, can undoubtedly reduce the symptoms of advanced, and advancing, prostate cancer.

The recent demonstration that high-dose estrogens can also exert a cytotoxic effect at this stage of the disease has led to their increasing use systemically, via plasters or by intramuscular injections.[2] In addition, corticosteroids on their own have been shown on a number of occasions to have a beneficial effect on subjective progression and symptomatology in this advanced metastatic stage.[3]

Management of pain in advanced prostate cancer

The majority of pain is caused by skeletal metastases. However, patients may experience severe pain from upper or lower urinary tract obstruction, rectal involvement, or direct involvement of the nerve plexuses in the pelvis. The cause of pain needs to be identified, in order that adequate analgesia may be given. The World Health Organization (WHO) have issued a pain ladder for the management of cancer-related pain and in this respect, prostate cancer is no different from other cancers and the general principles should be followed[4] (Figure 45.1).

The first step on this so-called pain ladder is the use of simple analgesics such as paracetamol or aspirin, or other nonsteroidal anti-inflammatory drugs. If pain persists, or increases, the second step would be the use of a weak opioid plus a non-opioid. For persistent pain after that then a strong opioid such as morphine itself plus a non-opioid should be used. Cancer related pain is continuous, and analgesia should be given in a continuous manner. Once the top rung of the ladder is reached, there is probably little point in increasing the dose of morphine by less than 30% of the existing dose. Only then will the analgesia be adequate.[5] In the presence of excess nausea and/or vomiting, thought should be given to administering the opioid by a systemic or intrathecal route. The giving of opioids should be accompanied by the administration of suitable laxatives.

Ancillary therapy—such as the use of radiotherapy for individual sites of bone pain, the use of systemic radiotherapy via radioactive nucleotides such as strontium-89 (^{89}Sr), and if necessary the use of nerve blocks or rhizotomy—should be considered.[6,7]

The adequacy of analgesia can be improved by the treatment of related disorders such as muscle spasm. The use of anticonvulsants and muscle relaxants, the use of anxiolytics and antidepressants, which can relieve the distress caused by the pain, can also potentiate the activity of many analgesic drugs. For pain caused by a rising intracranial pressure or spinal cord compression, dexamethasone is an important and necessary adjunct.

The various contributing factors to the pain felt by prostate cancer sufferers is summarized in Figure 45.2.

Urinary tract obstruction

Upper urinary tract

Local advancement of prostate cancer will frequently involve compression of the lower ureters, dilatation of the upper tract, and impending uremia. With the advent of JJ stents and the simplicity of

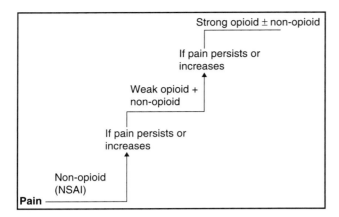

Figure 45.1
World Health Organization pain ladder (NSAI, nonsteroidal anti-inflammatory.)

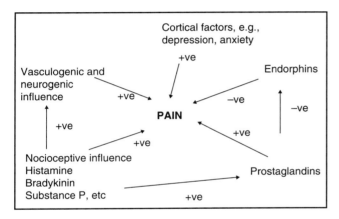

Figure 45.2
Factors contributing to the pain felt by prostate cancer sufferers.

bringing in nephrostomy tubes, it is tempting to suggest that upper urinary tract obstruction should always so be treated. However, if the general condition of the patient is deteriorating rapidly, and particularly if he has severe pain from other metastatic lesions, the dulling of the sensorium consequent upon the onset of uremia may be a blessing and diminish the need for large doses of strong analgesics and other similar drugs.[10] JJ stents can usually only be left in situ for 6 months and very frequently will block earlier. It may then be necessary to substitute these internal splints for external nephrostomies with accompanying deterioration in the patient's mobility and quality of life. Recently metal stents have been developed that can be inserted into the renal pelvis at the one end and into the bladder at the other end. These can be brought in via a laparoscopy and do not necessarily mean a long operative procedure. They can frequently be left in for longer than 6 months.[11]

Lower urinary tract

If the patient's general condition is good, lower urinary tract obstruction may be relieved by a simple transurethral procedure. Removing large quantities of malignant tissue may often impair

sphincter activity and lead to incontinence. The alternative is the use of a transurethral catheter or suprapubic catheter if incontinence is not a problem.[12]

Skeletal-related events

Skeletal-related events such as fracture are associated with pain and the danger of neurologic damage involving spinal cord compression and paralysis. The greatest hazard exists in the lower thoracic cord where the spinal canal is narrower than elsewhere. When a skeletal-related event such as fracture or nerve compression occurs, it is important that action is taken as quickly as possible in order to diminish the long-term effects. This may require local radiotherapy or surgery with or without radiotherapy. The use of high-dose steroids such as dexamethasone is recommended. Recently the incidence of skeletal related events in bony metastases has been shown to be lessened by the use of second and third generation bisphosphonates. These can be given in an intermittent manner once every 3 weeks until the situation is under control, and possibly in smaller doses than have been used in the recent past. In addition to bisphosphonates, endothelium A receptor antagonists diminish the activity of osteoblasts and can, therefore, limit new bone formation stimulated by prostate cancer metastases.[13]

Rectal symptoms

Direct invasion from the primary prostate tumor into the rectum is not an infrequent occurrence. Occasionally the tumor can cause obstruction of the rectum. A transanal resection of the tumor is sometimes necessary under these circumstances.[14] If the tumor encircles the rectum causing complete obstruction, then a diverting colostomy may become necessary. This is also a useful palliative tool in the presence of a fistula or fecal incontinence caused by direct involvement of the nerves involved in anal sphincter control. Occasionally the local spread of tumor is so ferocious that the sacral plexus is involved, giving rise to very severe pain and often necessitating the placement of a colostomy, a suprapubic catheter, and neurolysis.[13]

Bone marrow failure

In prostatic cancer, bone marrow failure is caused by direct infiltration of the marrow with depletion of myeloid and erythroid lines. There may also be severe platelet reduction and dysfunction. Apart from direct infiltration by tumor cells, the castrate levels of testosterone give rise to a reduction of at least 10% in the average hemoglobin of patients with prostate cancer. The platelet dysfunction can be so severe as to give rise to disseminated intravascular coagulation, and this may necessitate the paradoxical use of anticoagulants in the short term.[15] For total bone marrow failure blood transfusion will be necessary, but again the use of transfusions must be weighed against the likely prognosis for individual patients. Where the predominance is of anemia, the use of recombinant erythropoietin is an attractive, though expensive, substitute for blood transfusion.[16]

Lymph edema

In the first instance, lymph edema, which is often very troublesome in the genital region, may be relieved by elevation of the bed at night and of a settee during the day. Sometimes the edema is so severe that it is necessary to pass a catheter to enable adequate voiding to take place. Graduated compression with stockings of the lower limbs is an alternative, and intermittent pneumatic compression is recommended if the lower-limb edema is very severe. Lymph edema may occur together with venous edema. Where there is a clear indication that venous obstruction plays a significant role, then anticoagulant therapy may be indicated.[17]

Incontinence

Diagnosis of incontinence must be adequately made. The differentiation between overflow incontinence due to outflow obstruction and incontinence caused by neurogenic or muscular damage either caused iatrogenically or by the disease process itself must be made. If overflow incontinence is the problem and the patient's general condition is good, then a transurethral resection is the best alternative. Neurogenic incontinence or incontinence caused by direct involvement via the tumor should probably be managed by a transurethral catheter. A suprapubic catheter is not to be recommended apart from in the management of overflow incontinence.[18]

Psychosocial disorders and their management

There are four stages during the development and progression of prostate cancer where there is major psychosocial trauma, frequently accompanied by the appearance of psychological or even psychiatric disturbance.[19]

The diagnosis of a malignancy is always a life-shattering event. At the beginning of the disease, the patient and his family must be given realistic prognoses and a logical and clear description of the various treatment options at their disposal. If the initial therapy, as

is most frequent, is to be carried out with curative intent then the next psychological blow will occur when the patient develops rising prostate-specific antigen (PSA) levels or can be clearly told that the disease has recurred. The decision, at this point in time, of whether to introduce palliative therapy in the form of hormonal treatment will vary from patient to patient and from one tumor to another. Once the second line treatment has been started, there will probably be a period of 18 months to 2 years before "hormone escape" occurs. Ultimately, the tumor will progress, and this will be the third blow to the patient's psyche and that of his family. In the past, the fourth shock came when patients were told that we had no further therapeutic options. In the present treatment climate, this is never to be said. It is almost always possible for the symptoms of the disease to be controlled even if the disease itself is rampant.

Prostate cancer is a disease that affects the whole family and, therefore, the decision process, if the patient so wishes, should be shared. From the beginning, it is often wise to involve the patient and his family in the care process whether by modifications of diet or physical activity or simply by broadening the consultation process.

Sadly, the psychiatric care of the elderly with psychiatric disturbances has often been inadequate because of the fear of side effects of treatment.[20,21] The patient with prostate cancer who develops psychological or psychiatric disturbances should be treated exactly the same way as someone who does not have the cancer. If the disturbance is iatrogenic then modification of their medication is the first and most important step. Depression, anxiety, and fear are the three most common psychological disturbances, and each should be managed on its own merit. The use of anxiolytic drugs and antidepressants is to be encouraged, not only to relieve the psychological disturbance, but also to improve the effectiveness of analgesia and other therapeutic maneuvers. Care must be taken with the use of some antidepressants, such as the tricyclics, which can have a deleterious effect on urinary control.[22] It is important to remember that, because many of the patients at this stage of their disease are elderly, communication may become increasingly difficult, particularly in the presence of psychotropic or neurotropic drugs and in the presence of strong analgesia. It is important that a clinician knows the patient has received and understood the messages and suggestions.

The patient sits in the middle of a circle of carers including the primary care team, palliative care team, the lead care team (Urology) and the oncology team (Figure 45.3). Just as important in this circle

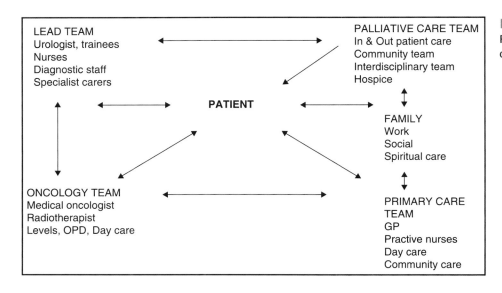

Figure 45.3
Patient-centered multidisciplinary cancer care.

is the family and the needs of the family before, during and after the death of the patient must be considered.[23]

Patients with an advancing malignancy often go through a number of psychological disturbances throughout the course of the disease. There is always an element of confusion at the beginning, associated with a certain amount of resentment and often attempts to find a cause involving other people or his environment. Once progression of the disease has been confirmed, there is often a tacit acceptance, which may lead to a reluctance to try further therapeutic measures. As the end approaches, the patient often experiences considerable fear, which may include fear of the method of his demise, fear of losing control either physically, of bowel or bladder, or mentally, with an inability to control his emotions and other thought processes, but also an intense fear for those that he is leaving behind who may also be elderly and infirm. These factors must all be addressed appropriately by members of the teams, and the patient and his family must know that, at the end, his symptoms will be adequately controlled and his family and those others he leaves behind will be adequately looked after.[24]

Conclusions

The progress of prostate cancer is much slower than with other malignant tumors, and, therefore, the prognosis is longer and sometimes more complicated. This means that the quality of care for the patient needs to be carefully maintained throughout, involving multi-disciplinary teams and sensible and logical use of the therapeutic modalities available. Although the greatest responsibility for the management of these patients lies with the lead team, that team must be prepared at all stages to involve other teams who could help individual aspects of the patients condition. The Association of Palliative Medicine defines palliation as the appropriate medical care of patient's with advanced and progressive disease for whom the focus of care is quality of life and in whom the prognosis is limited. In the case of prostate cancer this prognosis may be limited but may last many years giving the clinician and those who work with him/her the opportunity at all stages to optimize therapy ensuring the best quality of life, where the quantity cannot be increased, and the highest possible quality of death for the patient and those around him.

References

1. Petrylak DP. Chemotherapy for androgen independent prostate cancer. Semin Urol Oncol 2002;3:31–35.
2. Ockrim JL, Lalani E-N, Laniado ME, et al. Transdermal Estradiol Therapy for Advanced Prostate Cancer – Forward to the Past?, Departments of Surgical Oncology and Technology, Histopathology, Faculty of Medicine, Imperial College and Department Urology, Hammersmith Hospitals NHS Trust.
3. Hanks GW, Trueman T, Twycross RG. Corticosteroids in terminal cancer – a prospective analysis of current practice. Postgrad Med J 1983;59:702–706.
4. World Health Organization, Cancer Pain Relief. Geneva: WHO, 1994.
5. Hanks G, Expert Working Group EAPC. Morphine in cancer pain: modes of administration. Br Med J 1996;312:823–826.
6. Soerdjbalie-Maikoev V, Pelger RC, Lycklama A, et al. Strontium-89 (Metastron) and the bisphosphonate olpadronate reduce the incidence of spinal cord compression in patients with hormone-refractory prostate cancer metastatic to the skeleton. Eur J Nucl Med Imaging 2002;29:494–498.
7. Lacovou J, Marks JC, Abrams PH, et al. Cord compression and carcinoma prostate: is laminectomy justified. Br J Urol 1985;57:733–736.
8. Holland JC. Psycho-oncology: overview, obstacles and opportunities. Pscyho Oncol 1992;1:1–13.
9. Moorey S, Greer S, Bliss J, et al. Comparison of adjuvant psychological therapy and supportive counselling in patients with cancer. Psycho Oncol 1998;7:218–228.
10. Paul AB, Love C, Chisholm GD. The management of bilateral ureteric obstruction and renal failure in advanced prostate cancer. Br J Urol 1994;5:642–645.
11. Jabour ME, Desgrandchamps F, Angelscu E, et al. Percutaneous implantation of subcutaneous prosthetic ureters: long term outcome. J Endo Urol 2001;15:611–614.
12. Mazur AW, Thompson IM. Efficacy and morbidity of 'channel' TURP. Urology 1991;38:562–628.
13. Clarke NW. The management of hormone-relapsed prostate cancer, Christie Hospital NHS Trust and Salford Royal Hospitals NHS Trust, Manchester, UK. BJU Intl 2003;92:860–868.
14. Chen TF, Eardley I, Doyle PT, et al. Rectal obstruction secondary to carcinoma of the prostate treated by trans-anal resection of the prostate. Br J Urol 1992;70:643–647.
15. Gobel BH. Bleeding disorders. In Groenwald S, Grogge M, Goodman M, Yarbro C eds, Cancer Nursing—Principles and Practice. Boston, MA: Jones Bartlett, 1993, pp 575–607.
16. Albers PH, Cappell R, Schwaibold H, et al. Erythropoietin in urologic oncology. Eur Urol 2001;39:1–8.
17. Brennan MJ. Lymphoedema following the surgical management of breast cancer. J Pain Sympt Manage 1992;2:110–116.
18. Fossa SD. Quality of life in advanced prostate cancer. Semin Oncol 1996;23:32–34.
19. Derogatis LR. The prevalence of psychiatric disorders among cancer patients. J Am Med Assoc 1983;249:751–757.
20. Cleary JF, Carbonne PP. Palliative medicine in the elderly. Cancer 1997;80:1335–1347.
21. Lynch M. The assessment and prevalence of affective disorders in advanced cancer. J Palliat Care 1995;11:10–18.
22. Massie MJ, Holland JC. Depression and the cancer patient. J Clin Psychiatry 1990;51:12–17.
23. Grzybowska P. What are the palliative care needs of prostate cancer patients? In Bowsher W (ed.): Challenges in Prostate Cancer. Oxford: Blackwell Science, 2000.
24. Stjernswald J. Palliative medicine: a global perspective, In Doyle D, Hanks GWC, MacDonald N (eds): Oxford Textbook of Palliative Medicine. Oxford: Oxford University Press, 1996, pp 805–816.

46

The promise of immunotherapy in prostate cancer: from concept to reality

Vasily J Assikis, William Jonas, Jonathan W Simons

Introduction

Significant progress has been made since the mid 1990s in our ability to treat patients with advanced prostate cancer. Most prostate cancer patients now present with localized disease and mortality rates are dropping.[1] Despite the fact that the vast majority of men with prostate cancer are diagnosed with localized disease, current therapies for localized disease will cure only 50% to 85% of patients.[2–4] For patients with widespread prostate cancer the disease remains incurable with the currently available agents. Historically, metastatic disease has been treated with androgen deprivation therapy. Despite the extremely high response rates with this modality (>85%), patients universally progress once the cancer transitions to a castration-independent phenotype. Castration-independent prostate cancer (CIPC) is currently treated with cytotoxic chemotherapy. Work done over the past decade has clearly established that: 1) chemotherapy offers superior palliation (over steroids alone) and improvement of quality of life[5]; and 2) taxane-based chemotherapy offers a statistically significant, albeit modest, overall survival benefit.[6–7] This minor survival benefit achieved with taxanes has been met with great enthusiasm—since it is the first time ever any systemic therapy has been shown to affect overall survival in the CIPC setting. Nonetheless, a median survival of 1.5 years (as reported in the phase III registration trials with docetaxel) can not be seen as the goal but, rather, the starting line for further improvement. New concepts for treatment of advanced prostate cancer are urgently needed.

Currently, over 200 novel therapies are being tested in patients with prostate cancer. In addition to novel cytotoxic agents, interest has also focused on immunologic modulation (vaccines), targeted therapies (based on prostate-specific antigen [PSA] or prostate-specific membrane antigen [PSMA]), overcoming antiapoptotic and proliferative signaling (vitamin D analogs, PPARγ agonists, anti-BCL2), and disruption of key intracellular circuitry (signaling through epidermal growth factor receptor [EGFR], PI3/Akt, insulin-like growth factor 1 receptor [IGF1R], mitogen-activated protein kinase [MAPK], and interleukin 6 [IL6], just to name a few).[8] An expanding body of literature is developing over the merit and clinical benefits of targeting the host for metastatic prostate cancer, namely the bone. We now have well-described pairs of targets/therapeutic agents: osteoclasts/bisphosphonates, osteoblasts/endothelin 1 inhibitors, cancer-stroma interface/radiopharmaceuticals. Finally, targeting of the prerequisite new blood vessel formation, namely angiogenesis, has led to a number of investigational options currently tested in large scale trials.

It is the scope of this chapter to review recent advances in emerging therapies with a special focus on immunotherapy for prostate cancer.

Immunotherapy

The origins of immunotherapy as a treatment for cancer were first given credence when surgeons in the late nineteenth century observed spontaneous tumor regressions in patients. Noting that these were often preceded by infections, Coley et al were challenged in reproducing this phenomenon by treating patients with bacterial extracts.[9] Spontaneous remissions following intense inflammatory reactions are a known phenomenon reported in current literature as well.[10] In the early 1970s, the hypothesis of immune surveillance was presented. At its crux, the hypothesis held that the immune system maintained a role in protecting the host against tumors.[11] This hypothesis was later discounted with observations that the incidence of cancer in athymic mice was no different than that observed in wild-type mice.[12] In support of the above preclinical finding is the epidemiologic observation that immunosuppressed individuals do not appear to be more susceptible to common malignancies including prostate, colon, breast, and lung cancer, (although there is a higher incidence of Epstein–Barr virus-associated lymphomas, Kaposi's sarcoma and cervical cancer[13]). Subsequent research has demonstrated that tumors are not lacking potential antigens, but rather fail to activate the immune system to respond to them.[14] Tumors are, therefore, successful in inducing immune tolerance, hence circumventing the innate mechanisms of defense. It is now felt that it is not lack of appropriate nonself antigens that prevents a robust activation of the immune effector arm against tumor, but rather an unsuccessful discrimination between self and nonself.[15] Therefore, there is a role for the immune system in surveillance. In fact, the goal of therapy has shifted towards how to 1) most effectively present antigens to T cells; 2) enhance activation of cytotoxic immune effector cells as well as maximize humoral response; and 3) optimize delivery/trafficking of immune effector cells/cytokines to the tumor.

Pertinent issues to prostate cancer, with regard to immunomodulatory approaches, include the type and number of antigens employed as targets, various methods to generate either an in-vivo or an ex-vivo activation of specific anti-prostate immunity. A unique advantage is the lack of need for specificity for malignant prostate tissue: attack of benign prostatic tissue by use of antigens not restricted to cancer cells is, by and large, without clinical implications (of note, inflammation of benign prostatic tissue secondary to immune activation may lead to PSA elevation). In the following paragraphs we will review several methods of active and passive immunotherapy that have been tested in clinical trials.

Active immunotherapy

Prostate cancer vaccines

In designing a vaccine, there are two basic categories of antigens to take advantage of, those that have been identified and those that have not.[16] As one would expect, there are numerous antigens that have not been identified and there are over 500 sequences, unique to prostate cancer, known already. When a vaccine is developed from a whole cancer cell lysate, the underlying principle is that myriads of antigens, both known and unknown, would be present. This, in turn, would present more antigens for priming to the immune system and, as prostate cancer cells are known to downregulate antigens to evade immune recognition, it would make it more difficult for them to do so. There are advantages and disadvantages to approaches using defined and undefined antigens; some of these are listed in Table 46 .1.

Since the mid-1990s, one of the preferred platforms for active immunotherapy has been the use of autologous dendritic cells. Such an approach has a number of advantages. Dendritic cells (DCs) are the most efficient antigen-presenting cells (APCs) that initiate an antigen-specific immune response via uptake, processing, and presentation of antigens to T cells. Dendritic cells migrate to draining lymph nodes, where they present antigens to resting lymphocytes. When fully activated, DCs express high levels of cell surface major histocompatibility antigen complexes (MHC). For optimal activation of the effector arm it is crucial that co-stimulatory molecules (CD80,86/CD28; or the CD40 ligand/CD40 pairs) bind as well. Autologous dendritic cells can be harvested by leukapheresis, treated ex vivo with protocols that maximize maturation and activation, and then used as vehicles for carrying antigens to selected targets.[17] Antigen delivery to DCs can employ peptides, whole proteins, or even tumor mRNA; or, alternatively, viral vector systems can be used to transfect DCs with DNA encoding tumor associated antigens. In the next paragraphs we will provide a review of some DC-based vaccines for prostate cancer that have been tested in the clinic.

Prostate-specific membrane antigen vaccines

The first published report on a DC vaccine in prostate cancer involved the intravenous administration of autologous DCs pulsed with synthetic PSMA peptides. A phase I trial using DCs looked at human leukocyte antigen A2 (HLA-A2)-specific PSMA peptides (PSM-P1 and PSM-P2). Autologous DCs pulsed with these PSMA peptides were administered to 51 patients with CIPC.[18] All patients received four infusions of the preparations at 6-week intervals. There was no dosing limit achieved, and there were no significant toxicities. Cellular responses to the appropriate PSMA peptides were monitored. Subjects who were positive for HLA-A2 and who received DCs pulsed with PSM-P1 and PSM-P2 had increased cellular responses. There were 7 patients who achieved a greater than 50% reduction in their serum PSA levels; and 11 patients had stable disease. A subsequent phase II trial recruited 95 men with either locally recurrent (n = 37) or metastatic (n = 58) CIPC.[19] Six infusions of dendritic cells pulsed with either PSM-P1 or P2 were administered at 6-week intervals. This time, half of the patients also received 7 days of subcutaneous granulocyte-macrophage colony-stimulating factor (GM-CSF) with each infusion. Using the same response criteria as in the phase I study, three complete and 16 partial responses were reported; 11 responses were still ongoing at the time of the report. The addition of GM-CSF was not reported to significantly improve the clinical or immune response to vaccination. One of the major criticisms of the early work with this approach was the lack of correlation of peptide specific T-cell cytotoxicity with favorable outcome.[20] Furthermore, many patients were not HLA-A2-positive, and five of the responders were in fact HLA-A2-negative, an observation that called into question the specificity of the response to this peptide-based intervention. More recently, preliminary clinical data with a modification of the initial PSMA-targeted vaccine were presented. In a phase I/II trial, 24 patients with metastatic CIPC underwent a dose escalation of DCVax™ (Northwest Biotherapeutics), an autologous DC vaccine loaded with recombinant whole PSMA.[21] While only two patients had a greater than 50% reduction in their PSA, a total of 38% (nine) had an improvement in their post-treatment PSA slope. Of note, favorable clinical outcome was correlated with humoral response (development of anti-PSMA antibodies) but not with markers of cellular response.

Provenge

Provenge™ (Dendreon, Seattle, Washington) is a vaccine consisting of autologous dendritic cells exposed ex vivo to PA-2024

Table 46.1 Comparison of defined and undefined antigens for prostate cancer

	Defined antigens (e.g., PSA, PSMA)	Undefined cell-based vaccine antigens
Advantages	Potential to monitor immune response Easier biotechnology for manufacture and FDA review Prostate specificity	Available to larger patient population Enhance tumor immune surveillance Polyclonal immune responses Prostate specificity
Disadvantages	Genetically unstable tumors can easily evade immune surveillance through single antigenic loss Expression of antigen only in a fraction of cancer cells	Difficulty in assessing specific immune response in trials Requires autologous or allogeneic cells More complex biotechnology for manufacture and FDA review

PSA, prostate-specific antigen; PMSA, prostate-specific membrane antigen.

(a recombinant fusion protein of human prostatic acid phosphatase and GM-CSF). In a phase I/II study, 31 men with metastatic CIPC received escalating doses of intravenous Provenge during weeks 0, 4, 8, and 24.[22] There were no significant adverse events and the only toxicity reported was minor infusional reactions (fever, chills). Three of 19 men treated on the phase II portion had a decline in PSA of more than 50%, and time to progression was significantly longer in immune responders compared with non-responders (34 versus 13 weeks).These promising results led to a placebo-controlled phase III trial that randomized 127 men with asymptomatic metastatic CIPC to Provenge or placebo every 2 weeks for three doses.[23] In a preliminary report, the longer time to progression in the treated group did not reach the level of statistical significance (16 versus 9 weeks; p = 0.085), but those receiving the vaccine had a significantly higher chance of remaining free of cancer-related pain. A subset analysis found a significant clinical benefit for patients with Gleason score 7 or less and led the foundation for a second randomized phase III trial that is currently ongoing. Provenge is currently being tested also in the setting of PSA rise after prostatectomy in a prospective fashion.

Prostate-specific antigen vaccines

There are many reasons to consider using mRNA as a basis of a DC vaccine strategy including: 1) the generation of mRNA is relatively easy; 2) there is very little risk of the mRNA inserting itself into the host DNA; and 3) the production of an antigen by RNA will present multiple epitopes.[24] This approach will also be available to a wider range of patients as HLA-typing will not be necessary. In a phase I clinical trial, autologous DCs transfected with mRNA encoding PSA were used to treat 13 patients with metastatic CIPC.[25] They were treated with escalating doses of the vaccine, with the maximum dose being determined by the level of obtained DCs. There were no dose limiting toxicities with only grade 1 toxicity being reported including four patients with fever and influenza-like symptoms and four patients with injection site erythema. Nine patients had PSA-reactive T-cells measured pre- and post-treatment, all of whom initially had low or undetectable levels of PSA-reactive T-cells, and all had measurable levels after vaccination. There was no cross-reactivity against negative control proteins including human serum kallikrein or keyhole limpet hemocyanin (KLH). Prostate-specific antigen serum levels were also monitored. Seven patients were evaluable (the other 6 proceeded with therapies that could affect PSA levels including radiation for progressive disease or use of herbal medications). One of seven patients had a minor decrease in PSA. Interestingly, five additional patients were observed to have a decrease in their PSA velocity. While this does not provide evidence for clinical benefit, the measurable immune responses are promising.

Carbohydrate vaccines

Taking a very different approach, Slovin et al, have worked on vaccines that target epithelial surface carbohydrates: the idea is based on the observation that malignant cells express a different carbohydrate pattern on their cell surfaces than normal cells.[26]

Alpha-N-acetylgalactosamine-O-serine/threonine (Tn), is a monosaccharide that is found to be highly expressed by mucins on most epithelial cancers. Slovin et al conjugated the mucin-related O-linked glycopeptide Tn to KLH to give Tn(c)-KLH and to palmitic acid (PAM) to give Tn(c)-PAM, both with the saponin

adjuvant QS21 so as to boost immune response. In a phase I study, they treated 25 patients with biochemically relapsed prostate cancer.[27] Three groups of five patients received separate dosing regimens of the Tn(c)-KLH vaccine and, in the fourth group, 10 patients received Tn(c)-PAM. Administration was at random sites subcutaneously on patients' extremities at weeks 1, 2, 3, 7, 19, and a booster at week 50. All patients were able to complete the series. Side effects were mainly limited to pain and irritation at the injection sites. As the target here was not isolated to malignant cells only, there was a concern for autoimmunity, which was not observed. Interestingly, the lower dose of Tn(c)-KLH appeared to be optimal, with the suggestion that higher doses may in fact confer a suppression of antibody responses. At 50 weeks, of the 15 patients treated with Tn(c)-KLH, 5 had a greater than 50% decrease in their PSA slopes. Of the 10 Tn(c)-PAM recipients, only one had a greater than 50% PSA slope reduction.

Human telomerase reverse transcriptase vaccines

Human telomerase reverse transcriptase (hTERT) is overexpressed in more than 85% of solid tumors.[28] Due to its presence in solid tumors and its role in tumor growth, hTERT is an attractive molecular target.[29] It has been demonstrated that autologous DCs transfected with mRNA encoding hTERT are potent inducers of cytotoxic T lymphocytes (CTLs) and antitumor immunity.[30] Having established antitumor efficacy in models, a phase I trial was undertaken in 18 patients with CIPC.[31] Patients were vaccinated with DCs trandsfected with either hTERT or both hTERT and lysosome-associated membrane protein (LAMP) RNA. Lysosome-associated membrane protein was included as it has been shown previously that it leads to a greater stimulation of CD4+ T cells without negatively affecting the CTL response.[32] All 18 patients were found to have high frequencies of hTERT-specific CD8+ and CD4+ T cells. The vaccine was associated with clearance of circulating tumor cells and a positive impact on PSA velocity in a few patients. Those receiving hTERT/LAMP were found to have higher frequencies of CD4+ T cells and, additionally, their CTLs were found to exhibit a greater cytolytic activity against their targets.

Another group investigating hTERT conducted a phase I trial evaluating cancer patients.[33] Seven patients, five with hormone refractory prostate cancer and two with metastatic breast cancer resistant to conventional cytotoxic therapy, were vaccinated with HLA-A2-restricted hTERT 1540 peptide presented with keyhole limpet hemocyanin by ex-vivo generated DCs. Researchers recognized that certain normal cells, including the bone marrow, express telomerase activity and, therefore, followed the bone marrow by aspirations at the initial and at the third vaccine. There were no grade 3 or 4 adverse events, and no histologic changes were noted in the marrow. Serum immunoglobulin levels and absolute peripheral B-lymphocyte counts were monitored with no significant changes observed. Four of the prostate cancer patients had stable disease by standard radiographic assessment post-vaccination whereas one patient with breast cancer had progressive disease. Prostate-specific antigen levels were found to fall slightly during the vaccine schedule in two patients, before rising again. Important in this study was the demonstration of the induction of hTERT-specific CD8+ T cells without significant toxicity. In addition, after vaccination, there was one patient who experienced partial tumor regression, and with biopsy demonstrated infiltrating CD8+ lymphocytes.

Miscellaneous vaccines

Utilizing identified antigens for a peptide vaccine, a phase I trial was conducted with 10 patients with CIPC who were positive for HLA-A2.[34] After a prevaccination measurement of peptide-specific CTL precursors, a vaccine was individually designed based on each patient's positivity to a panel of 16 identified peptides. The median number of positive peptides administered was three (range 1–5). There were no major adverse reactions, but all developed grade I or II local erythema/edema at the injection site. Of the 10 patients, three were found to have a minor (<50%) PSA response. Recognizing that immune response did not translate into clinical benefit, Noguchi et al combined their vaccine with chemotherapy (estramustine).[35] Release of antigens by cells dying due to chemotherapy should allow cross-priming and, thus, enhance the activation of the effector arm. Results were very promising with 10 of 11 patients experiencing a decrease in PSA level, with eight of them experiencing a reduction of more than 50%. Six patients had an augmentation of peptide-specific CTL precursors, while peptide-specific IgG was observed in 10 of 11. There are plans for phase II studies.

Gene transfer biotechnologies for prostate cancer immunotherapy

Gene therapy involves the insertion of DNA into a cell to replace, or otherwise affect, gene expression of that cell. The goal of gene therapy, as it relates to cancer, is to reverse the malignant phenotype of the cell, trigger apoptosis, or for the altered cell to be marked for immune disposal by way of increasing the tumor cell's immunogenicity and/or by increasing the immune system's responsiveness to the tumor cell. Great strides in the field of gene therapy research have been made since the first human gene therapy trial was performed in 1990.[36] While the simplicity of the concept is elegant, it is a complex process.

Gene therapy requires a delivery vehicle (vector) to carry the therapeutic genetic information. A vector needs only to contain the gene of interest and a promoter to drive its expression.[37] There are many considerations when choosing the optimal vector: the ideal vector would be able to deliver its product specifically to the target cell, deliver it efficiently, not be toxic to the host, not be immunogenic, and not be mutagenic. On top of that, it would need to be reproducible, widely applicable, and of a reasonable cost. Vectors can be separated into two general categories: viral and nonviral (liposomes, naked DNA, DNA polymer complexes). Viral vectors are further subdivided to either DNA- or RNA-based platforms. Viral vectors utilize the inherent ability of viruses to carry foreign DNA into cells, and they are known to deliver genes much more efficiently than their nonviral counterparts. DNA vaccines are often preferable because they are easier to make, are not pathogenic, and the vectors are nonreplicating.[38] In the early experience with viral vectors, modified replication-deficient adenoviruses were employed: in an effort to curtail uncontrolled pathogenic replication, the price was transient expression of the therapeutic gene. More recently, replication-competent viruses (such as retroviruses) have been employed; they have the unique advantage of incorporating into the DNA of rapidly dividing (i.e., cancer) cells so that they are continuously expressed in the original target cell, and in any subsequent cells after mitosis. The efficiency of this approach is hindered by the low proliferative rates typically seen in prostate cancer.[38]

While the technology of DNA transporters continues to advance, some of the issues remain unresolved:

- Should the vector require a synthesizing target cell for integration of the delivered gene?
- If the vector provides incorporation of the delivered gene into the DNA of the target cell or into its cytoplasm, is it necessary for the gene to be expressed transiently or continuously?
- In a viral vector, is the desired effect for the vector to be replication deficient, attenuated, such that it enters only permissive cells, or competent?

Table 46 .2 lists various vectors with their advantages and disadvantages. Additional considerations include whether the vector is used to deliver DNA into cells removed from the patient (ex-vivo approach) that are subsequently re-administered upon genetic manipulation, or delivered to the subject directly (in-vivo approach). In the next paragraphs we will review some approaches that have been of particular interest to prostate cancer

Granulocyte-macrophage colony-stimulating factor gene therapy

Initial investigations in gene therapy for prostate cancer consisted of ex-vivo approaches, in which the patient's own prostate cancer cells (typically obtained at the time of prostatectomy) were manipulated to overexpress the cytokine GM-CSF via retroviral transfer. When the irradiated cells were then reintroduced into the patient, in-vivo secretion of GM-CSF was postulated to promote the uptake of tumor antigens by the patient's dendritic cells.[39]

Granulocyte-macrophage colony-stimulating factor is a cytokine that regulates granulocyte and macrophage stimulation, proliferation, differentiation, and survival. Mulligan et al used a relatively nonimmunogenic tumor model to identify specific gene products that could induce antitumor immunity that could not be achieved with the tumor cells alone.[40] They found GM-CSF to be the most potent product they studied, later attributed to its most potent stimulation and activation of antigen uptake by DCs.[41] This laid the framework for using GM-CSF as vaccine therapy. Using an ex-vivo approach, as demonstrated in Figure 46 .1, a vaccine was generated where a patient's own prostate cancer cells, usually collected at the time of prostatectomy, were engineered by way of a retrovirus to incorporate a gene, which led to the overexpression of GM-CSF. The cells were then irradiated and reintroduced into the patient: in-vivo secretion of GM-CSF should promote uptake of antigens by DCs. In a phase I trial, eight patients, who underwent a radical prostatectomy with curative intent but at surgery were found to have metastatic disease to the regional lymph nodes, were treated with an autologous, GM-CSF-secreting, and irradiated tumor vaccine prepared ex vivo from surgically obtained autologous prostate cancer cells.[39] The number of administered courses was limited to the amount of prepared vaccine. The main side effects were limited to local irritation at the injection site. Using untransduced autologous prostate cancer cells, a delayed-type hypersensitivity (DTH) reaction, only present in 2 of 8 patients prior to vaccination, was present in 7 of 8 patients after treatment. In addition, biopsies of reactive DTH sites demonstrated degranulated eosinophils consistent with both helper 1 and 2 T-cell activation. This phase I proof-of-concept trial was able to demonstrate an inducible immune response against the patient's own prostate cancer cells.[39] An attempt to broaden the applicability of this approach

Table 46.2 Advantages and disadvantages of some vectors for gene therapy

Vector	Advantage	Disadvantage
RNA retroviruses		
Oncovirus	Transmit to offspring, possible long-term expression	Only infects actively dividing cells, risk of insertional mutagenesis, low efficiency, inactivated by complement
Lentivirus	Can infect nondividing cells, long-term expression, not inactivated by complement	Possible recombination with other viruses
Human foamy virus	Can infect nondividing cells, not inactivated by complement, nonpathogenic	Low titers
DNA viruses		
Vaccinia virus	Large size, replicates	Low efficiency, immunity develops
Herpes simplex virus	Large size, can infect nondividing cells, episomal therefore no risk for insertional mutagenesis	Low titers, transient expression
Adenovirus	Can infect nondividing cells, episomal therefore no risk for insertional mutagenesis	Transient expression
Adeno-associated viruses	Can infect nondividing cells, nonpathogenic	Limited size, insertional mutagenesis
Synthetic vectors		
Naked DNA	Low cost, simple preparation, nontoxic	Poor efficiency
Liposomes	Large insertion size, safe for repeated use, low cost, nontoxic	Poor efficiency, short expression
DNA–protein complex	Large insertion size, safe for repeated use, low cost, nontoxic	Poor efficiency, short expression

Adapted from Mabjeesh NJ, Zhong H, Simons JW. Gene therapy of prostate cancer: current and future directions. Endocrine-related cancer 2002;9:115–139.

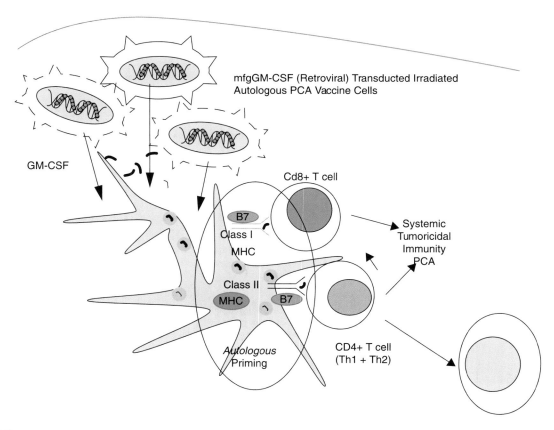

Figure 46.1
Autologous prostate cancer cells ex-vivo engineered to secrete GM-CSF.

involved the ex-vivo transduction of the GM-CSF gene into allogeneic rather than autologous prostate cancer cells. In a phase II trial, 96 men (55 with castration-independent and 41 hormone-naive metastatic prostate cancer) were treated with the prostate cancer vaccine GVAX™(Cell Genesys), which consists of irradiated allogeneic human prostate cancer cell lines PC-3 and LNCaP ex-vivo transduced to secrete human GM-CSF.[42] Eighty-six patients received a priming dose of 500 million cells followed by 12 booster doses (100 million cells each) at 2-week intervals, while the remaining 10 patients (all with CIPC) received higher booster doses (300 million cells each). Toxicity was restricted to minor local skin reactions at the injections site, and there was no autoimmunity. Only two patients met NCI Consensus PSA Panel criteria for biochemical response.[43] In the group of CIPC patients there was a trend towards a prolonged median time to progression (defined by radiologic imaging criteria) in the 10 patients who received the higher booster doses (140 days versus 85 days, p = 0.095). A follow-up presentation on the 34 CIPC patients with asymptomatic bone metastases showed a median overall survival of 26 months.[44] To increase the efficacy of GM-CSF transduction, the retroviral vector was substituted by a an adeno-associated viral vector and another phase I/II study was done investigating different schedules and various doses of vaccination. At the time of presentation, 80 patients had been treated on this study and median overall survival had not been reached at a median follow up of 12 months.[45] In this study, there was a correlation of escalating dose of vaccine with humoral response. Of interest there was stabilization or improvement in the serum levels of type I carboxyterminal telopeptide (ICTP), a known marker of osteolytic activity, raising the possibility of the vaccine targeting the bone microenvironment as well as the prostate cancer cells. These exciting preliminary results led to a currently ongoing phase III trial that randomizes men with asymptomatic metastatic CIPC to the bone to either GVAX or cytotoxic chemotherapy.

Interleukin 2 gene therapy

Another gene-therapy vaccine designed to enhance the immune system's response, utilizes interleukin 2 (IL2). A phase I trial treated 24 patients with locally advanced prostate cancer with Leuvectin, a DNA–lipid complex encoding for the IL2 gene.[46] Leuvectin was directly injected into the prostate twice, 1 week apart. Biopsies were obtained at baseline and again after Leuvectin administration. There was demonstrable response in the injected sites by way of increased intensity of T-cell infiltration. In addition, there were some transient decreases in PSA.

Prostate-specific antigen-based gene therapy

Prostate-specific antigen is, by and large, a protein specific to the prostate, and thus offers itself as a prime antigen for vaccination. A number of approaches have been investigated with this platform. PVAX/PSA is a plasmid vector DNA vaccine encoding recombinant PSA. In a phase I trial of pVAX/PSA, three cohorts of three patients received separate doses of the vaccine (100, 300, or 900 μg), maintained for five cycles. Granulocyte-macrophage colony-stimulating factor and IL2 were provided as vaccine adjuvants.[47] Two of three patients who received the highest dose had a measurable cellular

immune response against recombinant PSA. Given that PSA is a secreted protein, it would follow that PSA is a target for the activation of cellular immunity rather than the humoral arm of the immune system. While not membrane bound, (thus negating the conventional activation of the humoral arm), the expression of PSA by MHC class I on APCs would trigger the cellular immune response. This hypothesis has been eloquently demonstrated in mice, where the expression of human PSA by a mouse tumor cell line was able to elicit a PSA-specific CTL response and effect tumor cell death.[48] In the initial phase I study, a recombinant vaccinia virus encoding human PSA (Prostvac [Therion Biologics]) in metastatic prostate cancer was administered to five groups of patients.[49] The first two groups received Prostvac by dermal scarification; however, the remaining groups received the vaccine subcutaneously due to the increased dose levels. They all received GM-CSF subcutaneously as an adjuvant. Complications were mainly related to injection site irritation and vesicle formation with additional complications of fatigue, grades 2 and 3, in 5 (12%) patients, 2 patients (5%) with grade 2 elevated liver function tests, and 6 patients (14%) with grades 2 and 3 fevers. Evidence of an increased proportion of PSA-specific T cells after vaccination combined with the fairly safe toxicity profile are expected to lead to further studies. In another study, 33 men with biochemical progression received Prostvac along with GM-CSF.[50] There were only minor local skin reactions and promising clinical activity. Currently, Prostvac has been modulated to add costimulatory molecules (B7.1 ICAM1, LFA3) and as PROSTVAC-VF/TRICOM™ (Therion Biologics) is currently in phase II trials in metastatic CIPC. In a similar strategy, an ECOG phase II clinical trial was conducted to evaluate the feasibility and tolerability of a prime/boost vaccine strategy using vaccinia virus and fowlpox virus expressing human PSA in patients with biochemical progression after local therapy for prostate cancer.[51] The induction of PSA-specific immunity was also evaluated. The endpoint was PSA progression. Twenty-nine (45.3%) patients remained free of PSA progression at 19.1 months and 78.1% patients were found to have clinical progression-free survival. Of the subset of patients who were HLA-A2-positive, 46% were found to have an increase in PSA-specific T-cell response. Currently, an ongoing trial is addressing the question of optimal sequencing of the two pox viral vectors (fowlpox and vaccinia) and the role of adjuvant GM-CSF.

Suicide gene therapy

Suicide gene therapy, as the name implies, involves altering of the prostate cancer cell so that a newly incorporated gene, when expressed, will lead the cancer cell to apoptosis. BCL2 (an antiapoptotic gene) overexpression has been shown to be associated with resistance to radiation therapy and androgen deprivation.[52] BAX is a proapoptotic gene that counteracts the BCL2 antiapoptotic effects. Using an adenoviral vector, BAX was combined with a prostate-specific promoter.[53] Cancer cell lines treated with the vector had high levels of Bax expression and an 85% reduction in cell viability. Apoptosis was confirmed, as was specificity as cancer cells other than prostate were subjected to the vector. This study demonstrated tissue specificity for the vector and confirmed apoptosis of prostate cancer cells.

Adenoviruses have received much unfavorable attention after the death of a study patient with ornithine transcarbamylase deficiency when he received intravascular administration of an adenoviral agent.[54] This has served notice that, while most common side effects of vaccines are related to the injection site, serious reactions can still occur. Injecting the adenovirus-based therapy construct directly into the tumor may alleviate some of these concerns. Adenoviruses can be used as vectors for tumor-specific gene therapy that will impart apoptosis. Such oncolytic viruses have been produced by inserting a prostate-specific enhancer and a promoter coupled to the E1A gene, into a replication-competent adenovirus.[55] Expression of the E1A viral gene allows the virus to reproduce and enter the lytic cycle. Proof of specificity is provided by the observation that the oncolytic construct replicates 100 times better in PSA-positive than in PSA-negative cells. A phase I trial was performed to evaluate the safety and activity of CV706, a PSA selective replication-competent adenovirus.[56] Twenty patients who had locally recurrent prostate cancer after radiation therapy were treated in five groups with various doses of viral particles delivered intratumorally under guidance by TRUS. CV706 was found to be safe. Post-treatment biopsies as well as circulating virus copies demonstrated intraprostatic replication. The five patients who received the highest dose of CV706 achieved more than a 50% reduction in PSA. CV706 has also been studied in combination with radiation therapy in animal models yielding a synergistic effect.[57]

A similar oncolytic virus was constructed in an effort to further enhance affinity for prostatic tissue. CV787 is a replication-competent adenovirus that contains the prostate-specific rat probasin promoter, driving the adenovirus type 5 (Ad5) E1A gene, and the human prostate-specific enhancer/promoter, driving the E1B gene. CV787 was shown to destroy PSA-expressing prostate cancer cells 10,000 times more efficiently than PSA negative cells.[58] CG7870, a replication-selective, PSA-targeted oncolytic adenovirus, was administered to 23 patients with CIPC as a single intravenous infusion.[59] The treatment was well tolerated with flu-like symptoms being the most common adverse event. All patients developed antibodies to CG7870. Five patients had a minor decrease in serum PSA (25%–49%). This vaccine will be studied in combination with a taxane-based chemotherapy.

The most conventional approach to suicide gene therapy has been to deliver the herpes simplex virus–thymidine kinase (HSV-TK) gene: when expressed in the target cells it allows for targeted kill with ganciclovir. In a phase I/II study, 36 patients with local recurrence after radiotherapy were treated with doses of a replication-deficient adenoviral vector that coded for HSV-TK followed by ganciclovir.[60] Just one cycle of treatment caused a statistically significant prolongation of the PSA doubling time from 15.9 months to 42.5 months. Additionally, in 28 (77.8%) of the patients there was a mean reduction in PSA of 28%. An additional cycle of the therapy did not significantly alter the PSA doubling time; however, it did cause modest further decline PSA levels. The investigators also noted a correlation between the density of tumor infiltrating post-treatment CD8+ cells in biopsies with the number of apoptotic cells. The difficult question for future research is: what will be the most appropriate setting for this therapy as described? Besides the trial of 36 patients who had failed radiotherapy, two additional trials were conducted with this approach: one that enrolled 22 patients who received gene therapy prior to radical prostatectomy, and another that treated 27 patients concurrently with radiotherapy.[61] Activated CD8+ cells were measured as the endpoint. All three trials had significant elevations of CD8+ cells most prominently seen in conjunction with radiation therapy.

A novel approach of the same concept is to fuse HSV-TK with the gene for cytosine deaminase.[62] Cytosine deaminase activates the prodrug flucytosine (5-fluorcytosine) to fluorouracil. In a phase I

trial, 16 patients, in four cohorts, with locally recurrent prostate cancer received under TRUS visualization an intraprostatic injection of replication-competent adenovirus containing the fused gene in an escalating dose fashion.[62] Two days after injection with the gene therapy, patients were given flucytosine and ganciclovir for 1 week (cohorts 1–3) or 2 weeks (cohort 2). There were no dose limiting toxicities and the maximum tolerated dose was not defined. Seven of the 16 (44%) patients demonstrated a 25% or more decrease in PSA and three experienced a reduction of 50% or more. Transgene expression and tumor destruction were confirmed by biopsy of the prostate at 2 weeks. Two patients were negative for prostate cancer at 1 year. Although the transgene DNA could be detected in blood as far out as 76 days, there was no adenovirus detected in serum or urine.

In an effort to regain control of cell cycling, another approach focused on reintroducing wild-type p53 in prostate cancer cells. INGN 201 (Ad-p53) (Introgen Therapeutics) is a replication-defective adenoviral vector that encodes a wild-type p53 gene. Thirty patients with clinical stage T3, or T1c to T2a with a Gleason score of 8 to 10, or T2a to T2b with a Gleason score of 7 and a PSA of more than 10 ng/mL, were administered TRUS-guided intraprostatic injections of INGN 201.[63] There were no grade 3 or 4 adverse events. Twenty-six patients went on to have a prostatectomy. Ten of 11 patients who had negative immunostaining for p53 protein at baseline were subsequently positive for p53 after the first injection of INGN 201.

Clearly, this line of investigation carries great promise. As the technology continues to mature we hope to see various platforms of oncolytic gene therapy being further developed.

Active cytokine immunotherapy

Granulocyte-macrophage colony-stimulating factor

There have been studies that demonstrated that IL2 can induce prostate tumor cell regression in animals.[64] Granulocyte macrophage colony-stimulating factor has also been demonstrated to have antitumor properties and has been shown to cause a reduction in PSA.[65] In a phase II trial that comprised 36 patients who had progressive disease after androgen deprivation and antiandrogen withdrawal, 23 patients received a subcutaneous dose of GM-CSF at 250 μg/m^2/day for 14 days of a 28 day cycle.[66] Declines in PSA were seen during the first 2 weeks on therapy, but they dissipated in the 2 weeks following GM-CSF. Based on the observed oscillating PSA responses in the first cohort, the second cohort (n = 13) also received GM-CSF 250 μg/m^2 3-times weekly maintenance doses. In cohort 1, 10 patients (45%) had a decline in PSA while on therapy, with a resultant rise while off treatment. In cohort 2, 12 of 13 patients had a response with a median decline of 32%. Of note, no evidence that GM-CSF was interfering with PSA measurement or secretion was detected. The same type of therapy has been investigated in men with biochemical, nonmetastatic prostate cancer (D0).[67] Thirty patients with rising PSA after failure to be cured with either surgery or radiation therapy received GM-CSF at 250 μg/m^2/day for 14 days of a 28 day cycle. Only three (10%) patients achieved a reduction in PSA of 50%.[67] The biologic effect was reflected by an increase in the PSA doubling time (PSA-DT): the median PSA-DT increased from 8.4 to 15 months (p = 0.001).

Passive (antibody-based) immunotherapy

Prostate-specific membrane antigen

Tissue-specific targeting for prostate cancer has been achieved with monoclonal antibodies against a prostate-specific, nonshed surface antigen: PSMA. A second generation antibody (J591), targeting the extracellular domain of PSMA has been employed either as a single agent or as a platform for radioimmunotherapy (RIT) or targeted cytotoxic therapy. Use of J591 as single agent is based on the potential benefits from activation of antibody-dependent cellular cytotoxicity (ADCC). Early reports of clinical use with anti-PSMA single agent antibody have not shown very promising results.[68,69] On the other hand, when PSMA is used as a platform for targeted therapy, results appear to be more promising. MLN-2704 (Millenium) is an immunoconjugate consisting of the chemotherapeutic agent DM1 (Drug Maytansinoid-1) linked to the monoclonal antibody J591. MLN-2704 binds to the external portion of PSMA, is rapidly internalized, delivering DM1 directly to prostate cancer cells. DM1 inhibits microtubule formation, disrupting cell division and other cellular survival processes. MLN-2704 is currently being investigated in a phase I/II trial at Memorial Sloan-Kettering Cancer Center. As mentioned earlier, PSMA can also be employed to guide RIT to prostate cancer cells. Lutetium-177 and yttrium-90 are two radiopharmaceuticals that have been investigated in combination to J591 antibodies.[70] Both have shown promising clinical activity in pilot studies and are currently actively investigated.

Cytotoxic T-lymphocyte antigen 4-based therapy

One of the primary mechanisms of failure of CTLs to eradicate tumor cells is the inability to express adequate amounts of co-stimulatory molecules. When specific epitopes are presented by the MHC complex of the APCs to the T-cell receptor (TCR) optimal activation requires the expression of additional co-stimulatory molecules CD80,86 which will bind to CD28 on the TCR or signaling through the CD40/CD40-ligand pathway. The TCR also expresses CTLA-4 that may bind to CD80,86. The function of the CD28/CD80,86 pair is to promote activation of T-cell stimulation, whereas CTLA-4 mediates inhibitory signals. By preventing binding to CTLA-4 through the use of a neutralizing monoclonal antibody, it may be possible to sustain and augment immune responses.[71] A recent phase I trial reported on 14 men with metastatic CIPC treated with a single dose of a human anti-CTLA-4 antibody (MDX-101, Medarex).[72] Two patients sustained grade 3 toxicities (pruritus, rash) while two patients had a decline of more than 50% PSA. In a follow up study, MDX-101 was combined with GM-CSF and eight men with CIPC were treated in a phase I study without any clinical or laboratory evidence of autoimmunity[73]

Conclusions

Immunotherapy for prostate cancer offers much promise. The field has gone from no publications in 1993 to global clinical trials. New concepts are being integrated into immunotherapy clinical development, for example, the activation of DCs with prostate-associated antigens followed by the treatment of patients with co-stimulatory molecules such as the CTLA-4a antibody. As Eli Gilboa pointed out "from early excitement to total disillusionment" immunotherapy is gaining the momentum again.[14] Review of results outlined above suggests that several techniques can lead to relevant immune responses. Correlation of immunologic surrogates to clinical outcome has been problematic. Measurement of clinical response has traditionally been based on PSA measurements. While criteria of an association of PSA with clinical outcome have been defined for response to cytotoxic chemotherapy, they may not apply to immunotherapy. Early clinical experience suggests that activation of immune effector mechanisms initially leads to a deceleration of cancer growth followed by stabilization of disease progression, which, in select patients, may be followed by a conventionally measurable response. Also, it should be pointed out that, although most early clinical work has been in the androgen independent setting (proof-of concept and assessment of safety), immunotherapy is most likely to be successful in lower tumor burden states as therapy aiming to eradicate micrometastatic disease. The evolution of technology and the ever better understanding of the mechanisms governing an effective and sustainable immune response will pave the way for more efficacious applications of immunotherapy principles. It may be that combination of different approaches may be superior to any single modality. "Co-targeting" DC antigen presentation and augmentation of B-cell and T-cell anti-neoplastic immune responses are likely to have the highest probability of favorably increasing time to progression, overall survival. Lessons on the immunobiology of prostate cancer immune response learned from patients who participated in early clinical trials need to be integrated in the design of future translational investigations to further refine selection of patients, administration of therapy, and assessment of outcome.

References

1. Jemal A, Murray T, Ward E, et al. Cancer Statistics 2005. CA Cancer J Clin 2005;55:10–30.
2. Han M, Partin AW, Zahurak M, et al. Biochemical (prostate specific antigen) recurrence probability following radical prostatectomy for clinically localized prostate cancer. J Urol. 2003;169:517–523.
3. Roehl KA, Han M, Ramos CG, et al. Cancer progression and survival rates following anatomical radical retropubic prostatectomy in 3,478 consecutive patients: long-term results. J Urol 2004;172:910–914.
4. Kattan MW, Wheeler TM, Scardino PT. Postoperative nomogram for disease recurrence after radical prostatectomy for prostate cancer. J Clin Oncol 1999;17:1499–1507.
5. Tannock IF, Osoba D, Stockler MR, et al. Chemotherapy with mitoxantrone plus prednisone or prednisone alone for symptomatic hormone-resistant prostate cancer: a Canadian randomized trial with palliative end points. J Clin Oncol 1996;14:1756–1764.
6. Petrylak DP, Tangen CM, Hussain MH, et al. Docetaxel and estramustine compared with mitoxantrone and prednisone for advanced refractory prostate cancer. N Engl J Med 2004;351:1513–1520.
7. Tannock IF, de Wit R, Berry WR, et al. Docetaxel plus prednisone or mitoxantrone plus prednisone for advanced prostate cancer. N Engl J Med 2004;351:1502–1512.
8. Assikis VJ, Simons JW. Novel therapeutic strategies for androgen-independent prostate cancer: an update. Semin Oncol 2004;31:26–32.
9. Nauts HC. Bacteria and cancer: antagonisms and benefits. Cancer Surv 1989;7:713–723.

10. Krikorian J, Portlock C, Conney D, et al. Spontaneous regression of non-Hodgkin's lymphoma. A report of nine cases. Cancer 1980;46: 2093–2099.

11. Burnet FM. The concept of immunological surveillance. Prog Exp Tumor Res 1970;13:1–27.

12. Rygaard J, Povlsen CO. The mouse mutant nude does not develop spontaneous tumors. An argument against immunological surveillance. Acta Pathol Microbiol Scand Microbiol Immunol 1974;82: 89–98.

13. DeVita Jr V. Principles of chemotherapy. Cancer principles & practice of oncology. Philadelphia: Lippincott, 1997, p 276.

14. Gilboa E. The promise of cancer vaccines. Nature Rev Cancer 2004; 4:401–411.

16. Hurwitz AA, Yanover P, Markowitz M, et al. Prostate cancer, advances in immunotherapy. Biodrugs 2003;17:131–138.

17. Ragde H, Cavanagh WA, Tjoa BA, et al. Dendritic cell based vaccines: progress in immunotherapy studies for prostate cancer. J Urol 2004; 172:2532–2538.

18. Murphy G, Tjoa B, Ragde H, et al. Phase I clinical trial: T cell therapy for prostate cancer using autologous dendritic cells pulsed with HLA-A0201-specific peptides from prostate-specific membrane antigen. Prostate 1996;29:371–380.

19. Tjoa BA, Simmons SJ, Elgamal A, et al. Follow-up evaluation of a phase II prostate cancer vaccine trial. Prostate 1999;40:125–129.

20. Lodge PA, Jones LA, Bader RA, et al. Dendritic cell-based immunotherapy of prostate cancer: immune monitoring of a phase II clinical trial. Cancer Res 2000;60:829–833.

21. Assikis VJ, Elgamal AA, Daliani D, et al. Immunotherapy for androgen independent prostate cancer: results of a Phase I trial with a tumor vaccine of autologous dendritic cells loaded with r-PSMA Proc AACR 2002 [abstract 3352].

22. Small EJ, Fratesi P, Reese DM, et al. Immunotherapy of hormone-refractory prostate cancer with antigen-loaded dendritic cells. J Clin Oncol 2000;18:3894–3903.

23. Small EJ, Rini B, Higano C, et al. A randomized, placebo-controlled phase III trial of APC8015 in patients with androgen-independent prostate cancer. Proc ASCO 2003 [abstract 1534].

24. Gilboa E, Vieweg J. Cancer immunotherapy with mRNA-transfected dendritic cells. Immunol Rev 2004;199:251–263.

25. Heiser A, Coleman D, Dannull J, et al. Autologous dendritic cells transfected with prostate-specific antigen RNA stimulate CTL responses against metastatic prostate tumors. J Clin Inv 2002;109: 409–417.

26. Slovin SF, Kelly WK, Scher HI. Immunological approaches for the treatment of prostate cancer. Semin Urol Oncol 1998;16:53–59.

27. Slovin S, Govindaswani R, Musselli C, et al. Fully synthetic carbohydrate-based vaccines in biochemically relapsed prostate cancer: Clinical trial results with a-N-Acetylgalactosamine-O-Serine/Threonine conjugate vaccine. J Clin Oncol 2003;21:4292–4298.

28. Kim NW, Piatyszek MA, Prowse KR, et al. Specific association of human telomerase activity with immortal cells and cancer. Science 1994;266:2011–2015.

29. Shay JW, Wright WE. Telomerase: a target for cancer therapeutics. Cancer Cell 2002;2:257–265.

30. Nair SK, Heiser A, Boczkowski D, et al. Induction of cytotoxic T cell responses and tumor immunity against unrelated tumors using telomerase reverse transcriptase RNA transfected dendritic cells. Nat Med 2000;6:1011–1101.

31. Su Z, Vieweg W, Dannull J, et al. Vaccination of metastatic prostate cancer patients using mature dendritic cells transfected with mRNA encoding hTERT or an MHC class II targeted hTERT/LAMP fusion protein: Results from a phase I clinical trial. Proc ASCO 2004 [abstract 2507].

32. Su Z, Vieweg J, Weizer AZ, et al. Enhanced induction of telomerase-specific CD4+ T cells using dendritic cells transfected with RNA encoding a chimeric gene product. Cancer Res 2002;62:5041–5048.

33. Vonderheide RH, Domchek SM, Schultze JL, et al. Vaccination of cancer patients against telomerase induces functional antitumor CD8+ T lymphocytes, Clin Cancer Res 2004;10:828–839.

34. Noguchi M, Itoh K, Suekane S, et al. Phase I trial of patient-oriented vaccination in HLA-A2-positive patients with metastatic hormone-refractory prostate cancer. Cancer Sci 2004;95:77–84.

35. Noguchi M, Itoh K, Suekane S, et al. Immunological monitoring during combination of patient-oriented peptide vaccination and estramustine phosphate in patients with metastatic hormone refractory prostate cancer. Prostate 2004;60:32–45.

36. Anderson WF. Human gene therapy. Nature 1998;392:25–30.

37. Mahzar D, Waxman J. Gene therapy for prostate cancer. BJU Intern 2004;93:465–469.

38. Mabjeesh NJ, Zhong H, Simons JW. Gene therapy of prostate cancer: current and future directions. Endocr Relat Cancer 2002;9:115–139.

39. Simons JW, Mikhak B, Chang J, et al. Induction of immunity to prostate cancer antigens: Results of a clinical trial of vaccination with irradiated autologous prostate tumor cells engineered to secrete granulocyte-macrophage colony-stimulating factor using ex vivo gene transfer. Cancer Res 1999;59:5160–5168.

40. Mulligan RD. The basic science of gene therapy. Science 1993;260: 926–932.

41. Nelson WG, Simons JW, Mikhak B, et al. Cancer cells engineered to secrete granulocyte-macrophage colony-stimulating factor using ex vivo gene transfer as vaccines for the treatment of genitourinary malignancies. Cancer Chemother Pharmacol 2000;46:S67–S72.

42. Simons JW, Small E, Nelson W, et al. Phase II trials of a GM-CSF gene-transduced prostate cancer cell line vaccine (GVAX®) demonstrate anti-tumor activity. Proc ASCO 2001 [abstract 1073].

43. Bubley GJ, Carducci M, Dahut W, et al. Eligibility and response guidelines for phase II clinical trials in androgen-independent prostate cancer: recommendations from the Prostate-Specific Antigen Working Group. J Clin Oncol 1999;17:3461–3467.

44. Simons J, Nelson W, Nemunaitis J, et al. Phase II trials of a GM-CSF gene-transduced prostate cancer cell line vaccine (GVAX) in hormone refractory prostate cancer. Proc ASCO 2002 [abstract 729].

45. Small EJ, Higano C, Smith D, et al. A phase 2 study of an allogeneic GM-CSF gene-transduced prostate cancer cell line vaccine in patients with metastatic hormone-refractory prostate cancer. Proc ASCO 2004 [abstract 4565].

46. Belldegrun A, Tso CL, Zisman A, et al. Interleukin 2 gene therapy for prostate cancer: phase I clinical trial and basic biology. Hum Gene Ther 2001;12:883–892.

47. Pavlenko M, Roos AK, Lundqvist A, et al. A phase I trial of DNA vaccination with a plasmid expressing prostate-specific antigen in patients with hormone-refractory prostate cancer. Br J Cancer 2004;91: 688–694.

48. Wei C, Storozynsky E, McAdam AJ, et al. Expression of human prostate-specific antigen (PSA) in a mouse tumor cell line reduces tumorigenicity and elicits PSA-specific cytotoxic T lymphocytes. Cancer Immunol Immunother 1996;42:362–368.

49. Gulley J, Chen AP, Dahut W, et al. Phase I study of a vaccine using recombinant vaccinia virus expressing PSA (rV-PSA) in patients with metastatic androgen-independent prostate cancer. Prostate 2002;53:109–117.

50. Eder JP, Kantoff PW, Roper K, et al. A phase I trial of a recombinant vaccinia virus expressing prostate-specific antigen in advanced prostate cancer. Clin Cancer Res 6:1632–1638.

51. Kaufman HL, Wang W, Manola J, et al. Phase II randomized study of vaccine treatment of advanced prostate cancer (E7897): A trial of the Eastern Cooperative Oncology Group. J Clin Oncol 2004;22: 2122–2132.

52. Mackey TJ, Borkowski A, Amin P, et al. Bcl-2/bax ratio as a predictive marker for therapeutic response to radiotherapy in patients with prostate cancer. Urology 1998;52:1085–1090.

53. Lowe SL, Rubinchik S, Honda T, et al. Prostate-specific expression of Bax delivered by an adenoviral vector induces apoptosis in LNCaP prostate cancer cell. Gene Ther 2001;8:1363–1371.

54. Reid T, Warren R, Kirn D. Intravascular adenoviral agents in cancer patients: lessons from clinical trials. Cancer Gene Therapy 2002;9:979–986.

55. Rodriguez R, Schuur ER, Lim HY, et al. Prostate attenuated replication competent adenovirus (ARCA) CN706: a selective cytotoxic for

prostate-specific antigen-positive prostate cancer cells. Cancer Res 1997;57:2559–2563.

56. DeWeese Tl, van der Poel H, Li S, et al. A phase I trial of CV706, a replication-competent PSA selective oncolytic adenovirus, for the treatment of locally recurrent prostate cancer following radiation therapy. Cancer Res 2001;61:7464–7472.

57. Chen Y, DeWeese T, Dilley J, et al. CV706, a prostate cancer-specific adenovirus variant in combination with radiotherapy produces synergistic antitumor efficacy without increasing toxicity. Cancer Res 2001;61:5453–5460.

58. Yu DC, Chen Y, Seng M, et al. The addition of adenovirus type 5 region E3 enables calydon virus 787 to eliminate distant prostate tumor xenografts. Cancer Res 1999;59:4200–4203.

59. Wilding G, Carducci M, Yu DC, et al. A phase I/II trial of IV CG7870, a replication-selective, PSA-targeted oncolytic adenovirus, for the treatment of hormone-refractory, metastatic prostate cancer. Proc ASCO 2004 [abstract 3036].

60. Miles BJ, Shalev M, Aguilar-Cordova E, et al. Prostate-specific antigen response and systemic T-cell activation after in situ gene therapy in prostate cancer patients failing radiotherapy. Hum Gene Ther 2001;12:1955–1967.

61. Satoh T, Teh BS, Timme TL, et al. Enhanced systemic T-cell activation after in situ gene therapy with radiotherapy in prostate cancer patients. Int J Rad Oncol 2004;59:562–571.

62. Freytag SO, Khil M, Stricker H, et al. Phase I study of replication-competent adenovirus-mediated double suicide gene therapy for the treatment of locally recurrent prostate cancer. Cancer Res 2002;62:4968–4976.

63. Pisters LL, Pettaway CA, Troncoso P, et al. Evidence that transfer of functional p53 protein results in increased apoptosis in prostate cancer. Clinical Cancer Res 2004;10:2587–2593.

64. Triest JA, Grignon DJ, Cher ML, et al. Systemic interleukin 2 therapy for human prostate tumors in a nude mouse model. Clin Cancer Res 1998;4:2009–2014.

65. LeBlanc G, Small EJ, Bok RA, et al. Granulocyte Macrophage Colony-Stimulating Factor (GM-CSF) therapy for prostate cancer patients with serologic progression after definitive local therapy. Proc ASCO 2001;20:724.

66. Small EJ, Reese DM, Um B, et al. Therapy of advanced prostate cancer with granulocyte macrophage colony-stimulating factor. Clin Cancer Res 1999;5:1738–1744.

67. Rini BI, Weinberg V, Bok R, et al. Prostate-specific antigen kinetics as a measure of the biologic effect of granulocyte-macrophage colony-stimulating factor in patients with serologic progression of prostate cancer. J Clin Oncol 2003;21:99–105.

68. Bander NH, Nanus D, Goldsmith S, et al. Phase I trial of humanized monoclonal antibody (mAb) to prostate specific membrane antigen/extracellular domain (PSMAext). Proc ASCO 2001 [abstract 722].

69. Morris MJ, Pandit-Tasker N, Divgi C, et al. Pilot trial of anti-PSMA antibody J591 for prostate cancer. Proc ASCO 2003 [abstract 1634].

70. Milowsky MI, Nanus DM, Kostakoglu L, et al. Phase I trial of yttrium-90-labeled anti-prostate-specific membrane antigen monoclonal antibody J591 for androgen-independent prostate cancer. J Clin Oncol 2004;22:499–500.

71. Thompson CB, Allison JP. The emerging role of CTLA-4 as an immune attenuator. Immunity 1997;7:445–450.

72. Davis TA, Tchekmedyian S, Korman A, et al. MDX-010 (human anti-CTLA4): a phase I trial in hormone refractory prostate carcinoma (HRPC). Proc ASCO 2002 [abstract 74].

73. Fong L, Rini B, Kavanaugh B, et al. CTLA-4 blockade-based immunotherapy for prostate cancer. Proc ASCO 2004 [abstract 2590].

47

Role of the primary care professional in the care of the patient with prostate cancer: a UK perspective

Michael Kirby

There is growing recognition of the importance of the primary care physician in decision-making, diagnosis and management of patients with prostate cancer. This chapter describes the general practitioners' perspective within the UK in the context of international advances. With growing numbers of men diagnosed with this cancer and their increasing life expectancy, there is an increasing need for primary care health providers to be actively involved in shared care programs.

Prostate cancer is one of the most common forms of cancer among men in Western societies and, after lung cancer, is the second most common cause of death in men in the UK, accounting for 20,000 new cancer cases and about 10,000 deaths per year.[1] Prostate cancer is identified microscopically in 30% to 50% of men at postmortem,[2] so clearly some men are dying with, rather than as a result of, prostate cancer. Prostate cancer occurs rarely in men under 50 years of age, but the incidence increases rapidly in men between 60 and 80 years of age. More than 75% of cases are diagnosed in men over 65 years of age.[3]

Prostate cancer has a relatively high survival rate, approximately 50% at 5 years[4]; however, it still rates second in male cancer mortality in both Europe and the US.[5-7] A general practice in the UK with a list size of 7000 patients can expect at least two new diagnoses of prostate cancer each year.[8] Also, with the death rates for competitive mortalities falling and the incidence of clinical prostate cancer rising, the challenge in primary care is to identify and treat the life-threatening lesions in the most effective manner.

The causes of prostate cancer remain largely unknown and no single risk factor can explain the majority of cases. It is known that the tumor requires the presence of testosterone to grow, and the overall risk of developing the disease may be affected by hereditary, race, and environmental and dietary factors.[9]

Survival rates in patients with prostate cancer vary widely according to the stage and grade of disease at diagnosis. Favorable treatment outcomes, including cure or long-term disease-free survival, are more likely if the disease is detected and treated early. Unfortunately, men are notoriously reticent about seeking help for their health problems, especially any they consider embarrassing, and many men do not seek medical attention until the disease has spread beyond the prostate.

Increasing awareness of the symptoms of early prostate cancer, and the importance of seeking medical attention for these symptoms, is a major public health challenge, and those of us working in primary care have an important role to play in this. Men who are at risk of developing prostate cancer are likely to visit their primary healthcare practitioner (PHCP) for routine health checks or for the treatment of chronic conditions such as hypertension. PHCPs are likely to be the first point of contact in the event of any health concerns. They are, therefore, in an ideal situation to be proactive in providing advice about prostate cancer, its prevalence, symptoms, and treatment, as well as being in a prime position to detect the disease in its early stages.

PHCPs will refer patients with suspected prostate cancer to a urologist to confirm diagnosis. Tumor grade, established by biopsy, determines prognosis. If a patient is particularly frail, there are strong contraindications to transurethral biopsy, the prostate-specific antigen (PSA) is less than 10 ng/ml, there are no bothersome symptoms, and life expectancy is less than 10 years, nonreferral is an option. However, if a firm diagnosis would alter management, the patient should be referred.

Diagnostic dilemma

The diagnostic challenge for the PHCP is distinguishing prostate cancer from benign prostatic hyperplasia (BPH), because they commonly coexist. Both the PHCP and patient may initially consider prostate cancer as a cause of the lower urinary tract symptoms (LUTS) and many cancers of the prostate in the UK are diagnosed after presentation with LUTS. Studies have shown minimal association between BPH and cancer.[10-12] A man with obstructive urinary symptoms, such as frequency, hesitancy, and poor stream, is most likely to have BPH or detrusor instability.[13]

Because most men presenting to their PHCP with LUTS will have a rectal examination and their PSA tested, some cancers will be found, even though the tumors in these cases are often not responsible for the symptoms. Having BPH may be protective in that it increases the chances of discovering an incidental tumor.[14]

It is probable that T1 and T2 tumors may be symptomless and BPH is more likely to be the cause of LUTS. However, no urinary symptoms are sufficiently sensitive and specific to enable the PHCP to diagnose prostate cancer from these alone.[15]

It is not possible to distinguish precisely between the tumors that will progress to clinical disease and those that will remain latent for the patient's lifetime. Studies of carcinomas found by chance and diagnosed following transurethral resection of the prostate (TURP) indicate that the average time to progression for T1a tumors (well differentiated, low volume tumors) is 13.5 years, compared to 4.75 years for T1b tumors (moderately or poorly differentiated tumors of high volume). Therefore, a younger man with T1b disease is likely to benefit from more aggressive, potentially curative therapy, whereas an elderly man with T1a tumors may be best managed by watchful waiting alone.[16]

Screening

The introduction of screening programs to aid early detection, when the chances of survival are greatest, would have considerable resource and training implications for any healthcare service. To cope with this situation in the UK, the National Screening Committee has recognized that many men are now asking for a PSA test and that previous policies have not given clear guidance on how to respond. As a result health ministers made the decision that men who ask for a PSA test are now eligible to have it performed, together with any subsequent follow-up deemed necessary within the NHS. The National Screening Committee has recommended, therefore, that the first response to a request for a test should be to provide the patient with full information to ensure an informed choice. A website has been developed for those who wish to explore the subject in depth (www.nelh.nhs.uk/psatesting).

The value of screening asymptomatic men for prostate cancer is controversial because there is much discrepancy between the incidence of clinically significant disease and the presence of microscopic disease. In addition, the science for identifying patients in whom disease progression is probable is imprecise. The positive aspects of screening include the availability of simple tests (PSA and digital rectal examination [DRE]), detection of early lesions, reassurance of those screened as negative, and in theory, reduction in prostate cancer morbidity and mortality. The negative aspects of screening are that it may detect slow-growing tumors and some of the cancers detected may have never presented clinically. The efficacy of screening in reducing mortality is not proven, false-positive tests create stress and anxiety, it is expensive and time-consuming, and the transrectal ultrasound (TRUS)-guided biopsy carries a small risk of serious infection.

Screening rate in England and Wales

There are no routinely collected data in the UK with which to monitor or study the extent to which men are being tested for prostate cancer. An independent investigation of the rate of PSA measurement in primary care in England and Wales was funded by The Policy Research Programme of the Department of Health. The study was conducted by the Cancer Screening Evaluation Unit at The Institute of Cancer Research in association with 28 pathology laboratories and over 300 general practices.[17]

The aim of the study was to investigate the rate of PSA testing in asymptomatic men and to study factors associated with variation in the rate of testing within general practice. Taking part in the study were 443 practices (32% of which were potentially eligible). These practices had a total male population of 1,483,937. Retrospective data on PSA tests were collected from each laboratory's computerized database over a 2-year period, November 19, 1999 to November 18, 2001. Prospective data on PSA tests were collected from each laboratory and general practice from November 19, 2001 to May 31, 2002.

There were a total of 65,258 and 18,545 PSA records in the retrospective and prospective periods, respectively. The overall annual rate of testing in men with no prior diagnosis of prostate cancer was estimated to be 6.0 per 100 men, of which the annual rates of asymptomatic testing, symptomatic testing, and retesting were 2.0, 2.8, and 1.2 per 100 men, respectively, after adjusting for missing values. The rate decreased with increasing social deprivation and increasing proportions of black and Asian populations.

The overall rate of PSA testing increased significantly from 1999 to 2002. The number of PSA requests submitted to the researchers by laboratories (from general practices not participating in the study, but not the total number), rose from 35,695 (November 1999–May 2000) to 50,703 (December 2001–May 2002), a 42% rise.

If the NHS Prostate Cancer Risk Management Programme recommendations were applied, 14% of the asymptomatic tests and 23% of the symptomatic tests would be referred. Because the rate of PSA testing is rising and the benefits of screening are still unclear, monitoring of the workload and costs in primary care must be performed.

Clinical best practice guidelines have been issued to ensure there is a specific quality standard of PSA testing and a systematic and standardized pathway of follow-up available for those whose test result is above the threshold.

Prostate cancer risk management program (PCRMP)

As part of the NHS prostate cancer program, the prostate cancer risk management program (PCRMP) was officially launched on July 4, 2001 by Yvette Cooper, Health Minister. Because more and more men are requesting PSA tests from their PHCP, the program was initiated to ensure that all men considering a PSA test are given an informed choice and information on the benefits, risks, and limitations of the test. General practitioners, practice nurses, urologists, and pathologists received information packs containing evidence-based material to aid this.

The packs are a useful aid for general practitioners and practice nurses to use in counseling men who do not have symptoms but are worried about prostate cancer. The packs contain a tear-off pad which men can take home to read in their own time, allowing them to make an informed choice about whether or not to proceed with a PSA test. If they decide they would like a test, it is available free on the NHS.

PCRMP nurse project

Practice nurses are often ideally placed to advise the often difficult-to-assess older male population through chronic disease clinics. Hence, the program encourages the use of PCRMP packs among practice nurses in primary care. It is hoped that practice nurses will enquire about LUTS, especially urine outflow obstruction, in men over 45 years, exclude urinary tract infection (UTI) (recheck after treatment if positive), and discuss the pros, cons, and limitations of the PSA test using the information pack. The program also includes nurses taking blood from those requesting a PSA test as part of an informed choice, and discussing with them the results of the test, arranging repeat tests if necessary, or a DRE or urgent urologic referral. Practice nurses will also be involved in informing, educating, and advising younger, asymptomatic men about prostate cancer.

Table 47.1 Symptoms of prostate cancer

Localized or locally advanced	Advanced (additional symptoms)
Prostatism (obstructive or irritative)	Loin pain, anuria and/or uremia due to obstruction of the ureters by lymph nodes
Cystitis	Impotence (neurovascular bundle involvement)
Urinary retention	General malaise or nausea
Hematuria (seminal vesicle involvement)	Bone pain (metastases and/or pathologic fracture)
Painful ejaculation	Spinal cord compression
Reduced ejaculatory volume	Paraplegia secondary to spinal cord compression
Blood in semen	Hypercalcemia (constipation, dehydration, confusion, low mood)
Perineal and suprapubic pain	Thrombosis or phlebitis
	Lymph node enlargement
	Anorexia
	Weight loss
	Incontinence
	Renal failure
	Rectal symptoms, including tenesmus
	Lymphoedema, especially in lower limbs

Diagnosis

Symptoms

Because prostate tumors are relatively slow growing, men may live with the disease for many years without experiencing any symptoms. Symptoms may only occur once the disease has progressed beyond the periphery of the prostate gland, when the cancer has grown to compress the urethra or invade the sphincter or neurovascular bundle (Table 47.1).[18,19]

History

The first step in making a diagnosis is taking a good history. Because men may feel embarrassed to raise the issue, early symptoms of prostate disease may be revealed by asking the patient three questions as part of a well-man check:

- Are you bothered by any urinary symptoms?
- Have you noticed any deterioration in your urinary flow?
- Do you get up at night to pass urine?

African men appear to be at highest risk of prostate cancer, whereas Asian men have the lowest incidence. Family history is important as an affected first-degree relative raises the chance of clinical disease by two- to three-fold; if two first-degree relatives are affected, the risk is raised four-fold. Increasing age parallels an increased risk of prostate cancer. Men under 40 years of age have a 1 in 10,000 chance of invasive prostate cancer, whereas in men aged 60 to 79 years the risk rises to 1 in 8.[1]

For the man with LUTS, the initial enquiry may then lead on to a structured approach to investigation and treatment.[20]

Investigation

Diagnosis of prostate cancer requires a methodical and multitechnical approach. Although not perfect, modern techniques provide useful information that helps distinguish between benign conditions and those more likely to be malignant.

A general physical examination, including blood pressure measurement, is important in patients with prostatic disease, as men beyond middle age often suffer from other co-morbidities, such as hypertension, diabetes, and chronic obstructive airways disease. The abdomen should be examined in all patients with suspected prostate cancer to detect a palpable bladder or kidneys. Other symptomatic areas should also be examined, such as vertebral tenderness, and a focused neurologic examination will identify most significant neurologic diseases, which may be causing lower urinary tract symptoms. A number of techniques are used to detect the presence of prostate cancer, with the four most common being DRE, PSA, TRUS, and prostate biopsy.

Digital rectal examination

The DRE is the cornerstone of the physical assessment for prostate disease. It is the most simple and cost-effective method of assessing prostate health and has almost no morbidity. Studies have shown high levels of interobserver agreement for DRE which increases its value in diagnosis.[21,22]

The normal prostate is roughly the size of a chestnut and has the same rubbery consistency as the tip of the nose. BPH results in symmetrical enlargement with little alteration in consistency and preservation of the midline sulcus. Prostate cancer, by contrast, results in stony induration of the prostate that often starts as a palpable nodule and progresses to asymmetry of one lobe of the gland, with eventual involvement and fixation of adjacent structures, especially the seminal vesicles which are normally impalpable (Table 47.2).

Prostate-specific antigen test

PSA is not a definitive test for prostate cancer and elevated levels may also be found in men with prostatitis and BPH, hence the debate regarding the use of the test as a screening tool. The PSA test can often be justified by the fact that prostate cancer will be treated differently from BPH and in some cases it will lead to the accurate diagnosis and treatment of locally advanced cancers. However, one

Table 47.2 Clinical parameters that may be assessed by digital rectal examination[23]

Size	Transverse and longitudinal dimension estimated, as well as posterior protrusion. The normal gland is the size of a chestnut (20 g). In benign prostatic hyperplasia, the gland progressively enlarges to the size of a satsuma (>50 g)
Consistency	Slight pressure applied smoothly while gliding over the surface of the gland to detect whether: Smooth or elastic (normal) Hard or woody (may indicate cancer) Tender (suggests prostatitis)
Mobility	Attempts to move the prostate up and down or to the sides. A malignant gland may be fixed to adjacent tissue
Anatomic limits	Finger used to try and reach lateral and cranial borders; medial sulcus palpated carefully. The seminal vesicles should be impalpable; induration of these suggests malignancy

disadvantage is that, like screening, it may detect early, stage T1 cancers that would not have given rise to symptoms in the patient's lifetime.[24] The use of age-related PSA, free/total PSA, PSA velocity, and PSA density may provide more precise methods to aid diagnosis, but the relative merits of these measures are still debated. However, PSA measurements are useful for monitoring response to treatment and can act as an early warning of tumor recurrence. Patients should receive counseling with respect to the pros and cons of PSA testing, prior to requesting the investigation.

Transrectal ultrasonography

This procedure serves several purposes:

- Imaging of the internal structure of the gland and periprostatic tissues and the seminal vesicles.
- Estimation of prostate volume.
- Facilitation and aiming of ultrasound-guided prostate biopsy.

TRUS sometimes allows estimation of the local stage of a prostate cancer because asymmetry and irregularity of the capsule are associated with extracapsular spread of adenocarcinoma,[25] and prostatic blood flow can be evaluated with color Doppler ultrasound imaging incorporated into TRUS technology. Following the administration of a covering dose of antibiotics, which should be continued for several days, TRUS-guided biopsy of the prostate may be done, usually under local anesthesia.

Management decisions

Knowledge of the treatment options is essential when counseling the patient with prostate cancer, and discussion should include possible side effects and complications.

Early disease

The management of early prostate cancer remains controversial and many patients will attend their general practitioner to discuss the therapeutic options. Patients with clinically localized prostate cancer, i.e. biopsy-proven disease with no evidence of extraprostatic

extension, should be informed about the advantages and disadvantages of the following options.

Watchful waiting

Active surveillance is most appropriate for men with low volume, less aggressive disease and in those with a life expectancy of less than 10 years. Regular PSA checks are recommended and active treatment initiated if the disease progresses.

Radical prostatectomy

This is considered by many to be the gold standard of treatment. Radical prostatectomy involves the removal of the entire prostate gland. Provided that all cancer tissue is excised, and all surgical margins, seminal vesicles, and lymph nodes are clear, then life expectancy is equivalent to that of an age-matched individual who has never had cancer. Side effects include a low risk (<2–3%) of stress incontinence and a higher risk (>50%) of erectile dysfunction. However, both these problems improve with time and can often be treated effectively. If the entire prostate and all cancer has been excised the postoperative PSA should fall to less than 0.1 ng/ml, which aids follow-up and early identification of tumor recurrence. More recently, laparoscopic radical prostatectomy has been developed which, in expert hands, results in less bleeding and shorter hospital stays.

External beam radiotherapy

External beam radiotherapy (EBRT) is an effective form of therapy in early disease. Neoadjuvant androgen ablation, usually with a luteinizing hormone-releasing hormone (LHRH) analog, enhances results. Side effects include proctitis and rectal bleeding due to the anterior rectal wall being included in the treatment field. However, side effects may be reduced by focusing more accurately on the prostate with the use of conformal technology.

Brachytherapy

This involves the transperineal implantation of radi oactive seeds into the prost ate under light anesthesia.[26] LUTS may worsen for some time following this procedure due to swelling of the gland, so it should be used with caution in patients with preexisting severe bladder outflow obstruction. Brachyth erapy may be used in conjunction with EBRT in patients who are considered at high risk of disease recurrence. Men who have previously undergone TURP are generally not suitable for brachytherapy because the seeds are not satisfactorily retained in the prostate.

Cryotherapy

Growing in popularity but still regarded as experimental, so-called third-generation cryotherapy involves the insertion of between 10 and 20 needles into the prostate and the creation of an ice ball within the gland.[27]

Advanced disease

Patients are considered to have advanced disease if they have prostate cancer involving lymph nodes, other soft tissues or the skeleton. In these cases cure is not possible but androgen withdrawal will, in most cases, result in a remission that may be maintained for 24 to 36 months, depending on the extent of the metastatic burden at presentation.

A proportion of patients with prostate cancer present with extraprostatic extension, but no evidence of distant metastases. Radical surgery is inappropriate because of the high local and distant recurrence rates. Radiotherapy is usually the preferred treatment option.

Treatment of metastases

The proportion of patients with localized disease at the time of diagnosis is now rising, probably as a result of PSA testing. Depriving the cancer cells of the androgens necessary for their growth can be accomplished by a variety of means, both medical and surgical.

Four antiandrogenic agents have been extensively evaluated clinically for the treatment of metastatic prostate cancer: cyproterone acetate, flutamide, nilutamide, and bicalutamide. The addition of such an agent to achieve maximal androgen blockade may possibly increase both the time to disease progression and provide a survival advantage in some patients with good performance status and less advanced metastatic disease, although this is still controversial. Some aspects of sexual function may be preserved with the use of antiandrogens such as bicalutamide. However, the Committee on Safety of Medicines recommends that bicalutamide is not used as a primary treatment of clinically organ confined in prostate cancer. This is because data has suggested a possible increased mortality rate in men with localized prostate cancer treated with bicalutamide alone compared to placebo (5-year mortality 25.5% vs 20.5% with placebo; hazard ratio 1.2; 95% CI 1.0–1,5).[28] Androgen ablation can be achieved either by bilateral orchidectomy or the use of depot LHRH analog.

Potential side effects

Potential side effects of prostate cancer treatments include:

- Complete or partial loss of sexual functioning.
- Erectile dysfunction.
- Bladder problems.
- Bowel problems.
- Reduction of bone mineral density.
- Change in body shape/weight gain.
- Breast enlargement/tenderness.
- Hot flushes.
- Lethargy.

Palliative care

Considerable distress is experienced by the majority of cancer patients and their carers before death.[29] This aspect is often unrecognized or overlooked by services focusing on the terminal phase of the illness and it is important to identify and alleviate this suffering as much as possible.

One important initiative is gaining momentum within primary care. The Gold Standards framework is a resource for organizing proactive palliative care in the community. It is supported by funding from the National Lottery, Cancer Services Collaborative, and Macmillan Cancer Relief.[30] The framework provides a detailed guide to providing patient-centered care and facilitates effective, holistic care in the community. Other recently initiated mechanisms for the improvement of primary palliative care include the training of general practitioners with a special interest in palliative care and the new end of life initiative in England to improve palliative care provision.[31] Because primary care teams often know patients over long periods of time, they may be in a prime position, using chronic disease or cancer registers, to identify patients who would benefit from an early palliative care approach. PHCPs may be able to identify such patients by asking themselves one simple question, "Would I be surprised if this patient were to die in the next 12 months?"[32] This proactive approach in the early identification of such patients would facilitate active treatment and patient-centered support, through a team with which many patients and their carers establish a valued long-term relationship. For such an approach to be initiated, the goals of care need to be established and agreed, and management plans adjusted to suit the patent's specific situation. The effective control of symptoms and the maintenance of quality of life must be prioritized.

Looking to the future

The optimal management of prostate cancer now requires care to be shared between urologist and family practitioner. The initial treatment strategy should be devised by a specialist on the basis of tissue diagnosis and careful staging. Radiotherapy or prostatectomy are obviously the province of the hospital-based team but the initial diagnosis and follow-up may be the joint responsibility of the urologist and family practitioner. Metastatic disease is increasingly managed by monthly or 3-monthly depo injections of LHRH analogs, and there is now evidence to support the early introduction of endocrine therapy at the time of diagnosis rather than waiting for symptoms to develop.[33]

In future it may be possible to predict a subgroup of patients in whom total androgen blockade rather than antiandrogen therapy may offer a definite survival advantage. Newer and more effective first- and second-line curative pharmacotherapies also need to be developed.

These challenges may be added to the many others that must be overcome to reduce the morbidity and mortality of this prevalent and insidious disease. Measures for the future might include:

- Early detection—using more accurate tumor markers to improve the ability of clinicians to distinguish early prostate cancer from BPH.
- Better staging—enhanced imaging and molecular staging.
- Prognostic indicators—molecular prognostic indicators, e.g. E-cadherin expression, are currently the subject of intense research.
- New therapies—laparoscopic radical prostatectomy, cryosurgery, high-intensity focused ultrasound, specific inhibitors of growth factors, and possibly gene therapy.

Antiprostate cancer vaccines are also now a not too distant prospect. Eventually, oncogenes could be neutralized or deleted or tumor suppressor genes reinserted by any of the several vector methods currently under development.

References

1. Office for National Statistics. Registrations of cancer diagnosed in 1994–1997, England and Wales. Health Statistics Quarterly 2000;7:71–82.
2. Selby M. Prostate cancer. Urology Update 2004;24 Sept:110–117.
3. Reis LAG, Eisner MP, Kosary CL, et al (eds). Seer Cancer Statistics Review 1973–1998, Bethesda, MD: National Cancer Institute, 2001.
4. Quinn M, Babb P, Brock A, et al. Cancer trends in England and Wales 1950–1999. London: The Stationary Office, 2001. http://www.statistics.gov.uk/statbase.
5. Lu Yao GL, Greenberg ER. Changes in prostate cancer incidence and treatment in the USA. Lancet 1994;343:251–254.
6. Edwards B, Howe H, Reis L, et al. Annual report to the nation on the status of cancer, 1973–1999 featuring implications of age and aging on US cancer burden. Cancer 2002;94:2766–2792.
7. Chu K, Tarone RE, Freeman H. Trends in prostatic cancer mortality among black men and white men in the United States. Cancer 2003;97:1507–1516.
8. Gronberg H. Prostate cancer epidemiology. Lancet 2003;361:859–364.
9. Steinberg GD, Carter BS, Beaty TH, et al. Family history and the risk of prostate cancer. Prostate 1990;17:337–347.
10. Guess HA. Benign prostatic hyperplasia and prostatic cancer. Epidemiol Rev 2001;23:152–158.
11. Coley CM, Barry MJ, Fleming C, et al. Early detection of prostate cancer. Part II: Estimating the risks, benefits and costs. American College of Physicians. Ann Intern Med 1997;126:468–479.
12. Greenwald P, Kirmss V, Polan AK, et al. Cancer of the prostate among men with benign prostatic hyperplasia. J Natl Cancer Inst 1974;53:335–340.
13. Verhamme K, Dieleman J, Bleumink G, et al. Incidence and prevalence of lower urinary tract symptoms suggestive of benign prostatic hyperplasia in primary care—The TRIUMPH Project. Eur Urol 2002;42:232–328.
14. Hamilton W, Sharp D. Symptomatic diagnosis of prostate cancer in primary care: a structured review. Br J Gen Pract 2004;54:617–621.
15. Department of Health. Referral Guidelines for Suspected Cancer. London: Department of Health, 2000. http://www.dh.gov.uk/assetRoot/04/01/44/21/04014421.pdf.
16. Kirby RS, Oesterling JE, Denis LJ. Prostate Cancer: Fast Facts. Oxford: Health Press, 1996.
17. Melia J, Moss S, John L, and contributors in the participating laboratories. Rates of prostate specific antigen testing in general practice in England and Wales in asymptomatic and symptomatic patients: A cross sectional study. BJU Int 2004;94:51–56.
18. Horwich A, Waxman J, Abel P, et al. Tumours of the prostate. In: Souhami R, Tannock I, Hohenberger P, Horiot JC (eds): The Oxford Textbook of Oncology, 2nd ed. Oxford. Oxford University Press, 2001, pp 1939–1971.
19. Guess HA. Benign prostatic hyperplasia and prostate cancer. Epidemiol Rev 2001;23:152–158.
20. Speakman M, Kirby R, Joyce S, et al. Guidelines for the primary care management of male lower urinary tract symptoms. BJU Int 2004;93:985–990.
21. Herranz Amo F, Verdu Tartajo F, Diez Cordero JM, et al. Variability of rectal examination of the prostate among various groups of observers. Actas Urol Esp 1996;20:873–876.
22. Roehrborn CG, Sech S, Montoya J, et al. Interexaminer reliability and validity of a three-dimensional model to assess prostate volume by digital rectal examination. Urology 2001;57:1087–1092.
23. Kirby R, Fitzpatrick J, Kirby M, et al. Shared Care for Prostatic Diseases, 2nd ed. ISIS Medical Media, Oxford, 2000.
24. Etzioni R, Cha R, Feuer EJ, et al. Asymptomatic incidence and duration of prostate cancer. Am J Epidemiol 1998;148:775–785.
25. Ohori M, Egawa S, Shinohara K, et al. Detection of microscopic extracapsular extension prior to radical prostatectomy for clinically localised prostate cancer. Br J Urol 1994;74:72–79.
26. Ragde H, Elgamal A, Snow PB, et al. Ten year disease free survival after transperineal sonography-guided iodine 125 brachytherapy with or without 45 Gray external beam irradiation in the treatment of patients with clinically localised, low to high Gleason grade prostate carcinoma. Cancer 1998;83:989–1001.
27. Donnelly BJ, Saliken JC, Ernst DS, et al. Prospective trial of cryosurgical ablation of the prostate: 5 year results. Urology 2002;60:645–649.
28. Committee on Safety of Medicines. Casodex 150 mg (bicalutamide): no longer indicated for treatment of localised prostate cancer. http://www.mca.gov.uk/ourwork/monitorsafequalmed/safetymessages/casodex.
29. Murray SA, Kendall M, Boyd K, et al. Exploring the spiritual needs of people dying of lung cancer or heart failure: a prospective qualitative interview study of patients and their carers. Palliat Med 2004;18:39–45.
30. Thomas K. Caring for the Dying at Home: Companions on a Journey. Oxford: Radcliffe Medical Press, 2003.
31. Murray SA, Boyd K, Sheikh A, et al. Developing primary palliative care. BMJ 2004;329:1056–1057.
32. Lynn J. Serving patients who may die soon and their families: the role of hospice and other services. JAMA 2001;285:925–932.
33. The Medical Research Council Prostate Cancer Working Party Investigators Group. Immediate versus deferred treatment for advanced prostate cancer. Initial results of the Medical Research Council Trial. Br J Urol 1997;79:235–246.

Index